Oral Microbiology
& Infectious Disease

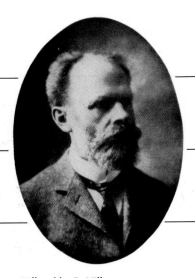

Willoughby D. Miller
A.B., D.D.S., M.D., Ph.D., Sc.D.
(1853–1907)

The father of oral microbiology.
As the formulator of the
chemico-parasitic theory of
dental caries he was the first
to apply a basic science to
the solution of dental disease.
Dr. Miller was a great leader
as an investigator, practicing
dentist, teacher, and prolific
author in all phases of
dentistry. He wrote the
first comprehensive textbook
of oral microbiology,
*Die Mikroorganismen der
Mundhöhle,* published in Germany
in 1889 and in the
United States in 1890 as
*The Micro-Organisms of the
Human Mouth.* (From School
of Dentistry, University
of Michigan.)

Oral Microbiology & Infectious Disease

Third Edition

Edited by

George S. Schuster, D.D.S., M.S., Ph.D.

Ione and Arthur Merritt Professor,
Department of Oral Biology,
School of Dentistry;
Associate Professor of Cell
and Molecular Biology,
School of Medicine;
Medical College of Georgia,
Augusta, Georgia

1990   B.C. Decker, Inc.   Philadelphia · Toronto

Publisher

B.C. Decker Inc
3228 South Service Road
Burlington, Ontario L7N 3H8

B.C. Decker Inc
320 Walnut Street
Suite 400
Philadelphia, Pennsylvania 19106

Sales and Distribution

United States and Puerto Rico
Mosby—Year Book Inc.
11830 Westline Industrial Drive
Saint Louis, Missouri 63146

Canada
Mosby—Year Book Ltd.
5240 Finch Ave. E., Unit 1
Scarborough, Ontario, M1S 5A2

Australia
**McGraw-Hill Book Company Australia
Pty. Ltd.**
4 Barcoo Street
Roseville East 2069
New South Wales, Australia

Brazil
Editora McGraw-Hill do Brasil, Ltda.
rua Tabapua, 1.105, Itaim-Bibi
Sao Paulo, S.P. Brasil

Colombia
**Interamericana/McGraw-Hill de Colombia,
S.A.**
Apartado Aereo 81078
Bogota, D.E. Colombia

Europe
McGraw-Hill Book Company GmbH
Lademannbogen 136
D-2000 Hamburg 63
West Germany

France
MEDSI/McGraw-Hill
6, avenue Daniel Lesueur
75007 Paris, France

Hong Kong and China
McGraw-Hill Book Company
Suite 618, Ocean Centre
5 Canton Road
Tsimshatsui, Kowloon
Hong Kong

India
Tata McGraw-Hill Publishing Company, Ltd.
12/4 Asaf Ali Road, 3rd Floor
New Delhi 110002, India

Indonesia
P.O. Box 122/JAT
Jakarta, 1300 Indonesia

Italy
McGraw-Hill Libri Italia, s.r.l.
Piazza Emilia, 5
I-20129 Milano MI
Italy

Japan
Igaku-Shoin Ltd.
Tokyo International P.O. Box 5063
1-28-36 Hongo, Bunkyo-ku
Tokyo 113, Japan

Korea
C.P.O. Box 10583
Seoul, Korea

Malaysia
No. 8 Jalan SS 7/6B
Kelana Jaya
47301 Petaling Jaya
Selangor, Malaysia

Mexico
**Interamericana/McGraw-Hill de Mexico,
S.A. de C.V.**
Cedro 512, Colonia Atlampa
(Apartado Postal 26370)
06450 Mexico, D.F., Mexico

New Zealand
McGraw-Hill Book Co. New Zealand Ltd.
5 Joval Place, Wiri
Manukau City, New Zealand

Panama
**Editorial McGraw-Hill Latinoamericana,
S.A.**
Apartado Postal 2036
Zona Libre de Colon
Colon, Republica de Panama

Portugal
Editora McGraw-Hill de Portugal, Ltda.
Rua Rosa Damasceno 11A-B
1900 Lisboa, Portugal

South Africa
Libriger Book Distributors
Warehouse Number 8
"Die Ou Looiery"
Tannery Road
Hamilton, Bloemfontein 9300

Southeast Asia
McGraw-Hill Book Co.
348 Jalan Boon Lay
Jurong, Singapore 2261

Spain
McGraw-Hill/Interamericana de Espana, S.A.
Manuel Ferrero, 13
28020 Madrid, Spain

Taiwan
P.O. Box 87-601
Taipei, Taiwan

Thailand
632/5 Phaholyothin Road
Sapan Kwai
Bangkok 10400
Thailand

United Kingdom, Middle East and Africa
McGraw-Hill Book Company (U.K.) Ltd.
Shoppenhangers Road
Maidenhead, Berkshire
SL6 2QL England

Venezuela
McGraw-Hill/Interamericana, C.A.
2da. calle Bello Monte
(entre avenida Casanova y Sabana Grande)
Apartado Aereo 50785
Caracas 1050, Venezuela

NOTICE

The authors and publisher have made every effort to ensure that the patient care recommended herein, including choice of drugs and drug dosages, is in accord with the accepted standards and practice at the time of publication. However, since research and regulation constantly change clinical standards, the reader is urged to check the product information sheet included in the package of each drug, which includes recommended doses, warnings, and contraindications. This is particularly important with new or infrequently used drugs.

Oral Microbiology and Infectious Disease, 3rd Edition

ISBN 1-55664-181-8

Library of Congress catalog card number: 90–81207

10 9 8 7 6 5 4 3 2 1

Contributors

Editor

George S. Schuster, D.D.S., M.S., Ph.D.
Ione and Arthur Merritt Professor
Department of Oral Biology
School of Dentistry
Medical College of Georgia
Augusta, Georgia

Contributing Authors

Gretchen B. Caughman, Ph.D.
Associate Professor
Oral Biology/Microbiology
School of Dentistry
Medical College of Georgia
Augusta, Georgia

Virginia A. Merchant, D.M.D., M.S.
Associate Professor
Department of Biomedical Sciences
School of Dentistry
University of Detroit
Detroit, Michigan

Benjamin F. Hammond, D.D.S., Ph.D.
Professor
Department of Microbiology
School of Dental Medicine
University of Pennsylvania
Philadelphia, Pennsylvania

Chris H. Miller, M.S., Ph.D.
Professor and Chairman
Department of Oral Microbiology
Indiana University School of Dentistry
Indianapolis, Indiana

John A. Molinari, Ph.D.
Professor and Chairman
Department of Biomedical Sciences
School of Dentistry
University of Detroit
Detroit, Michigan

Eugene A. Pantera, Jr., D.D.S., M.S.
Associate Professor
Department of Endodontics
School of Dentistry
Medical College of Georgia
Augusta, Georgia

Mark R. Patters, D.D.S., Ph.D.
Professor and Chairman
Department of Periodontics
College of Dentistry
University of Tennessee
Memphis, Tennessee

Charles F. Schachtele, Ph.D.
Professor and Director
Dental Research Institute
School of Dentistry
University of Minnesota
Minneapolis, Minnesota

George S. Schuster, D.D.S., M.S., Ph.D.
Ione and Arthur Merritt Professor
Department of Oral Biology
School of Dentistry
Medical College of Georgia
Augusta, Georgia

Keith R. Volkmann, D.M.D., Ph.D.
Associate Professor
Oral Biology/Microbiology
School of Dentistry
Medical College of Georgia
Augusta, Georgia

John T. Wilson, D.M.D., Ph.D.
Associate Research Professor
Department of Genetics
Yale University
School of Medicine
New Haven, Connecticut

Preface

Oh that one would hear me!
behold, my desire is,
that the Almighty would
answer me,
and that mine adversary
had written a book.

Job XXXI:35

The previous editions of *Oral Microbiology and Infectious Disease* were intended to serve as reference texts for students as well as reference books in the field of oral microbiology. Subsequently such editions became too large and costly for typical student use, and as a result the student edition evolved. In that form the book was reduced in size and content, by reducing the text and illustrations and eliminating certain topics. The current edition combines features of both versions. Some sections have been expanded to provide more detail, in order to clarify concepts. Others have been expanded to take into account new knowledge that enhances our understanding of oral diseases and their control. Added to this are the sections covering diseases and related problems unrecognized a few years ago. For example, the impact of acquired immunodeficiency syndrome is felt throughout the medical field. Not only is the disease itself a problem that must be discussed, but the concurrent changes in disease patterns pose an additional burden. These are manifest as a resurgence of mycobacterial infections in immunocompromised patients and in infections resulting from members of the normal microbial flora. These pose new diagnostic and therapeutic challenges. Infection control, previously honored in the breach, has assumed significant proportions and consumes considerable amounts of time and money. Thus, a text must provide the student and the practitioner with a sound understanding of the fundamental problem and of its clinical significance. This we have attempted to do in the new edition. The basic information on microbiology and infectious disease, as well as the implications for dentistry, are presented, along with additional information and background for those who desire to go deeper into a subject.

As in the prior edition of *Oral Microbiology and Infectious Disease* we have used multiple authors. All are individuals who are active in teaching and research in oral microbiology. This provides a depth and strength to the coverage of a field that is becoming steadily more complex.

While a broad microbiology and infectious disease background is important to the clinician, he or she must be particularly knowledgeable in the relationships of these to the oral cavity. Not only do local and systemic diseases have an impact on the patient's treatment, but the converse is also true; the treatment may affect the disease process and its manifestations. Therefore, examples involving the oral cavity and its microbiota are used whenever possible, and special attention has been given to oral infectious diseases, diseases with oral manifestations, and systemic infections with special implications for dental personnel.

All chapters have been rewritten or revised. Literature references have been updated but the numbers somewhat reduced, with an emphasis on review articles. New illustrations and tables have been added to clarify some of the complex concepts and to provide more information in a limited space. By these changes we hope to provide the dental practitioner with a sound background on which to add more in-depth knowledge.

As we move into a new phase with this text we wish to acknowledge the first author and editor of *Oral Microbiology and Infectious Disease,* George W. Burnett, D.D.S., M.S., Ph.D. It was his vision that there be a microbiology text specifically directed toward dentistry, and that it would apply basic principles of microbiology to the clinical discipline. This edition is a tribute to that vision. He was a scientist, a scholar, and above all a gentleman in every sense of the word.

GEORGE S. SCHUSTER

Contents

Part VIII   Oral Microbiota and Oral Disease

To the memory of
George Wesley Burnett
1914–1989
His expertise as a dentist,
a scientist, and a teacher
will continue to influence this text
through subsequent editions

Part I

Microbiological Classification and Techniques

1

Microbial Taxonomy

Chris H. Miller

Microbiology is a branch of the biological sciences that is concerned with the study of life that is ordinarily too small to be seen with the unaided human eye. Microorganisms included in the field of microbiology are listed in Table 1.1. Those that are known to cause infectious diseases in animals are the pathogenic fungi, protozoa, bacteria, rickettsiae, chlamydiae, and viruses. The macroscopic metazoa and microscopic protozoa that are parasites or pathogens are usually grouped in the branch of biology known as parasitology.

Taxonomy

The present concepts of evolution seem to indicate that microbes were derived from primitive ancestors of the plant and animal kingdoms and are, in fact, in a position somewhere between them. This led Haeckel in 1866 to propose that the acellular or unicellular microbes, because of their apparent relative simplicity, should be placed in a separate kingdom designated as Protista (Gr. *prōtista,* the very first).

As techniques and the necessary apparatus (chiefly the electron microscope) became available, the cellular organization of microbes was revealed in more detail. It became evident that protozoa, fungi, and most algae could be described as eukaryotic (possessing a true nucleus) because, like the cells of plants and animals, their distinctive nucleus, which is enclosed by a nuclear membrane, contains multiple chromosomes and an apparatus that equally divides their chromosomes during cell division. In contrast, the bacteria and the blue-green algae belong to a group of cells termed prokaryotic (prenuclear; lacking a true nucleus). The nucleus or genophore of these cells consists of a single, circular, naked chromosome not separated from the cytoplasm by a nuclear membrane. Major features that differentiate eukaryotes from prokaryotes are presented in Table 1.2.

Bacterial Classification

Differentiation within the kingdom Procaryotae became necessary as more and more different microbes

3

Table 1.1: The Microbial World

Algae	Bacteria
Fungi	True bacteria
Yeasts	Rickettsiae
Molds	Chlamydiae
Protozoa	Viruses

were discovered. Bacterial classification stems from work by the Swedish botanist Carolus Linnaeus (Carl von Linné) in 1753 and provides an overall scheme into which bacteria are inserted on the basis of specific properties (see Chap. 2). Bacterial classification is used to describe different microbes responsible for causing different processes in nature, or in humans; to diagnose infectious diseases and institute appropriate therapy; and to ensure proper cataloging of identical microbes as they are isolated and studied at different locations throughout the world.

Table 1.3 lists some of the microbes important in dentistry and medicine as they appear in the 1984 edition of *Bergey's Manual of Systematic Bacteriology* and the eighth edition of *Bergey's Manual of Determinative Bacteriology*. The classification system used in *Bergey's Manual* and adapted for use here is the product of over 50 years of development with periodic revisions. Like the classification schemes for plants and animals, it is organized into Division, Class, Order, Family, Genus and Species. The actual designation of a bacterium consists of genus and species names, which are derived from Latin and usually reference some characteristic of the bacterium or the name of the person who first described the bacterium.

Bacterial classification is an ongoing process that reflects the isolation of previously unrecognized bacteria and the reclassification of known organisms at the species, genus, and sometimes lower levels. As technological advances permit study of microorgan-isms in greater and greater detail, more opportunities for differentiation of closely related bacteria occur. For example, bacteria grouped together as *Bacterium melaninogenicum* in 1928 are now placed in one of six different species of the genus *Bacteroides* (see Chap. 49). Reclassification may involve the temporary use of subspecies names (e.g., *B. melaninogenicus* subsp. *melaninogenicus,* now known as either *B. melaninogenicus, B. loescheii,* or *B. denticola*). Differentiation within a species may also entail classification based on biotype (the set of biochemical properties), serotype (the set of antigenic properties), or phagotype (ability to be lysed by certain bacteriophages).

The basic taxonomic group in bacterial systematics is the species. A bacterial species may be regarded as a collection of strains that share many features in common and differ considerably from other strains. A strain consists of the descendants of a single isolate in a pure culture. One strain of a species, designated as the type strain, serves as the permanent example of the species. Different isolates are differentiated by assigning a different strain identification to each isolate. This is important for cataloging purposes, to identify specific isolates for which an exact classification has not yet been confirmed, and to ensure the use of the same isolate in studies attempting to confirm or extend previous scientific work. The system used to identify strains is not standardized but usually includes the initials of the person who isolated the bacterium or an abbreviation indicating where the bacterium can be obtained, along with numbers. For example, *Actinomyces viscosus,* ATCC 15987, is a specific isolate maintained by the American Type Culture Collection (ATCC) in Rockville, Maryland. Stock cultures of specific bacterial strains are maintained (by procedures described in Chap. 2) by several commercial firms such as ATCC, by clinical and hospital laboratories, by microbiology research laboratories,

(Text continues on page 11)

Table 1.2: Comparison of Prokaryotic and Eukaryotic Cells*

Feature	Prokaryotic	Eukaryotic
Cell wall	Complex with glycopeptide	Not as complex, no glycopeptide
Cell membrane	No sterols	Sterols
Mesosomes	Present	None
Nucleus	DNA; no membrane	DNA complexed with histones; membrane
Cell division	Binary fission; budding	Mitosis; meiosis
Ribosomes	70S	80S
Chromosomes	Single	Multiple
Mitochondria	None	Present
Chloroplasts	None	Present
Chromatophores	Present in some organisms	None

*Reproduced with permission from J. A. Molinari and M. J. Phillip: Microbiology and Sterilization. In *Review of Dental Assisting,* edited by B. A. Ladley and S. A. Wilson. C. V. Mosby, St. Louis, 1980.

Table 1.3: Outline of the Principal Bacterial Genera of Dental and Medical Importance

Kingdom: Procaryotae

Single cells or cells in a simple association that do not have a nuclear membrane and are generally but not always enclosed by a rigid cell wall. One or more of these microorganisms inhabit almost every moist environment.

Division II. *The Bacteria.* Division consists of prokaryotic microorganisms that are unicellular or in simple association. They usually divide by binary fission or by budding. Some are motile, others are not; some form endospores, others do not. With the exception of the *Mollicutes* the cells are enclosed in relatively rigid cell walls. The cells may be aerobic or anaerobic, or facultative.

Spirochetes

Order 1. *Spirochaetales.* Gram-negative, unicellular, slender helical bacteria that are nonsporulating, motile, variably aerobic, facultatively anaerobic, or anaerobic. They are either free-living, commensal, or parasitic; some are pathogenic.

Family I. *Spirochaetaceae.* Free-living spirochetes found in sewage, polluted water, and in fresh and salt water. Anaerobic or facultatively anaerobic. The family contains four genera.

Genus III. *Treponema* (a turning thread). Gram-negative, motile, unicellular, helical rods. Fermentative metabolism. Strictly anaerobic. Some have not been cultivated. Found in the oral cavity, intestinal tract, and genital regions of man and other animals. The genus contains 11 recognized species. The more important pathogenic species are *Treponema pallidum* (syphilis), *Treponema pertenue* (yaws), and *Treponema carateum* (pinta or carate). Oral residents of man and other animals include *Treponema macrodentium, Treponema denticola, Treponema orale, Treponema scoliodontum,* and *Treponema vincentii.*

Genus IV. *Borrelia* (after A. Borrel). Gram-negative, helical cells that are generally parasitic, living on mucous membranes. Some species are pathogenic for man, other animals and birds, causing such diseases as avian borreliosis and relapsing fever. Nineteen species are recognized. The type species is *Borrelia anserina.*

Family II. *Leptospiraceae.* Gram-negative, flexous, helical, motile cells that have one or both ends bent.

Genus I. *Leptospira* (a fine coil). Description as above. The genus is represented by two species, *Leptospira interrogans* and *Leptospira biflexa.* Some strains are pathogenic (leptospirosis); others are free-living saprophytes.

Spiral and Curved Bacteria

Gram-negative, rigid, helical cells that are motile by flagella. Variably aerobic and anaerobic. Do not ferment carbohydrates. Some are inhabitants of fresh and salt water, others are saprophytes or parasites. Some are pathogenic.

Genus *Spirillum* (a small spiral). Cellular description as above. *Spirillum voluntans* is the only species.

Genus *Campylobacter* (a curved rod). Gram-negative, nonsporulating, spirally curved rods that do not ferment or oxidize carbohydrates. Several recognized species. *Campylobacter fetus* is the type species. Others are *Campylobacter jejuni, Campylobacter sputorum* and *Campylobacter concisus.* The various species are found in the oral cavity, intestinal tract, and reproductive organs of man and other animals. Some species are pathogenic for cattle and sheep, causing abortion and human infections.

Gram-Negative Aerobic Rods and Cocci

Family I. *Pseudomonadaceae.* Gram-negative curved or straight aerobic rods that are motile. Type genus is *Pseudomonas.*

Genus I. *Pseudomonas* (false monad). Description as above. Strictly aerobic with respiratory metabolism. Type species is *Pseudomonas aeruginosa.* The genus is divided into four sections with 12 species in Section I, 7 species in Section II, 8 species in Section III, and 3 species in Section IV. Generally the species are found in the environment in soil and water. Some are pathogenic for mammals and plants. *Pseudomonas aeruginosa* has been isolated from a wide variety of human infections and is occasionally a plant pathogen. *Pseudomonas fluorescens* is associated with the spoilage of foods; *Pseudomonas pseudomallei* is a cause of meliodosis. *Pseudomonas mallei* causes glanders and farcy in horses. *Pseudomonas salanacearum* is an important plant pathogen.

Family VII. *Legionellaceae.* Gram-negative, aerobic, motile rods that do not ferment carbohydrates. One genus is recognized.

Genus I. *Legionella* (after legion or army). Description as above. There are six species. *Legionella pneumophila,* the type species, was first recognized after an outbreak of pneumonia at a Legionnaires' convention in 1976. The species are isolated from surface water, mud, and thermally polluted lakes. There is no known soil or animal source. The species are pathogenic for humans.

Family VIII. *Neisseriaceae.* Gram-negative, nonmotile, spherical bacteria that are aerobic and have complex growth requirements. Organisms are heterotrophic, utilizing organic nitrogen and carbohydrates. Cells occur in pairs or masses with adjacent sides flattened, or as rod shapes in pairs or chains. Obligate parasites of the mucous membrane of man. The family consists of *Neisseria, Moraxella, Acinetobacter,* and *Kingella.*

Genus I. *Neisseria* (after A. Neisser). Aerobic or facultatively anaerobic bacteria that occur in pairs with interfaces flattened. The genus consists of recognized species, of which *Neisseria gonorrhoeae* (gonococcus) and *Neisseria meningitidis* (meningococcus) are most important medically.

Genus II. *Moraxella* (after V. Morax). Gram-negative short rods that occur in pairs and short chains. Bacterium carries out oxidative metabolism. There are two subgenera: *Moraxella (Moraxella),* which has six species, such as *M. (M.) lacunata,* and *Moraxella (Branhamella),* which has four species, such as *M. (B.) catarrhalis.* All of the species inhabit the mucous membranes of humans and other warm-blooded animals.

continued on next page

Table 1.3 continued

Genus III. *Acinetobacter* (nonmotile rod). Gram-negative, nonmotile, nonsporulating, short and plump rods. Genus contains one species, *Acinetobacter calcoaceticus,* an inhabitant of healthy and diseased man and other animals. Probably an opportunistic pathogen in debilitated individuals.

Genus IV. *Kingella* (after E. O. King). Gram-negative to gram-variable, nonmotile, aerobic to facultatively anaerobic straight rods. Three species exist. *Kingella kingae* is the type species. Their natural habitat is the upper respiratory tract of humans.

Genera of Uncertain Affiliation

Genus *Brucella* (after Sir David Bruce). Gram-negative, nonmotile, nonsporulating, coccobacilli (short rods) that are strictly aerobic and are mammalian parasites and pathogens. *Brucella melitensis* is the type species. Six recognized species occur. *Brucella melitensis* is pathogenic for goats, sheep, cattle, and man. *Brucella abortus* is pathogenic for cattle and man. *Brucella suis* is pathogenic for swine, hare, reindeer, and man. *Brucella neotoma* is found in rats. *Brucella ovis* infects sheep, and *Brucella canis* infects dogs.

Genus *Bordetella* (after Jules Bordet). Gram-negative, variably motile minute coccobacilli that are strictly aerobic. The members of the genus are parasites and pathogens of mammals. Three recognized species occur, with *Bordetella pertussis* as the type species. *Bordetella pertussis* causes whooping cough in man, while *Bordetella parapetussis* produces a whooping cough-like disease in man. *Bordetella bronchiseptica* causes bronchopneumonia in dogs and other mammals.

Genus *Flavobacterium* (a yellow bacterium). Gram-negative, nonsporulating, motile cells that are pigmented, with hues ranging from yellow to brown, and are fastidious in their nutritive requirements. Twelve species have been isolated, of which *Flavobacterium breve* is pathogenic for laboratory animals and *Flavobacterium meningosepticum* is pathogenic for man. Species are commonly isolated from fresh and salt water.

Genus *Francisella* (after Edward Francis). Gram-negative, nonmotile, nonsporulating rods and cocci that are extremely pleomorphic. Two species are recognized, with *Francisella tularensis* as the type species. *Francisella tularensis* is found in natural waters and in species of wild animals in North America, Europe, Russia, Turkey, and Japan, where it is the cause of tularemia. *Francisella novicida* can induce a tularemia-like disease in white mice, guinea pigs, and hamsters, but it does not affect man.

Gram-Negative Facultatively Anaerobic Rods

Family I. *Enterobacteriaceae.* Gram-negative, motile and nonmotile, facultatively anaerobic rods that have both a respiratory and fermentative metabolism. The type genus is *Escherichia.*

Genus I. *Escherichia* (after Theodor Escherich). Cells are as described above.

The genus contains two species. The more important is *Escherichia coli,* which has several hundred antigenic specificities whose different combinations allow for several thousand serotypes.

Genus II. *Shigella* (after K. Shiga). Gram-negative, nonmotile rods that cannot utilize citrate as a sole carbon source. Ferments carbohydrates with the production of acid but no gas. Four recognized species occur; *Shigella dysenteriae* is the type species. All species inhabit the intestinal tracts of man and higher monkeys and all species produce dysentery in man.

Genus III. *Salmonella* (after D. E. Salmon). Gram-negative, usually motile rods that can use citrate as a source of carbon. The species of this genus have been named at different times according to the disease they produce or by the animal from which they were isolated, the geographic site at which they were first isolated, or the antigenic formula as established by the Kaufmann-White scheme, which designates by numbers and letters the different O, V, and H antigens of a given strain. The genus has now been divided into five subgenera that contain over 2,100 serotypes.

Genus IV. *Citrobacter* (citrate-using rod). Motile, gram-negative rods that can use citrate as the sole carbon source. The genus contains three recognized species, *Citrobacter freundii, Citrobacter diversus,* and *Citrobacter amalonaticus.*

Genus V. *Klebsiella* (after Edwin Klebs). Gram-negative, nonmotile capsulated rods that can use citrate and glucose as the sole carbon source. Three recognized species occur. *Klebsiella pneumoniae* is widely distributed in the environment, is a normal inhabitant of the intestinal tract of man and animals, and may be associated with infections of the intestinal and respiratory tracts. *Klebsiella ozaenae* is found in chronic diseases of the respiratory tract and ozena. *Klebsiella pneumoniae* subsp. *rhinoscleromatis* causes rhinosclerma.

Genus VI. *Enterobacter* (intestinal small rod). Gram-negative, motile rods that can utilize citrate and acetate as the sole carbon sources. Five species are recognized. *Enterobacter cloacae* is found in the feces of man and other animals and in the environment in sewage, soil, and water; it is found in pathological material from animals. *Enterobacter aerogenes* is found in sewage, soil, water, dairy products, and human and animal species.

Genus VII. *Erwinia* (after Erwin F. Smith). Gram-negative, motile, facultatively anaerobic rods. Several of the 12 species cause plant diseases. Some have been isolated from humans.

Genus VIII. *Serratia* (after Serafuno Serrati). Gram-negative, motile, capsulated rods that form pink, red, or magenta pigments. The genus contains six species. *Serratia marcescens* is widely distributed in food, soil, and water; and is an opportunistic pathogen in humans.

Genus IX. *Hafnia* (old name for Copenhagen). Gram-negative, motile, encapsulated rods that can use citrate and acetate as sole sources of carbon. The genus is represented by *Hafnia alvei,* which is found in human and animal feces, dairy products, sewage, soil, and water.

Genus X. *Edwardsiella* (after P. R. Edwards). Motile, gram-negative rods. The genus contains three species. *Edwardsiella tarda* is found in water, the intestinal tract of snakes, and the human intestinal tract, blood, and urine.

Table 1.3 continued

Genus XI. *Proteus* (a god who could transform himself into many forms). Gram-negative, pleomorphic, motile, nonencapsulated, straight rods that form involuted forms, coccoids, filaments, and spheroplasts. The genus has three recognized species. The species are found variously in human, chicken, and animal feces, sewage and soil, decomposing protein, urine, and human clinical specimens.

Genus XII. *Providencia* (after Providence, Rhode Island). Gram-negative, motile, facultatively anaerobic rods. Three species are recognized and have been isolated from diarrhetic stools, urinary tract infections, wounds, burns, and bacteremias.

Genus XIII. *Morganella* (after H. de R. Morgan). Gram-negative motile rods. *Morganella morganii* is the only species and is an opportunistic secondary invader isolated from bacteremias and from respiratory tract, wound, and urinary tract infections.

Genus XIV. *Yersinia* (after J. E. Yersin). Gram-negative, nonencapsulated, variously motile ovoid cells or rods. The genus is divided into seven recognized species. *Yersinia pestis,* the type species, causes plague in humans and rodents. *Yersinia pseudotuberculosis* causes a form of pseudotuberculosis in animals, generally in the mesenteric lymph nodes. *Yersinia enterocolitica,* while not pathogenic, is widely distributed in sick and healthy humans and animals and in dairy products.

Family II. *Vibrionaceae.* Gram-negative, motile, short rods that have a respiratory and fermentative metabolism and are facultatively anaerobic. Organisms inhabit fresh and salt water and the intestinal tracts of animals. Some species are pathogenic for man and fish.

Genus I. *Vibrio* (that which vibrates). Gram-negative, motile, nonsporulating rod that is facultatively anaerobic and has a respiratory metabolism. It is found in fresh and salt water and the intestinal tract of man and animals. Some species are pathogenic for man and fish. Twenty recognized species occur, with *Vibrio cholerae* as the type species. *Vibrio cholerae* is present in the intestines of normal and diseased man and animals, and classic cholera is related to certain strains of *Vibrio cholerae*. Other species are found in water and fish and other marine animals. Some are found in brine and cured meat.

Genus II. *Aeromonas* (gas-producing monad). Gram-negative, motile, rod-shaped cells that are both respiratory and fermentative. The genus has four recognized species, with *Aeromonas hydrophila* as the type species. The various species infect frogs and salmon, and *Aeromonas hydrophila* infects humans.

Genus III. *Plesiomonas* (neighbor monad). Gram-negative, motile, rod-shaped cells that have a respiratory and fermentative metabolism and are facultative anaerobes. The genus is represented by one species, *Plesiomonas shigelloides,* which inhabits the gastrointestinal tracts of man and animals and causes an infectious gastroenteritis in humans.

Family III. *Pasteurellaceae.* Gram-negative, nonmotile, straight rigid coccoid to rod-shaped cells that are aerobic with varying degrees of microaerophilia, or are facultatively anaerobic. Some are pathogenic for humans.

Genus I. *Pasteurella* (after Louis Pasteur). Gram-negative spherical, ovoid, or rod-shaped cells that are facultatively anaerobic. Six species occur, with *Pasteurella multocida* as the type species. They are widely distributed in nature, principally causing diseases in domesticated animals.

Genus II. *Haemophilus* (blood lover). Gram-negative, nonsporulating, parasitic rod-shaped or coccobacillary cells that are facultatively anaerobic and require growth factors present in the blood. There are 16 species, with *Haemophilus influenzae* as the type species. Species are found in the upper respiratory tract of man and other animals and in the oral cavity of man, where they cause a variety of infections. *Haemophilus ducreyi* is associated with soft chancre. *Haemophilus vaginalis* is found in the human genital tract but is not pathogenic for laboratory animals.

Genus III. *Actinobacillus* (ray bacillus). Gram-negative, nonmotile, nonsporulating cells that are spherical, oval, or rod-shaped and have a fermentative metabolism. There are five species. *Actinobacillus lignieresii,* the type species, is pathogenic for cattle and sheep but only slightly pathogenic for man and dogs. *Actinobacillus equuli* is pathogenic for horses and pigs. Evidence has been accumulating to assign a role to *Actinobacillus actinomycetemcomitans* in the development of juvenile periodontitis.

Genera of Uncertain Affiliation

Genus *Chromobacterium* (colored rod). Gram-negative, motile, nonencapsulated rods that have respiratory or fermentative metabolism and are strict aerobes or facultative anaerobes. They produce a violet pigment and are common inhabitants of fresh water and soils. The genus has two recognized species. *Chromobacterium violaceum* is found in soils and fresh water and causes serious pyogenic or septicemic infections in man and other mammals. *Chromobacterium lividum* has a similar distribution but is not pathogenic in man or other mammals.

Genus *Cardiobacterium* (bacterium of the heart). Gram-negative, nonmotile, nonsporulating, pleomorphic rods that have a fermentative metabolism and are facultatively anaerobic. The genus has one species, *Cardiobacterium hominis,* which is also the type species. It is a normal inhabitant of the human nose and throat and causes endocarditis in man.

Genus *Streptobacillus* (twisted or curved small rod). Gram-negative, nonmotile, nonsporulating rods that spontaneously convert to L phase. The cells are facultatively anaerobic and have a fermentative metabolism. The genus contains one species, *Streptobacillus moniliformis,* which is also the type species. Its activities range from parasitic to pathogenic in rats and other mammals, including man. A cause of rat-bite fever and arthritis.

Genus *Calymmatobacterium* (sheathed rodlet). Gram-negative, nonmotile, nonsporulating, encapsulated rods. The genus contains one species, *Calymmatobacterium granulomatis,* which is also the type species. The organism causes granuloma inguinale in man but is not pathogenic in laboratory animals.

Genus *Gardnerella* (after H. L. Gardner). Gram-negative to gram-variable pleomorphic rods that are nonmotile and facultatively anaerobic. Considered to be a major cause of bacterial nonspecific vaginitis.

continued on next page

Table 1.3 continued

Genus *Eikenella* (after M. Eiken). Gram-negative, nonmotile, facultatively anaerobic straight rods that do not produce acids from carbohydrates. *Eikenella corrodens,* the only recognized species, is found in the human mouth and intestine.

Gram-Negative Anaerobic Bacteria

Family I. *Bacteroidaceae.* Gram-negative, variably pleomorphic, variably motile, obligately anaerobic rods that are present in the cavities of man and other animals and the intestinal tracts of insects. Some species are pathogenic for man and animals.

    Genus I. *Bacteroides* (rod-like). Gram-negative, nonsporulating, nonmotile, obligately anaerobic rods that ferment sugars to produce organic acids. The genus contains 20 or more species, of which *Bacteroides fragilis* is the type species. The various species are found in the oral cavity, upper respiratory tract, genital tract, appendix, lacrymal gland, intestinal tract, and feces of man; the rumen of cattle and wild animals; the intestines of poultry, turkeys, and termites; and the infected hoofs of sheep and goats.

    Genus II. *Fusobacterium* (small spindle-shaped rod). Gram-negative, nonsporulating, variably motile rods that metabolize carbohydrates to produce organic acids and are obligately anaerobic. The genus contains 16 recognized species, of which *Fusobacterium nucleatum* is the type species. The species are common residents of the cavities of man and other animals. Some are pathogenic and they appear in various human infections.

    Genus III. *Leptotrichia* (fine hair). Gram-negative, nonmotile, anaerobic, straight or curved rods that produce acid but not gas from carbohydrates. One species is recognized, *Leptotrichia buccalis,* which is also the type species. An inhabitant of the oral cavity of man.

    Genus VIII. *Wolinella* (after M. J. Wolin). Gram-negative, motile, helical, curved or straight unbranched rods that are anaerobic. Carbohydrates are not fermented and do support growth. *Wolinella succinogenes* and *Wolinella recta* are the recognized species and occur in the bovine rumen and the human mouth. These bacteria have been isolated from periodontal disease sites and infected root canals.

    Genus IX. *Selenomonas* (moon-shaped monad). Gram-negative, motile, anaerobic, curved to helical rods. The genus contains two species. *Selenomonas sputigena,* the type species, is an inhabitant of the human mouth.

Gram-Negative Anaerobic Cocci

Family I. *Veillonellaceae.* Gram-negative, nonmotile, anaerobic cocci that have complex nutritional requirements. A common inhabitant of the intestinal tract of man, ruminants, rodents, and pigs, and a predominant species in the human oral cavity. The family is composed of three genera, of which *Veillonella* is the type genus.

    Genus I. *Veillonella* (after A. Veillon). Gram-negative, nonmotile, nonsporulating, anaerobic cocci that are unable to ferment carbohydrates and have complex nutritional requirements. Seven recognized species occur; *Veillonella parvula* is the type species. An abundant inhabitant of the human, rat, and hamster mouth, respiratory, and intestinal tracts.

Gram-Positive Cocci

Family I. *Micrococcaceae.* Gram-positive spheroidal cells that form regular or irregular clusters or packets. Motile or nonmotile. Chemoorganotrophs. The family consists of *Micrococcus, Staphylococcus,* and *Planococcus.*

    Genus II. *Staphylococcus* ("grapelike coccus"). Nonmotile cocci that tend to form irregular clusters. Respiratory or fermentative metabolism. Facultative anaerobes that prefer aerobic conditions. The genus consists of *Staphylococcus aureus,* a potential pathogen that is an obligate parasite of the respiratory and intestinal tracts of warm-blooded animals; *Staphylococcus epidermidis,* primarily an inhabitant of skin and mucous membranes of warm-blooded mammals as commensals or parasites; and *Staphylococcus saprophyticus,* a nonpathogen found in the environment, dairy products, and urine.

Family II. *Streptococcaceae.* Gram-positive spherical or ovoid cells that tend to form chains. Usually nonmotile and nonsporulating. Facultatively anaerobic with a fermentative metabolism and complex nutritional requirements. The family consists of five genera: *Streptococcus, Leuconostoc, Pediococcus, Aerococcus,* and *Gemella.*

    Genus I. *Streptococcus* (pliant coccus). Gram-positive cells, typically occurring in pairs or chains. Fermentative metabolism and facultatively anaerobic, with complex nutritional requirements. Twenty-one species are recognized, divided into a hemolytic pyogenic group, subdivided by immunological criteria (e.g., *Streptococcus pyogenes*); a viridans group (turns blood green), of which *Streptococcus salivarius, Streptococcus mitis,* and *Streptococcus sanguis* constitute a major part of the oral microbiota; an enterococcus group, represented by *Streptococcus faecalis,* that contains primarily intestinal parasites but is also found in the mouth; and a lactic group of primarily plant parasites, also used for the manufacture of dairy products (e.g., *Streptococcus lactis*). Not included in these four groups are some 80 types of *Streptococcus pneumoniae* (the pneumococcus), primarily an obligate parasite of the nasopharynx and an important pathogen of the respiratory tract, causing pneumonia.

Family III. *Peptococcaceae.* Gram-positive cocci that occur in pairs, tetrads, irregular masses, and cubic packets or in chains. Nonsporulating and nonmotile, with complex nutritional requirements. Inhabitants of the oral cavity and the intestinal and respiratory tracts of man and other animals and the human female urogenital tract.

    Genus I. *Peptococcus.* Consists of six species of spherical bacteria (type species, *Peptococcus niger*) that do not require carbohydrates but obtain energy from protein decomposition products. Inhabitants of the human female urogenital tract, the human oral cavity, the human intestinal and respiratory tract, tonsils, skin, and infected areas, but of uncertain pathogenicity.

    Genus II. *Peptostreptococcus.* Gram-positive, nonmotile, nonsporulating spherical or ovoid cells. Anaerobic and

Table 1.3 continued

generally ferment carbohydrates to form organic acids. Inhabitants of the normal and infected oral cavity and female genital tract and often found in septic wounds, gangrene, osteomyelitis, and appendicitis. There are five recognized species; *Peptostreptococcus anaerobius* is the type species.

Endospore-Forming Rods

Family I. *Bacillaceae.* Gram-positive, motile or nonmotile, aerobic facultative or anaerobic sporulating rods with one genus having spherical cells.

Genus I. *Bacillus* (rodlet). Gram-positive, sporulating, motile, rod-shaped cells that are aerobes or facultative anaerobes. Some 48 species occur in the genus, with *Bacillus subtilis* as the type species. *Bacillus anthracis* causes anthrax in animals and humans.

Genus III. *Clostridium* (small spindle). Generally gram-positive, occasionally nonmotile, sporulating, generally strictly anaerobic rods. Inhabitants of marine and freshwater sediments, soil, and the intestinal tract of man and other animals and animal products. The genus contains more than 60 species. *Clostridium butyricum* is the type species. Various species infect wounds and cause gas gangrene, tetanus, and botulism.

Gram-Positive, Asporogenous Rod-Shaped Bacteria

Family I. *Lactobacillaceae.* Gram-positive, nonmotile, anaerobic or facultative straight or curved rods with complex nutritional requirements. Metabolize carbohydrates to produce lactate. Widely distributed in plant and animal products. A common organism in the oral cavity, vagina, and intestinal tract of man and other animals.

Genus I. *Lactobacillus* (milk-rodlet). Gram-positive rods that vary from long and slender to short coccobacilli that are generally nonmotile. Metabolize sugars to terminally produce lactate. The genus has 25 recognized species, with *Lactobacillus delbrueckii* as the type species. The species are widely distributed in dairy products, grain, meat products, water, sewage, pickled fruit and vegetables, beer, wine, and silage. Particularly common in the oral cavity, intestinal tract, and vagina of humans and other animals.

Genera of Uncertain Affiliation

Genus *Listeria* (after Lord Lister). Gram-positive, motile, nonsporulating, small coccoid rods that are found on vegetation, silage, and in the intestinal tracts of man and other animals. The genus has four recognized species; *Listeria monocytogenes* is the type species. Diseases produced include abortion, local abscesses, endocarditis, septicemia, encephalitis, and meningitis. Pathogenicity is variable among the species.

Genus *Erysipelothrix* (erysipelas thread). Gram-positive, nonsporulating, nonmotile, aerobic, rod-shaped organisms that form filaments. Parasites of birds, mammals, and fish. One species exists, *Erysipelothrix rhusiopathiae,* which is also the type species. This microbe causes swine erysipelas and is occasionally pathogenic for man.

Actinomycetes and Related Organisms

Coryneform Group of Bacteria. Pleomorphic, mostly nonmotile rods that are frequently banded with metachromatic granules. Generally gram-positive. Includes the genera *Corynebacterium, Arthrobacter, Microbacterium, Cellulomonas,* and *Kurthia.*

Genus I. *Corynebacterium* (club bacterium). The cells frequently show club-shaped swelling and "snapping division" that produces palisade arrangement of cells. The genus has been divided into three sections: I—Human and animal parasites and pathogens. II—Plant pathogenic corynebacteria. III—Nonpathogenic corynebacteria. Section I is divided into nine recognized species, with *Corynebacterium diphtheriae,* the cause of diphtheria, as the type species.

Order I. *Actinomycetales.* Gram-positive, acid-fast bacteria that form branching filaments that fragment to coccoid, elongate, or diphtheroid elements. Some forms reproduce by spores on aerial hyphae.

Family I. *Actinomycetaceae.* Gram-positive, non-acid-fast bacteria that form filaments that fragment into diphtheroid-shaped or coccoid cells.

Genus I. *Actinomyces* (ray fungus). Gram-positive, non-acid-fast, nonmotile, nonsporulating bacteria that occur as filaments that fragment into diphtheroids. Mostly anaerobic, but some are facultative anaerobes. Five species are recognized, with *Actinomyces bovis* as the type species. All species are found in the oral cavity of man and other animals.

Genus II. *Arachnia* (filamentous microcolonies). Similar to, but distinct from, the genus *Actinomyces.* Represented by a single species, *Arachnia propionica,* which is pathogenic for man and mice, causing a disease similar to actinomycosis.

Genus IV. *Bacterionema* (thread-shaped long rod). Gram-positive, nonsporulating, nonmotile, pleomorphic filaments and bacilli. Facultative anaerobe that ferments carbohydrates. Represented by a single species, *Bacterionema matruchotii,* that is found in the oral cavity of primates and man in calculus and dental plaque.

Genus V. *Rothia* (after G. D. Roth). Gram-positive, non-acid-fast, nonsporulating, nonmotile bacteria that can occur singly or as a mixture of coccoid, diphtheroid, or branched filaments. Represented by the species *Rothia dentocariosa,* a normal inhabitant of the oral cavity.

Family II. *Mycobacteriaceae.* Cells composed of curved or straight rods that also branch or form filaments. Gram-positive, nonmotile, nonsporulating. Aerobic. Slow or rapid growth. Found in the soil, water, and in warm-blooded and cold-blooded animals. Contains one genus, *Mycobacterium.*

Genus I. *Mycobacterium* (fungus rodlet). Cells as described above with a high lipid content. Composed of 30 recognized species. *Mycobacterium tuberculosis,* the cause of tuberculosis, is the type species. Many of the other species are pathogenic. *Mycobacterium leprae,* the cause of leprosy, is another important species.

continued on next page

Table 1.3 continued

Family VI. *Nocardiaceae.* Gram-positive, variably acid-fast, nonsporulating, obligate aerobes. Cells vary among filaments, coccoids, and bacillary fragments. Reproductive spores are produced on differentiated hyphae.

  Genus I. *Nocardia* (after E. Nocard). Cells similar to those described above. The genus consists of some 31 recognized species, with *Nocardia farcinica* as the type species. Common inhabitant of soils and humans and other animals. Some species cause nocardiosis, which resembles actinomycosis.

Family VII. *Streptomycetaceae.* Resemble fungi, with vegetative hyphae that produce branched mycelia that do not fragment easily. Forms aerial spores. Gram-positive, aerobic. Four genera.

  Genus I. *Streptomyces* (pliant or bent fungus). Forms slender coenocytic hyphae and aerial mycelia that bear reproductive spores. Many strains are sensitive to antibacterial agents. There are more than 400 recognized species that are widely distributed in the environment. Many of these species and strains produce antibacterial, antifungal, antiviral, antialgal, antiprotozoal, or even antitumor antibiotics.

The Rickettsias

Order I. *Rickettsiales.* Gram-negative, nonmotile, pleomorphic, rod-shaped, coccoid, small microorganisms that can multiply only in the cells of a suitable host. These procaryotic microorganisms are not related to viruses.

Family I. *Rickettsiaceae.* Small pleomorphic organisms, intracellular parasites that, with one exception, have not been cultured in cell-free media. The organisms occur as parasites of man and other animals and are transmitted by insect vectors such as mites, ticks, fleas, and lice.

  Tribe I. *Rickettsieae.* Small, pleomorphic, intracellular microorganisms that are obligate parasites and pathogens.

  Genus I. *Rickettsia* (after H. T. Ricketts). Gram-negative short rods that have not been cultivated without the presence of living host cells. Growth occurs in the cytoplasm of such cells. Man may be the reservoir or the incidental host of *Rickettsia* species. Small rodents and other vertebrates also serve as reservoirs and disseminate rickettsia. Arthropods, the principal reservoirs, regulate transmission to and from susceptible vertebrates. There are 10 recognized species. The type species is *Rickettsia prowazekii.* The various strains of the genus *Rickettsia* can be divided into biotypes that cause either typhus, spotted fever, or scrub typhus.

  Genus II. *Rochalimaea* (after H. da RochaLima). Similar to the genus *Rickettsia,* this genus depends on vertebrates and arthropods for survival. The genus contains one species, *Rochalimaea quintana,* which is also the type species. The organism causes trench fever, which is transmitted to the primary human host by the human louse.

  Genus III. *Coxiella* (after H. R. Cox). Resembles the genus *Rickettsia* but is more resistant. The genus contains one species, *Coxiella burnetii,* which is the type species. *Coxiella burnetii,* the cause of Q fever, is widely distributed throughout the world in domestic animals and their ectoparasites, as well as the ectoparasites of rodents and marsupials. While such vectors transmit the disease, it is also an aerosol infection.

Family II. *Bartonellaceae.* Gram-negative, pleomorphic, rod-shaped, coccoid, and disc-shaped cells that are parasites of human and vertebrate erythrocytes but can be cultivated on nonliving media.

  Genus I. *Bartonella* (after A. L. Barton). Gram-negative but stain poorly. Found in the host in fixed tissue cells and erythrocytes but can be grown in cell-free media. The genus has one species, *Bartonella bacilliformis,* which is the type species. It is the cause of human bartonellosis, which occurs as either an anemia (Oroya fever) or as cutaneous eruptions (verruga peruana).

Order II. *Chlamydiales.* Gram-negative coccoid microorganisms that require an intracellular mode of reproduction involving an infectious phase (elementary body) and a noninfectious form (initial body).

Family I. *Chlamydiaceae.* Coccoid organisms that have a developmental cycle within the cytoplasm of the host. Cause various diseases.

  Genus I. *Chlamydia* (cloak). Gram-negative, nonmotile, obligate intracellular parasites that undergo a developmental cycle in the cytoplasm of the host's cells. Greatly dependent on the host cells for metabolic activity. Of the two recognized species, *Chlamydia trachomatis* is the type species. *Chlamydia trachomatis* causes trachoma, inclusion conjunctivitis, lymphogranuloma venereum, urethritis, and proctitis. The other species, *Chlamydia psittaci,* causes psittacosis; ornithosis; pneumonitis in several domestic animals; polyarthritis in cattle, sheep, and pigs; abortion in cattle and sheep; enteritis in cattle; conjunctivitis in cattle and sheep; intestinal infections in cattle and sheep; and encephalomyelitis in cattle.

The Mycoplasmas

Class *Mollicutes.* Prokaryotic organisms that lack a true cell wall and are incapable of synthesizing certain cell wall precursors. Cells are gram-negative and consist of small, highly pleomorphic coccoids or filaments that are small and sometimes ultramicroscopic. All recognized species are capable of growth in cell-free media. These organisms may be either saprophytic, parasitic, or pathogenic. Pathogenic species cause diseases in both animals and plants.

Order I. *Mycoplasmatales.* Description of the order similar to the class. Only one order, *Mycoplasmatales,* occurs in the class *Mollicutes;* two families occur in the order *Mycoplasmatales.*

Family I. *Mycoplasmataceae.* Description similar to that of the class and order. Require sterols.

  Genus I. *Mycoplasma* (fungus form). Gram-negative, extremely pleomorphic cells with alternate means of replication. The organisms, which lack a true cell wall, form very small colonies (up to 600 μm) on solid media. Generally they have a fermentative metabolism, and all species require sterols for growth. They range from aerobes to facultative anaerobes. They may be either parasites or pathogens in a wide range of mammals and birds. The principal diseases are contagious pleuropneumonia of cattle and goats, pink-eye in cattle, chronic respiratory diseases in poultry, infectious synovitis in chickens and turkeys, "rolling disease" in mice, atrophic rhinitis, pneumonia in pigs, primary atypical pneumonia in man, mastitis in cattle, and purulent polyarthritis in rats. More than 36 species are recognized; *Mycoplasma mycoides* is the type species.

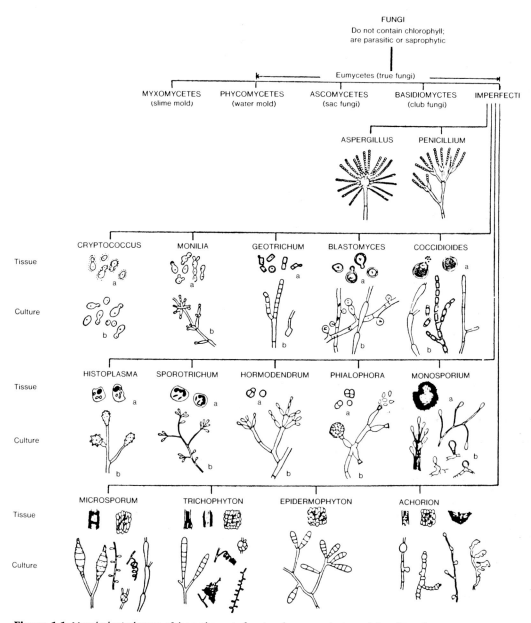

Figure 1.1: Morphological types of the pathogenic fungi as they occur in tissue (*a*) and in culture (*b*). (Adapted with permission from chart prepared by N. E. Conant: In *Musser's Internal Medicine,* Ed. 5, edited by M. G. Wohl. Lea & Febiger, Philadelphia, 1951.)

and by various industrial firms that use microorganisms in their manufacturing processes (e.g., breweries, wineries, pharmaceutical houses, food manufacturers and processors, chemical manufacturers).

Eumycetes (True Fungi)

The true fungi may be defined as nonphotosynthetic thallophytes that typically grow in filaments and re-

produce by sporulation, i.e., each unit plant produces a large number of spores, whereas most of the sporulating bacteria produce only one spore per cell and can multiply indefinitely without sporulation. Most fungi have well-defined sexual modes of sporulation, involving nuclear fusion and reduction in chromosome number, but they form spores asexually most of the time (Fig. 1.1).

On germination, the spore enlarges and puts forth one or more processes called germ tubes, which elongate at the distal end to become filaments, called hyphae. In many cases, each hypha lays down cross walls (septa) to form a chain of cells. The cell walls are typically well defined, relatively thick, and extraordinarily resistant chemically, resembling the chitin of the outer coat of crustaceans and insects. As the hyphae grow, they branch and form a tangled mat of filaments called the mycelium, examples of which are familiar to everyone as the growth of molds. A part of the mycelium penetrates the substrate to absorb nourishment and is called a vegetative mycelium; another part extends into the atmosphere and is called an aerial mycelium. When an aerial mycelium begins to bear spores, it is a reproductive mycelium.

A considerable group of fungi, the yeasts, are quite primitive and do not form true filaments but grow instead as single spheroid cells. Yeasts reproduce asexually by putting forth spheroid buds, called blastospores, which break off, enlarge, and reproduce as the parent does. One group of yeasts can also form spores asexually. With nuclear fusion and reduction of chromosome number, the cell enlarges to form a spore sac (ascus) containing one to eight spores, which are termed ascospores. An intermediate yeast, the genus *Candida,* forms a pseudomycelium consisting of chains of elongated buds. Quite a few pathogenic fungi can grow either in a yeastlike or moldlike filamentous form, depending on cultural conditions. In vivo, the yeastlike forms predominate. Such fungi are said to be false yeasts.

Unlike bacteria, most fungi are large enough and exhibit sufficient differentiation of structure to permit classification along standard botanical lines without resorting to physiological and biochemical characteristics. They are classified by the type of colony produced (yeast types, resembling bacterial colonies, or mold type); by the presence or absence of mycelia; by the character of the mycelium (septate or not); by the size, structure, and color of the spores; and, most important, by the characteristic mechanisms of sexual and asexual spore formation. On these bases, eumycetes are divided into four classes:

I. Phycomycetes ("seaweed fungus"). A diverse, widely distributed group but of negligible medical importance.

II. Ascomycetes ("sac fungus"). A diverse and widely distributed group; a few genera occasionally infect man and animals.

III. Basidiomycetes. Except for the species that form powerful poisons, they are not medically important.

IV. Fungi imperfecti (imperfect fungi). Hyphae septate; no sexual stage known; asexual spores formed in various typical ways as conidia (see Ascomycetes) or directly within, upon, or from the thallus (= mycelium or body of the fungus) as thallospores. Practically all of the fungi pathogenic for man fall in this class. Many of these grow yeastlike in vivo and under appropriate culture conditions, and moldlike under other culture conditions.

Classification and Nomenclature of Viruses

It is generally agreed that four characteristics distinguish a virus. 1) It contains either DNA or RNA but not both, in contrast to other microorganisms and higher forms. 2) It lacks enzymes to convert substrates into high-energy compounds needed to drive biosynthetic reactions, and also lacks the enzymes requisite for biosynthesis. 3) It cannot grow and then divide by binary fission. 4) Its reproduction consists essentially of the replication of its nucleic acid genetic material by the metabolic mechanisms of the infected host cell. The incidental production of a proteinaceous coat (capsid) serves primarily to stabilize the nucleic acid component and protect it from nucleases during passage of the virus to a fresh host cell.

In biological terms, a virus is a rudimentary subcellular genetic entity that is capable of gaining entrance into a limited range of living cells and capable of reproduction only within such cells. Intracellularly, after conversion into a noninfective form, its genetic information specifically directs biosynthetic pathways of the host cell to replicate the viral genome and its associated capsid. This process does not necessarily impair the infected cell seriously—in some systems the cell survives and liberates new virus indefinitely; in others, the cell and its progeny maintain a persistent infection without the appearance of extracellular virus.

A completely satisfactory definition of viruses is hardly possible at present, let alone a description of their natural relationships to each other and to more familiar microorganisms. The criteria of filterability and size ceased to be definitive with the discovery of free-living organisms smaller than many viruses. The property of obligate intracellular parasitism is relevant but is not peculiar to viruses, being characteristic of occasional protozoa and bacteria. The property of producing disease is of methodological value only, since many viruses are maintained in their hosts for long periods without producing discernible pathological change.

The modern classification of viruses relates largely to the physicochemical properties of the virus particle. The principal components involved are nucleic acids and proteins, although larger virions may contain carbohydrates and lipids.

As for other organisms, the basis for viral nomenclature is varied and often arbitrary. Many names are based on clinical, pathological, or epidemiological features, e.g., Eastern equine encephalomyelitis virus. Others are descriptive, being based on some outstanding characteristic of the virus, e.g., orbivirus group (L. *orbis* = ring), derived from their large doughnut-shaped capsomeres. Some names are acronyms, e.g., reovirus, from *r*espiratory-*e*nteric-*o*rphan, while others reflect the name of the individual who first described the virus, such as the Rous sarcoma virus. Finally, some describe the region where the virus was located or predominates, such as Colorado tick fever virus.

Virus classification is based on common, genetically stable properties that include nucleic acid type, strandedness, and molecular weight; virus shape; capsomere number; site of production or maturation; and presence or absence of an outer envelope. These and other major characteristics are summarized for the major families of RNA and DNA viruses in Table 34.2.

ADDITIONAL READING

Buchanan, R. E., and Gibbons, N. E. (Eds.) 1974. *Bergey's Manual of Determinative Bacteriology.* Williams & Wilkins, Baltimore.

Fenner, F. 1974. The Classification of Viruses; Why, When and How. Aust J Exp Biol Med Sci, **52**, 223.

Krieg, N. R., and Holt, J. G. (Eds.) 1984. *Bergey's Manual of Systematic Bacteriology.* Williams & Wilkins, Baltimore.

Melnick, J. L. 1980. Taxonomy of Viruses. In *Manual of Clinical Microbiology,* edited by E. H. Lennette, A. Balows, W. J. Hausler, and J. P. Truant. American Society for Microbiology, Washington, D.C.

Molinari, J. A., and Phillip, M. J. 1980. Microbiology and Sterilization. In *Review of Dental Assisting,* edited by B. A. Ladley and S. A. Wilson. C. V. Mosby, St. Louis.

Ravin, A. W. 1960. The Origins of Bacterial Species. Genetic Recombination and Factors Limiting It between Bacterial Populations. Bacteriol Rev, **24**, 201.

Skerman, V. V. D. 1959. *A Guide to the Identification of the Genera of Bacteria.* Williams & Wilkins, Baltimore.

Society of General Microbiology. 1959. Symposium: The Principles of Microbial Classification. J Gen Microbiol, **12**, 314.

2

Isolation and Systematic Examination of Pathogenic Microorganisms

Chris H. Miller

The isolation of pathogenic microorganisms from man and their identification are of primary importance in determining the diagnosis and in recommending therapy for infectious diseases. In addition, the techniques used are important in determining the types and numbers of microorganisms present at various body sites under various conditions. (For example, in research studies on the "anticaries" effects of an antimicrobial agent, effects on both caries-inducing and less pathogenic oral microorganisms must be measured.) During the isolation and identification of microorganisms from the human body, consideration must be given to many procedures, each of which can influence the final results: specimen collection, transport, and initial processing; selection, inoculation, and incubation of growth media; and identification of the isolated microorganisms. The specific procedures depend on the type of specimen, the suspected types of microorganisms present in the specimen, and the specific types of re- sults desired. Of particular procedural importance in all phases of microbial isolation, identification, and manipulation is the use of aseptic technique—procedures that prevent or reduce unwanted microbial contamination.

Collection of Specimens

Sampling Sites

The site of specimen collection is usually dictated by the pathogenesis of the disease. Specimens that are usually free of indigenous microorganisms are needle or surgical biopsy tissues, blood, spinal fluid, and exudates or other unnatural accumulations of fluid within various internal body cavities. Contaminating indigenous microorganisms are usually found in specimens associated with mucous membranes and skin. It is necessary to avoid as much as possible contamination of a clinical specimen by normal body flora. This is a constant problem when sampling oral sites. The oral lesions from which microbial specimens are often obtained include periodontal lesions, including pericoronitis, acute necrotizing ulcerative gingivitis, and periodontitis; lesions of the oral tissues such as might occur in syphilis, oral gonorrhea, denture stomatitis, candidiasis, herpes, and other fungal and viral infections; abscesses with suppuration; postoperative infections from extractions or soft tissue surgery; sinus drainage through the oroantral fistula from perforations of the maxillary sinus; salivary gland infections; biopsy tissues; and infected root canals.

Sampling Methods

When fluid or biopsy tissue is collected by needle aspiration through the skin or a mucous membrane, the surface must be disinfected with an antiseptic to reduce or prevent entry of organisms into the tissues and contamination of the specimen by normal body flora. Blood, spinal fluid, midstream urine specimens, bronchial washings, sputum, saliva, and feces are best collected directly into sterile containers which are transported to the laboratory. Tissue specimens and dental plaque are collected with aseptic technique and commonly placed into small containers of stabilizing or transport fluid to preserve microbial viability. Swabbing of specific lesions or other sites should involve as little contamination as possible from adjacent sites. For example, a sample of purulent drainage from an excised oral abscess or opened tooth pulp must not be contaminated with saliva. Since plain cotton swabs may contain antibacterial fatty acids, it is best to use sterile swabs made of calcium alginate or Dacron or Fortrel polyesters. Commercially available swabs include those which are packaged in a receptacle containing a transport fluid.

If strictly anaerobic bacteria are highly likely to be present, such as in oral infections, samples may be collected under anaerobic conditions. The sample is collected as usual and then immediately placed into a prereduced fluid that has low oxygen tension and a low oxidation-reduction potential. Such fluids are commercially available. To avoid entrance of air, a stream of oxygen-free gas may also be used when the container of prereduced fluid is opened. Other devices have been described for use during the sampling of anaerobic organisms such as might be found in periodontal pockets. The samples are taken through cannulas modified so that the site can be continually flushed with oxygen-free gas while the sample is taken. Such samples are then placed in a prereduced medium from which oxygen has been excluded; they may be dispersed and cultured in an anaerobic environment.

Transport of Specimens

Specimens should be transported to the microbiology laboratory for analysis as quickly as possible to prevent overgrowth of contaminating microorganisms and the death of potential pathogens. When specimens are collected in a hospital or research setting, a common time limit between collection and delivery to the laboratory is 2 hours. Specimens collected in the dental office should be taken to the laboratory immediately. If the specimens must be mailed, they should be placed in a transport medium, preferably in an unbreakable tube sealed with waterproof tape, wrapped with absorbent material, placed in a second container sealed with waterproof tape, and finally placed in a sealed, properly labeled shipping container. Shipping with dry ice may help preserve the specimen.

Each clinical specimen must be fully described so that the laboratory will be able to select the proper procedures for analysis. The description should include the type of specimen, site of collection, attempts taken to avoid contamination, patient symptoms or suspected diagnosis, suspected types of microorganisms present, and need for antibiotic sensitivity testing on the predominant or unusual isolates.

Initial Processing of Specimens

Some specimens such as feces and dental plaque must be diluted before culturing so that workable numbers of microorganisms can be obtained. In addition, dental plaque samples must first be dispersed by controlled sonic oscillation or vortexing with glass beads to facilitate the separation of the many types of bacterial cells present in this adherent mass. Precautions must be taken during dispersion and dilution procedures to preserve the strictly anaerobic microorganisms.

General information on the microbial content of a raw specimen can frequently be obtained by performing various types of bacterial staining and microscopic procedures (e.g., gram stain, capsular stain, dark-field examination). A great deal of research is being conducted on the rapid identification of microorganisms including methods analyzing for specific microbial products and components directly in raw specimens. Advances in this field are of particular importance to the dentist and physician because the sooner the microorganisms can be identified, the sooner the diagnosis can be made and appropriate therapy instituted.

Bacteria

The presence of some specific bacteria can be detected directly in mixed cultures using DNA probes. However, the identification of most bacteria still requires that they be separated from all other microorganisms and maintained in pure culture. Since this type of identification entails working with a population of like cells rather than with a single cell (due to the small size), a pure culture is commonly defined as an isolated colony of more than 1 million bacterial cells that are direct offspring of a single cell or colony-forming unit (CFU).

Methods of Isolation

Specimens from the human mouth and other body sites contain mixed populations of microbes, and characterization of the different bacteria present requires that each type be separated from the others. The isolation of a pure culture of bacteria can be accomplished with a suitable agar-containing medium by either the streaking method or the pour plate method. Samples are placed on or in a suitable nutrient broth that is made semisolid by the addition of agar. Agar is a polysaccharide from seaweed that is nontoxic and not affected by bacteria. When placed in an aqueous nutrient broth and boiled prior to steam sterilization, the agar liquefies (at about 100°C). When the medium is cooled to about 40°C, the agar solidifies and will not melt again until temperatures of 100°C are reached.

Streak Plate Method. A suitably diluted specimen containing a mixture of bacterial types or species is spread or "streaked" on the surface of a suitable solidified agar medium in a sterile Petri dish. Spreading or streaking is performed with a sterilized bacteriological inoculating loop, a sterilized bent glass rod, or by automatic plating. As the inoculum passes over the surface of the agar, individual or small groups of bacterial cells (CFU) are deposited, and after appropriate incubation each develops into an isolated colony if the sample was diluted sufficiently and spread properly (Fig. 2.1). Each isolated colony, now usually visible to the naked eye, can be counted (if one is determining numbers of CFU in the original specimen) and subcultured for further tests leading to identification.

Pour Plate Method. This is an alternative to the streak plate method. Sterile, melted agar medium is cooled to about 48°C and the properly diluted specimen is added and gently mixed. The medium is poured into a Petri dish and allowed to cool and solidify. After appropriate incubation, visible, isolated colonies develop throughout the agar.

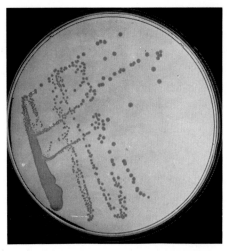

Figure 2.1: Open view of Petri dish containing nutrient agar upon which a bacterial inoculum has been spread with an inoculating loop to give distinct and separate colonies.

Aerobic and Anaerobic Culturing

Bacteria have varying requirements for oxygen and carbon dioxide, and bacteria from the human body may be aerobic, facultatively anaerobic, microaerophilic, or anaerobic. Plating and culturing of anaerobic bacteria may be carried out in an anaerobic environment using anaerobic chambers or glove boxes in which the air has been replaced with an oxygen-free gas mixture (e.g., 85% N_2, 10% H_2, 5% CO_2). Growth media also may be inoculated under a stream of oxygen-free gas and the vessels sealed or placed in an anaerobic holding jar until ready for incubation. Cultures in sealed anaerobic tubes are incubated in the usual fashion. Unsealed cultures may be incubated in temperature-adjusted anaerobic chambers and glove boxes or they may be placed in sealed, reduced-oxygen jars and placed in a regular incubator. Oxygen can be removed from a closed container by a catalytic process in which hydrogen reacts with the oxygen in the presence of a platinized asbestos catalyst to form water. Commercially prepared units are available in which water is added to an exact mixture of chemicals and placed in jars that contain the catalyst. The oxygen is removed and carbon dioxide is produced, yielding an anaerobic environment. The media used to culture strict anaerobes should also contain reducing agents (e.g., dithiothreitol, thioglycollate) to lower the oxidation-reduction potential. Reduced media also may be prepared and stored under oxygen-free conditions prior to inoculation.

Bacterial Growth Media

Media used for the isolation of bacteria by the streak or pour plate methods can be divided into two types, nonselective and selective. In general, both types contain basic growth nutrients in the form of protein digests, extracts of yeasts or plant and animal tissues, salts, and frequently blood and sugars. The nonselective media (e.g., blood agar) support the growth of many commonly encountered pathogenic and nonpathogenic bacteria. Selective media contain either inhibitors of undesired bacteria or growth promoters of desired bacteria, or both. Rogosa's medium, selective for the aciduric lactobacilli, contains acetate and other salts to suppress most oral bacteria and enrichments for lactobacilli. Crystal violet and potassium tellurite are used to select for certain oral streptococci (e.g., Mitis-Salivarius medium) and facilitate the isolation of *Streptococcus mitis, Streptococcus salivarius,* and other streptococci. In other selective media, dyes, bile, antibiotics, and high salt content are typical inhibitors.

In most microbial analyses of mixed culture specimens a combination of nonselective and selective media is used for primary isolation. Use of only a nonselective medium may result in the masking or interspecies inhibition of important bacteria. Such bacteria may be present in the sample at lower concentration, and thus would appear only on plates that have a large total number of colonies, making isolation and/or enumeration difficult or impossible. The use of appropriate selective media permits the isolation of bacteria that are masked or inhibited on nonselective media. On the other hand, the use of selective media for enumeration of specific bacteria in a given specimen must be done with caution, since this type of medium can select against as well as for the desired bacterium.

Not all pathogenic bacteria can be cultured in vitro, and some have few or no animal hosts. Fully pathogenic *Treponema pallidum* apparently has not been cultured in vitro but can be maintained by serial transfer in rabbit testes. *Mycobacterium leprae* has not been cultured in vitro and has only one apparent animal host, the armadillo. Nevertheless, animal inoculation is an important means for isolating and, in a few instances, for maintaining pathogenic bacteria. In addition, microscopic studies coupled with microbial isolation and identification suggest that microorganisms are present in the mouth and alimentary canal of man that have never been cultured or identified.

Maintenance of Pure Cultures

While awaiting identification or further study, pure cultures of bacteria must be maintained in such a way as to preserve their viability without significantly changing their properties. Lyophilization is widely used to preserve bacteria. Suspensions in sterile protein solution are quick-frozen in dry ice and alcohol, their water is removed under a high vacuum, and the tubes are sealed and stored under refrigeration. Lyophilized bacteria survive for a long time but die slowly so that after prolonged storage the surviving population may be selected for some particular characteristic. When lyophilization is not available, pure cultures may be stored at 4°C in sealed tubes of agar media or frozen in broth media to which a 10% final concentration of sterile glycerin has been added.

Enumeration of Bacteria

It is frequently necessary to determine the concentration of bacteria present in clinical specimens or laboratory cultures. For example, the microbiological diagnosis of a urinary tract infection is commonly based on demonstration that the urine specimen contains more than 100,000 organisms per 1 ml. Recovery of 10,000 to 100,000 per 1 ml with three or more bacterial species represented usually denotes contamination of the urine during collection rather than infection. Enumeration of the different types of bacteria in dental or crevicular plaque or saliva samples has been used to determine the predominant bacteria present during different stages of periodontal disease and dental caries. This approach is also used to measure shifts in the proportions of pathogenic oral bacteria during the testing or use of various preventive or treatment regimens for caries and periodontal diseases. Additionally, bacterial enumeration is important in the quality control of drinking water and milk, since certified milk is limited to 10,000 bacteria per 1 ml and drinking water to 1 coliform per 100 ml in the United States. Counting bacteria is also important in the determination of growth requirements, measurement of virulence, or standardization of reference cultures and whole-cell vaccines.

The most useful counting procedures are the direct count and the viable count. A direct count, usually carried out in a counting chamber under the microscope, indicates the total number of cells, whether living or dead. The viable count gives the number of bacterial cells that will grow under given culturing conditions. For a viable count, measured amounts of various sample dilutions are plated by the streak or pour plate method and the colonies that develop after incubation are counted. Each colony theoretically represents a single cell originally deposited on or in the agar medium. In reality, a single colony may be derived from 1 to 25 or more cells (a CFU), owing to cell aggregation or natural associations (e.g., chains of streptococci) in the inoculum.

Systematic Examination of Bacteria

Once a bacterium has been isolated and established as a pure culture, it is necessary to determine enough of its properties to identify and classify it. In general the systematic examination involves determining colony characteristics, cell morphology, staining reactions, biochemical properties, and occasionally its antigenic properties, virulence in animals, susceptibility to specific bacteriophages, cell wall chemistry, and DNA chemistry (e.g., guanine and cytosine content, hybridization characteristics). In identifying bacteria it must be kept in mind that most bacteria experience mutations, as well as many physiological variations according to age, the type of culture medium, the time and temperature of incubation, and other environmental factors. The establishment and the reliability of bacterial characteristics are dependent on the control and standardization of such factors.

Colony Characteristics. Colony morphology is an important characteristic of bacteria and is one of the first properties of a freshly isolated strain to be observed. It is commonly determined by examination of colonies by the unaided eye or with a stereoscopic binocular dissecting microscope (Fig. 2.2).

The most important colony characteristics of bacteria and typical terms used to describe them are:

1. *Size:* diameter in mm.
2. *Form:* punctiform, circular, filamentous, irregular, rhizoid, spindle.
3. *Elevation:* flat, raised, convex, pulvinate, umbonate, umbilicate.
4. *Margin* (edge of colony): entire, undulant, lobate, erose, filamentous, curled.
5. *Color:* white, yellow, black, buff, orange, etc.
6. *Surface:* glistening, dull, other.
7. *Density:* opaque, translucent, transparent, other.
8. *Consistency:* butyrous, viscid, membranous, brittle, adherent.
9. *Changes in medium:* hemolysis, discoloration.

Cellular Morphology. Cellular characteristics important in defining a bacterial species are microscopically observed on stained bacterial cells fixed by heat to glass slides. Staining is usually done with gram stain, acid-fast stain, metachromatic stain, or special stains to demonstrate some specific part of a cell, such as capsules or flagella. Dark-field or phase-contrast microscopy can be used to observe living, unstained bacteria. Electron microscopy, utilizing electrons rather than light, will reveal many of the finer details of bacteria but is not always used for bacterial identification. Cellular characteristics used in describing bacteria are size, overall shape (sphere, rod, filament, curved, or spiral), arrangement in aggregates or chains, presence and arrangement of spores, staining affinities, presence or absence of capsules, and the presence or absence of flagella (motile or nonmotile).

Phenotypic Properties. After determination of colony and cellular morphologies from nonselective and selective growth media along with the gram stain reaction, many isolates can be placed in a "suspected" bacterial group (e.g., streptococci, gram-negative bacilli, gram-positive bacilli). Further identification of the isolates at the genus and species levels usually requires characterization of their biochemical properties and sometimes their immunochemical characteristics. Of the numerous tests available, only some are important in differentiating organisms within a "suspected" group. The common types of biochemical tests used include those that measure oxygen requirements, nutritional requirements, sensitivity to specific growth inhibitors or lysing agents, production of specific enzymes, adherence in the presence of certain nutrients, actions on proteins, and production of specific components or products. The biochemical nature of the isolates is sometimes reflected in the immunological properties. Antibodies produced by the body in response to a given bacterium are used to detect and identify homologous bacteria. Immunological techniques have been greatly expanded by the conjugation of antibodies with fluorescent dyes, such as fluorescein. This procedure is a valuable and sensitive tool for identifying bacteria and other microorganisms in a variety of specimens and tissues.

Genotypic Properties. One of the most specific kinds of test used in identification of bacteria entails analysis of the bacterial genome to determine its genotypic properties. The most common test is determination of the mole percent of guanine plus cytosine (mol% G + C) in the bacterial genome DNA. Although the amount of G + C varies among species, it is quite constant within the same species. The mol% G + C is commonly measured during attempts to classify a new isolate or to reclassify a known strain but not in the routine identification of bacteria in clinical specimens. The techniques involved are relatively complex, and the isolate to be identified must be subcultured to purity, the cells disrupted, and the genome DNA purified. The mol% G + C is calculated after determining the increase in ultraviolet (UV) light absorbance while heating the DNA or after determining the DNA buoyant density resulting from gradient centrifugation.

Other examinations of the bacterial genome involve DNA-DNA hybridization tests. Bacteria with identical DNA basepair nucleotide sequences in their genomes are likely to be members of the same species. The basis for these hybridization tests is the

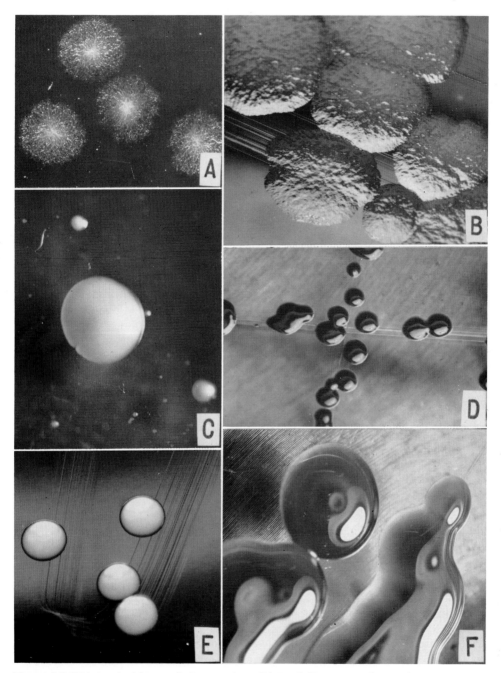

Figure 2.2: Various colonial types of microorganisms. **(A)** Rough filamentous colonies of *Lepto-trichia* species. **(B)** Rough colonial forms of *Escherichia coli* grown on beef heart infusion agar. **(C)** The largest colony is that of an oral yeast species, showing a creamy smooth surface, an entire margin, and a heaped-up contour. The medium-sized smooth colonies are those of oral *Lactobacillus* species. The smaller pinpoints are those of oral streptococcal species. **(D)** Mucoid colonies of *E. coli* growing on eosin-methylene blue agar. **(E)** Flattened, smooth colonies of *Staphylococcus epidermidis* growing on beef heart infusion agar. **(F)** Mucoid colonies of *Klebsiella pneumoniae* growing on beef heart infusion agar. **(A** courtesy of B. G. Bibby.)

ability of separated strands of double-stranded DNA to reassociate (hybridize) with homologous (complementary) strands. Thus, if the separated strands of DNA from a known species (called a DNA probe) can be shown to hybridize with separated strands of DNA from an unknown bacterium, then both bacteria are likely to be closely related or of the same species. The degree to which the known and unknown strands hybridize is a measure of the relatedness of the two bacteria, with identical species exhibiting 100% hybridization. More and more species-specific DNA probes are being developed to aid in definitive identification and as tools to detect specific species in mixed-culture clinical specimens. For example, such probes are used to detect periodontal pathogens like *Bacteroides gingivalis, Bacteroides intermedius,* and *Actinobacillus actinomycetemcomitans* directly in material collected from periodontal pockets, which avoids the rigorous tasks of culturing, isolating, and analyzing a variety of phenotypic properties.

As the systematic examination continues, the reactions of the isolate are compared with the known reactions of previously characterized reference bacteria until identification is confirmed. Some bacteria can be identified from only a few characteristics; others require extensive testing. Some isolates do not fit into any known species classification because of changes in their properties or because they have not been previously identified.

Rickettsiae and Chlamydiae

Like viruses, rickettsiae and chlamydiae are obligate intracellular parasites, but their structure and chemical composition indicate that they are specialized forms of gram-negative bacteria. The rickettsiae, which cause such diseases as typhus, Rocky Mountain spotted fever, and Q fever, reproduce by transverse binary fission only within a host cell, and most (exception: Q fever agent) are transmitted to man through the bite of an infected arthropod. Chlamydiae, which cause diseases such as psittacosis, trachoma, inclusion conjunctivitis, and nongonococcal urethritis, also reproduce by binary fission within host cells. However, unlike rickettsiae, they develop into a specialized form for survival when released from the host cell and do not require vectors for transmission.

Both rickettsiae and chlamydiae can be cultured in the yolk sac of embryonated chicken eggs or in specific types of tissue cultures (e.g., mouse lymphoblasts for the scrub typhus rickettsiae and mouse fibroblasts for chlamydiae). Bacterial contamination is suppressed by use of appropriate antibiotics. The systematic examination of these specialized forms of bacteria is mainly based on the clinical and epidemiological features of the diseases produced in animals and man, demonstration of tissue forms of the organisms, immunological properties, and/or the effects of physical and chemical agents on growth.

Viruses

Viruses, like rickettsiae and chlamydiae, are obligate intracellular parasites and require living cells for growth and reproduction. The isolation and identification of viruses is more difficult than for bacteria because of their small size, obligate parasitism, and greater lability. Viral specimens include nasal washings, nasal or pharyngeal swabs, throat washings or swabs, mouth swabs, vesicular fluid and scrapings, exudates, urine, stools and rectal swabs, blood, spinal fluid, or biopsy specimens. Before propagating the specimen, as many bacteria as possible should be removed by centrifugation, filtration through a membrane filter, or by the addition of antibacterial agents (e.g., antibiotics). Viruses are commonly propagated in the host system, in cell culture, by animal inoculation, or in embryonated eggs. Characteristics commonly sought in tissue cultures are cell destruction and cell alterations (cytopathic effects). In properly inoculated animals, observations are made of the signs of the disease that develops or of the immunological response. Growth of a virus in an embryonated egg frequently will produce lesions that can be detected visually. Also, viruses may be isolated from the membranes, sac fluids, or homogenates of the embryos. Purification of viruses (e.g., filtration, partition, differential centrifugation) is required before they are examined systematically.

After purification, virus particles are examined for their form, stability, infectivity, host cell specificity, and animal interaction. The viral nucleic acid of the particle is examined for type and form, molecular weight, and molar base ratio. Viral proteins are examined for enzyme activity, antigenic nature, and hemagglutinating ability. Viral lipids, if present, are examined for composition and relation to infectivity. Particle stability is examined in relation to pH, temperature, presence of various ions, and response to lipid solvents. Particle form is described according to size, capsid shape, capsomere number, and the presence or absence of envelope or accessory structures. Host interactions are described according to sites of synthesis, assembly, maturation, and mode of release.

Fungi

Fungi are eukaryotic organisms that grow as single cells, the yeasts, or as multicellular filamentous forms, the molds and mushrooms. Most fungi are saprophytic but some can cause serious disease in humans. Molds reproduce by spores which germinate into long filaments called hyphae. The hyphae grow and branch, forming a mat called a mycelium. Yeasts commonly divide by budding or by fission. Some pathogenic fungi are dimorphic, existing as yeasts or molds, while others exist only in one form or the other.

Fungi have relatively simple nutritional requirements and are not sensitive to antibiotics that inhibit bacteria. These characteristics allow the development of selective media for isolation of fungi that do not support the growth of bacteria (e.g., Sabouraud dextrose agar and Littman oxgall agar). Cornmeal agar is often used to stimulate sporulation and the development of fungal characteristics. Temperature, humidity, age, nutrition, and strain variation affect fungal morphology during in vitro culture.

The systematic examination of pathogenic fungi often requires the demonstration of tissue and lesion forms as well as their examination in culture. In culture, colonial morphology, pigmentation, and cellular characteristics are important in identifying and describing species and strains. Spores, formed by aerial mycelia, exhibit species differences in size, shape, and arrangement—properties useful in identification. Other characteristics required for more detailed identification are biological, biochemical, and immunological, including the development of hypersensitivity in fungal infections.

ADDITIONAL READING

Aranki, A., Syed, S. A., Kenney, E. B., and Freter, R. 1969. Isolation of Anaerobic Bacteria from Human Gingiva and Mouse Caecum by Means of a Simplified Glove Box Procedure. Appl Microbiol, **17,** 568.

Buchanan, R. E., and Gibbons, N. E. (Eds.) 1974. *Bergey's Manual of Determinative Bacteriology,* Ed. 8. Williams & Wilkins, Baltimore.

Cowen, S. T., and Steel, K. J. 1974. *Manual for the Identification of Medical Bacteria.* Cambridge University Press, Great Britain.

Koneman, E. W., Allen, S. D., Dowell, V. R., Jr., and Sommers, H. M. 1979. *Color Atlas and Textbook of Diagnostic Microbiology.* J. B. Lippincott, Philadelphia.

Lennette, E. H., Balows, A., Hausler, Jr., W. J., and Shadomy, H. J. 1985. *Manual of Clinical Microbiology,* Ed. 4. American Society for Microbiology, Washington, D.C.

Manganiello, A. D., Socransky, S. S., Smith, C., Propas, D., Oran, V., and Dogon, I. L. 1977. Attempts to Increase Viable Count Recovery of Human Supragingival Dental Plaque. J Periodont Res, **12,** 107.

Rogosa, M., Mitchell, J. A., and Wiseman, R. F. 1951. A Selective Medium for the Isolation and Enumeration of Oral Lactobacilli. J Dent Res, **30,** 682.

Tanner, A. R. C., and Goodson, J. M. 1986. Sampling of Microorganisms Associated with Periodontal Disease. Oral Microbiol Immunol, **1,** 15.

Part II

Cellular and Molecular Microbiology

3

Bacterial Structure and Function

Benjamin F. Hammond

Bacteria are prokaryotic (prenuclear) cells and by definition have a distinctive pattern of cellular organization. In general, the internal structure of prokaryotic cells is simpler than that of eukaryotic cells since prokaryotes lack a membrane-bound nucleus, an extensive endoplasmic reticulum, mitochondria, and structures associated with mitosis. However, a number of structures are common to all cells, as dictated by universal biological functions—the transmission of genetic material (extremely primitive nucleus), protein synthesis (ribosomes), and osmotic regulation (cytoplasmic membrane). The nuclear DNA exists as a covalently closed circular structure that is folded back upon itself many times to give a highly twisted form called a supercoil. If the DNA of a typical bacterium—say, *Escherichia coli*—were opened and linearized, it would be about 1 mm long. This amount of DNA corresponds to about 4.2×10^6 basepairs and is consistent with the known molecular weight of the *E. coli* genome (2.7×10^9 daltons). Although this amount of DNA is sufficient to specify all the major genetic information of the cell, it is much less (600 times less) than

the amount of DNA found in a typical eukaryotic cell (5×10^{-15} g vs. 3×10^{-12} g per mammalian cell). In the amorphous cytoplasm surrounding the nucleus there are numerous 70S ribosomes in which protein synthesis occurs. There are also a number of cytoplasmic inclusions (often referred to as reserve energy storage granules) which may be present in some bacteria under appropriate cultural conditions. Other cytoplasmic structures, such as endospores and chloroplasts, occur in only a few bacteria and have specific functions associated with the survival and maintenance of these organisms in their environment.

The external or surface structure of the bacterial cell is much more complex than the internal structure. A rigid cell wall surrounds the underlying cytoplasmic membrane. Additional components of the cell envelope may include filamentous appendages known as flagella and pili, external surface layers (capsules or slime layers), and other specific surface macromolecules. Considerable is known about the structure-function relationships of these surface components, making it possible to relate function to

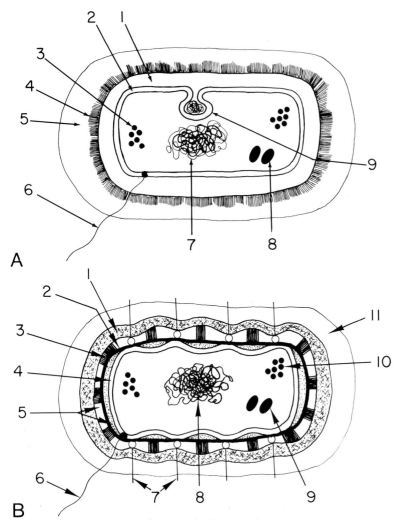

Figure 3.1: Diagram of typical bacterial cells, showing most of the structures seen in the cells.
(A) Gram-positive cell: *1,* cell wall peptidoglycan; *2,* cytoplasmic membrane; *3,* ribosomes; *4,* surface proteins; *5,* capsule; *6,* flagellum; *7,* chromosome; *8,* inclusion body; *9,* mesosome. **(B)** Gram-negative cell: *1,* outer membrane; *2,* peptidoglycan; *3,* lipoprotein; *4,* cytoplasmic membrane; *5,* periplasmic space; *6,* flagellum; *7,* pili; *8,* chromosome; *9,* inclusion body; *10,* ribosomes; *11,* capsule.

chemical architecture. Schematic representations of two prototype bacterial cells are shown in Figure 3.1.

This chapter examines bacterial structure with an emphasis on structure-function relationships as they relate to oral bacteria.

Bacterial Morphology and Size

Morphology

There are two principal morphological forms of bacteria: cocci or spheres (L., modified from the Gk. *kokkus,* berry), and rod-shaped organisms or bacilli (L. *baculus,* rod). Many different variants of these two forms are known (Fig. 3.2). Cocci may occur as pairs (diplococci), in chains (streptococci), in clusters (staphylococci), or in tetrads (sarcina). Similarly, bacilli may be quite short (coccobacilli), have tapered ends (fusiform bacilli), grow as long threads (filamentous forms), or grow in a curved or S configuration as vibrios or spirilla. The spiral forms may be considered as rod-shaped organisms twisted into a helix of variable rigidity. If the helix is flexible the organism is referred to as a spirochete (*Treponema, Leptospira, Borrelia*); if the helix is rigid the organism is probably a member of the genus *Spirillum.*

Bacteria are grouped according to 1) the geometry of successive planes of cell division and 2) the ease with which daughter cells pull apart after division. If

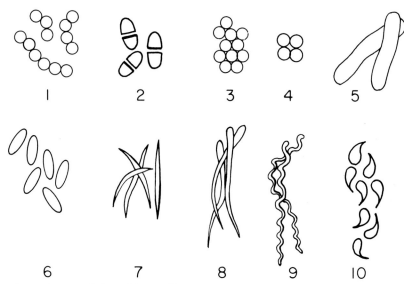

Figure 3.2: Morphological forms of bacteria: *1,* streptococci; *2,* diplococci; *3,* staphylococci; *4,* sarcina; *5,* bacilli; *6,* coccobacilli; *7,* fusiform bacilli; *8,* filamentous bacilli; *9,* spirochetes; *10,* vibrios.

the successive planes of division are perpendicular, tetrads will result; if parallel, the cells will occur singly, in pairs, or in chains, depending on their tendency to pull apart. The postdivisional separation of cells (pulling apart) may be determined by a number of factors, including specific enzymes that dissolve cellular material at the point of contact between two daughter cells, flagellar activity in motile cells, and the production of certain adherent macromolecules.

The shape of individual cells is genetically determined and characteristic of the various genera and species of bacteria. It is generally agreed that the primary regulator of bacterial shape is the rigid cell wall component (the peptidoglycan or murein), since removal of the wall or the prevention of wall synthesis results in cells, even rod-shaped cells, acquiring a balloon or spherical configuration (see Bacterial Cell Walls, p. 32). Other factors that have been implicated in this complex and quite variable process include

1) the differential rate controls of envelope assembly and 2) asymmetric architecture in certain parts of the bacterial cell envelope.

Size

The small size of bacteria is one of the earliest and most important properties of the group (Table 3.1). Their dimensions place them at the upper levels of the size of colloidal matter (0.01 to 0.5 μm). In many respects the behavior of bacterial cells is analogous to the behavior of colloids (Brownian movement, light scattering via the Tyndall effect, migration in an electric field). Another important aspect of the small size of bacteria involves their surface/volume relationships. The growth of most organisms, large or small, depends in part on the amount of available surface area, since it is at the surface that the transfer of metabolites into the cell and the elimination of waste

Table 3.1: Sizes of Various Microorganisms

Cell Type/Structural Unit	Biological Group	Volume (V) (μm³)	Surface (S) (μm²)	S/V (μm)
Eukaryotic cells	Unicellular algae	6.5×10^{13}	7.8×10^9	1.2×10^4
	Yeast (*Saccharomyces cerevisiae*)	110	110	1
Prokaryotic cells	*Escherichia coli*	0.52	3.1	6
	Lactobacillus casei	1.6	7.85	5
	Mycoplasma sp.	0.00818	0.196	23.9
Viruses	*E. coli* phage	2.5×10^4	0.02	80

products occur. It is often stated that the larger the surface area per unit volume, the greater is the cell's metabolic rate. *E. coli* with a surface/volume (S/V) ratio of 6 can catabolize up to 10,000 times its weight of lactose in 1 hour, whereas it has been estimated that a 70-kg man would need 28 years or 250,000 hours to catabolize a comparable weight of lactose. This generalization, however, is valid only up to a point: there is a lower limit to the S/V ratio beyond which viable cells cannot exist. This lower limit reflects the amount of space needed to accommodate the metabolic machinery (enzyme proteins, cofactors, organic substances, etc.) and the genetic apparatus of a biologically functional cell.

The mycoplasmas or pleuropneumonia-like organisms (PPLO) (diameter of 0.25 μm) are often referred to as the "theoretically minimum cell." The cell volume is approximately 0.01 μm^3 and the cell consists of a cytoplasmic membrane, ribosomes, and a nuclear body. The small amount of DNA is just sufficient to code for all the products needed for self-reproduction at the expense of nutrients in an artificial medium. The cells, therefore, appear to be at or very close to the molecular limit of cellular function. The S/V ratio for these cells is approximately 20, although their metabolic rate is considerably less than the rate for *E. coli*. The smallest viable reproductive units of mycoplasmas range from 125 to 250 nm in diameter. As is evident from Table 3.1, viruses also have very high S/V ratios, yet their metabolic rates are negligible or nonexistent.

Surface Structures of Bacteria

There is enormous variation in surface architecture among the different bacterial genera and species. Moreover, as a result of the large surface area provided by cultures of bacterial cells, numerous opportunities exist for chemical and physical modifications in surface structure due to environmental stresses. In addition, a number of well-known genetic mutations can produce major changes in bacterial cell surfaces so that within a single population, it is possible to see several subpopulations with different surface structures and properties. The following section describes some of the major surface structures of bacteria, but it must be remembered that not all cells have every structure and that considerable variation in the chemical and physical properties of each structure is common.

Capsules

Most bacteria produce a hydrophilic, gel-like structure of low optical density; this structure, usually located just outside the cell wall, is variously termed a microcapsule, capsule, or slime layer. It is easily demonstrated by negative staining (India ink suspension); the capsular layer will appear as a clear zone between the opaque background and the more refractile cell body. Most capsules are relatively simple polysaccharides composed of repeating units of two or three sugars that may or may not be present in the cell wall. Other bacteria are known to produce capsules of different chemical composition—for example, *Bacillus anthracis* forms a capsule of poly-D-glutamic acid linked by a δ peptide bond, while the outer layer of the tubercle bacillus (*Mycobacterium tuberculosis*) is composed of protein, polysaccharide, and mycolic acid. Capsular materials are usually antigenic and can be detected on cells by exposure to specific antibody; the resultant increase in refractility gives the appearance of capsular swelling (quellung reaction) (Fig. 3.3). The specificity of the quellung reaction is often used in the identification of certain pathogenic bacteria, e.g., the pneumococcus where over 80 different capsular serotypes have been demonstrated. Many oral bacteria are also known to produce extracellular polysaccharides (dextrans and levans of *Streptococcus mutans* and *Streptococcus salivarius*), which may give the appearance of capsular material but are more often found in the medium rather than as well-defined surface layers. Other oral bacteria (*Lactobacillus casei, Neisseria* species, and many other gram-negative bacteria) produce well-defined capsules, which may be of significance in the survival and maintenance of these and other species in the oral milieu. The polysaccharide capsule of *L. casei* is known to prevent phage adsorption and possibly to serve as a reserve nutrient supply under conditions of nutrient limitation.

Ordinarily the biological significance of capsules in bacteria is limited to a consideration of their antiphagocytic properties. Since capsules are hydrophilic polysaccharides and since the surfaces of phagocytic cells are generally hydrophobic, the engulfment or phagocytic process is usually prevented. Thus, there is a positive association between capsule formation and the virulence of some bacteria because capsules interfere with one of the host's first line of defense, phagocytosis.

The ability of *Bacteroides gingivalis* and other black-pigmented *Bacteroides* species to survive in diseased periodontal tissues and experimental abscesses despite the large numbers of polymorphonuclear leukocytes has been attributed in part to the production of an antiphagocytic capsular layer. Another periodontopathic bacterium, *Actinobacillus actinomycetemcomitans,* produces a ruthenium-red heteropolysaccharide capsule, but its relationship to virulence has not been precisely defined.

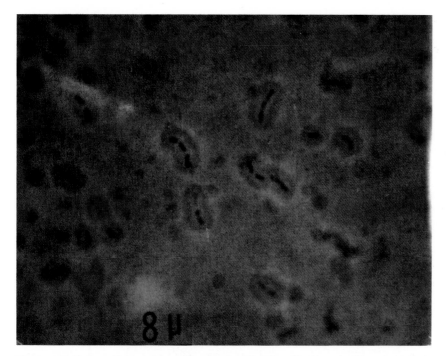

Figure 3.3: The specific capsular swelling reaction ("quellung") of *Lactobacillus casei* cells (strain L324M) exposed to specific antibody to the capsular material.

In a more restricted sense the capsule can be thought of as a product of metabolism rather than as a structure per se. Capsular size, for example, usually depends on the rate of formation and secretion of capsular material (e.g., microcapsule). In other instances capsules may not be detectable at all unless there is a specific nutrient in the growth medium, indicating, perhaps, the nonessentiality of capsule formation in the biological economy of the cell.

Surface Appendages

Flagella. Bacterial cells often have one or more filamentous appendages termed flagella (L. *flagellum,* whip). The flagellum (Fig. 3.4) is a long (3 to 12 μm), thin (12 to 25 nm) structure that originates in the cell membrane basal body and terminates outside the cell. Because of their narrow diameter, flagella are not seen with the ordinary light microscope unless coated with stains containing a precipitating agent (tannic acid). In living cells the structure is coded in the form of a cylindrical helix but in dried preparations it appears as regular sinusoidal curves (or more appropriately as flattened helices) whose wave length is characteristic for a species. Bacteria with a single polar flagellum are *monotrichous,* those with two or more polar flagella are *lophotrichous,* and those with a random arrangement of flagella all over their surface are called *peritrichous.* On this basis the common bacteria are separated into two orders, Eubacteriales (peritrichous flagella) and Pseudomonadales (polar flagella).

Purified flagella (obtained by differential centrifugation) consist of a globular protein, flagellin (approximate molecular weight = 40,000 daltons), whose chemical composition appears to be the same in different genera of bacteria although differences in primary structure are known and account for serologic differences. The protein is antigenically different from the rest of the cell body, and these differences form the basis for the serological identification of many flagellated gram-negative bacteria. For example, the combination of flagellar antigens (H, from the German *hauch,* meaning breeze or whiff) and somatic antigens (O, or *ohne hauch*—without flagella) provides the basis for serological typing of salmonellae in the Kauffman-White schema.

The primary function of flagella is to provide bacteria with a mechanism for motility. There are a few exceptions, such as spirochetal motility due to alternate contractions of the axial filament which is attached to each end of the cell, and the gliding movement of certain nonflagellated *Capnocytophaga* and *Mycoplasma* on solid surfaces due to cell binding and pili. However, in the main, bacterial motility is a direct function of flagellar activity. Motility occurs when there is a rotation of the rigid, helically coiled flagellum after a torque is created in the basal body. At the

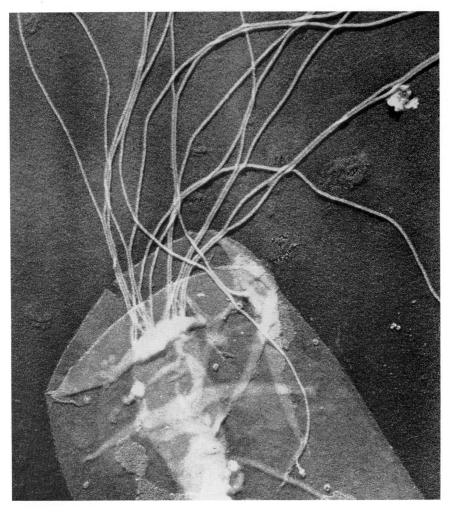

Figure 3.4: *Spirillum serpens* cell autolyzed and digested by trypsin. Note flagella attached to basal granules inside the cell. (Reproduced with permission from M. R. J. Salton: The Anatomy of the Bacterial Surface. *Bacteriol Rev,* **25,** 77, 1961.)

base of the flagellum within the cytoplasmic membrane there are two sets of rings surrounding the flagella cylinder: an inner set, which rotates, and an outer set, which serves as bearings to minimize friction and leakage. As the inner set of rings rotates the flagellum begins to move in propeller-like motion. The energy for the process is thought to come from oxidative phosphorylation in the cytoplasmic membrane.

Fimbria or Pili. Bacterial cells, both gram-positive and gram-negative, often have as many as 150 filamentous appendages called fimbria or, more recently, pili, that are shorter, thinner, and less rigid than flagella. They are 75 to 100 nm in diameter and up to 2 μm long (Fig. 3.5). Like flagella, they also arise in the cytoplasmic membrane and are composed of a serologically distinct protein (pilin). They can be eas-

ily removed from bacterial cells without affecting vitality and they reform rapidly. Based on the known functions, there are two varieties of pili: a sex pilus, once thought to be a tube through which DNA was transferred during the process of conjugation between two bacterial cells, and a somatic pilus, which has adhesive properties that aid in the adherence of bacterial cells to mucosal and other cell surfaces as a first step in bacterial colonization of the host. Recent evidence suggests that the real function of the sex pilus is to serve as a recognition device between mating cell types, followed by the formation of some kind of cytoplasmic bridge between cell envelopes. The significance of the somatic pili in adherence and colonization was first established by oral microbiologists who demonstrated most convincingly that the selective localization of certain oral bacteria depended on

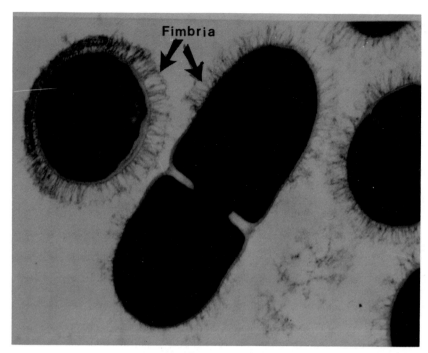

Figure 3.5: Fimbria on an oral streptococcus (× 60,000). (Courtesy of Dr. Chern Lai, University of Pennsylvania.)

the presence of these fibrillar coatings. Studies of numerous other investigators have established the universality of the phenomenon; adherence mechanisms, mediated by pili or other "adhesins," play a fundamental role in the natural ecology of pathogenic and nonpathogenic bacteria. The colonization of *Actinomyces viscosus,* one of the first organisms shown to produce periodontal disease and root surface caries in gnotobiotic ("germ-free") animals, is dependent on pili. Avirulent mutants of *A. viscosus* lack pili and are unable to colonize the oral cavity (Fig. 3.6). Pili have been implicated in the gliding motion of nonflagellated bacteria on solid surfaces, a phenomenon known as surface translocation.

Other Surface Appendages. Certain bacteria (stalked, prosthecate, budding bacteria) produce extrusions termed stalks, hyphae, and buds, which are smaller in diameter than the mature cell and contain cytoplasm bounded by a cell wall. Apart from these purely morphological structures and their different environments, the primary difference between these bacteria and conventional bacteria is the formation of a new cell wall from a single point (polar growth) rather than throughout the cell (intercalary growth).

In addition, many gram-negative bacteria produce numerous ball-like eversions of the outer membrane and a small amount of cytoplasm called *vesicles* (microvesicles or blebs) (Fig. 3.7). Because the outer membrane contains endotoxin, these appendages

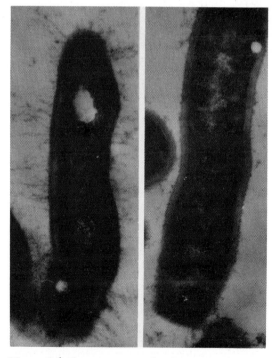

Figure 3.6: Electron micrographs of *Actinomyces viscosus* strains T14V (virulent) and T14AV (avirulent) (× 52,650). Note the presence of numerous fimbria-like projections on virulent cells (*left*) and the absence of such projections on avirulent cells (*right*). (Courtesy of Dr. Dale Birdsell and Dr. Werner Fischlschweiger, University of Florida.)

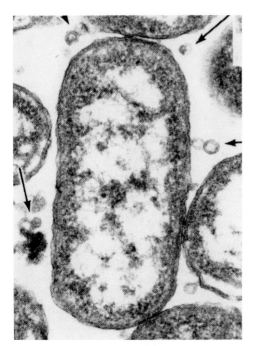

Figure 3.7: Electron micrograph of *Actinobacillus Actinomycetemcomitans,* strain Y4, showing extracellular membranous vesicles (blebs) with arrows (× 68,000). (Reproduced with permission from Chern Lai, Max Listgarten, and Benjamin Hammond, *J Periodont Res,* **16,** 379, 1981. © 1981 Munksgaard, Copenhagen.)

were once associated with the "free endotoxin" concept. Their presence in several periodontal bacteria, including *Actinobacillus actinomycetemcomitans* and *Bacteroides gingivalis,* has been correlated with virulence. In the *Actinobacillus* it has been shown that the vesicles have several potent toxins in addition to the endotoxin, including a bone-resorbing factor and a leukotoxin. Since these microvesicles are produced in large numbers during growth, it is possible that they could facilitate the interaction of host cells with the pharmacologically active mediators assumed to be of importance in the pathogenesis of periodontal disease.

Bacterial Cell Walls

One of the most important characteristics of prokaryotic cells (bacteria and blue-green algae) is the presence of a rigid cell wall containing the unique peptidoglycan (PG or murein) moiety. All bacteria except the mycoplasmas and certain halophilic bacteria have rigid cell walls and some variation of the peptidoglycan serving as the basic structural unit of the wall. The significance of the PG is best illustrated by the numerous functions it serves:

1. It is responsible for the strength and rigidity of the wall. The walls of some bacteria can withstand pressures of up to 400,000 g without rupture or distortion of shape.

2. The inertness of the wall to a variety of chemical agents derives from the resistance of PG to such agents. Equally important is the concept that agents that affect the integrity or synthesis of the wall are almost always bactericidal in nature. Any compromise in wall structure, function, or synthesis usually leads to cell death.

3. Associated with its strength and rigidity, the PG is essentially (although not exclusively) responsible for the shape of the cell. If the PG layer is digested by lysozyme or if its synthesis is blocked by an antibiotic, the cell loses its characteristic shape and becomes a spherical body. (The cell will be lysed unless it is placed in a hypertonic medium, such as 20% sucrose.) Thus, a rigid rod-shaped bacillus in hypertonic medium will become a flexible spherical body if the wall is lost. (Since the free energy of a system tends toward a minimum, a flexible body will assume the smallest possible surface area, and the smallest possible surface area for any given volume is a sphere.) The wall-less forms are called protoplasts or spheroplasts. The difference between them and their significance will be discussed later.

It is possible to isolate and purify cell wall preparations of various bacteria by cell rupture, enzymatic treatment, and differential centrifugation. The isolated PG is now known to be a single, giant, bag-shaped macromolecule that may account for 10% to 40% of the cell's dry weight. The PG consists of three parts (Fig. 3.8): 1) a backbone chain made up of repeating units of two amino sugars (*N*-acetylglucosamine and muramic acid) joined by a β-1,4 linkage; 2) a set of identical tetrapeptide units joined at the CO end of muramic acid and with an alternating D/L configuration of amino acids and a diamino acid in position 3; and 3) a set of identical cross-bridges to hook the backbone chains together.

The basic PG unit is essentially the same for all bacteria, but there are variations in the number and nature of the cross-bridges and in the diamino acid in position 3 of the tetrapeptide unit. Some of the taxonomic and other implications of these differences in wall structure are discussed in the sections on Gram-Positive and Gram-Negative Walls.

There are certain similarities in the bacterial PG and the rigid cell walls of the few eukaryotic cell walls. The β-1,4 linkage provides a strong and thermodynamically stable polysaccharide chain; it is also found in cellulose (β-1,4-glucose) of algal cell walls, in chitin (poly-β-1,4-*N*-acetylglucosamine) of fungal cell walls, and in the xylans (β-1,4-xylose) of certain woody plant cells. These similarities explain in part the strength and resistance to rupture of these rigid cell walls.

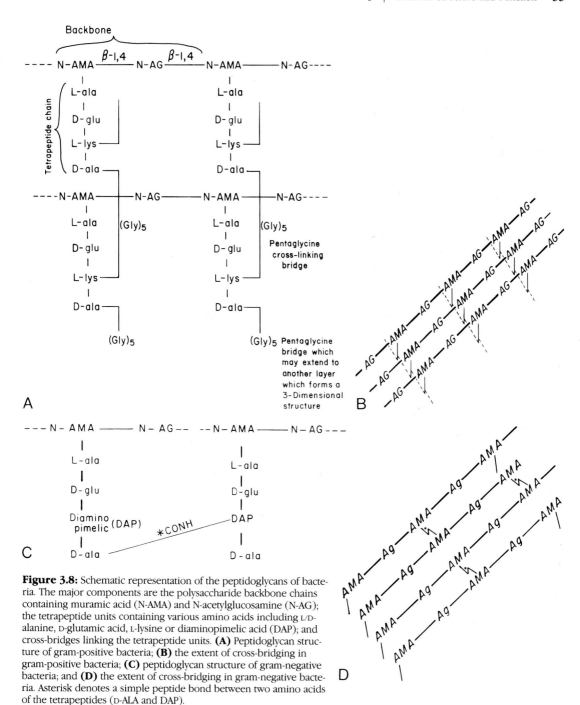

Figure 3.8: Schematic representation of the peptidoglycans of bacteria. The major components are the polysaccharide backbone chains containing muramic acid (N-AMA) and N-acetylglucosamine (N-AG); the tetrapeptide units containing various amino acids including L/D-alanine, D-glutamic acid, L-lysine or diaminopimelic acid (DAP); and cross-bridges linking the tetrapeptide units. **(A)** Peptidoglycan structure of gram-positive bacteria; **(B)** the extent of cross-bridging in gram-positive bacteria; **(C)** peptidoglycan structure of gram-negative bacteria; and **(D)** the extent of cross-bridging in gram-negative bacteria. Asterisk denotes a simple peptide bond between two amino acids of the tetrapeptides (D-ALA and DAP).

There are other chemical explanations for the toughness of the PG, including the alternation of D- and L-amino acids in the tetrapeptide (greater strength of structure than L- or D-homopolymers) and the extensive amount of hydrogen bonding between peptide groups. Where there is an extensive amount of crossbridging to produce a meshlike structure of interlacing strands of disaccharide chains, the PG assumes an even greater structural strength. The overall picture of PG is of a giant, bag-shaped, covalently linked molecule with marked ability to protect the cytoplasmic membrane and other parts of the cell from many physical and chemical forces in the external environment of the cell.

Table 3.2: Some Differences Between Gram-Positive and Gram-Negative Bacteria

Property	Gram-Positive	Gram-Negative
Cell wall thickness	Greater	Less
Amino acids in cell wall	Few	Numerous kinds
Lipids in cell wall	None or low	Present
Bacterial action of saliva	Resistant	Susceptible
Digestion by gastric/pancreatic juices	Resistant	Susceptible
Lysozyme lysis	Susceptible	Less susceptible
Inhibition by penicillin	Susceptible	Usually resistant
Inhibition by sulfonamides	Usually susceptible	Usually resistant
Inhibition by streptomycin	Usually resistant	Usually susceptible
Inhibition of basic dyes (crystal violet)	Susceptible	Usually resistant
Lysis by anionic detergents	Very susceptible	Much less susceptible
Autolysis	Less common	More commonly noted
Isoelectric range	pH 2–3	pH 4–5
Nutritional requirements	Complex generally, none autotrophic	Relatively simpler, many autotrophic
Nature of toxins produced	Exotoxins	Endotoxins
Lysis by antibody + complement	Resistant	Some susceptible

Gram Stain

Bacteria can be differentiated into two large groups by a stain developed in the early 1880s by the Danish bacteriologist Christian Gram. The procedure consists of four basic steps:

1. Primary staining with a slightly alkaline solution of a triphenyl methane dye, such as crystal violet.

2. Mordanting with aqueous iodine solution to form a water-soluble complex in both cell wall and cell cytoplasm.

3. Differential decolorizing with an organic solvent, usually ethanol. This step is critical, for all bacteria are decolorized by this treatment if exposed long enough. On brief exposure, however, many kinds of bacteria retain much of the iodine complex. These are designated gram-positive. The kinds of bacteria that decolorize completely are designated gram-negative. Some bacteria (diphtheroids, *Neisseria*) retain varying amounts of the dye-iodine complex and are termed gram-variable.

4. Counterstaining with a dye of contrasting color and chemical character, usually aqueous safranin or basic fuchsin (red). This step is necessary to make gram-negative bacteria visible. It has no effect on gram-positive bacteria except for a darkening of the normal purple color.

The mechanism of the gram stain appears to be critically related to the intactness of the cell wall and to the permeability properties of the intact cell envelope. Gram-positive bacteria stain gram-negative on autolysis, or on loss of osmotic integrity, as occurs in old or dying cells. A unique bacterial cell wall component does not appear to explain the reaction since no specific gram-positive substrate has been isolated. Whatever the precise mechanism, two facts are clearly established:

1. The difference in their reactions to the gram stain is but one manifestation of fundamental differences between gram-positive and gram-negative bacteria—differences in susceptibility to various chemical and physical agents, metabolic potential, chemical composition, and structure. These differences in turn are reflected in pathogenic potential (nature of toxins produced, role of antibody in defense, etc.). A summary of these differences is presented in Table 3.2.

2. The cell wall structures of gram-positive and gram-negative cells are clearly different with respect to chemical composition, ultrastructure, physical properties, and serological properties.

Some of the chemical and structural differences between the two kinds of cell wall are described in the following paragraphs.

Gram-Positive Walls. From the standpoints of chemical components, size, and major physiochemical properties, the PG dominates the structure of virtually all gram-positive walls. Most of the thickness of the wall and the dry weight of isolated wall preparations is due to the PG, and the susceptibility to the various chemical and physical agents reflects the importance of the PG as the primary structural unit in gram-positive walls. Early ultrastructural and chemical studies showed that the thickness of the PG layer was due to the presence of numerous disaccharide chains joined together by extensive cross-bridges between the tetrapeptide units, giving a heavily intertwined meshlike structure of considerable strength. There is considerable diversity in terms of some of the individual components of the PG in gram-positive bacteria such as the amino acids in tetrapeptides, the nature of the cross-bridges, etc., but two factors are constant: the high total amount of PG (40% to 90% of dry weight) in the wall and the extensive cross-bridging between chains.

The high percentage of PG in the cell wall of gram-positive bacteria increases the availability of the β-1,4 linkage of the backbone chains to lysozyme, a naturally occurring substance found in tears and salivary secretions. This enzyme is able to cleave the β-1,4 linkage between the two amino sugars, muramic acid and β-acetylglucosamine, breaking the chain, destroying the integrity of the PG structure, and ultimately causing cell lysis. Resistance to lysozyme, although more common among the gram-negative bacteria because of the outer membrane cover, also occurs in some gram-positive bacteria as well. Many gram-positive oral bacteria appear to be resistant to lysozyme, a fact that would explain their high numbers in a milieu such as saliva where lysozyme is known to be present. The basis for this resistance is probably related to modification of PG structure (*O*-acetylation of muramic acid) or the inability of lysozyme to gain access to the wall PG (steric interference of surface macromolecules or structures). The lethal effect of penicillins on growing populations of bacteria is similarly related to an effect on PG structure, i.e., penicillins block the terminal step of PG synthesis in which the peptide chains are cross-linked.

In addition to PG, there are other components of the gram-positive wall. The teichoic acids (Gk. *teichos,* wall) are water-soluble polymers of ribitol or glycerol linked covalently to PG via phosphodiester linkages (usually C_6 hydroxyl of *N*-acetylmuramic acid residues). Membrane teichoic acids (lipoteichoic acids, LTA) usually contain only glycerophosphate polymers and terminate in the membrane glycolipid. These polymers, both wall and membrane teichoic acids, are major surface antigens of gram-positive cells and are probably important in a number of other surface-related phenomena such as adherence and regulation of ion passage through the PG layer. The membrane teichoic acids (LTA) are amphipathic molecules (both polar and nonpolar ends) that can interact with a variety of other biologically active molecular species such as lipids in erythrocyte membranes to produce hemagglutination, or divalent cations, particularly in the regulation of intracellular Mg^{2+}. In many respects, LTA is analogous to the lipopolysaccharide of the gram-negative cell wall.

Other wall-associated substances of gram-positive cells include antigenic polysaccharides (e.g., group- and type-specific streptococcal polysaccharides); teichoic acid polymers covalently attached to the PG and generally formed under conditions of phosphate limitation; and antigenic proteins which are not identical with pili or flagella but which may be associated with adherence. The M protein of group A streptococci is an illustration of such a wall-associated protein. In general, it has been said that the gram-positive wall is devoid of proteins because the procedures used in wall isolation often employ proteolytic enzymes (trypsin, etc.) that would destroy ordinary D- or L-homopolymers. However, the tetrapeptides composed of the alternating D- and L-amino acids are resistant to these proteolytic enzymes.

Gram-Negative Walls. The gram-negative cell wall is considerably more complex than its gram-positive counterpart in terms of structural heterogeneity, chemical composition, and functional activities. Also, the wall PG is intimately connected with other surface layers of the cell and with membrane-associated functions. Because of the structural complexity of the wall in gram-negative bacteria, the term "cell envelope" may be preferable to "cell wall" when applied to these bacteria.

The unique three-layered envelope consists of an outer membrane overlying a thin PG layer, which in turn is separated from the underlying cytoplasmic membrane by a periplasmic space (Fig. 3.9). The outer membrane (6 to 8 nm thick) consists of two layers of protein separated by a layer of phospholipids. The outer membrane structure plays a vital role in the biology of the cell since it contains receptors for antibodies, bacterial viruses, and bacteriocins (see Chap. 4) and performs a number of permeability-related functions consistent with the designation of membrane. The outer membrane serves as a barrier to the passage of many antibiotics (notably some of the penicillins), detergents, and other chemicals (dyes, bile salts). Part of the barrier effect is due to the presence of outer membrane matrix proteins such as porins which selectively inhibit permeation of molecules with a molecular weight greater than 800 daltons. Porins also serve as receptor sites for viruses and bacteriocins.

Another major component of the outer membrane is lipopolysaccharide (LPS or endotoxin), which is unique to gram-negative bacteria, including spirochetes. LPS consists of three regions: a lipid portion, termed lipid A; a core polysaccharide common to most LPS molecules; and an O-specific polysaccharide side chain. The O-specific side chains may be visualized as projections from the surface of the outer membrane; their function may be to prevent the harmful interaction of antibody and complement with the outer membrane. The structure of the different O residues exhibit considerable variation based on the differences in the nature and arrangement of the individual sugars, thereby making it possible to classify different organisms or strains of an organism on the

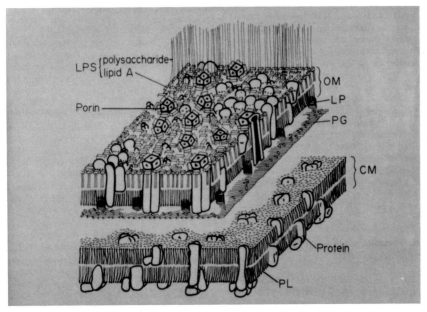

Figure 3.9: An interpretive diagram of the gram-negative envelope structure. *LPS,* lipopolysaccharide; *OM,* outer membrane; *LP,* lipoprotein; *PG,* peptidoglycan; *CM,* cytoplasmic membrane; *PL,* phospholipid. (Adapted with permission from J. M. DiRienzo et al.: *Annual Review of Biochemistry,* **47,** 481, 1978, and presented in *Zinsser Microbiology,* Ed. 17, edited by W. Joklik, H. P. Willett, and D. B. Amos. Appleton-Century-Crofts, New York, 1980.)

basis of these somatic antigens. When the O antigen is lost by mutation, the normally "smooth" colony formation changes to "rough." There appears to be a selective advantage associated with the presence of the O side chains since they tend to make the bacterium resistant to many host defenses (phagocytosis, complement, antibody interaction, etc.). The polysaccharide portions of the LPS are responsible for the antigenic properties of the molecule, while lipid A, a glycophospholipid, is responsible for the toxicity of the molecule.

There are a number of similarities between this characteristic molecule of gram-negative cells and the lipoteichoic acids of gram-positive cells. Both are amphipathic surface macromolecules and both share a number of common biological properties (immunogenicity, hypersensitivity, bone-resorbing capacity, erythrocyte stimulation, Shwartzman reaction). They differ in that only LPS is pyrogenic, mutagenic, and lethal to mice. Of considerable interest in dental medicine are recent reports on the potential significance of LPS preparations obtained from oral bacteria associated with periodontal disease. Known periodontopathic bacteria, especially those associated with juvenile periodontitis (*Actinobacillus actinomycetemcomitans*), produce potent endotoxins with marked ability to cause in vivo bone resorption and other inflammatory changes due to cell systems known to be involved with the disease process (com-

plement activation, release of lysosomal enzymes from inflammatory cells, platelet aggregation).

Some of the major differences in gram-positive and gram-negative cell walls are summarized in Table 3.3.

The one additional kind of bacterial cell wall requiring attention is the cell wall of the acid-fast bacteria (members of the genus *Mycobacterium,* including the tubercle bacillus *Mycobacterium tuberculosis,* and some species of *Nocardia*). They are called acid-fast because once they are stained with carbolfuchsin, they resist decolorization with acid-alcohol. This staining property is correlated with the presence of cell wall–bound mycolic acids, a group of α-branched, β-hydroxy-fatty acids (C_{30} to C_{90} chain lengths). The wall of *M. tuberculosis* contains roughly equal amounts of lipid, peptidoglycan, and arabinogalactan (a polymer of arabinose and galactose). The arabinogalactan is bound to the PG at muramic acid and the mycolic acid via the C_5 hydroxyl group of arabinose. The lipids in the cell wall and elsewhere in the envelope of the tubercle bacillus have a profound effect on the surface properties of this organism and its pathogenic potential (see Chap. 23).

Protoplasts and Spheroplasts

As indicated earlier, protoplasts (usually grampositive in origin) and spheroplasts (usually gramnegative in origin) arise when the structural integrity

Table 3.3: Differences in Gram-Positive and Gram-Negative Cell Walls

	Gram-Positive	Gram-Negative
Peptidoglycan	Thick layer	Thin layer
Disaccharide chain	Numerous, intertwined mesh in three dimensions	Few chains and in a two-dimensional layer
Cross-bridges	Extensive (up to 100% in *S. aureus*) Combinations of one or more amino acids or a single amino acid, e.g., glycine	Minimal (30% in *E. coli*) Simple peptide bonds often
Tetrapeptide amino acids	Alternating L- and D-forms with a diamino acid in position 3 (L-lysine usually but also DAP, ornithine, DAB)	Same except L-lysine is usually substituted for by DAP
Other		
Teichoic acids	Yes	No
Endotoxin (LPS)	No	Yes
Amino acids	Few in number	Numerous
Membrane lipids	No (but lipoteichoic acids)	Yes (outer membrane)
Surface antigens	Yes (polysaccharides, teichoic acids, protein appendages)	Yes (of many kinds but usually do not cross-react with gram-positive antigens)

Note: DAP = diaminopimelic acid, DAB = 2,4-diaminobutyric acid.

of the cell walls is compromised. Protoplasts are devoid of cell wall, whereas incomplete removal of the wall (usually occurring in gram-negative bacteria because of the intimate association between the wall and the membranes) results in spheroplasts. Protoplasts and spheroplasts can be produced by exposing sensitive vegetative cells to antibiotics (e.g., penicillin) that inhibit cell wall formation or to an enzyme (e.g., lysozyme) that disrupts the wall. Both protoplasts and spheroplasts are osmotically fragile and their cytoplasmic membranes are easily ruptured, but they can be maintained in a hypertonic solution if they are protected from mechanical shock. Many protoplasts and spheroplasts cannot divide normally or reform cell walls. Those resulting from the action of penicillin can often grow, divide, and resume formation of cell walls if the antibiotic is removed. The mycoplasmas previously discussed lack the ability to form cell walls but are capable of growth and cell division. Another group of prokaryotic wall-less cells (or cells with impaired cell walls) are the L-forms. L-Forms are bacterial mutants of gram-positive or gram-negative parents in which PG synthesis has been severely deranged but they have developed compensatory changes in the membrane that allows them to grow and divide. Although most L-forms are osmotically fragile, some can grow at the osmolality of serum. Their role in human infectious disease is unclear even though they have been cultured from the lesions of pyelonephritis and oral aphthous ulcers. What is clear and disturbing about them is the threat that they pose in view of their resistance to most wall inhibitory antibiotics. Some of the characteristics of protoplasts, spheroplasts, L-forms, and mycoplasmas are summarized in Table 3.4.

Table 3.4: Characteristics of Prokaryotic Bacteria without Cell Walls or with Defective Cell Walls

Microorganism	Origin	Osmotic Fragility	Cell Division	Cell Wall Status
Mycoplasma	Mycoplasma	±	+ (slow)	Absent
Protoplasts	Known gram-positive bacterium	+ +	− to ±	Absent
Spheroplasts	Known gram-negative bacterium	+ +	− to ±	Part of wall remains
L-forms	Known gram-positive or gram-negative bacterium	±	+ (slow)	Absent or part of wall may remain

Eukaryotic Cell Walls

In contrast to prokaryotic cells, eukaryotic animal organisms do not have cell walls; only the eukaryotic plant and algal cells have rigid cell walls, and these are quite different from the prokaryotic peptidoglycan structures. Plant and algal cell walls contain a network of cellulose fibers arranged in a strong amorphous matrix. Cellulose is a linear polymer of glucose joined by β-1,4 linkages. Other polysaccharides found in this matrix include hemicellulose (branched polymers containing glucose and other sugars) and pectins (hydrated polymers containing galacturonic acid with smaller amounts of rhamnose). Fungi also contain rigid cell walls in which the principal chemical component is chitin, a polymer of *N*-acetylglucosamine. Smaller amounts of other carbohydrate polymers (mannans, galactans, etc.) are also part of this rigid structure, with still lesser amounts of protein, lipid, polyphosphates, and inorganic salts making up the remainder of the wall.

Cytoplasmic Structures

Cytoplasmic Membrane

Internal to the cell walls of all bacteria is a cytoplasmic membrane, the principal osmotic barrier of the cell. It is composed of a phospholipid bilayer into which membrane proteins are intercalated (unit membrane). The polar regions of the phospholipids are found in the outer surfaces of the bilayer while the hydrophobic fatty acid chains extend into the center of the membrane (Fig. 3.10; see also Fig. 3.1A). The membrane (approximately 4 to 5 nm thick) makes up 10% of the cell dry weight and 20% of the total cellular protein. As is true for virtually all prokaryotic cells, bacteria and their cell membranes do not contain or synthesize sterols. (Some *Mycoplasma* species can incorporate exogenous sterols from the medium into their surface layer but lack the ability to synthesize sterols.) The absence of sterols in prokaryotic cells explains their resistance to polyene antibiotics (nystatin, candicidin), which are known to react with sterols of eukaryotic cells and mycoplasma species, destabilizing the membranes.

Membranes may be observed with both light and electron microscopy by placing bacterial cells in hypertonic solutions, which results in plasmolysis, or shrinkage of the membrane and cytoplasm as a result of the osmotic pressure. In gram-positive bacteria the membrane is in close association with the peptidoglycan cell wall layer, whereas in gram-negative bacteria it lies a little below the peptidoglycan (see Fig. 3.9).

The osmotic barrier function of the membrane is indicated by the ability of bacteria to selectively trans-

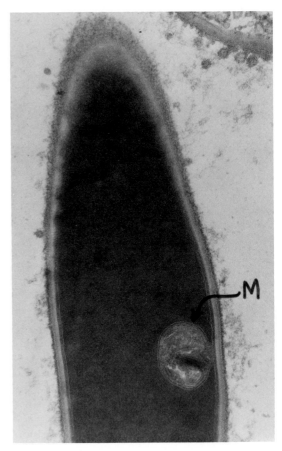

Figure 3.10: A transmission electron micrograph of the oral bacterium *Bacterionema matruchotii* (strain 100) showing mesosome (*M*) and its attachment to the cell membrane (× 68,000). (Courtesy of Dr. Chern Lai, University of Pennsylvania.)

port many organic and inorganic nutrients into the cell. Several membrane protein transport systems are known to exist in various bacteria and are responsible for the accumulation of many amino acids, inorganic nutrients, and other organic molecules against a concentration gradient. The activity of these enzyme-like proteins (*permeases*) is rapid (more rapid than passive diffusion) and exhibits considerable substrate specificity (discrimination between enantiomorphs of optically active compounds—e.g., D- vs. L-amino acids). Of particular interest to oral microbiologists is the transport of sugars into cariogenic bacteria, such as *Streptococcus mutans,* and sucrose transport. The sugar may be transported either by the carrier-mediated active transport (permease) system or by a group translocation (phosphotransferase, PTS) system. Active transport releases the sugar unmodified in the cytoplasm, unlike group translocation, where the sugar is first phosphorylated before it enters the cell. The phosphorylation involves the participation of four functional components, including 1) phosphoenol pyruvate (high-energy phosphate bond/phosphate donor); 2) a heat-stable protein, designated HPr, which acts as a carrier of high-energy phosphate, and 3) and 4) the enzyme proteins necessary to catalyze the reactions involving both a) and b):

$$\text{Phosphoenolpyruvate} + \text{HPr} \rightarrow \text{HPr-P} + \text{pyruvate}$$
$$\text{(in cytoplasm);}$$

$$\text{HPr-P} + \text{sugar} \rightarrow \text{Sugar-P} + \text{HPr}$$
$$\text{(in membrane).}$$

The membrane is also a major metabolic center for the cell since many of the enzymes involved in biosynthesis, electron transport, DNA replication, and membrane permeability are found here. Many of the biosynthetic reactions involved in cell wall assembly occur in or on the membrane, as do the energy-yielding reactions associated with electron transport and coupling mechanisms employed in active transport of substrate molecules. The assembly of extracellular polysaccharide units that form capsules and other extracellular polymers (dextrans, levans, etc.) occurs in the membrane when a phosphorylated lipid carrier molecule translocates these units to the exterior surface where they are covalently bound to the growing extracellular polymer.

Mesosomes

The cytoplasmic membranes of some bacteria, particularly gram-positive cells, may be invaginated to form internal structures called mesosomes (see Fig. 3.1A, item 9). They are connected to the membrane and do not occur as free membrane-bound organelles in the cytoplasm (e.g., mitochondria) (Fig. 3.10). The only known exceptions to this rule among the prokaryotes are the thylakoids found in some photosynthetic bacteria in which these chloroplast-like, membrane-bound organelles are distinct and separate from the membrane. Mesosomes appear to be associated with cell wall synthesis, segregation of nucleic acid during cell division, and secretion of exoenzymes, e.g., penicillinase; they also increase the surface area of the membrane and its transport systems.

Ribosomes

The cytoplasm of bacterial cells is filled with a large number of small (18 nm in diameter), dense, roughly spherical inclusions termed ribosomes whose primary if not sole function is protein synthesis. Ribosomes contain RNA (60% to 70%) and protein (30% to 40%) and make up about 40% of the cell's dry weight and 80% to 90% of the cellular RNA. When grouped together by attachment to a single strand of messenger RNA they are called polysomes or polyribosomes. The RNA of bacterial cells consists of ribosomal RNA (rRNA), transfer RNA (tRNA), and messenger RNA (mRNA). Twenty to 30 individual proteins are also present in the ribosomes. There are one to four kinds of tRNA for each of the 20 amino acids. There are also many kinds of mRNA, each acting as the template for synthesis of individual proteins. *E. coli* is estimated to contain between 2,000 and 3,000 different proteins and approximately 1,000 different kinds of mRNA.

All of the ribosomes of bacteria are of the 70S variety (based on their sedimentation rate in the ultracentrifuge; S = Svedberg units) and are therefore different from the 80S ribosomes characteristic of eukaryotic cells. This difference in ribosome structure forms the basis of selective toxicity of several antibiotics known to inhibit protein synthesis—in other words, it is possible to selectively prevent protein synthesis in a prokaryotic bacterial cell without substantially affecting the eukaryotic host cell. Unfortunately, some of these antibiotics, notably chloramphenicol, also inhibit the 70S ribosomes found in eukaryotic mitochondria and chloroplasts. Thus, selective toxicity is not absolute for this antibiotic.

Nucleus (Nuclear Region, Nucleoid)

One of the primary reasons that bacteria are grouped with prokaryotic cells is that they have a primitive nucleus, a repository for the DNA that serves as genetic material but is not enclosed by a nuclear membrane. Since no clear structural distinction is evident between nucleus and cytoplasm, the term nuclear region is often used. This term, however, is a misnomer since it is possible to isolate discrete masses of biologically active DNA by gentle lysis of cells, indicating that one is dealing with a structural entity rather than some indefinite space. Moreover, the physical and cytological properties of the material are complementary to and consistent with genetic data. It is difficult to demonstrate the nucleus in ordinary staining reactions because the presence of large amounts of RNA throughout the cytoplasm obscures the nucleus. One or more chromatin bodies (chromosomes) can be demonstrated and they serve as the functional equivalents of the eukaryotic nucleus. Bacterial DNA appears as a fibrillar network that often runs parallel to the cell axis. The bacterial chromosome usually exists as a single circular DNA molecule from 100 to 1,400 μm long. The fibrillar appearance arises from the considerable amount of folding of this extremely long DNA molecule (see Fig. 3.1).

Although the bacterial nucleus serves as the principal repository for DNA and carries all the genetic information ordinarily associated with the growth, metabolism, and survival of the cell, there are other repositories for DNA, termed plasmids. Most bacteria harbor these extrachromosomal, circular DNA molecules, capable of autonomous replication and carrying the determinants for several phenotypic characters (e.g., drug resistance, pilus formation, bacteriocin formation, enzyme synthesis, etc.). The amount of DNA in a plasmid is 0.1% to 0.5% of that found in chromosomal DNA, supporting the view that plasmids may be lost from the cell without any real impairment of cell viability. Several oral bacteria (*Streptococcus mutans, S. faecalis, Capnocytophaga* spp., etc.) have been reported to contain plasmids but their roles in oral disease and oral microbial ecology have not been clearly established. The plasmid in *S. mutans* is considered by some to be a virulence plasmid since it codes for enzymes associated with the production of dextrans necessary for adherence and colonization of this organism in the oral cavity. Plasmids for which there is no known phenotypic property are called cryptic.

Cellular Inclusions

Most if not all bacteria are capable of forming some kind of cytoplasmic inclusion if the appropriate cultural or environmental conditions are present. Until recently the full significance of these inclusions in the overall biological economy of the cell was not recognized. A few general facts about their synthesis have been known for a long time: 1) Most are high molecular weight polymers (no osmotic energy is required to keep them inside the cell). 2) Most inclusions are formed under conditions of unbalanced growth (carbohydrate excess, nitrogen limitation, phosphate excess). 3) Not all inclusions are formed by any one organism at any one time. However, very little information was available about the catabolism of these inclusions and their possible significance in cellular physiology. Most of these inclusions are found in various oral bacteria and their roles in oral microbial ecology have been investigated in some detail.

Glycogen.   During the later phases of growth, when the synthesis of nucleic acids and proteins is decreased (i.e., nitrogen limitation), and in the presence of residual carbohydrate (e.g., glucose, sucrose), a large number of bacteria accumulate large amounts of an α-1,4-linked glucose polymer (glycogen). This material is produced by a large number of plaque-forming bacteria, including most oral streptococci, *Lactobacillus casei,* diphtheroids, *Veillonella,* and other plaque-related bacteria (Fig. 3.11). In several cases this intracellular iodophilic polysaccharide (IPS) amounts to 50% to 60% of the cell dry weight and is

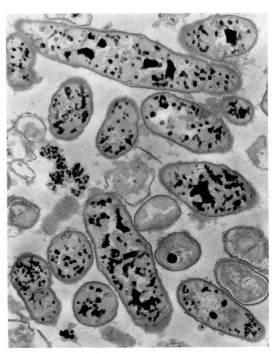

Figure 3.11: Transmission electron micrograph of *Streptococcus sanguis* G9B showing large amounts of intracellular glycogen (stained for polysaccharide) (× 29,800). (Courtesy of Dr. Chern Lai, University of Pennsylvania.)

used as a reserve storage material that can be stoichiometrically converted to lactic acid in the absence of exogenous carbohydrate (Fig. 3.12). This could account for the sustained production of acid by human dental plaque in the absence of dietary carbohydrate (i.e., during sleep). This hypothesis received additional support when it was found that IPS-producing bacteria were more numerous in plaques and carious lesions from caries-active persons than in similar material from caries-inactive individuals. Moreover, the in situ production of glycogen was demonstrated in freshly stained supragingival plaque—bacteria in plaque samples could be stained directly to show this intracellular polymer. However, studies using IPS-defective mutant strains were less clear in demonstrating a positive correlation between IPS production and cariogenicity: some mutants produced fewer carious lesions, and some mutants produced higher caries scores than uninfected controls. Other roles for glycogen catabolism in oral ecology have included a possibly enhanced survival since glycogen-producing cells of *Streptococcus mitis* have a much higher viability upon prolonged storage than non-glycogen-producing cells. Also, IPS catabolism provides the cell with utilizable energy for enzyme induction (β-galactosidase induction was much faster in IPS-positive cells than in IPS-negative cells under otherwise identical conditions).

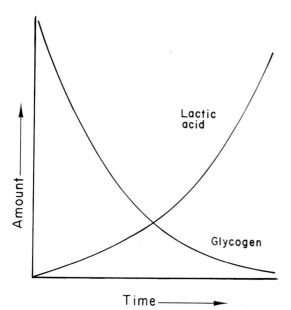

Figure 3.12: Catabolism of intracellular glycogen to lactic acid by washed cells of *Lactobacillus casei* (strain 32-1l). Note that there is an almost stoichiometric conversion of glycogen to lactic acid when there is no exogenous substrate.

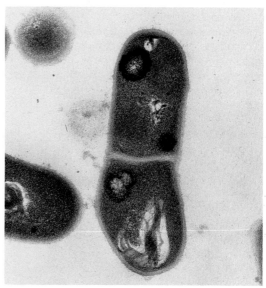

Figure 3.13: Transmission electron micrograph of *Corynebacterium diphtheriae* 19409 showing intracellular metachromatic granules (*arrows*) ($\times 68{,}000$). (Courtesy of Dr. Chern Lai, University of Pennsylvania.)

Poly-β-hydroxybutyrate.   Poly-β-OH-butyric acid is a polymer of the C_4 fatty acid. Whereas glycogen-type polymers are found in both eukaryotic and prokaryotic cells, PβHB is uniquely found in prokaryotes such as species of *Pseudomonas, Bacillus,* and *Spirillum.* Prokaryotes use this material as a reserve storage compound, in contrast to the neutral fat stored by eukaryotes. Catabolism of PβHB occurs after the material is activated by a Ca^{2+}-requiring enzyme and the final products include acetoacetate and β-OH-butyrate. In the presence of coenzyme A (CoA) the synthesis of PβHB may be recycled with the formation of acetoacetyl CoA. Accumulation of PβHB ranges from 7% to 40% of the cell's dry weight.

Volutin Granules (Babès-Ernst or Metachromatic Granules).   Volutin granules are acid-insoluble polymetaphosphates characteristically seen in *Corynebacterium diphtheriae, Mycobacterium tuberculosis,* and *L. casei.* They are called metachromatic because they appear red when stained with a blue dye (metachromasy = color change) (Fig. 3.13). The granules form under starvation conditions and appear to function as intracellular phosphate reserves that can be mobilized as a phosphorus source for nucleic acids. The degradation of polymetaphosphate has also been considered as a possible source of ATP, although this function is currently in considerable doubt.

Other Inclusions.   Many other inclusions have been reported in bacteria. Several are associated with specific metabolic or physiologic functions, such as sulfur granules, associated with sulfur oxidation; gas vacuoles, associated with movement of cells in a vertical plane; carboxysomes, associated with CO_2 fixation; and chlorosomes, associated with photosynthesis.

Bacterial Spores and Spore Formation

The ability of some bacteria to produce the highly refractive and resistant internal structures known as endospores represents an extraordinary example of differentiation. The process leads to the production of a new type of cell that is structurally, antigenically, and physiologically different from the parent cell (sporangium) from which it is formed and ultimately released (Figs. 3.14 and 3.15). Considerable work has been done to define in mechanistic terms the nature of sporulation, not only because it presents a series of fascinating problems related to cellular differentiation, but also because of medical and public health implications. Although spore formation is uncommon among most pathogenic bacteria, the two genera in which it occurs, *Bacillus* (aerobic) and *Clostridium* (anaerobic), are highly important. *Bacillus anthracis* is the etiological agent of anthrax and its spores are the single most important factor in disease prevention and transmission of the infectious agent. Members of the genus *Clostridium* are responsible

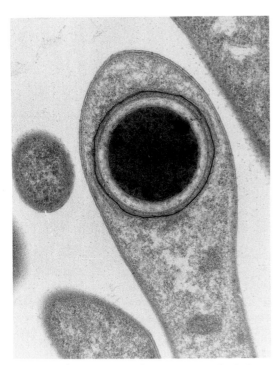

Figure 3.14: Transmission electron micrograph of *Clostridium malenominatum* 25776 showing endospore (×68,000). (Courtesy of Dr. Chern Lai, University of Pennsylvania.)

for tetanus (*C. tetani*) and botulism (*C. botulinum*); again, the spores of both organisms play a critical role in the production of disease. Most sterilization procedures also use spore destruction as one of the principal criteria for sterilizing efficiency (see Chap. 13).

Spores are formed by an invagination of the double layer of cell membrane (*spore septum*) within which is enclosed part of the host cell genome and a small amount of cytoplasm (*forespore*). The process usually begins at the end of exponential growth in the presence of a limited supply of an essential nutrient (e.g., glucose or other energy source). In general, growth and sporulation are opposing processes since sporulation, induced by exhaustion of glucose, is inhibited if more glucose is subsequently added to the sporulating culture. It is probable that glucose inhibits the synthesis of specific enzymes required for sporulation through the process of catabolite repression (see Chap. 6). Spore integument forms between the double membranes, and the cytoplasm condenses to complete the inner core, which is enclosed by a thin membrane (*spore wall*). Surrounding the spore wall is a layered *cortex*, which in turn is surrounded by two relatively impervious coats that account for much of the resistance of spores to heat, drying, or chemicals. The coats are composed of keratin-like protein, which

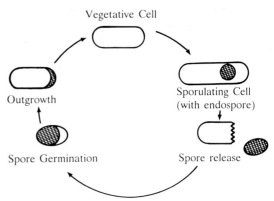

Figure 3.15: Life cycle of a spore-forming bacterium.

is associated with resistance to chemicals and ultraviolet and ionizing radiation. Inside the cortex is the *core*, which contains the nuclear DNA, ribosomes, etc. The chemical substance that is characteristic of endospores but not found in vegetative cells is the calcium salt of dipicolinic acid (Fig. 3.16). This substance, found in the core, is probably responsible for the heat resistance of bacterial endospores. The completion of sporulation requires about 6 to 8 hours.

Spores have very little metabolic activity. Selective synthesis and uptake of metabolites do occur, but to a very limited extent. At germination, physiologic activity resumes, usually in three stages: 1) *Activation* by some agent that damages the spore coat (heat, sulfhydryl groups, acidity, abrasion). This step probably involves some reversible denaturation of some specific macromolecule. 2) In the *Initiation* phase, most of the characteristic properties of the spore are irreversibly lost, as demonstrated by a loss of refractility, increased stainability, and a marked decrease in resistance to deleterious physical and chemical agents. As expected, there is a loss of calcium dipicolinate, an uptake of water, and hydrolytic breakdown of several spore components. 3) The *outgrowth* phase is marked by lysis of the cortex and outer layers of the spore and the development of a new vegetative cell. During this period of intense biosynthesis the spore coat membrane develops into the peptidoglycan cell wall of the

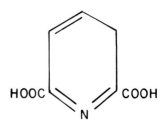

Figure 3.16: Dipicolinic acid (pyridine 2,6-dicarboxylic acid).

vegetative cell and most of the other morphological features characteristic of vegetative cells are produced. Because of all these changes this phase is inhibited by antibiotics known to inhibit various metabolic processes (cell wall, protein synthesis, or nucleic acid synthesis).

ADDITIONAL READING

Brock, T. T., and Madigan, M. T. 1988. *Biology of Microorganisms,* Ed. 5. Prentice Hall, Englewood Cliffs, N.J.

Gibbons, R. J., and van Houte, J. 1975. Bacterial Adherence in Oral Microbial Ecology. Annu Rev Microbiol, **29,** 19.

Hamilton, I. R. 1976. Intracellular Polysaccharide Synthesis by Cariogenic Microorganisms. In *Microbial Aspects of Dental Caries* (H. M. Stiles, W. J. Loesche, and T. C. O'Brien, eds.), Microbiol Abstr Spec Suppl **3,** 683.

Lamanna, C., Mallette, M. F., and Zimmerman, L. N. 1973. *Basic Bacteriology,* Ed. 4. Williams & Wilkins, Baltimore.

Leive, L. (Ed.). 1973. *Bacterial Membranes and Walls.* Marcel Decker, New York.

Lin, E. C. C. 1970. The Genetics of Bacterial Transport Systems. Annu Rev Genet, **4,** 225.

Meynell, G. G. 1973. *Bacterial Plasmids.* The M.I.T. Press, Cambridge, Mass.

Shively, J. M. 1974. Inclusion Bodies of Procaryotes. Annu Rev Microbiol, **28,** 167.

Stanier, R. Y., Adelberg, E. A., and Ingraham, J. L. 1986. *The Microbial World,* Ed. 5. Prentice-Hall, Englewood Cliffs, N.J.

Watson, J. D. 1987. *The Molecular Biology of the Gene,* Ed. 4. W. A. Benjamin, Inc., Menlo Park, Calif.

Wicken, A. J., and Knox, K. 1977. Biological Properties of Lipoteichoic Acids. In *Microbiology—1977,* pp. 360–365, edited by D. Schlessinger. American Society for Microbiology, Washington, D.C.

4

Bacterial Genetics

John T. Wilson

An orderly mechanism of inheritance in bacteria is implied by the fact that they "breed true." If the distribution of genetic material at bacterial cell division were not uniform, progeny identical with the parent bacteria would only occur by chance. In general, the morphological and physiological identity of most bacteria is maintained from one generation to the next. This constancy in properties is the basis for the routine identification of unknown organisms in nature. Similarly, the control of infectious diseases would be greatly compromised if the genetic stability of microorganisms was not so common. Antigenic variation would nullify the benefits of vaccines, and variation in drug susceptibility would create chemotherapeutic nightmares. Indeed, one of the early considerations about the efficacy of the proposed caries vaccine was the possibility of antigenic drift in the serotypes of *Streptococcus mutans*. Thus, genetic stability in microorganisms is not absolute and gene mutations do occur. The natural antibiotic resistance in bacteria is well known and has caused serious prob-

lems. Moreover, the evolution of microorganisms is predicated on change and the ability to change.

One of the more positive aspects of these genetic changes in microorganisms, especially bacteria, is that is has provided the molecular biologist with a powerful tool to study various aspects of cell biology in a rapid and easily reproducible way. The significance of a property (A) can be determined by using mutant pairs (A+ and A−) of otherwise identical organisms, many of which have doubling times (generation times) of less than 30 minutes. Thus, many generations of a population can be studied in a very short time to determine the significance of a single property.

Typical genetic processes and molecular mechanisms operate in prokaryotic microorganisms even though their organization is simpler than that of the eukaryotic cell. The basic structure of DNA and mechanisms for replication, transcription, and translation of genetic information should be familiar to most readers. However, a brief summary of genetic structures and mechanisms as they relate to bacteria will be presented. Additional information will be provided concerning recent work on the genetics of oral bacteria and how the application of basic genetics is clearly relevant and necessary in dental medicine.

The Bacterial Chromosome

The chromosome of all bacteria thus far reported is a single circular DNA molecule. The *E. coli* chromosome has an estimated molecular weight of 3×10^9 daltons and contains about 5×10^6 basepairs. The bacterial chromosome does not have histones attached to it, but small polyamines may serve similar functions (stabilize the DNA molecule and increase resistance to strand separation). As is true for eukaryotes, bacterial DNA is a polymer of the deoxyribonucleotides of adenine (A), guanine (G), thymine (T), and cytosine (C), connected by phosphodiester linkages to form a chain. The DNA molecule takes the form of two adjacent chains arranged in a double helix and stabilized by hydrogen bonds between pairs of bases on the two side chains. Pairing occurs between adenine and thymine and between guanine and cytosine.

DNA replication in the bacterial chromosome occurs in a semiconservative fashion so that progeny chromosomes consist of one chain from the parent molecule and one newly formed chain. The latter chain is the result of enzymatic polymerization of a sequence of nucleotides arranged on a template consisting of one strand of a parental DNA molecule.

The genetic information encoded in the order of the nucleotides and divided into hereditary units known as genes is transcribed into messenger RNA (mRNA), then translated into proteins by reactions typical of this process. Bacterial mRNA is polygenic, that is, it contains information from more than one gene. The information contained in such a molecule generally specifies proteins whose functions are related, such as the enzymes for a specific pathway.

Mutation

Mutation and recombination are the two major sources of genetic variation in any species. Mutation may be defined as any change in the nucleotide sequence of the DNA molecule. Changes in nucleotide sequence can conceivably occur in two ways: 1) basepair substitution (one pair is substituted for another basepair as the result of an error during replication) and 2) breakage of the sugar-phosphate backbone of DNA with subsequent deletion, inversion, or insertion of old/new segments.

An alteration in the nucleotide sequence of a gene may change the structure and therefore the function of the protein coded for by that gene. The expression of such mutations (phenotypic change) can occur for any property of the cell (nutrition, morphology, drug susceptibility, etc.). Besides producing recognizable changes in structure or function, mutations may be lethal to the cell, may produce no visible effects, or may go unrecognized until the organism is placed under conditions of a selective or permissive environment, e.g., the absence of a metabolite or at an abnormal temperature. Mutations may be spontaneous or caused by mutagens that specifically alter DNA structure. In all instances, however, mutations are random events and occur irrespective of environmental factors and pressures. Resistance to an antibiotic among bacterial cells in a culture occurs in the complete absence of the antibiotic and at the same rate as would have occurred if the antibiotic was present.

Mutations can be broadly categorized as microlesions or macrolesions. Microlesions are changes that result from the addition, subtraction (base deletion), or substitution of a single base within the DNA molecule. Macrolesions are inversions, duplications, and deletions and generally affect many genes or large blocks of DNA.

Substitution is the simplest type of mutation to understand and probably the most prevalent in nature. Within the DNA molecule there are four bases, each of which can be exchanged for any of the other three, for a total of 12 possible substitutions. These substitutions are subdivided into two types: 1) transitions, where a purine is substituted for a purine or a pyrimidine is substituted for a pyrimidine, and 2) transversions, where a purine is substituted for a pyrimidine or a pyrimidine is substituted for a purine.

Substitutions change only one codon. Often these mutations do not result in a change in the amino acid sequence of the protein and are called silent mutations. When the mutation does result in the substitution of one amino acid for another, it is called a missense mutation. Finally, if a single base substitution results in the early termination of mRNA, then it creates a terminator and is called a nonsense mutation.

Frameshift Mutations

The consequence of the addition or subtraction (deletion) of a single base is much more drastic to the organism than is a simple substitution. Such mutations are also called frameshift mutations because they alter the reading frame of the mRNA. All of the codons following the mutation generally code for a different sequence of amino acids than that which was found in the original protein. The amount of change (usually the amount of damage) that a given frameshift mutation causes is dependent on where the mutation occurs with respect to the end of the transcriptional unit. In some cases, a single mRNA may code for as many as ten different gene products. Should a frameshift mutation occur early in the first gene, all ten genes would be inactivated. If a mutation in one gene affects other genes that are on its distal side, it is called a polar mutation.

Spontaneous Mutations

Mutations that arise in the absence of a known mutagen are called spontaneous mutations. They occur at a frequency of 10^{-7} to 10^{-10} per organism per cell division. The most likely mechanism for spontaneous point mutations is thought to be errors in pairing at the replication fork as the wrong tautomeric form of a base is incorporated. The Watson-Crick model for the structure of DNA shows that each of the four bases may exist in tautomeric forms due to a shift of electrons. Cytosine and adenine can exist in either the common amino or rare imino states, whereas thymine and guanine can exist in either the normal keto or rare enol state. In nature, an equilibrium is established between the keto and enol forms and between the amino and imino forms. This equilibrium generally favors the keto and amino states. However, when the bases exist in the rare forms, they can be incorporated into the DNA molecule during replication. Following incorporation, these bases will mispair, and the result will be the incorporation of the wrong base during subsequent rounds of replication. For example, thymine in the enol form (rather than the normal keto state) will hydrogen bond with guanine instead of adenine and change the base sequence and triplet code.

Other postulated mechanisms for the occurrence of spontaneous mutations include 1) production of mutagens from normal metabolites, 2) loss of a segment of DNA, or 3) alteration in activity or synthesis of enzymes involved in DNA replication or repair.

Mutagens and Induced Mutations

A number of agents and techniques can increase the errors a cell makes in DNA replication. Many of these errors lead to cell death (lethal mutations), but proper selection methods can permit isolation of nonlethal mutants.

There are numerous agents known as mutagens, so called because they are capable of raising the spontaneous mutation rate. These mutagens can be broadly classified into those caused by light energy and those caused by chemical energy.

1. Light Energy. In the study of mutations resulting from ionizing radiation, it becomes evident that there is a direct relationship between the wavelength of light and the mutation rate: the shorter the wavelength, the higher the mutation rate.

The most common way to produce mutations from ionizing radiation is to expose the sample to x-rays. The x-rays collide with the atoms in the DNA molecule and produce ions, which results in breakage of the DNA molecule. A plot of the number of mutations vs. the dosage would show a linear relationship. This is explained by the target hypothesis, which states that the gene is a target for mutation. The greater the dosage, the higher the probability of a hit, and therefore the greater the mutation rate. The mutations caused by ionizing radiation are generally macrolesions, such as chromosomal aberrations.

Ultraviolet (UV) light radiation has also been shown to cause chromosomal aberrations. However, the most common mutations that result from UV radiation are point mutations. One important point to remember about UV radiation is that it is too mild to produce ions and affects only compounds that absorb it (only organic ring compounds such as the bases found in DNA). When DNA is exposed to UV radiation, the most common result is the formation of thymine dimers: T^T. These dimers are hypothesized to distort the DNA molecule and therefore cause errors in replication. A most unusual aspect of UV radiation effects is that they are often reversed by exposure to visible light (blue light). This process, called photoreactivation, is believed to be due to the activation of repair enzymes which remove the T^T.

2. Chemical Energy. Various chemicals are known to increase the mutation rate. The most common chemical mutagens used in the laboratory are base analogues, nitrous acid, hydroxylamine, and alkylating agents (ethyl methanesulfonate, EMS) and acridine dyes. The proposed mechanism for these various chemical mutagens is as follows:

Generally, base analogues are believed to increase the mutation rate by increasing the incidence of tautomeric shifts such that mispairing occurs. For example, 5-bromouracil (5-BU) is an analogue of thymine. It is usually in the keto form but undergoes a tautomeric shift to the enol form, which allows it to pair with guanine. This results in an A-T to G-C substitution. Occasionally, 5-BU may be incorporated in the rare enol form (pairing with guanine) and revert back to the keto form, which pairs with adenine to give a G-C to A-T transition.

The base analogue 2-aminopurine shows similar mutational properties as 5-BU, enabling it to be incorporated as a substitute of adenine but to pair with

Table 4.1: Common Mutagens and Their Primary Effects

Mutagen	Mutations Induced
Base analogues:	Transitions
5-bromouracil (5-BU)	
2-aminopurine (2-AP)	
Hydroxylamine	C to T transitions only
Nitrous acid	Transitions
Alkylating agents:	
Ethyl methanesulfonate (EMS)	Transitions, transversions
Nitrosoguanidine (NTG)	Transitions, transversions, deletions
Ultraviolet radiation	Frameshift, transitions, transversions
X-rays	Primarily macrolesions
Acridine dyes	Frame shift, deletions
Spontaneous	Transitions, transversions, deletions

cytosine, or to pair initially with cytosine and subsequently with thymine.

Nitrous acid acts primarily through the removal of the amino group (deamination) from adenine and cytosine, thereby converting these bases to hypoxanthine and uracil, respectively. Hypoxanthine now pairs with cytosine (A-T to G-C) and uracil pairs with adenine (G-C to A-T), resulting in transitions.

Hydroxylamine also produces transitions within the DNA molecule. It adds an OH group to the amino group of cytosine, which enables the base to undergo a tautomeric shift so that it can pair with adenine.

Alkylating agents such as nitrogen mustard and ethyl methanesulfonate (EMS) may produce mutations in at least two ways: 1) by adding methyl or ethyl groups to guanine, causing it to behave as a base analogue of adenine and thereby produce pairing errors, and 2) by depurinating the DNA of guanine bases resulting in deletions.

Acridine dyes such as proflavin and acridine orange cause mutations in the DNA molecule by inserting themselves between two neighboring purine bases. These chemical mutagens generally cause either insertions or deletions during subsequent rounds of replication.

Table 4.1 shows some of the common mutagens and their primary effects.

Effects of Mutation on the Cell

The set of genetic determinants carried by a cell is its genotype. The observable properties of the cell are called its phenotype. A gene mutation can only be recognized if it causes an observable phenotypic change. When studying phenotypic change with respect to enzyme function, we can categorize these changes into either gain mutations or loss mutations. A gain mutation confers on the cell the ability to synthesize an active enzyme, and there is no lag between the time of the mutation and the beginning of enzyme synthesis. A loss mutation is a mutation that results in the loss of synthesis of an enzyme. However, since most enzymes present in the cell exist for a period of time, there is a phenotypic lag associated with loss mutations, owing to the presence of functional enzyme within the cell prior to the mutational event.

Effects of Mutation on Cell Populations

The proportion of mutants within a cell population is the mutant frequency and is dependent on three factors: 1) the mutation rate—the probability that a cell will mutate during a given interval, 2) the time distribution of mutational events—mutations that occur early in the growth of a culture will have more mutant progeny than those that occur late, and 3) the growth rate of the mutant cells as compared to the parental type—if a mutation severely inhibits the growth rate, the number of progeny of that cell over a given period of time will be much less than that found for a normal cell. In addition, if the mutant cell has a different death rate than the parental cell, this will also affect the population shift.

Microbial populations are commonly subjected to constant selection, either consciously or unconsciously. Since most mutants are present in low frequency, absolute selection is often necessary for their detection.

In a number of cases the genetic damage due to mutation may be circumvented by two other processes, suppression and complementation.

Suppression

The loss of activity by a protein as a result of a mutation may be partially or completely offset by a second mutation at a different site. The second mutation, called a suppressor mutation, may occur in the same gene as the primary mutation (intragenic suppression) or in a different gene (extragenic suppression). Intragenic suppression may result from the substitution of an amino acid that compensates for the first change. An example of extragenic suppression is the suppression of mutations by mechanisms involving alterations in the anticodon portion of the tRNA molecule. The anticodon region is a three nucleotide sequence in the tRNA that pairs with a compatible sequence, the codon, in the mRNA molecule. The change in the anticodon permits it to read a mutated codon resulting from an alteration in DNA structure. However, since the change is limited to the anticodon loop of tRNA, it is still able to bind the correct amino acid and insert it into the correct place in the polypeptide chain. The primary mutation occurred in the gene that specified the codon, resulting in an incorrect codon, while the second mutation occurred in the tRNA, which permitted the tRNA to read the altered codon. Other possible mechanisms of suppression involve an alternate pathway for production of a product that cannot be synthesized, owing to a primary mutation, or production of a product that replaces the product of the mutated gene.

Complementation

A mutation that produces an altered polypeptide chain with decreased activity can sometimes be reversed by changes not in genetic structure, but rather in the functional aspects of the protein. This occurs by complementation, wherein genetic material from an organism which has normal function is introduced into the mutated one and supplies the missing components—those the first organism lost by mutation—so that a functional protein is produced.

Results of Mutation

Since genes regulate protein structure, which determines the structural and metabolic properties of the cell, mutations cause changes in various cell properties. Loss of certain functions is not critical in certain cases: if an alternate pathway is available, or if the synthesis of a polymer (e.g., capsule) will not affect the viability of the cell. However, some gene products are indispensable, for the cell dies if they are lost through mutation (lethal mutations). Another form is the conditional lethal mutation, which is expressed under one set of environmental conditions but not another. Conditions where the lethal mutation is expressed are called nonpermissive, while those where they are not expressed are called permissive. One of the more common conditional mutations is that affecting temperature sensitivity, where protein structure is altered so that it is nonfunctional at one temperature but functional at another. If this change occurs and affects an indispensable protein, the cell dies when it is placed at nonpermissive temperatures.

Gene Transfer

In eukaryotic cells, new gene combinations arise by gamete fusion. Diploid cells are formed and recombinant chromosomes result from the transfer of genetic material from one cell to the other. A similar process may occur in bacteria whereby a recombinant chromosome is formed from genetic material of two different parental cells. For this process to occur in bacteria, the genetic material from one parent must be transferred to the other. Transfer may occur by transformation, conjugation, or transduction; the result is that part of the donor cell genetic material is transferred to the recipient, making the latter a partial diploid. The original genome of the recipient is called an endogenote, while the donor DNA is called the exogenote. In transformation, a single-stranded piece of donor DNA replaces a strand of the endogenote DNA; in transduction, a small fragment of donor DNA is transferred to the recipient by a bacterial virus, a bacteriophage; and in conjugation, the donor DNA is transferred between cells that are in direct contact. If the exogenote has a base sequence homologous to a segment of the endogenote, pairing occurs and a recombinant chromosome is formed, a step that is called integration. If integration does not occur, the exogenote may be segregated upon subsequent cell division, it may replicate independently, or it may be degraded. Recombination occurs by breakage of the parental DNA followed by reunion of the broken ends with the donor DNA, producing a chromosome with the exogenote DNA incorporated into it.

Several generalizations can be made about all these mechanisms of gene transfer:

1. The transfers are always unidirectional—from DNA donor to DNA recipient. There is not a genetic exchange in the sense that both partners receive part of the genetic material; only one partner is the recipient.

2. The transfer of genetic material is usually incomplete. Except in a very few instances, only part of the donor DNA is transferred; *meromixis* (from Greek roots meaning partial mixing) is used to describe the bacterial process of genetic transfer. Similarly, the term merozygote is substituted for zygote to indicate a recipient (partial zygote) without the complete complement of the donor's haploid genome.

3. Not all organisms are capable of all of the genetic transfer mechanisms. In some instances specific cultural or environmental conditions prevent transfer (e.g., "competency" in transformation); in other instances the presence of a specific surface structure (sex pilus in conjugation) appears to be a prerequisite. Thus, the mechanism of gene transfer depends in large measure on the individual properties of the bacterium in question.

4. The successful completion of gene transfer (incorporation and integration of the donor DNA into recipient DNA) requires some positive level of DNA homology. DNAs with low homology (i.e., very few similar nucleotide sequences) do not hybridize and therefore cannot be integrated. Some of the various mechanisms of gene transfer in bacteria are described below and summarized in Table 4.2.

Conjugation

Conjugation is mediated by small extrachromosomal DNA elements called plasmids. Plasmids are dispensable under ordinary conditions but are detected when they confer new properties on the host cell. The most common types of plasmids and their associated properties are as follows: 1) Sex factors. Sex factors, or F plasmids, mediate conjugation. 2) Colicin factors. These factors carry genes that cause their host to produce colicins, proteins that are lethal toxins to coliform bacteria. 3) Resistance factors. These carry genes that confer antibiotic resistance on the host cell. Some R plasmids may carry several genes that confer resistance to many antibiotics. 4) Penicillinase plasmids of staphylococci. These special plasmids contain a gene for penicillinase that renders the host resistant to penicillin. Penicillinase plasmids differ from R plasmids in that they cannot be transferred by conjugation. 5) Degradative plasmids of *Pseudomonas*. These plasmids carry genes for enzymes of catabolic pathways, such as the enzymes for the degradation of camphor, toluene, octane, or salicylic acid.

All plasmids are circular, double-stranded DNA molecules with a molecular weight in the range of 3,000,000 to 100,000,000 daltons. This size range is sufficient to code from 5 to 160 average-sized proteins. Plasmids regulate their own DNA replication; however, most use the host cell machinery. DNA replication is generally bidirectional, but unidirectional replication is known. Plasmids can be classified into a number of compatibility groups, and members within each group are closely related, as indicated by DNA hybridization experiments. Two members of the same group cannot coexist in the same cell. This incompatibility may be due to the necessity of binding to a specific receptor, of which there is only one per cell for each group. Plasmids undergo recombination with each other and with the host chromosome. If there is an equal number crossover (i.e., 2, 4, 6), then the plasmid becomes integrated into the chromosome. Once integrated, it replicates as part of the host chromosome. Once a plasmid is integrated it is called an episome. The ability to integrate is generally solely a function of DNA sequence homology between the plasmid and the chromosome. Once integrated, the hybrid chromosome has two replicators, the plasmid site and the chromosome site. Generally, replication originates at the chromosomal site, and it is thought of as dominant. However, if replication cannot initiate at the chromosomal site (e.g., under nonpermissive temperatures in temperature-sensitive mutants), it often will initiate at the plasmid site. No matter which site is used, when DNA replication is initiated, the whole structure (chromosome + plasmid) is replicated. One of the most important aspects of some plasmids is their ability to self-transfer.

In gram-negative organisms, many plasmids are conjugative in that they carry genes called *tra* genes that mediate their transfer via conjugation. Some of the *tra* genes code for the sex pili, which are protein threads several times the length of the cell. During the process of conjugation, the pili from one cell attach to receptor sites in the cell wall of another gram-negative cell, and shortly thereafter the cells come into direct contact. The plasmid in the donor cell then replicates and the replicated strand of DNA is transferred to the recipient cell. Experiments that measure DNA transfer prior to the cell-cell contact indicate that DNA transfer occurs by way of the sex pilus. No cytoplasm or other cell material is transferred from the donor to the recipient via conjugation.

Self-transfer of plasmids is not as common in gram-positive organisms as in gram-negative bacteria. The best-known example of plasmid-mediated transfer in a gram-positive organism is the SCP1 plasmid found in *Streptomyces*. This plasmid contains the genes for producing the antibiotic methylneomycin and the genes necessary for its transfer. Gene transfer in this system also requires cell-cell contact; however, no sex pili are formed. The molecular details of gene transfer in this system are not well understood but have some similarities to those of gram-negative bacteria.

Gene Transfer of *E. coli* K12. The difference in sexual behavior between donors and recipients is caused by a small transmissible factor called F, the sex or fertility factor. Donor cells containing F (F^+) can transmit this factor in high frequency to recipient cells (F^-), which in turn become donors. The transmission of F is independent of the transmission of chromosomal genes. However, a small fraction of recipient cells (about 1/100,000) do receive chromosomal genes. The transfer of chromosomal genes is probably due to recombination events in which genetic material is exchanged between the F factor and the chromosome.

Studies on conjugation have shown some F^+ cell populations which can transfer chromosomal genes at a high frequency (1/1,000) and have been designated high-frequency recombination (Hfr) cells. One major difference in the transfer of genes by an F^+ cell and an Hfr cell is the frequency with which each transfers a

Table 4.2: Summary of Genetic Transfer Mechanisms

Genetic Process	Representative Organisms	State of DNA as Transfer Agent	Direction of Transfer	Frequency	Amount of Transfer	Other
Transformation	*Streptococcus pneumoniae, Haemophilus influenzae, Bacillus* species, *Neisseria* spp., oral streptococci (*Streptococcus sanguis, Streptococcus mitior*)	"Naked" DNA	DNA donor → DNA recipient	10^{-3} up to 25%	Few genes (1/200 of chromosome)	1. "Competency" of cell surfaces 2. Environment plays a major role in transfer process 3. Historically, the first mechanism of gene transfer reported in bacteria
Transduction	*Salmonella* spp., *Escherichia coli, Shigella*	Bacteriophage carrier	Phage donor → phage recipient	10^{-5} to 10^{-6}	Small linkage groups	1. Two kinds of transduction: restrictive and generalized 2. Nature of infective phage (lytic/lysogenic)
Lysogenic conversion	*Corynebacterium diphtheriae* and other exotoxin-producing bacteria	Phage/prophage	Lysogenic → nonlysogenic	100%	1 or 2 genes	
Conjugation	*E. coli, Shigella, Salmonella, Proteus, Bacillus, Streptococcus mutans, Bacteroides* spp., *Streptococcus faecalis*	DNA via cytoplasmic bridge	Hfr → F$^-$ (F$^+$ → F$^-$)	10^{-3} 10^{-6} to 10^{-7}	Large linkage group	1. Requirement for fertility factor (F) 2. Cell–cell contact required 3. Oriented transfer of linkage group (origin → end)

particular gene. Let the genes on a chromosome be designated as A, B, C, . . . , X, Y, Z. An F$^+$ cell can transfer any gene (A to Z) at about the same frequency. However, with an Hfr cell, there appears to be a gradation in recombination frequencies so that A is most frequently transferred, D less frequently, and J even less frequently than A or D. Some genes, such as X, Y, and Z, are almost never transferred by an Hfr cell. Furthermore, in contrast to F$^+$ recombinants, most recombinants produced by Hfr cells remain F$^-$ recipients; only a very few become Hfr. Those that do become Hfr also have recombinants for the genes that are generally transferred at the lowest frequency (X, Y, and Z). Not all Hfr strains initiate transfer of the bacterial chromosome at the same point (i.e., in some strains, E is transferred with the highest frequency and B, C, and D with the lowest frequency). These findings have been explained on the basis of integration of the F factor. In F$^+$ strains, the sex factor lies in the cytoplasm. From there it is free to recombine (at a very low frequency) at random sites with the chromosome and transfer a small segment of the chromosome to the recipient cell. In contrast, in the Hfr cell the F factor has integrated (randomly) into the donor chromosome and directs the transfer of the donor chromosome first and itself last to the recipient cell.

A third class of recombinants has also been recognized whose members transfer genes at a rate equivalent to that of an F factor. This class, called F$'$, is the result of an F factor in a Hfr cell which has lost its integrated state on the bacterial chromosome and reenters the cytoplasm as a free F particle, but in doing so has incorporated a part of the bacterial chromosome.

A major use of conjugation is in gene mapping. Since the transfer of the chromosome is polar (i.e., each gene is transferred in sequential order) and the mating process can be disrupted, various genes can be mapped with respect to one another through conjugation. In fact, most *E. coli* gene maps list the genes in order, with units referred to as minutes. For example, if gene A is our standard reference, and gene B is always transferred 5 minutes after gene A, then the *E. coli* map lists gene B 5 minutes from gene A. If gene C is always 10 minutes after gene B, then its position is 15 minutes (B is 5 minutes from A and C is 10 minutes from B, therefore C is 15 minutes from our reference A).

Transformation

Transformation is the uptake of DNA molecules, such as plasmids, from the surrounding medium by a bacterial cell. If the transforming DNA is a plasmid, the process is usually called transformation. If the DNA molecule is a bacterial virus (bacteriophage)

DNA, the process is sometimes referred to as transfection, but that term is losing its popularity in bacterial genetics. Instead, transfection is more commonly used to denote the uptake of DNA (plasmid or virus) by a eukaryotic cell. The uptake of phage DNA by a bacterial cell is then called transformation. In either case, the transforming DNA is probably the major means of gene exchange.

The overall process of transformation can be divided into several common steps: 1) the cells develop a state of "competence" (i.e., the ability to take up DNA); 2) the DNA binds to the cell; 3) the DNA is taken up by the cell; 4) a preintegration complex forms; and 5) the DNA is integrated into the host chromosome.

Transformation can occur in nature in both gram-positive and gram-negative bacteria, but with slightly different procedures. In addition, certain bacterial cells as well as eukaryotic yeast cells can be transformed in the laboratory by artificial means. However, laboratory transformation differs significantly from the naturally occurring process. In comparing the process of transformation in various organisms, it is convenient to do so with respect to the various common steps.

Transformation in Gram-Positive Bacteria

1. Competence development. In the laboratory, development of competence has been shown as the ability of bacteria to take up DNA in a DNAse-resistant form. DNA cannot be removed from the bacteria by simple washing procedures. Competence is an induced state, and most bacteria become competent only under special conditions of growth. For example, when *Streptococcus* is grown in an acceptable medium, the culture develops competence at a critical cell density of 10^8 or 10^9 cells per ml.

The development of competence is achieved by the cellular secretion of a small protein called a competence factor. This protein has a molecular weight of 5,000 to 10,000 daltons and is continually released from growing cells. Its action within the bacterial cell is similar to a hormone in that it induces high levels of competence when given to noncompetent cells. The proposed mechanism for the development of competence is the binding of the competence factor to cell surface receptors, which in turn render the cell competent. Another 68,000-dalton protein has been isolated that has been shown to be a competence factor–inhibiting protein, thereby inactivating the competence factor. In liquid cultures, only a small percentage (10% to 20%) of cells ever develop competence.

2. DNA binding. The second step in transformation is the binding of the DNA molecules to the cell. This binding can be either reversible or irreversible. The bound DNA is in a double-stranded state and contains nicks (breaks in one strand) that are spaced about 6,000 basepairs apart. A competent pneumococcal cell contains 30 to 80 receptor sites at which the DNA can bind. A binding factor protein has been isolated, but its activity has yet to be characterized.

3. **DNA uptake.** The uptake of DNA from the medium, also called absorption, is defined as the conversion of DNA into a DNAse-resistant and nonelutable form. DNA uptake has an absolute requirement for Ca^{2+} in pneumococcal cells and Mg^{2+} in *B. subtilis* cells. Also, it requires an endonuclease (endonuclease I), which cleaves the DNA opposite nicks. One of the major factors in the uptake of DNA is that one of the two strands is degraded and therefore only a single-stranded molecule is taken up. Which strand is degraded and which strand is taken up is a purely random process.

4. **Eclipse complex.** When single-stranded DNA is isolated from a transforming cell, this DNA no longer contains transforming activity and is said to be in eclipse. However, transforming activity can be restored following its conversion to a double-stranded form by integrating into the chromosome. The formation of an eclipse complex is an active process and is characterized by DNA–protein interactions.

Several roles have been proposed for the formation of an eclipse complex. One proposal is that the degree of free energy associated with the complex formation could promote the transfer of DNA into the cell. Another proposed role is that this complex protects the DNA from nucleases during the process of transfer into the cell and integration. A third proposed role is that the eclipse complex promotes integration by stabilizing the nucleotides.

5. **Integration.** The mechanism of integration is a nonselective recombinational event that involves a double-stranded chromosome and a single-stranded donor DNA. It begins with the formation of a heteroduplex formation, and more than one donor DNA can be integrated at a time. Often the size of the integrated DNA is as large as 10,000 basepairs.

6. **Correction of mismatched bases.** Following integration, mismatched bases are repaired. Experimental evidence suggests that cells have some mechanism for recognizing donor and recipient strands. Often the recipient strand is corrected, as opposed to the donor strand. This in turn can lead to a change in the genotype of the organism. When one of two linked markers is corrected, the other marker is also corrected, which suggests that the correction process is probably a "sweeping" mechanism.

Transformation of Gram-Negative Bacteria

1. **Development of competence.** Competence development in gram-negative organisms is internally regulated. There are no known competence factors, and the process varies considerably between species. For example, *Haemophilus* develops competence when cell division is blocked under conditions that allow protein synthesis to continue. In *Neisseria gonorrhoeae,* only piliated cells can become competent.

2. **DNA binding and uptake.** The features of DNA binding and uptake in gram-negative bacteria differ considerably from those in gram-positive organisms. Probably the most striking difference is that gram-negative organisms take up double-stranded DNA whereas gram-positive organisms take up single-stranded DNA. Also, a specific DNA sequence (AAGTGCGGTCA) is associated with the gram-negative chromosome which the cell wall seems to recognize in order to take up the DNA from the medium. In *Haemophilus,* these DNA sequences occur once every 4,000 basepairs along the chromosome. In conjunction, gram-negative organisms have a high specificity for transforming only with homologous DNA. Foreign DNAs can be bound to the cell but are absorbed poorly and cannot compete with homologous DNA for uptake.

Other factors have been found to be important for DNA uptake in gram-negative organisms. It has been shown to require metabolism and to be both pH and temperature dependent. Ca^{2+}, Na^+, and/or K^+ ions have an effect on the uptake of DNA in gram-negative bacteria.

3. **Fate of transforming DNA.** DNA that is taken up from the medium is double-stranded, yet is integrated as a single-stranded molecule. Therefore, at some time, the DNA is converted to single-stranded molecules. Genetic studies have shown that *Haemophilus* has three integration sites on its chromosome.

Once the DNA is taken into the cell, it is not attacked by nucleases. This protection from nucleases is achieved by the formation of a protein–DNA complex which may be similar to the eclipse complex found in gram-positive bacteria. However, no eclipse activity is associated with transforming DNA in gram-negative bacteria as is found with gram-positive bacteria. The protection against nucleases may also be achieved by the compartmentalization of DNA into vesicle-like cell surface structures.

Transformation Involving Viral or Plasmid DNA. Transformation of cells with viral or plasmid DNA can occur both in nature and in the laboratory. In nature, transformation with viral or plasmid DNAs is very inefficient. In gram-positive cells, this inefficiency is probably due to the need to convert the DNA from double- to single-stranded molecules before transformation. In gram-negative bacteria, this inefficiency is probably due to the compartmentalization of the transforming DNA within the cell, which prohibits it from being replicated, or to the need for specific recognition sequences. In general, naturally occurring transformation of viral and plasmid DNAs is on the order of 1,000 to 10,000-fold less than chromosomal DNA.

In the laboratory, cells can be transformed by artificial means. Artificial transformation is defined as the introduction of DNA into the cell without the use of the highly evolved naturally occurring transformation process. Artificial transformation is generally achieved by treating the bacterial cells with $CaCl_2$. Very little is known about the mechanisms involved. However, it is known that the DNA uptake is nonselective (i.e., any DNA will be taken up) and that it is not converted to single-stranded molecules. The efficiency of artificial transformation is much greater than naturally occurring transformation.

The artificial transformation of bacteria with plasmid DNA is the basis for recombinant DNA technology. In recombinant DNA technology (gene cloning), bacterial plasmids are used as vectors or carriers for introducing other DNA molecules (such as human genes) into bacterial cells. The process involves the linearization of the plasmid by a single cleavage (cut) of the circular plasmid DNA and then attaching a "foreign" DNA to the ends of the plasmid. The "hybrid" DNA is then recircularized and used to transform bacterial cells. The transformed cells contain both the plasmid and the foreign DNA sequences. These "hybrid" plasmids replicate and produce large quantities of the "hybrid" DNA sequences. When the genes of the hybrid DNA are expressed by the bacteria containing them, the products that they code for may be produced in great quantity.

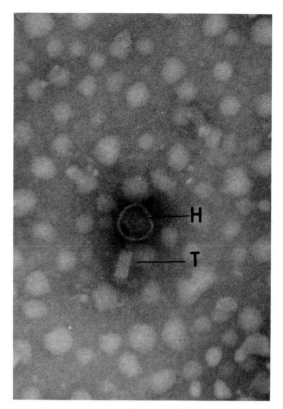

Figure 4.1: An electron micrograph of a bacteriophage against *Actinobacillus actinomycetemcomitans,* a well-known periodontal pathogen associated with juvenile periodontitis. Note the head (*H*), tail (*T*), and contractile fibers. The preparation was stained negative with 1% phosphotungstic acid. (Courtesy of Dr. R. H. Stevens and Dr. Chern Lai, University of Pennsylvania.)

Transduction

Transduction is the transfer of DNA from one bacterial cell to another by means of a bacterial virus (bacteriophage or phage) (Fig. 4.1). Transduction in which any chromosomal marker can be transferred is termed generalized transduction. If only certain genes can be transferred by a phage, the process is called restricted transduction. The ability of a phage to mediate transduction of one or the other type depends on the relationship of the phage to host DNA.

Host-Bacteriophage Relationships. Bacteriophages infect by attaching to bacterial cells into which they inject their DNA. If the phage is virulent, it goes through a vegetative cycle in which it replicates to produce new virus particles which are released by lysis of the host cell. A temperate phage, on the other hand, may follow alternate pathways after infection. It may go through a lytic cycle, or a repressor may be produced that prevents the lytic cycle. In the latter instance, phage DNA enters into a nonvirulent relationship with the host cell and is incorporated into the host chromosome. Such a relationship is called lysogeny, or the lysogenic state, and the phage DNA in this state is called prophage. With lysogeny the host cell acquires new properties. First, it is immune to infection by a homologous phage. Second, any genetic characteristics accompanying the phage DNA are imparted to the cell and may be expressed.

During assembly of phage particles in a host cell prior to release by lysis, host DNA may be packaged into the phage coat, forming a generalized transducing particle. The packaging is random with regard to which host DNA is packaged; it occurs at a low frequency, and the amount of DNA is equivalent to the size of the genome normally carried by the phage. In generalized transduction the transducing particles contain no detectable phage DNA, but when a generalized transducing phage infects a new host, the bacterial DNA it is carrying is transferred to the new host. On the other hand, production of phages for restricted transduction depends on formation of the lysogenic state. The integration of phage DNA is not irreversible, but it can be induced to come out of the host chromosome and initiate a lytic cycle. Induction is caused by UV light, changes in environment, or sometimes occurs "spontaneously." If this occurs and if the prophage carries a portion of host DNA with it, there may be production of specialized transducing particles. However, the amount of host DNA is limited since the total amount of DNA in a phage is limited. The reason that specialized transducing particles carry only specific genes is that the phage DNA integrates into a host at a very few specific sites, and thus the host genes it can take with it are only those adjacent to it. In this process a portion of the phage DNA is excluded, the amount depending on how much host DNA is present (analogous to F duction).

Abortive Transduction and Lysogenic Conversion. In many instances the exogenote pairs with the endogenote and recombination occurs, producing a recombinant-type organism. In other instances the exogenote may persist and function but not replicate so that when cell division occurs only one cell in the population contains the exogenote. In some cases a given suspension of phage will produce ten times more abortive transductions than the normal ones. Since abortive transduction results when recombination does not occur between the exogenote and the endogenote, it follows that procedures that stimulate recombination (e.g., exposure to UV light) will convert abortive transductions to normal transductions.

Certain properties of bacterial cells are controlled solely by phage genes and are manifested in lysogenic or phage-infected cells. For example, *Corynebacterium diphtheriae* produces toxin only if it is infected with a particular strain of phage (beta); phage-free cells do not produce toxin. This process in which a new property is acquired as the result of phage infection is lysogenic conversion. Several other examples of lysogenic conversion are well known: 1) antigenic changes in the cell surface of *Salmonella* strains, 2) toxin formation by major bacterial pathogens (*Streptococcus pyogenes* and its erythrogenic toxin, leukocidin of *Staphylococcus aureus* and the highly potent toxin of *Clostridium botulinum*), and 3) some virulence-associated properties of *Vibrio cholerae* (El tor biotype). In all of these cases a lysogenic phage is necessary for the expression of a property that is never expressed in the absence of phage infections.

Plasmids and Episomes

One of the primary differences between eukaryotes and prokaryotes is the absence in prokaryotes of membrane-bound organelles containing DNA (mitochondria, chloroplasts). The autonomously replicating centers were once thought to be analogous in many respects to the bacterial chromosome. With the discovery of the F factor it became clear that some bacteria do occasionally harbor extrachromosomal packets of DNA on a temporary basis. Unlike mitochondria and chloroplasts, these extranuclear bacterial elements 1) do not have membrane coverings, 2) lack the machinery for transcription and translation or organellar protein synthesis, and 3) are not essential to life. Two types of extrachromosomal DNA are known for bacteria: plasmids and episomes. Plasmids are autonomous genetic elements not capable of integration into the chromosome, while episomes can exist autonomously or can be integrated into the chromosome. Some elements are plasmids in one species and episomes in others (F′ is an episome in *E. coli* but a plasmid in *Proteus mirabilis,* indicating that episomes are host specific). Both may be eliminated from the cell by treatment wth various ("curing") agents, including acridine dyes, UV light, and heat. This criterion of elimination is further evidence that plasmids and episomes are dispensable, autonomous elements not coding for essential gene functions.

Extrachromosomal genetic elements have been divided into large and small factors. Large factors, composed of 100 to 200 genes, include F (fertility) factor, antibiotic resistance (R) factors, and a few bacteriocinogens. Small factors (only about 15 genes) include most bacteriocinogens and a number of cryptic plasmids (plasmids with no known gene function). Both kinds of factors can be recognized by standard genetic and physical techniques. Genetically, a plasmid is revealed if a gene function(s) can be shown *not* to be linked to the chromosome with respect to autonomous replication. The autonomous replication of such an extranuclear element is assumed if the factor is transferred at conjugation independent of the chromosome or by "curing" experiments with acridine dyes, in which case the plasmid function is irreversibly eliminated. Physical detection of plasmids is based on differences in the physicochemical properties of plasmid and chromosomal DNAs:

1. Plasmid DNAs are often less dense and show up as "satellite bands" on ultracentrifugation in a density gradient.
2. If the densities are similar, plasmid DNA can be differentiated from chromosomal DNA by the intercalation of various acridine dyes that increase the density of plasmid DNA but not chromosomal DNA. This method (dye–buoyant density) is based on the fact that plasmid DNA is a supercoiled, closed, circular molecule and much more likely to take up the dye molecules than the linear fragments of chromosomal DNA.

Replication of large factors is usually synchronous with replication of the bacterial chromosome. Mutations that prevent replication of the bacterial chromosome may also prevent replication of large plasmids. Replication of small plasmids is not synchronous with replication of the bacterial chromosome, and the replication rate of these small plasmids may differ widely from the replication rate of the chromosome under certain conditions, giving rise to numerous copies of the plasmid within a single cell. Many of the large plasmids are transmissible to other cells by formation of their own conjugation apparatus, whereas the small plasmids do not usually code for enough proteins to ensure self-replication and self-transfer.

Several cryptic plasmids have been detected among bacteria associated with oral disease. Particular attention has been directed toward *Streptococcus mutans* and other lactic acid bacteria with regard to the acquisition of pathogenic potential as a result of a plasmid-mediated gene transfer. A small plasmid from *S. mutans* LM7 was recently cloned in *E. coli* cells and shown to be associated with the production of a protein of unknown function, but no association with cariogenicity was demonstrated. Attempts to demonstrate a positive correlation between glycogen formation and the small plasmids in *Lactobacillus casei* were also unsuccessful. Conjugal transfer of a plasmid from a streptococcus (group F) to strains of *L. casei* has recently been demonstrated, although the biological significance of this transfer (antibiotic resistance) in the context of oral health is not clear. The original idea behind many of these investigations was to determine the extent to which genetic transfer between oral bacteria could explain the observed variations of clinical isolates. Since most of the plasmids are cryptic, the original question remains unanswered. Many possibilities seem quite reasonable in view of the known role of plasmids as critical determinants of pathogenicity in other infectious diseases, such as enterotoxin production in pathogenic strains of *E. coli,* pilus formation and adherence of the gonococcus, sucrose fermentation, antibiotic resistance, and bacteriocin formation.

Antibiotic Resistance

Resistance Involving Extrachromosomal Factors

One of the most important clinical implications of gene transfer is the ability of plasmids to transfer resistance to a number of antibiotics and chemicals in mixed populations of bacteria. Thus, a single bacterium can develop resistance to several antibiotics as a result of one plasmid transfer and, subsequently, can transfer this multiple resistance to yet another bacterium, often of another genus or species. This was shown when multiply resistant strains of *Shigella* were mixed with antibiotic-sensitive strains of *E. coli:* the multiple resistance was transferred to the sensitive organisms. The plasmids responsible for this type of multiple resistance to antibiotics and other antibacterial agents are termed R factors. The R factor consists of two parts: one part, the resistance transfer factor (RTF), carries the genes for replication and the conjugative transmission of the plasmid; the other part consists of one or more sequentially linked resistance determinants (genes for enzymes that inactivate or otherwise modify the antibiotics in question). These two components may exist as separate, autonomously replicating elements, in which case the resistance determinants appear to be incapable of undergoing transfer unless mobilized by RTF. In many respects R factors are analogous to the F factor in that both code for surface pili and other factors associated with their conjugative transmission—e.g., R and F pili—and both may exist as autonomously replicating units in the cytoplasm or may be integrated into the chromosome, i.e., they are in the strict sense episomes, although they are usually designated as plasmids.

Resistance Involving Chromosomal Mutation

It is to be remembered that resistance due to R factors and plasmids is different from resistance arising from spontaneous chromosomal mutations. First, there are enormous differences in the occurrence of chromosomal mutations responsible for drug resistance as compared to the en bloc conjugative transfer of resistance genes in plasmids. The likelihood of simultaneous chromosomal mutations to resistance to four or five antibiotics is infinitesimally small since the probability is the algebraic sum of the mutation frequencies for the universal drug. As an example:

Mutation rate to antibiotic X is 10^{-5}

Mutation rate to antibiotic Y is 10^{-6}

Mutation rate to antibiotic Z is 10^{-7}

Therefore, the likelihood of a simultaneous mutation to resistance to X, Y, and Z is 10^{-18}.

Furthermore, chromosomal mutations obviously do not require conjugation or some other means of genetic transfer. There are also differences in the mechanisms of resistance associated with R factors as opposed to chromosomal mutations. Plasmid genes encode enzymes that chemically inactivate the antibacterial agent (e.g., chloramphenicol transacetylase) whereas chromosomal resistance genes usually modify the cellular target of the drug (cell wall, ribosome).

Penicillinase Plasmids

Many bacteria produce a β-lactamase (a penicillinase) that hydrolyzes the β-lactam ring of the penicillin molecule, resulting in high levels of resistance to penicillin. The gene for this enzyme along with others is located on a plasmid and is responsible for almost all cases of penicillin resistance in clinical isolates. The penicillinase plasmid that has been studied most intensively is the one found in *Staphylococcus aureus,* an important human pathogen that causes skin and wound infections. Unlike the enterobacteria, *S. aureus* is unable to conjugate and its plasmids are transferred by transduction. There is considerable epidemiological evidence in human studies that *S. aureus* transduction occurs naturally and may be responsible for the widespread resistance so frequently observed in clinical isolates of this organism. Certainly, lysogeny is well documented in clinical isolates of staphylococci.

Bacteriocins

Many bacteria produce low molecular weight, heat-stable bactericidal proteins called bacteriocins. The genetic determinants for bacteriocins are carried on plasmids (bacteriocinogens) but may, under certain circumstances, be integrated into the bacterial chromosome. These proteins are very toxic at low doses. Their actions are very specific but differ among the various types of bacteriocins. They may, for example, halt nucleic acid synthesis, cause cell lysis, or inhibit respiration. The colicins are the most widely studied bacteriocins. One inhibits ATP formation in *E. coli,* another causes breaks in DNA. *Streptococcus mutans* strains produce bacteriocins (mutacins) that have proved useful in grouping or classifying strains of *S. mutans* and in epidemiological studies. Their possible role in the natural environment is not known, but the susceptibility of bacteriocins to proteolytic enzymes could compromise their activity in a salivary milieu.

ADDITIONAL READING

Danner, D. B., Deich, R. A., Sisco, K. L., and Smith, H. O. 1980. An Eleven-basepair Sequence Determines the Specificity of DNA Uptake in *Haemophilus Transformation.* Gene, **11,** 311.

Donowitz, G. R., and Mandell, G. L. 1988. Beta-Lactam Antibiotics. N Engl J Med, **318,** 419.

Elwell, L. P., and Shipley, P. L. 1980. Plasmid-mediated Factors Associated with Virulence of Bacteria to Animals. Annu Rev Microbiol, **34,** 465.

Gots, J. S., and Benson, C. E. 1974. Biochemical Genetics of Bacteria. Annu Rev Genet, **8,** 77.

Graves, J. F., Biswas, G. D., and Sparling, P. F. 1982. Sequence-Specific DNA Uptake in Transformation of *Neisseria gonorrhoeae.* J Bacteriol, **152,** 1071.

Hamada, S., and Slade, H. D. 1980. Biology, Immunology and Cariogenicity of *Streptococcus mutans.* Microbiol Rev, **44,** 331.

Hayes, W. 1968. *The Genetics of Bacteria and Their Viruses,* Ed. 2. Blackwell, Oxford, England.

Kelstrup, J., Richmond, S., West, C., and Gibbons, R. J. 1971. Fingerprinting Human Oral Streptococci by Bacteriocin Production and Sensitivity. Arch Oral Biol, **15,** 1109.

Riley, M., and Anilonis, A. 1978. Evolution of the Bacterial Genome. Annu Rev Microbiol, **35,** 519.

Stiles, H. M., Lowsche, W. J., and O'Brien, T. C. (Eds.). 1976. Microbial Aspects of Dental Caries; Vol. III. Biochemical and Genetic Determinants of Virulence. Microbiol Abstr Spec Suppl.

Watson, J. D. 1987. *Molecular Biology of the Gene,* Ed. 4. W. A. Benjamin, Inc., Menlo Park, Calif.

5

Metabolism of Bacteria

John T. Wilson

Bacterial growth and maintenance are the result of an extraordinary series of chemical and physical reactions that occur within the cell. Two general groups of reactions may be identified: 1) synthesis of cellular constituents (*anabolism*), which requires energy, and 2) the opposite process of *catabolism* (decomposition or breakdown) of cellular components, which is accompanied by the release of energy and the accumulation of breakdown products. Anabolic reactions are essentially similar in all cells, eukaryotic as well as prokaryotic—i.e., the synthesis of proteins, nucleic acids, lipids, and polysaccharides is governed by a few reactions common to all biological systems. Indeed, the concept of unity in biochemistry is derived from studies based on bacterial metabolism. Catabolic reactions in bacteria, while sharing a number of biochemical pathways with reactions in other cell systems, exhibit an extraordinary diversity as well. Thus, unity amid diversity is one of the hallmarks of bacterial metabolism and is fundamental to the taxonomy, classification, and physiology of bacteria. The catabolic mechanisms of bacteria range from the oxidation of inorganic compounds such as sulfides, ferrous salts, or hydrogen to the oxidation of carbohydrates, hydrocarbons, and many other compounds for energy sources. This metabolic versatility is especially important in the human oral cavity since variations in diet and other environmentally induced changes provide an enormous number of metabolizable substrates and possibilities for bacterial action.

This chapter will be concerned with some of the catabolic reactions of bacteria, with an emphasis on the metabolism of oral bacteria. It does not purport to be a detailed analysis or even a survey of bacterial metabolism. A more comprehensive and detailed coverage can be found in the supplemental readings listed at the end of this chapter.

Energy Liberation and Storage

The essential task of metabolism is to carry out thermodynamically possible chemical reactions that do not occur directly under the conditions of life, notably at neutrality and at temperatures from 10 to 45°C, or for which no direct path is known. We know, for example, that glucose can be oxidized directly to carbon dioxide and water:

$$C_6H_{12}O_2 + 6O_2 \rightarrow 6CO_2 + 6H_2O.$$
$$(\Delta G = 688,000 \text{ calories*})$$

This reaction occurs only at temperatures destructive to life, and the available chemical energy escapes as heat. Consider also the reactions by which glucose is converted to lactic acid:

$$C_6H_{12}O_6 \rightarrow 2CH_3\text{—CHOH—COOH.}$$
$$(\Delta G = 55,000 \text{ calories*})$$

However, no way is known to accomplish this conversion directly. Such a conversion is possible in many biological systems except that it involves a series of intermediate reactions, each of which entails only a modest exchange of energy. The process (called glycolysis) entails at least 11 steps, some receiving energy, others liberating energy. The free energy available from this conversion still totals − 55,000 calories. Much of this energy is captured and stored by the cell in the form of high-energy phosphate bonds of adenosine triphosphate (ATP).

There are three methods by which the energy released as a result of catabolic reactions can be trapped as ATP: 1) substrate level phosphorylation, 2) oxidative phosphorylation, and 3) the most complex of all, photosynthesis.

Substrate Level Phosphorylation

Substrate level phosphorylation is a term used to describe the process in which the energy released through oxidation is localized in a high-energy phosphate bond of the oxidized substrate. In this process organic compounds serve as both electron donors (being oxidized) and electron acceptors (becoming reduced). For example:

$$\text{3-Phosphoglyceraldehyde} + P_i \xrightarrow{\text{NAD \quad NADH}} \text{1,3-Diphosphoglyceric acid.}$$

*The symbol ΔG denotes the so-called free energy change, i.e., the energy available for work from the reaction of one gram molecule of reactant. A negative sign means that the starting materials release free energy and that the reaction should theoretically proceed spontaneously. A positive sign means that the reaction would go in the direction indicated only if energy were supplied. The ΔG values under physiological conditions have not been determined exactly. Revision of the values used here, however, would not change the outcome of the reactions described.

The best-known examples of substrate level phosphorylations occur in the fermentations. In fermentations the substrate (usually a carbohydrate) gives rise to a mixture of end products, some of which are more oxidized and some of which are more reduced—i.e., there is a balance in the oxidation and reduction levels of the products. Other fermentable compounds include organic acids, amino acids, purines, and pyrimidines. All fermentations occur under anaerobic conditions and result in the incomplete oxidation of the substrate. Pasteur referred to fermentation as *la vie sans l'air* and recognized its importance in the metabolism of many bacteria. Many bacteria are strict anaerobes (see Chap. 6 for a discussion of the mechanisms of strict anaerobiosis); others are facultative anaerobes and are able to grow in the presence or absence of air. Many of these facultative organisms in the presence of air are able to convert their mode of ATP generation to respiration (see below). However, one group of very important oral bacteria (the lactic acid bacteria—streptococci and lactobacilli) are exceptions since they continue to ferment even in the presence of air. The inefficiency of this method of energy generation is in sharp contrast to other ATP generative processes.

Oxidative Phosphorylation (Electron Transport)

In this process it is possible to get complete oxidation of a substrate with a much greater release of energy for growth and maintenance of the cells. Unlike fermentation and substrate level phosphorylation, the final electron acceptor is oxygen and the process is often referred to as respiration. Electrons are passed sequentially from one electron carrier to the next in an electron transport chain:

$$\text{Organic substrate} \rightarrow \text{NAD} \rightarrow \text{Flavoprotein} \xrightarrow{\text{quinone}} \text{Cytochrome b, c, a} \rightarrow O_2.$$

Redox potential: 0.32 V
$$0.20 \rightarrow\!\!\!\rightarrow + 0.01 \rightarrow 0.022 + 0.81.$$

The mechanism of ATP generation by the transport of electrons is not completely clear but the current explanation that has received the greatest amount of support is called the chemiosmotic hypothesis. This explanation suggests that the electron transport system is oriented in the cell membrane in such a way as to cause the outward flow of protons which cannot reenter the membrane except at a specific membrane site where ATP areas are found. As a consequence, a proton gradient (ΔpH) is created across the membrane. This gradient derives the following reaction, resulting in the generation of ATP:

Table 5.1: Fermentation Versus Respiration as an Energy Source

	Fermentation	Respiration
Electron donor	Organic compound	Organic compound
Final electron acceptor	Organic compound	Oxygen
Energy liberation from 1 mole of glucose	55 kcal	688 kcal
Method of ATP generation	Substrate phosphorylation	Electron transport (oxidative phosphorylation)
Oxygen requirement	Oxygen absent	Oxygen required

$$ADP + P_i + H^+ \xrightarrow{ATPase} ATP + H_2O.$$

In any event, the breakdown of one mole of glucose by this respiratory mechanism (i.e., oxidative phosphorylation involving electron transport) yields about 12 times more energy than the fermentative (anaerobic) breakdown to organic end products such as lactic acid. Some of the comparative differences between fermentation and respiration are shown in Table 5.1.

Photosynthesis

Photosynthesis, the third method of ATP generation, uses light as the energy source. This process is rarely if ever found in bacteria of medical importance but it is critically important in a context of ecology. Many photosynthetic bacteria occupy a wide range of habitats and are able to fix nitrogen and regulate the supply of dissolved oxygen in lakes where there is a high amount of nitrate and phosphate. The photosynthetic process is not unlike oxidative phosphorylation since ATP is once again formed by the passage of electrons through special electron transport chains. This photophosphorylative process begins when light is absorbed by a chlorophyll molecule. The excited chlorophyll molecule emits an electron that is accepted by an iron-containing electron acceptor called ferredoxin and then is passed through a series of cytochrome pigments where 2 moles of ATP are formed from ADP for each pair of electrons passed.

Overview

Cells are not capable of utilizing energy liberated in reactions outside themselves. Energy must be made available by a catabolic reaction within the cell and retained in one of its products, which is the energy-transferring link to the next reaction in the metabolic chain. In most cases only a fraction of the energy produced is captured and the rest is lost as heat. In a catabolic process, substrate is converted into products of lower energy content and the energy released is captured in various compounds. It can then be used to "prime" additional catabolic reactions and drive synthetic functions. Since carbohydrates occupy an important position in metabolism, the various relationships are best summarized by a consideration of its utilization.

In a context of oral ecology, however, it is important to point out that many of the organisms found in the human gingival crevice (*Bacteroides gingivalis, Vibrio* species, and other gram-negative anaerobes) are asaccharolytic and are unable to utilize carbohydrates, including any of the common dietary sugars (sucrose, fructose, maltose, or glucose). These organisms obtain their energy from other sources, e.g., amino acid fermentations, hydrogen, etc. Thus, while the centrality of carbohydrate metabolism is well established for all of the cariogenic lactic acid bacteria, carbohydrates are much less important for many other oral microorganisms.

Carbohydrate Metabolism

The discussion of carbohydrate metabolism will be divided into six parts, the first five related to carbohydrate breakdown, the sixth part a discussion of the carbohydrate metabolism of dental plaque and oral bacteria. Carbohydrate utilization may occur in the following six phases: 1) cleavage of hexoses and pentoses into three-carbon and two-carbon compounds, principally pyruvate or lactate and acetate or ethanol (plus carbon dioxide); 2) cleavage of pyruvate to carbon dioxide and a two-carbon fragment ("active acetyl") and conversion of other two-carbon compounds to "active acetyl"; 3) oxidation of the acetyl residue to carbon dioxide and water via the tricarboxylic acid cycle; 4) transfer of hydrogen from NADH and NADPH (formed in the preceding reactions) to oxygen via the cytochrome system; 5) utilization and synthesis of polysaccharides; and 6) carbohydrate metabolism of dental plaque. The various reactions in carbohydrate metabolism are presented from the viewpoint of dissimilation, but since many of

Table 5.2: Lactic Fermentation of Glucose (Embden–Meyerhof Pathway)

Glucose	
+ ATP $\quad$ Hexokinase, Mg^{++}	High energy phosphate transfer, practically irreversible
Glucose 6-phosphate + ADP	
$\quad$ Phosphohexose isomerase	Isomerization
Fructose 6-phosphate	
+ ATP $\quad$ Phosphofructokinase	High energy phosphate transfer, practically irreversible
Fructose 1,6-diphosphate + ADP	
$\quad$ Aldolase	Reversible aldol condensation
Glyceraldehyde-3-phosphate + dihydroxyacetone	
$\qquad\qquad$ phosphate	
+ 2 NAD$^+$ $\quad$ Triosephosphate isomerase	Isomerization
+ 2 H$_3$PO$_4$ $\quad$ Triosephosphate dehydrogenase	Dehydrogenation + phosphorylation → high energy phosphate; mechanism obscure
Two 1,3-diphosphoglycerate + 2 NADH	
+ 2 ADP $\quad$ Phosphoglycerate kinase	High energy phosphate transfer regenerates ATP
Two 3-phosphoglycerate + 2 ATP	
$\quad$ Phosphoglyceromutase	Phosphate transfer
Two 2-phosphoglycerate	
$\quad$ Enolase, Mg^{++}	Dehydration and creation of high energy phosphate
Two phospho-enol-pyruvate + H$_2$O	
+ 2 ADP $\quad$ Pyruvate kinase	High energy phosphate transfer regenerates ATP
Two pyruvate + 2 ATP	
+ 2 NADH $\quad$ Lactic dehydrogenase	Regeneration of NAD$^+$
Two lactate + 2 NAD$^+$	

Glucose + 2 phosphate + 2 ADP →
$\qquad\qquad$ 2 lactate + 2 H$^+$ + 2 ATP $\qquad$ Net reaction. ΔG = −34,000 calories

the intermediate steps are reversible, they may serve as well for the synthesis of carbohydrates. Many of the intermediate compounds may be diverted by interconnecting reactions into amino acid, nucleic acid, and fatty acid metabolism.

Embden–Meyerhof Pathway (Glycolysis)

The primary cleavage of sugars is best exemplified by the fermentation of glucose to lactic acid via the classic Embden-Meyerhof pathway. A condensed summary of the essential stages of this fermentation is shown in Table 5.2. Other hexoses, such as fructose, galactose, and mannose, enter this pathway at the hexose monophosphate stage through phosphorylations and, where necessary, isomerizations.

The conversion of the glucose molecule to two lactates in the Embden–Meyerhof pathway releases 55,000 calories of free energy, of which about 40% (21,000 calories) is captured in the high-energy phosphate groups of two ATPs, where it is available for cellular processes that require energy. When compared to the complete oxidation of glucose, which captures about two thirds of 688,000 calories of free energy, lactic acid fermentation is clearly not an efficient means of obtaining cellular energy. Never-

theless, homofermentative lactobacilli (homolactic bacteria) and streptococci rely almost entirely on lactate fermentation, even in the presence of oxygen.

Pentose Phosphate Pathway (Phosphogluconate; Hexose Monophosphate Shunt)

Heterofermentative organisms (heterolactic bacteria) proceed by an alternative route, sometimes called the pentose phosphate pathway, which yields equal molar quantities of lactate, ethanol, and CO$_2$ (Fig. 5.1).

The pentose–phosphate pathway for the primary splitting of hexoses via five-carbon compounds is used in part by some organisms, and wholly by others that lack aldolase. This process may be summarized as follows: glucose-6-phosphate is partially dehydrogenated via NADP to form 6-phosphogluconate, which is further dehydrogenated via NADP to keto-6-phosphogluconate, which is decarboxylated to form a ketopentose, ribulose-5-phosphate. The latter is the connecting link to the metabolism of pentoses, since it is reversibly isomerized enzymatically to ribose-5-phosphate, a common denominator in pentose dissimilation. This reaction provides pentose phosphate for nucleic acid synthesis. In dissimilation, pentose

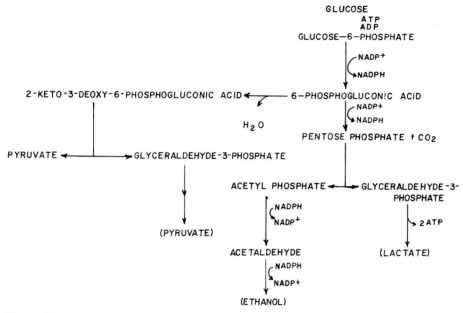

Figure 5.1: Entner-Doudoroff pathway.

phosphate is split into glyceraldehyde-3-phosphate, which follows the path to lactate indicated in Table 5.2, and a two-carbon fragment, "active glycolaldehyde," which accepts hydrogen from NADPH to form ethanol, or is rearranged to form acetate.

Entner–Doudoroff Pathway

A third method of bacterial dissimilation of glucose to pyruvate is known as the Entner–Doudoroff pathway. This pathway is found in certain groups of prokaryotic cells (notably the pseudomonads) and is unlike the Embden–Meyerhof and pentose phosphate routes, which are found in both eukaryotes and prokaryotes. Glucose-6-phosphate is the first intermediate in this pathway (see Fig. 5.1) and is oxidized to 6-phosphogluconic acid. The unique or "signature" intermediate in the pathway is 2-keto-3-deoxy-6-phosphogluconic acid (KDPG), which is formed by the dehydration of the 6-P-gluconic acid. KDPG is cleaved to 1 mole of pyruvate and 1 mole of glyceraldehyde-3-phosphate, which is subsequently metabolized via glycolysis to a second mole of pyruvate. The net yield of 1 mole of glucose through this pathway is 1 mole of ATP and 2 moles of NADH.

Further Metabolism of Pyruvate and Two-Carbon Fragments

The focal reaction of the next stage in biological oxidation is the formation of "active acetyl" directly from two-carbon fragments or from pyruvate by ox-

idative decarboxylation. Acetyl-CoA is the normal end product of this phase of the metabolism of pyruvate and two-carbon fragments. The various reactions coupled to these transformations yield three high-energy phosphates per molecule of pyruvate.

Depending on available cellular enzymes, acetyl is also converted to compounds such as acetate, ethanol, and butanol, either by transfer from acetyl-CoA, acetyl lipoate, or a presumed acetaldehydecarboxylase intermediate. Acetyl is a connecting link to fatty acid metabolism. Pyruvate is converted by other mechanisms to propionate, isopropanol, or acetone; or to lactate, butanediol, and formate. Some bacteria convert formate by hydrogenlyase to carbon dioxide and hydrogen. The direct path from pyruvate, however, leads to the oxidation of acetyl via the "tricarboxylic acid cycle." Pyruvate, through the reversible condensation of its methyl group with carbon dioxide, forms oxalacetate ($COOH$-CH_2-CO-$COOH$), a key compound that initiates the cycle.

Tricarboxylic Acid Cycle

Active acetyl, in the form of acetyl-CoA, is condensed through its methyl group with the carbonyl group of oxalacetate to form citrate. This initiates a remarkable series of reactions that convert acetyl into carbon dioxide and reduced hydrogen acceptors, and regenerate oxalacetate. The essential stages of the cycle are shown in Table 5.3. Because they are incompletely understood, the energy-capturing reactions are omitted. A part of this capture occurs during the

---

Table 5.3: Tricarboxylic Acid Cycle

Oxalacetate + acetyl-S-CoA		
+ H_2O ⇅ Condensing enzyme	$C_4 + C_2$ condensation → tricarboxylic acid	
Citrate + CoA-SH		
⇅ Aconitase	Dehydration to unsaturated acid	
cis-Aconitate + H_2O		
+ H_2O ⇅ Aconitase	Rehydration to citrate isomer	
Isocitrate		
+ NADP$^+$ ⏸ Isocitric dehydrogenase	Oxidation of —CHOH— to —C— with =O	
Oxalosuccinate + NADPH		
⇅ Oxalosuccinate decarboxylase	One carbon eliminated as CO_2	
α-Ketoglutarate + CO_2		
+ NAD$^+$ ⏸ α-Ketoglutarate oxidase	Second carbon eliminated as CO_2. Details uncertain	
+ CoA-SH		
Succinyl-S-CoA + CO_2 + NADH		
+ ADP ⏸ Enzyme	Phosphorylation, regeneration of CoA-SH	
+ phosphate		
Succinate + CoA-SH + ATP		
⇅ Succinic dehydrogenase	Dehydrogenation → double bond. Acceptor?	
Fumarate + acceptor·H_2		
+ H_2O ⇅ Fumarase	Addition of H_2O to double bond	
Malate		
+ NAD$^+$ ⇅ Malic dehydrogenase	Oxidation of —CHOH— to —C— with =O	
Oxalacetate + NADH		

CH_3CO-S-CoA + $3H_2O$ + 4 Acceptor → $2CO_2$ + CoA-SH + 4 Acceptor·H_2	**Net reaction**	

---

subsequent oxidation of the reduced hydrogen acceptors in the cytochrome pathway.

The tricarboxylic acid cycle is an essential part of aerobic metabolism in animal tissues but it seldom operates in its entirety in a microorganism. Intermediate reactions can be carried out by various bacteria that utilize an incomplete or modified version of the cycle. Since its reactions are reversible, the cycle serves synthetic as well as catabolic purposes. It is also a metabolic crossroads that serves as a bridge between carbohydrate and protein metabolism; through acetyl-CoA, it connects with fatty acid synthesis.

Terminal Path to Oxygen

Hydrogen is accepted by NAD$^+$, NADP$^+$, or another acceptor at four stages in the tricarboxylic acid cycle and in various other reactions involved in carbohydrate metabolism. In aerobic metabolism, hydrogen is eventually transferred to oxygen by a series of reactions apparently coupled so that 3 high-energy phosphates are created, making a total of 12 for the 4 acceptors in the tricarboxylic acid cycle.

In animal tissues, carbohydrates appear to be completely utilizable by the tricarboxylic acid cycle. Bacteria form a metabolic spectrum beginning with obligate aerobes such as *Neisseria* species. Intermediate in the spectrum are staphylococci, and the typhoid, dysentery, and colon bacilli, which possess cytochromes but are able to grow and multiply anaerobically. At the other end of the spectrum are the fermentative streptococci, pneumococci, and lactobacilli and the obligate anaerobes of the genus *Clostridium,* which lack cytochromes and are able to utilize only a small fraction of the free energy potentially available from nutrient.

Utilization and Synthesis of Polysaccharides

Many bacteria produce enzymes that release utilizable monosaccharides from nonutilizable polysaccharides. The intracellular formation of polysaccharides and their utilization as stores of energy have not played as prominent a role in bacterial metabolism as in animal and plant metabolism, although, as will be seen subsequently, production and degradation of intracellular polysaccharides seem to be im-

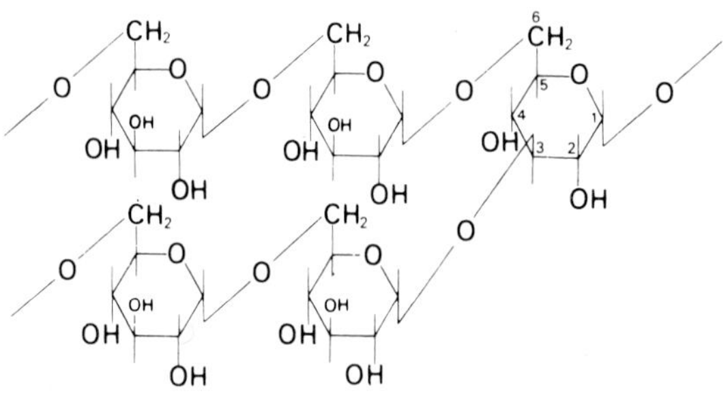

Figure 5.2: Chemical structure of a bacterial glucan molecule showing α-1,6 linkage and branching at C_3 in an α-1,3 linkage. *Straight lines* represent hydrogens.

portant in the metabolism of plaque bacteria. Many of these bacteria accumulate polysaccharides during growth on sugars that are consumed during sugar deprivation. When grown on glucose, 60% of the cultivable organisms from human carious material produced enough glycogen to stain deeply with iodine. Such carbohydrates may permit the bacteria to form extracellular acid in the absence of exogenous carbohydrate (see Chap. 3).

Of interest for the general problem of biochemical polymerization is the enzymatic synthesis of bacterial polysaccharides during dissimilation of disaccharides. *Streptococcus mutans* is capable of converting sucrose to water-soluble and water-insoluble glucans. The water-soluble glucans contain glucose primarily in α-1,3 linkages (Fig. 5.2). These polysaccharides are synthesized by enzymes, glucosyltransferases, which for the most part are extracellular or are bound to the cell surface. This extracellular synthesis transfers glucose units from sucrose to an acceptor, which usually is the growing dextran-like polymer. The enzyme conserves the energy of the link ($\Delta G = +6,600$ calories) between the C1 of glucose and the C2 of fructose present in sucrose and is used to create the new bond in the polymer. The reaction may be summarized as follows:

$$n\text{-Sucrose} + \text{acceptor} \xrightarrow{\text{glucosyltransferase}} (\text{glucan}) + {}_n\text{fructose}.$$

By similar reactions *Streptococcus salivarius* uses fructosyltransferase to make levan (fructose polymer) and glucose from sucrose. The monosaccharides released can be used by the organism as energy sources. In addition, sucrose can be hydrolyzed by extracellular and intracellular invertase activity to glucose and fructose, which are then metabolized mainly to lactic acid through the Embden–Meyerhof pathway. Apparently, these latter reactions are quite important and only a few percent of glucosyl moieties of sucrose find their way to glucan, particularly if the amount of sucrose is limited. This will be discussed more thoroughly in the context of dental caries production (Chap. 51).

The glucan formed by *Streptococcus mutans* in the presence of sucrose contributes importantly to the mucinous consistency of the dental plaque and cohesion of its bacterial cells, and to its tenacious adherence to the enamel surface.

The synthesis of plant, animal, fungal, and bacterial polysaccharides involves uridine triphosphate (UTP). Starting with glucose-6-phosphate, this reaction is exemplified by the synthesis of type 3 pneumococcus capsular polysaccharide, a polymer of glucose and glucuronic acid (see below):

$$\text{Glucose-6-phosphate} \xrightarrow{\substack{\text{phosphogluco-}\\\text{mutase}}} \text{glucose-1-phosphate.}$$

$$\text{Glucose-1-phosphate} + \text{UTP} \xrightarrow{\substack{\text{uridyl}\\\text{transferase}}} \text{uridine diphosphoglucose (UDPG)} + \text{pyrophosphate.}$$

$$\text{UDPG} + 2\ \text{NAD} \xrightarrow{\substack{\text{UDPG}\\\text{dehydrogenase}}} \text{uridine diphosphoglucuronic acid (UDPGA)} + 2\ \text{NADH.}$$

$$\text{UDPG} + \text{UDPGA} \xrightarrow{\substack{\text{type 3}\\\text{pneumococcal}\\\text{enzyme}}} (\text{glucose-glucuronic acid})_n + P_i.$$

Through the action of enzymes on other uridine diphosphate (UDP) sugars and uronic acids, a variety of polysaccharides have been synthesized, including bacterial cell wall polysaccharides. The capsular polysaccharides have great significance because they protect the bacterial cell against phagocytosis.

Carbohydrate Metabolism of Dental Plaque

The metabolism of carbohydrates by dental plaque is extraordinarily complex since it depends on the interactions of a number of constantly changing variables. The bacterial composition of plaque is the major variable and exhibits all the variation one would expect of a complex ecosystem. There are well over 100 different bacterial species isolable from various plaques representing a remarkable spectrum of biochemical possibilities. The expression and realization of these biochemical possibilities is influenced and in part controlled by numerous environmental and ecological factors (diet, salivary components, bacterial interactions). Moreover, the intraoral location of the plaque, the time of day, oral hygiene, and the patient's age are factors that contribute to the heterogeneity of plaque. Thus, plaque is not an entity but a heterogeneous series of bacterial communities attached to the tooth; the composition and biochemical activities of these communities vary from mouth to mouth, from tooth to tooth, even from one surface of the tooth to another surface of the same tooth. Changes in the bacterial composition of various plaques are especially important and are associated with specific pathogenic mechanisms and ecologic niches; e.g., some cariogenic, supragingival plaques contain a large percentage of lactic acid–forming streptococci, whereas a subgingival plaque associated with a form of periodontal disease may contain few or no streptococci but a majority of gram-negative anaerobes. The end product of the streptococcal plaque may be lactic acid, whereas the major end product of the gram-negative plaque may be butyric acid, e.g., a metabolic product of certain *Bacteroides* species.

Most of the recent research on plaque metabolism has concentrated on the metabolism of carbohydrates by supragingival plaque, in an attempt to relate the biochemical activities of plaque samples and pure cultures of plaque bacteria to various aspects of human dental caries. It has been known since the 1897 pioneering work of W. D. Miller and subsequently the 1899 work by G. V. Black that carious lesions on tooth surfaces are always preceded by the accumulation of adherent bacterial plaques. The isolation of lactic acid–forming bacteria from such plaques by numerous investigators over the years led to the notion that the carious dissolution of the enamel was due to the decalcification caused by accumulations of lactic acid in plaque. In the presence of a fermentable carbohydrate in the diet, certain bacteria would catabolize the carbohydrate via glycolysis to lactic acid and the critical pH necessary to initiate the carious lesion or "white spot." The homofermentative nature of plaque was assumed, since in vitro pure culture studies of known cariogenic bacteria (*Streptococcus mutans, Lactobacillus casei*) demonstrated that lactic acid was the sole (over 95%) end product of glucose breakdown by these organisms.

It is surprising that this belief persisted until recently, since Muntz in 1943 had shown that lactate was not the sole metabolic end product of plaque carbohydrate metabolism. More recently, Gilmour and associates showed that plaque and materia alba incubated with glucose resulted in the formation of acetate, propionate, and lactate. Furthermore, the concentrations of acetate and propionate were similar to or greater than that of lactate. Subsequent in vivo work showed that the addition of sucrose or glucose to in situ plaque resulted in the formation of butyrate as well as acetate, propionate, and lactate (both D(−) and L(+) forms). Moreover, and more complicating, the proportions of these acids varied with respect to time after exposure to the sugar—e.g., lactate was high immediately following sugar ingestion but declined with time. The decline in lactate (a nonvolatile acid) concentration was paralleled by an increase in volatile acids (acetate, propionate) and ethanol.

Other studies done on pure cultures of cariogenic streptococci, including *S. mutans,* have provided a possible explanation for the heterofermentative character of plaques dominated by these classically designated homofermenters. The primary reason for the variation in fermentation patterns of these oral streptococci is associated with the regulation of two enzymes: lactic dehydrogenase (LDH) and pyruvate formate lyase (PFL). LDH has an absolute requirement for an activator, fructose 1,6-diphosphate (FDP) in order to function (see discussion under Enzyme Regulation, Chap. 6). Under conditions of glucose/sucrose excess the cellular concentration of FDP was high while that of phosphoenolpyruvate (PEP) was low; under conditions of sugar limitation the reverse was true. The high level of FDP in glucose/sucrose-rich cells explains why lactate is the main end product, and the low level of FDP in glucose/sucrose-limited cells explains why there is a decrease in lactate. Pyruvate breakdown under carbohydrate limitation now proceeds via PFL to formate, acetate, and ethanol (Fig. 5.3).

The regulation of PFL is under the control of glyceraldehyde-3-phosphate (GAP). Unlike FDP, a positive effector (activator) for LDH, GAP is a negative effector for the enzyme PFL. Under glucose/sucrose-limiting conditions the cellular concentrations of both FDP and GAP are low, thereby inhibiting LDH and releasing the negative inhibition of pyruvate–formate lyase with the resulting formation of formate, acetate, and ethanol. Conversely, when cells are grown in excess glucose, the concentrations of FDP and GAP are high, and since PFL is inhibited by GAP, only LDH is activated and lactate is the sole end product. Under most conditions the organisms in plaque are limited with respect to a carbohydrate source and therefore carry on a heterofermentative metabolism *except* when there is a dietary intake of carbohydrate (e.g., candy ingestion), allowing the positive activation of LDH by FDP and the negative effect of GAP on PFL.

Other Aspects of Plaque Carbohydrate Metabolism

The endogenous carbohydrate metabolism of plaque bacteria will be discussed later in the context of cariogenic potential and the structure–function relationships of oral bacteria (glycogen granules). There are, however, two other aspects that merit discussion.

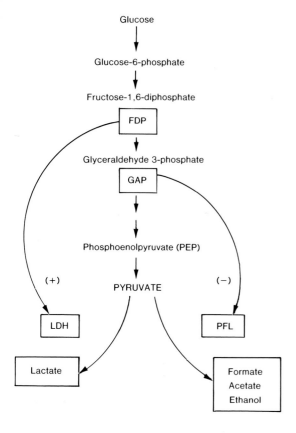

Glucose excess ⇌ Glucose limitation

Figure 5.3: Pathways of carbohydrate metabolism of *Streptococcus mutans* under conditions of glucose excess and glucose limitation. Lactic dehydrogenase (*LDH*) showing activation (+) by fructose = 1,6-diphosphate (*FDP*); pyruvate formate lyase (*PFL*) showing negative effect (−) of glyceraldehyde-3-phosphate (*GAP*). (Adapted with permission from T. Yamada and J. C. Carlsson: The Role of Pyruvate-Formate-Lyase in Glucose Metabolism of *Streptococcus mutans*. In *Microbio Abs,* Spec Suppl, **3,** 809, 1976.)

1. Acid utilization and the nature of the dietary carbohydrate source. One of the factors thought to modify the cariogenic potential of dental plaque is the ability of several plaque bacteria to utilize acids, particularly lactic acid. These include species of *Veillonella, Neisseria,* and *Bacterionema matruchotii.* Both aerobic and anaerobic mechanisms for acid utilization have been described, but because the microenvironment of most plaques is largely anaerobic, more interest has been shown in the anaerobic mechanism. Some of these mechanisms are summarized below:

Aerobic:
  Neisseria species
  B. matruchotii

$$\text{Lactate} \xrightarrow{\;+O_2\;} \text{acetate} + CO_2.$$

Anaerobic:
  Veillonella

$$\text{Lactate} \xrightarrow{\;-O_2\;} \text{propionate} + \text{acetate} + CO_2 + H_2.$$

Many *Veillonella* strains lack the enzyme hexokinase and therefore are unable to utilize sugars via the glycolytic pathway. Their ability to utilize lactate represents an attractive ecological possibility by which these numerically important members of the plaque microflora could convert lactate into weaker acids (propionate and acetate). Several suggestions have been made that the ratio of *Veillonella* to acidogenic bacteria might be related to cariogenic potential. "Germ-free" animal experiments have provided indirect support for this hypothesis since coinfections using *Veillonella* and known acidogenic and cariogenic streptococcal strains resulted in caries reductions as compared to animals inoculated with the streptococci alone.

Changes in dietary carbohydrate are also known to change plaque metabolism. Not only does the amount of lactic acid vary, but the rate of acid formation and the fermentative pathway are also known to depend on the nature of the carbohydrate substrate. More lactic acid is produced by—and the pH drops more rapidly in—plaque incubated with sucrose or glucose than with lactose or starch. Practical advantage is taken of the fact that sugar alcohols, although sweet in taste, are not metabolized in the same way as sugars; i.e., sorbitol and mannitol are used as sweetening agents in certain chewing gums and foods because they are metabolized to weak acids and ethanol. Another sugar alcohol with great sweetening power, xylitol, has the added advantage of not being fermented by most plaque microflora, including *S. mutans.* Xylitol was once considered to be an ideal sugar substitute because of this property, but side effects have compromised its widespread use for human consumption.

2. Inhibitors of carbohydrate metabolism in plaque. A variety of inhibitors of plaque metabolism are known to occur in the oral milieu and various attempts have been made to exploit these inhibitors to prevent or restrict plaque formation and the parallel biochemical activities of the plaque microflora. The major inhibitor receiving the largest amount of attention has been fluoride in its several forms. It is clear that fluoride inhibits microbial growth and metabolism in dental plaque and in saliva. The principal mechanism of fluoride's action on oral microorganisms is inhibition of acid formation via glycolysis. Inhibition of the glycolytic pathway is due to the inhibition of enolase activity. Enolase converts 2-phosphoglycerate to phosphoenol pyruvate (PEP). Not only is the glycolytic pathway blocked, but the cellular transport mechanism (PEP phosphotransfer-

ase system) is also inhibited. The inhibition of the transport system is crucially important in the caries process since the marked cariogenicity of certain bacteria (e.g., *S. mutans*) depends on the rapid entry of glucose into the cell, allowing for an equally rapid production of acid. The PEP phosphotransferase system of *S. mutans* is remarkably effective in glucose uptake and transport—and the glycolytic rate for this streptococcus is considerably more active than for other oral bacteria, such as *Actinomyces viscosus.* The third metabolic function inhibited by fluoride is the synthesis of glycogen, since the supply of glucose-6-phosphate is markedly diminished or absent as a result of the glycolytic shutdown. Of interest, endogenous glycogen breakdown by whole cells continues at an appreciable rate even in the presence of fluoride, once again reflecting the critical importance of glucose transport into the cell. (Catabolism of glycogen does not require phosphorylation of glucose to glucose-6-phosphate as part of the entry process.)

Protein Metabolism

Bacteria are unable to ingest intact proteins, but many species produce proteinases and peptidases that hydrolyze proteins successively to peptides and amino acids, which the cell can assimilate. Proteolytic bacteria generally cannot initiate growth on intact protein but require at least traces of amino acids or ammonia to get started. Amino acids are utilized as such for the synthesis of proteins, or they may be metabolized in several ways to produce intermediates such as pyruvate, α-ketoglutarate, and oxaloacetate, which interconnect with the pathways of carbohydrate metabolism.

Probably the most general reaction of this type is transamination between an amino acid and keto acid (Fig. 5.4). Since keto acids are available from carbohydrate metabolism or other reactions, transamination is an important source of the corresponding amino acids.

Another common reaction of amino acids is oxidative deamination (Fig. 5.5). The reverse reaction, reductive amination of keto acids by ammonia, may be a source of amino acids from carbohydrate metabolism.

Decarboxylation of amino acids to their corresponding amines is a common reaction. However, bacterial decarboxylases are formed most actively at about pH 5; their activity at neutrality has been doubted. Nevertheless, amines have been detected in the contents of the gingival sulcus.

Amino acids are derived through various biosynthetic pathways from a variety of precursors. For example, α-ketoglutarate gives rise to glutamate, which can then form glutamine. It can also form proline by

$$^-OOC-CH_2-CH_2-\overset{\overset{\displaystyle NH_3^+}{|}}{CH}-COO^-$$
Glutamate

$$+ {}^-OOC-CH_2-\overset{\overset{\displaystyle O}{\|}}{C}-COO^-$$
Oxalacetate

$$\text{transaminase} \updownarrow \text{pyridoxal phosphate}$$

$$^-OOC-CH_2-CH_2-\overset{\overset{\displaystyle O}{\|}}{C}-COO^-$$
α-Ketoglutarate

$$+ {}^-OOC-CH_2-\overset{\overset{\displaystyle NH_3^+}{|}}{CH}-COO^-$$
Aspartate

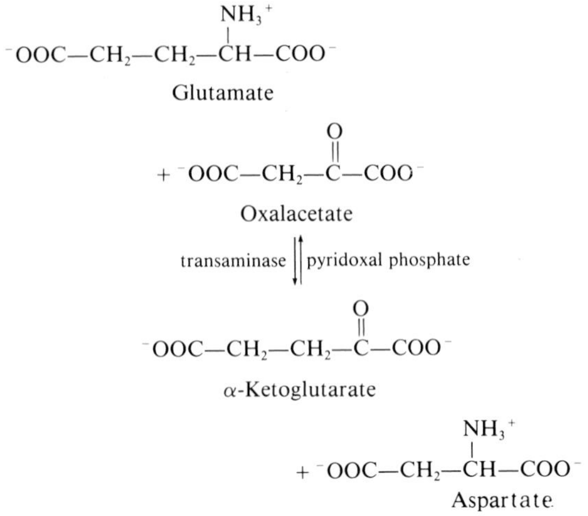

Figure 5.4: Transamination illustrated by the reaction between glutamate and oxalacetate.

another pathway or, through a series of reactions, go through ornithine or citrulline to arginine. Similarly, oxaloacetic acid can, by transamination, form aspartic acid, which can then form a whole group of other amino acids. Protein is synthesized by successive coupling of amino acids by peptide bonds in a definite sequence determined by DNA.

Lipid Metabolism

Bacterial lipids occupy intermediate positions in metabolism. They are made of building blocks from a variety of chemical classes; for example, phospholipids are derivatives of glycerol phosphate. Amines and amino acids can be attached to phos-

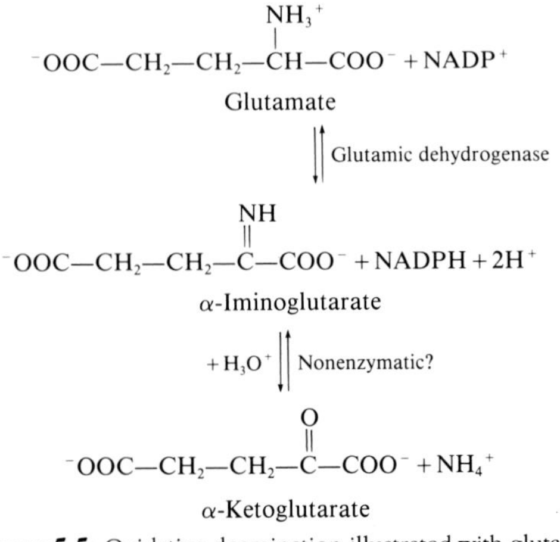

$$^-OOC-CH_2-CH_2-\overset{\overset{\displaystyle NH_3^+}{|}}{CH}-COO^- + NADP^+$$
Glutamate

$$\updownarrow \text{Glutamic dehydrogenase}$$

$$^-OOC-CH_2-CH_2-\overset{\overset{\displaystyle NH}{\|}}{C}-COO^- + NADPH + 2H^+$$
α-Iminoglutarate

$$+ H_3O^+ \updownarrow \text{Nonenzymatic?}$$

$$^-OOC-CH_2-CH_2-\overset{\overset{\displaystyle O}{\|}}{C}-COO^- + NH_4^+$$
α-Ketoglutarate

Figure 5.5: Oxidative deamination illustrated with glutamate.

phate, while hydroxyl groups of other glycerol carbons are linked to fatty acids or hydrocarbons. Glycerol can be metabolized by way of its connection with carbohydrate metabolism. Also, some amino acids can be transferred to fatty acids. Relatively few bacterial species are effective in attacking lipids, but most synthesize them to a significant degree. They may be utilized when the medium is low in oxidizable substrates. Internal storage may provide available lipids. For a more complete discussion of lipid metabolism, the reader is referred to Stryer (1988).

Nucleic Acid Metabolism

Nucleic acids make up an unusually high proportion of bacterial protoplasm, so that much of the bacterial cellular activity relates to nucleic acid biosynthesis and catabolism. In some bacterial species RNA seems to serve as a reserve food material.

The structural units of nucleic acids are the purines, adenine and guanine; the pyrimidines, cytidine, thymine, and uracil; and phosphates of the pentoses, D-ribose and D-deoxyribose. These substances derive from intermediates of amino acid and carbohydrate metabolism by a lengthy series of enzymatic reactions too detailed to present here (see Stryer, 1988). Transglycosidation converts the purines, pyrimidines, and pentose phosphates to the corresponding ribosomes (nucleosides) and inorganic phosphate. Nucleosides are phosphorylated with the aid of ATP to form nucleotides and nucleotide pyrophosphates (ATP is a nucleotide pyrophosphate), which are polymerized enzymatically to the nucleic acids. Nucleic acids can be returned to the metabolic pools whence they came by the successive actions of nucleases, nucleotidases, and nucleosidases.

ADDITIONAL READING

Bowden, G. H. W., Elwood, D. C., and Hamilton, I. R. 1979. Microbial Ecology of the Oral Cavity. Adv Microb Ecol, **3,** 135.

Hamada, S., and Slade, H. D. 1980. Biology, Immunology, and Cariogenicity of *Streptococcus mutans.* Microbiol Rev, **44,** 331.

Mandelstam, J., and McQuillen, K. (Eds.) 1973. *Biochemistry of Bacterial Growth,* Ed. 2. Wiley, New York.

Sanawal, B. D. 1970. Allosteric Controls of Amphibolic Pathways in Bacteria. Bacteriol Rev, **34,** 20.

Stanier, R. Y., Adelberg, E. A., and Ingraham, J. L. 1976. *The Microbial World,* Ed. 4, Ch. 6, 7, and 8. Prentice-Hall, Englewood Cliffs, N.J.

Stryer, L. 1988. *Biochemistry.* W. H. Freeman, New York.

Volk, W. A. 1982. *Essentials of Medical Microbiology,* Ch. 5, J. B. Lippincott, Philadelphia.

Yamada, T., and Carlsson, J. C. 1976. The Role of Pyruvate-Formate Lyase in Glucose Metabolism of *Streptococcus mutans:* Microbial Aspects of Dental Caries. Microbiol Abstr Spec Suppl, **3,** 809.

6

Physiology of Bacteria

Benjamin F. Hammond

In the previous chapter the chemical and physical architecture of the bacterial cell was described. This chapter considers the growth of bacterial cells and the various factors involved in growth measurement and regulation. The growth of a bacterial cell consists in the orderly increase in the chemical components making up the cell (cytoplasm, cell wall, surface appendages). The synthesis of these components from materials available in the immediate environment is followed by their organization and assembly to reproduce the original units and the subsequent multiplication of cells (cell division). Growth is therefore measured as an increase in the number of cells or an increase in cellular mass.

The requirements of bacterial growth are quite complex but can be divided into the following categories: 1) proper concentration of essential nutrients, 2) a suitable environment with specific physical and chemical factors, and 3) the availability of a continuous source of energy, usually obtained from a series of coupled oxidation–reduction reactions. If one con-

siders nutritional and energy requirements, most bacterial species fit somewhere between two extremes. At one extreme are the *autotrophic* or *lithotrophic* bacteria, which generally are not pathogenic for man. They require only simple nutrients such as inorganic salts and CO_2, and they obtain their energy from light (photosynthetic autotrophs) or by the oxidation of inorganic substances (chemosynthetic autotrophs) such as sulfur, iron, nitrite, or ammonia. At the other end of the spectrum are the *heterotrophic* or *organotrophic* bacteria, which include the common pathogens. These bacteria use organic compounds, such as glucose, as an energy source and convert a portion of their energy source to the other organic compounds they require.

The oral environment is capable of supporting the growth of a huge number of diverse bacteria in distinct ecological niches, each of which has specific nutrient sources and characteristic physicochemical milieus. Dental plaque reportedly contains more than 200 different bacterial species that exhibit an extraordinary range of physiological potentials and growth characteristics. A few examples of their growth and physiology are described in this chapter.

Effects of Environmental Factors on Growth

Temperature

Since the growth of bacteria depends on a series of chemical and enzymatic reactions, it is not surprising that these organisms are profoundly affected by variations in temperature. As the temperature rises, the metabolic reactions and the resultant growth proceed more rapidly. However, above a certain temperature many biological macromolecules and cellular components may be denatured, resulting in metabolic injury or cell death. As the temperatures decrease there is a corresponding decrease in some of the same metabolic reactions, but not with the same degree of predictability. Much of the metabolic injury related to freezing of bacterial cells is due to changes in the fluidity of the cell membrane and the loss of nutrient transport function. Most bacteria grow variably over a temperature range of 30°C or more but grow best at an optimum temperature that has a relatively narrow range. The optimum temperature for growth is a relatively stable characteristic that is widely used as a taxonomic criterion.

Bacteria can be divided into three groups according to the temperature range at which they grow. *Pyschrophiles* grow over a range of 0 to 30°C, with an optimum slightly below 29°C. However, such bacteria do grow and multiply at 0° C, so that they can grow in food or biologicals stored at refrigerator temperature. *Mesophiles,* which include common pathogens in mammalian bodies, grow at 10 to 45°C. Most bacteria that are human pathogens grow best at or near 37°C. *Thermophiles* grow over a range from 25 to 75°C, with an optimum of 50 to 55°C.

In general, prokaryotic bacteria grow over a much wider range than eukaryotic bacteria, which explains the presence of prokaryotes in such diverse habitats as the boiling springs of Yellowstone National Park and in refrigerated dairy and food products.

Acidity and Alkalinity

Bacterial growth extends over a wide range of hydrogen ion concentrations (3 to 4 pH units), with optimal growth usually occurring within a span of less than 1 unit. Most pathogenic bacteria grow best between pH 7.2 and 7.6. Some acid-forming (acidogenic) bacteria such as *Lactobacillus* and *Acetobacter* species produce and tolerate acids to pH 3 or even below. Organisms that function well in acidic environments are known as acidophilic (acid loving) or aciduric (acid tolerating). However, many organisms in the gingival crevice grow best at neutral to alkaline pH values. Other bacteria such as *Vibrio cholerae* and *Escherichia coli* can tolerate an alkalinity of pH 8 to 9.

Microbial production of acids and alkaline substances may profoundly alter the immediate environment. The acid decalcification of enamel by lactic acid–producing bacteria is essential for dental caries, and many dairy products result from similar microbial fermentations (see Chaps. 17 and 51). Moreover, the growth pH of a bacterial culture plays a major role in determining the biochemical activities and metabolic end products of that culture—i.e., certain enzymes are active at neutral pH, others at acid or alkaline pH values. There is also a pH effect on enzyme synthesis: homolactic streptococci produce considerable dehydrogenases at alkaline pH values, while at neutral or acidic pH the same organisms may produce transaminases or decarboxylases. In each case the products of the reactions are different.

Oxidation–Reduction Potential

Bacteria can be divided into groups according to their requirements for oxygen. *Obligate anaerobes* grow only in the absence of molecular oxygen or in a highly reduced medium. *Facultative* bacteria grow either in the absence of oxygen (reduced state) or in the presence of oxygen (oxidized state). *Obligate aerobes* require oxygen, although some species can grow at a very low oxygen tension. *Microaerophilic* bacteria require a reduced oxygen tension, for growth is suppressed at a high oxygen tension. The oxidation–reduction potential (E_h) of a medium is critical for initiating the growth of a given bacterial species. The E_h, expressed in volts or millivolts, may be positive (+ volts), indicating an oxidized state, or negative (− volts), indicating a reduced state. A typical aerobic culture broth has an E_h of + 0.3 V. Facultative or obligate anaerobes require a negative E_h for growth. The reduced state required by anaerobes can be achieved by culturing them in closed containers from which oxygen has been removed catalytically or by the chemical actions of chromous sulfate or pyrogallol. An anaerobic or reduced state can also be achieved even in a medium exposed to the atmosphere by the addition of an oxidation–reduction buffer such as sodium thioglycolate (0.1%) or glutathione (glutamyl–cyteinyl–glycine), which will poise the oxidation–reduction potential at the proper reduced level.

Aerobic bacteria require oxygen for growth. However, oxygen dissolved in culture media is rapidly used by such bacteria, and since atmospheric oxygen diffuses slowly across an air–medium interface, an oxygen insufficiency soon results in such cultures. Growth in aerobic cultures can be increased by forced aeration.

Oxygen Toxicity and Strict Anaerobes

Obligate or strict anaerobes grow only in the absence of molecular oxygen. In fact, oxygen is actually toxic to these cells. The toxicity of oxygen results from the formation of two toxic substances produced by the oxidations of flavoproteins and other enzymes by oxygen: hydrogen peroxide (H_2O_2) and the extremely toxic free radical,* superoxide (O_2^-). Aerobic and aerotolerant organisms produce an enzyme, superoxide dismutase, that catalyzes the following reaction:

$$O_2^- + O_2^- + 2H^+ \xrightarrow[\text{dismutase}]{\text{superoxide}} O_2 + H_2O_2.$$

These organisms also have one or more mechanisms for disposal of H_2O_2. The enzyme catalase decomposes H_2O_2 into oxygen and water:

$$H_2O_2 \xrightarrow{\text{catalase}} 2H_2O + O_2$$

and is found in most organisms able to grow in the presence of oxygen. One notable exception to this rule is the lactic acid bacteria that lack catalase but have a peroxidase system that reduces H_2O_2 to water at the expense of oxidizable organic substrates, e.g.,

$$NADH + H^+ + O_2 \xrightarrow[\text{oxidase}]{\text{NADH}} NAD^+ + H_2O_2,$$

$$NADH + H + H_2O_2 \xrightarrow[\text{peroxidase}]{} NAD^+ + 2H_2O.$$

Net reaction:

$$2NADH + 2H^+ + O_2 \longrightarrow 2NAD + 2H_2O.$$

The absence of catalase, peroxidase and superoxide dismutase from almost all obligate anaerobes provides an explanation (albeit not absolute) for the toxicity of oxygen to these organisms. *Bacteroides gingivalis,* although generally classified as a strict anaerobe, has been reported to be aerotolerant because some strains produce high levels of superoxide

dismutase and other enzymes that neutralize the toxic products of oxidative metabolism. It has been suggested that possession of these enzymes makes these strains more virulent because they are better able to survive in the periodontal pockets until the redox potential is lowered to permit growth and metabolism. Since the large majority of the oral microflora are anaerobic, it is not difficult to understand why H_2O_2 was used for years in reducing oral infection and sepsis.

Carbon Dioxide

All bacteria seem to require some CO_2 to initiate and even to continue growth. Many bacteria, particularly when first isolated, require a level of CO_2 greater than that found in the atmosphere (and culture medium) to initiate growth. For others, atmospheric CO_2 (about 0.03%) is sufficient. Once growth has begun, bacterial cultures may furnish sufficient CO_2 to meet most growth requirements. In practice, an increased CO_2 tension is provided by placing the cultures in a closed environment to which CO_2 is added. Of interest, many oral bacteria have an absolute requirement for increased levels of CO_2 in order to grow and metabolize. Two such organisms have been associated with the etiology of one form of periodontal disease: *Actinobacillus actinomycetemcomitans* and *Capnocytophaga* species. They are found in the gingival crevices of patients with localized juvenile periodontitis and are obligate *capnophiles* (*capno* = CO_2; *phile* = loving).

Inorganic Ions

The inorganic ions required by bacteria for growth are usually supplied by water or by ingredients that are used to make up the medium. Among these inorganic ions, Mg^{2+}, K^+, NH_4^+, SO_4^{2-}, and PO_4^{3-} are required by practically all bacteria. CO^{2+} is essential to vitamin B_{12}. When there is no organic sulfur or nitrogen, SO_4^{2-} and NH_4^+ or NO_3^- may be used for growth by some bacteria. Phosphates are related to the transport of energy in bacteria. K^+ is essential to protein synthesis. Mg^{2+} is an essential cofactor for many enzymes and for ribosomal activity. Iron (Fe^{2+} or Fe^{3+}) is considered an essential trace ion because it is required for heme proteins in the oxidative enzymes of aerobic bacteria; even anaerobic bacteria have iron-containing enzymes. Ca^{2+} is important to spore formation and to enzyme secretion from grampositive cells. Zn^{2+} and Mn^{2+} are important constituents of enzymes. Na^+ and Cl^- are not required by most bacteria and, in fact, with some exceptions, may be inhibitory as their concentration increases.

---

*A free radical is a compound with an unpaired electron. Superoxide, having gained an extra electron, carries a negative charge.

Organic Nutritional Requirements of Bacteria

The heterotrophic pathogenic bacteria require sources of carbon in organic forms. They also require growth factors, vitamins, as well as trace amounts of fats, lipids, and other organic compounds, depending on the particular requirements of a given bacterial species.

Carbon Requirements

Apparently, elemental carbon is not utilized by bacteria. However, all bacteria, including autotrophic and heterotrophic forms, require some CO_2 for the initiation of growth and for cell division. In addition to the CO_2 requirements, heterotrophic bacteria must have an organic source of carbon, which is usually supplied by a wide variety of mono- and disaccharides. Glucose is the most common source, but amino acids can serve alternatively in many cases, e.g., certain asaccharolytic gram-negative rods in the gingival crevice. A few bacteria and fungi (but not yeasts) can use starch as a source of carbon. Cellulose is utilized by some bacteria, particularly those associated with the alimentary tract of herbivorous animals and termites.

Nitrogen Requirements

Heterotrophic bacteria usually require a complex source of nitrogen, including amino acids, peptones, and peptides, and specific nitrogenous growth factors. At present these are primarily supplied by digests and infusions, and by extracts of plants, animal tissues, or in some cases yeasts, singly or in combination. Blood or serum is often used as a source of accessory growth factors for streptococci or *Haemophilus* species. Serum albumin is protective since it has an affinity for small molecules that may inhibit bacterial growth.

Vitamin Requirements

The vitamin requirements of bacteria vary widely, but in some species they are extensive. For example, some oral streptococci and lactobacilli require as many as nine B vitamins and 17 amino acids, as well as purines and pyrimidines. For many years it was difficult to explain how the oral environment could support their growth, given the limited nutrient sources of pure saliva and other oral fluids. It is now clear that the complex nutritional requirements of the more fastidious bacteria can be met from a variety of sources, including but not limited to exogenous dietary components, the lysis of shed cells (epithelial and phagocytic), and the bacteria themselves, via symbiotic interactions (see Chap. 50).

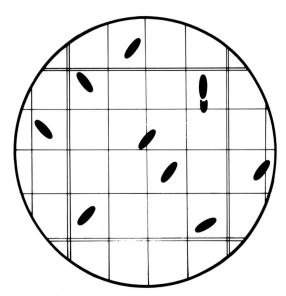

Figure 6.1: Direct microscopic count. Microscopic observation: Count only the cells in the large square (7 in this field). In practice, several such squares are counted and the numbers averaged.

Measurement of Growth

Growth is measured by determining increases in cell number or some parameter of cell mass, such as cell weight, cell nitrogen, or DNA content. There are several methods for using either approach and reasons for choosing one over the other.

Cell Number

Total Cell Count. The number of cells in a population may be counted directly under the microscope using the appropriate dilution; this method produces the *direct microscopic count*. A sample (usually in microliter amounts) containing bacteria is diluted in saline or other diluent and placed in a counting chamber (Petroff-Hausser) on a small grid of a known total area (1 sq mm) and covered with a cover slip, giving a total volume of 0.02 mm^3. The whole grid usually has 25 large squares, and the number of bacterial cells per square can be counted under the microscope and the numbers averaged (Fig. 6.1). To calculate the number of cells per mL one simply multiplies this average figure by a conversion factor based on the volume of the chamber sample. Apart from the tediousness of the procedure there are a number of other disadvantages, including:

1. Dead cells are counted the same as living cells under most conditions.
2. Precision is difficult to achieve, since very small

cells may not be seen or pairs may be counted singly. Moreover, the method will not work where cells exist in low density, for there will not be enough cells to be seen easily in a given microscopic field.

Viable Count.   One of the disadvantages of the total microscopic count is the inability to differentiate between living and dead cells. The viable count is the count of cells capable of dividing and forming offspring, i.e., capable of forming colonies on a suitable agar plate. The *plate count* or *colony count* is performed by pipetting a sample (usually no more than 0.1 mL) onto or into the surface of an agar medium which is then incubated to allow growth and colony formation. Knowing the dilutions of the original sample, one may extrapolate back to get the total number of viable organisms per mL. The accuracy of this method is compromised by the following disadvantages:

1. Some cells clump so that a single colony may represent the progeny of several individual cells.
2. Small colonies may not be seen because not all cells may be dividing synchronously.
3. The number of colonies depends on the suitability of the culture medium as well as the incubation time and temperature.

Cell Mass

In many instances it may be preferable to determine cell mass or some parameter thereof. *Cell weight* may be determined directly by weighing wet or dried centrifuged cells, or the very simple procedure based on turbidity measurement may be used. A cell suspension scatters light in proportion to the cell density of the suspension. With colorimetry or spectrophotometry, the turbidity (expressed as absorbance) can be used as a convenient substitute for counting, but again, it does not discriminate between viable and nonviable cells. Other measures include chemical determination of any of the major components of cell structure, such as cell nitrogen, cell DNA, RNA, protein, etc., or of cellular metabolism (oxygen consumption) (Fig. 6.2).

Growth Cycle of Bacterial Populations

For the purposes of the present discussion, growth refers to a progressive increase in cellular protoplasm by the synthesis of cell components and the imbibi-

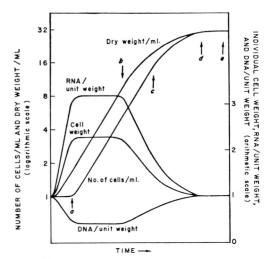

Figure 6.2: Diagram correlating typical changes in cell size, number, and chemical composition during bacterial growth in broth inoculated with a culture in early stationary phase (*e*). Initial values of all variables have been equalized as one arbitrary unit. (Reproduced with permission from D. Herbert: *Microbial Reaction to Environment,* p. 395. Cambridge University Press, New York, 1961.)

tion of water and electrolytes that eventuates in cellular division. Multiplication may then be regarded as a necessary response to the pressure of growth. Indeed, if multiplication is prevented without other injury to the cell, as can be done with certain antibiotics, the cell grows, becomes grossly distorted, and eventually perishes.

When a few quiescent bacteria are introduced into an environment that meets their requirements for growth and multiplication, they first pass through a period of adjustment, commonly called the *lag phase,* during which there is no multiplication or increase in number (up to point *a* in Fig. 6.2). The physiology of this phase of adaptation is not completely understood. A priori, there seems to be no reason that the cell should not grow and multiply promptly. Actually, growth of cells commences and becomes exponential after a much shorter phase of adjustment (dry weight per milliliter) than shown in Figure 6.2. Growth is evidenced also by a rapid increase in individual cell weight (dry weight per cell count) and by an even more rapid rise in RNA content per unit weight, reflecting intensive protein synthesis. Because each cell is larger and metabolically more active, there are corresponding increases in the rates per cell of oxygen consumption, carbon dioxide production, and heat evolution. In sum, cellular growth runs ahead of cellular division. However, as many as four nuclei (chromatinic bodies) per cell may accumulate because of nuclear division without cellular division. Although DNA per unit weight declines steadily and

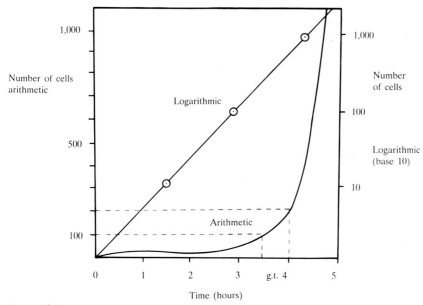

Figure 6.3: Growth curve of an organism growing exponentially, plotted arithmetically and semi-logarithmically. Generation time (*g.t.*), the time required for the population to double itself, is 30 min.

reaches a minimum at the end of the lag phase, the DNA content per nucleus remains nearly constant.

It is not certain what influences stimulate cellular division. Most theories have been based on the consideration that the cell should outgrow its ability to nourish itself, which is limited by its surface to volume ratio.

It is quite understandable that at some critical size the rate at which nutrients could be transported into the cell would become insufficient for maintenance of the enclosed volume of protoplasm, and division into smaller cells would become necessary. Alternatively, the need could be met from without by providing a greater concentration of nutrients, which would, up to a point, increase their rate of transport into the cell. Richer media should therefore support a population of larger cells, but in general, the reverse seems to occur.

Whatever may be the various factors that determine the lag in multiplication, it terminates after a period of a few hours in a transition period when the physiological activity per cell, RNA content per unit weight, and individual cell weight are greatest; DNA content per unit weight is least; and cellular division begins (*a* in Fig. 6.2). The population now enters what is termed the *exponential* or *logarithmic phase* of multiplication (*a* to *c* in Fig. 6.2), since the logarithm of the number of cells now increases linearly with time. Physiologically, the cells have reached a steady state in relation to their environment. Total bacterial mass increases exponentially, but individual cell weight, RNA content per unit weight, and DNA content per unit weight

remain constant. Cellular division occurs regularly at a definite time interval called the *mean generation time,* which is characteristic for each species under given conditions. For a wide variety of oral bacteria in optimal media at body temperature, it falls between 20 and 90 minutes (Fig. 6.3). An extreme example is the tubercle bacillus, which may not divide more than once a day, even under favorable conditions. Nuclear division typically occurs during the middle third of the interval between cell divisions. If the medium is regularly removed and replaced with a fresh sample of the same medium at the same temperature, the cells will continue to grow and multiply at the exponential rate indefinitely. This kind of growth is called *continuous culture.* Once the system is in equilibrium, cell number and nutrient status remain constant; i.e., the system is in steady state. Approximately these circumstances probably prevail in the mouth, for, except for the addition of extra nutriment at mealtimes and a period of stagnation at night, the culture medium is being renewed constantly, although at a variable rate.

If the medium is not renewed, the period of exponential multiplication commonly lasts from 3 to 24 hours to yield a total growth of 10^8 to 10^{10} cells per mL. The larger the original inoculum, the more limited the nutrients, and the faster the inherent rate of multiplication of the organism, the shorter is the period of exponential multiplication, and vice versa. The cells next enter a second transitional phase, during which first the growth rate (point *b* in Fig. 6.2) and then the multiplication rate (*c*) declines. Concur-

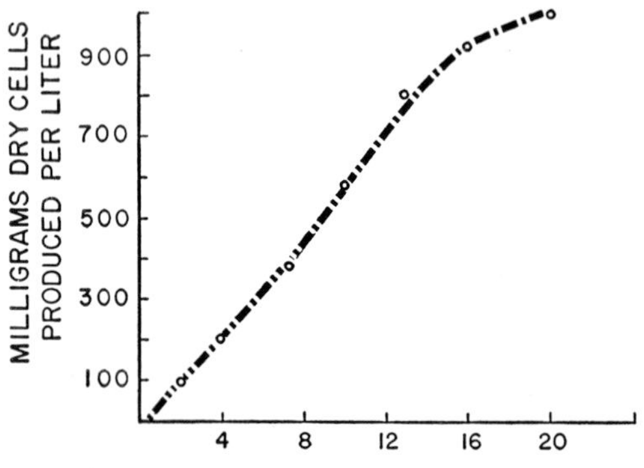

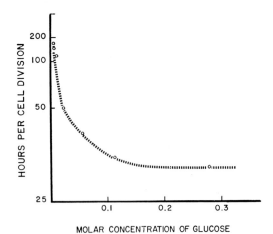

Figure 6.4: Limitation of total growth of a bacterium (*Lactobacillus casei*) by an insufficient supply of an essential nutrient (riboflavin) in an otherwise complete medium. Below 16 µg/L, growth is directly proportional to the concentration of riboflavin and is limited by exhaustion of the supply. Above 20 µg/L, additional riboflavin has less and less effect and total growth approaches the limiting M concentration for this organism in this medium. This form of curve is generally applicable to microbiological assay, whether the limited essential nutrient is a vitamin, amino acid, carbohydrate, mineral, or other substance. (Compiled from the data of E. E. Snell: Nutritional Requirements of the Lactic Acid Bacteria. *Wallerstein Laboratories Communications,* **11,** 81, 1948.)

rently, RNA synthesis and individual cell weight decrease. Finally, RNA per unit weight, DNA per unit weight, and cell size return to values characteristic of resting cells (*d*). Growth and multiplication cease and the cells enter the *stationary phase* (*e*). The total number of cells now remains constant for a considerable period, after which the *phase of decline* sets in, with progressive death and, in many cases, autolysis of the cells. Bacteria in the stationary phase are called resting cells. Although they have ceased to multiply, such cells retain their ability to carry on metabolic processes. It follows that microorganisms in general can continue to function in pathological processes long after they have passed the peak of their growth and multiplication. An example is continued acid production by nongrowing cariogenic bacteria in plaque.

The growth of bacteria may be limited by suboptimal concentrations of essential nutrients (Fig. 6.4), but even though all are provided in excess, the total number of cells per unit volume cannot exceed a maximal value called the *M concentration,* which is characteristic for each organism and medium. The first explanation of this limitation that comes to mind is that the medium has been "staled" by the accumulation of toxic metabolic end products of the organism. This explanation is certainly applicable in some cases. For example, the presence of utilizable carbohydrate greatly stimulates the growth of a microorganism

(Fig. 6.5), but it also limits growth, owing to the acidification of the medium. The situation is different in sugar-free broths in a number of instances. If the majority of the cells are removed from such a broth culture in the stationary phase and the supernatant fluid is reincubated, the typical multiplication cycle is repeated by the remaining cells. Obviously, such a medium was not "staled" by the first growth. It has been noted also that when equal amounts of two nonantagonistic species with the same M concentrations are inoculated together, each reaches only one-half its usual cell mass. This has given rise to the concept that growth is limited by the available biological space, which, although descriptive, does not explain the phenomenon. Since the volume of a typical bacterial cell is of the order of 10^{-12} mL, even in a dense culture containing 10^{10} cells per mL, the total cellular volume would not exceed 1% of the total volume of the medium. If the cells in such a culture are killed by heating but are not removed, the spatial constraint no longer exists, for a fresh inoculum will go through the usual multiplication cycle. Evidently we are dealing with an obscure antibiotic effect that occurs even between presumably identical living cells.

The duration of the stationary phase depends in part on the inherent tendency of the given organism to autolyze and in part on the nature of the medium. In general, the presence of fermentable carbohydrate is unfavorable for survival, since it leads to a bactericidal degree of acidification of the medium. If this is avoided, cultures of the gram-negative bacilli of the

Figure 6.5: Effect of changing the concentration of a nutrient (glucose) on the rate of division of a bacterium (*Mycobacterium tuberculosis* in Dubos medium). In 0.005 M glucose (1 g/L), there was only one division per week; in 0.3 M glucose (50 g/L), one in 30 hours. Further increase of the concentration of glucose would have little effect. (Compiled from the data of W. Schaeffer: Recherches sur la croissance du *Mycobacterium tuberculosis* en culture homogène. *Annales de l'Institut Pasteur,* **74,** 458, 1948.)

enteric group, for example, survive for months if refrigerated. Special requirements may be important, but if these are met, survival will be prolonged.

The typical S-shaped growth curve described for bacteria is by no means peculiar to them or even to microorganisms in general. Rather, it describes the course of events to be expected whenever a few self-reproducing units are introduced into a favorable environment.

Growth and Division of Single Bacterial Cells

Most data on the growth and division of bacterial cells have been obtained as averages of large unsynchronized bacterial populations, or, at best, from a population that is roughly synchronized for only a few generations. With the advent of the electron microscope and the attainment of longer periods of synchronized bacterial growth, considerable information has been obtained about the sequences and events involved in the reproduction cycle of individual bacterial cells.

Cell Division

The genetic requirement for the sequence of events necessary for bacterial cell duplication is found in the DNA of the bacterial chromosomes. The number of chromosomes in a bacterial cell is partly related to its physiological state at a given time. Bacterial cell division begins with the initiation of DNA replication, followed by its complete duplication.

When replication of the DNA is complete, the duplicate chromosomes separate from each other, resulting in a type of nuclear division. Separation of the duplicate chromosomes relates to a function of the cytoplasmic membrane. In gram-positive bacteria, the chromosomes are attached to an extension of the cytoplasmic membrane called a *mesosome*. When the chromosome has replicated, the mesosome splits and the two parts separate, each carrying one of the chromosomes with it. The separation of mesosomes is accomplished by the formation of new cell membrane in the area between the separated mesosomes. In gram-negative bacteria the mesosomes are not formed or are not so prominent in chromosome separation. In these bacteria the chromosomes seem to attach directly to the cell membrane (Fig. 6.6).

When the duplicate bacterial chromosomes have separated from each other, two daughter cells form and separate. These steps are achieved by the synthesis of a transverse equatorial septum, by cell membrane growth, and by cell wall synthesis. Initiation of septum formation depends on the completion of

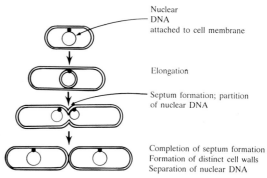

Figure 6.6: Cell division in a rod-shaped bacterium.

chromosome replication and the passage of time to allow for protein synthesis. The place and time of septum formation are essential for the proper division of the materials in the mother cell (Fig. 6.7). Cell wall formation follows septum formation. In gram-positive bacteria, the cell wall forms equatorially and by diffuse intercalation. In cell wall formation the mesosome moves toward the center of the cell, followed by the developing cell wall septum. After the transverse cell wall septum is completed the cells separate by a process mediated by hydrolases.

Microbial Regulatory Processes

In their independent existence in widely fluctuating environments, bacterial cells must be able to maintain an individual biological steady state (homeostasis) in order to metabolize, grow, and reproduce. The growth and survival of microorganisms depends on a variety of mechanisms, including 1) the structure and composition of their cell walls, 2) the regulation of the intake and outgo of metabolites, as well as their concentrations in microbial cells, and 3) the osmotic and specific transport activities of the cytoplasmic membranes. In addition, microorganisms, particularly bacteria, possess a number of intracellular regulatory mechanisms that allow them to adapt to a wide variety of environments. These regulatory mechanisms depend on factors involved in the synthesis and activities of enzymes and in the control and the synthesis of nucleic acid and protein.

Metabolic Uptake

Relatively early in the development of bacteriology, it was evident that permeability and osmotic barriers existed in bacterial cells. An enzyme that was present and active in the bacterial cytoplasm of an intact cell did not attack its specific substrate if the substrate was outside of the cytoplasmic membrane. It was also evi-

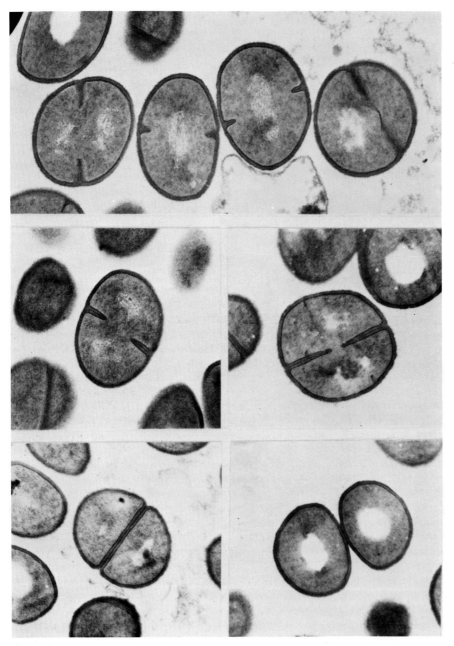

Figure 6.7: Successive stages of cross-wall formation and division in lag phase growth of a strain of *Staphylococcus aureus*. (Reproduced with permission from R. M. Cole, A. N. Chatterjee, R. W. Gilpin, and F. E. Young: Ultrastructure of Teichoic Acid-Deficient and Other Mutants of Staphylococci. *Ann New York Acad Sci,* **236,** 22, 1974.)

dent that cytoplasmic membranes took some active part in the transport of substances across such barriers. Bacterial cells exposed to a dilute concentration of amino acids accumulated a higher concentration of these amino acids inside the cell than existed outside the cell, indicating some form of active transport across the membrane.

The cell membrane has at least three main functions in regard to metabolism and growth (including cell division) of bacteria. For metabolism, growth, and cell division to occur in bacteria, their membranes must either transport or at least allow essential nutrients to come into the cell. The membranes must also transport or permit passage of the waste products from the cell to the environment, and must not allow essential metabolites to diffuse or be transported from the cell. The membranes that carry out these essential functions are thought to consist of two layers of lipid molecules surrounded on each side by layers of protein (Chap. 3).

Characteristics of Transport Systems

The transport systems of bacterial membranes have a specificity similar to that of enzymes. Transport systems also resemble enzymes in their stereospecificity, by requiring protein synthesis, and because their formation is subject to induction/repression and influenced by nutrition. Also, they usually do not follow diffusion kinetics. They do not resemble enzymes in that the material being transported does not undergo permanent enzymatic conversion.

The specificity of a transport system depends on membrane transport proteins. A given transport system can accept and transport only a limited number of different substances that have similar chemical structures. The rate of transfer of a substance is initially related to its concentration. As the concentration increases, the rate of transport reaches a steady state, indicating a limited number of adsorption sites. A given transport system may be at least partially involved in the transportation of substances both in and out of bacterial cells. Transportation across the cell membrane against a concentration gradient requires energy. In such instances active transport can be halted by chemical substances that interfere with energy metabolism.

Carrier-mediated cell membrane transport occurs in three stages. In the first stage, the substance being transported combines with a specific chemical group or molecule on the exterior of the membrane. The substance is then transported across the membrane. In the final step, the substance is released inside the cell and the transport system returns to its original state. Energy is supplied to the transport system at one of the steps in the transportation cycle. In such systems the concentration of the substance inside the cell may be 1,000 times greater than the concentration of that substance outside the cell. Also to be remembered is that the carrier-mediated process often shows saturation at low external concentrations (Fig. 6.8).

In *group translocation* the substance to be transported is chemically modified in the course of its transport across the membrane. This type of system has been described previously in discussions of cell membranes and sugar transport in certain cariogenic bacteria (sucrose phosphotransferase system of *Streptococcus mutans;* see Chap. 5).

Another example of the variety of transport functions is *Escherichia coli* growing in the presence of

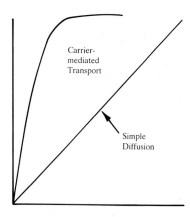

Figure 6.8: Comparison of uptake rate and external concentration in simple diffusion and carrier-mediated transport.

β-galactoside. This results in the formation of β-galactosidase by the cells, as well as the mechanism for the transport of β-galactoside into the cells. The transport of the substrate is not against a concentration gradient and hence does not require energy. On the other hand, *E. coli* can actively transport nonhydrolyzable analogues of β-galactoside against a concentration gradient if it is supplied energy. The same transport system is evidently used by both β-galactoside and its analogue, whether or not energy is required for their transfer. When a substance is utilized inside the cell more rapidly than it is transported, systems capable of active transport sometimes become uncoupled from their energy source and function as facilitated transport systems that shuttle back and forth without utilizing energy.

Enzyme Regulation

The preceding section examined how bacteria cope with their environment and maintain a biologically steady state through the regulatory activities of their cell membranes. Bacteria have, in addition, several equally important mechanisms for intracellular regulation of their metabolic activities that allow them to live in and adapt to many different environments.

Few, if any, bacterial enzymes are produced at a steady rate in all environments. The enzymes of bacteria vary widely both in presence and in concentration. The production of an enzyme in a given environment depends on the corresponding metabolites being present in the medium in which they are grown. Enzymatic regulation of metabolism may occur at the level of enzyme activity or enzyme synthesis.

Regulation of Enzyme Activity. Regulation at the level of enzyme activity is very rapid; no significant time lapse occurs before the effects of such regulatory action are manifest. Generally, the enzymes that are subject to control at the level of activity are those that occupy strategic points, particularly branch points, in the sequence of reactions of metabolism, so that changing their activity immediately affects the entire pathway beyond that enzyme. The enzymes involved are called *allosteric* (other shape) since they can change their configuration, and the type of regulation in which they are involved is called *end-product* or *feedback inhibition,* since their activity is subject to regulation by the end product of that pathway. Allosteric enzymes can be inhibited (or activated) by substances that are structurally dissimilar to their substrate. This can occur because these enzymes have two different kinds of combining sites, a site for the substrate and a site for the inhibitor or activator. The enzyme molecule is flexible, so its shape can be changed by combination with the substrate or the inhibitor. This ability to change shape influences the shape of the catalytic site. If this site is occupied by substrate, or if the other site is occupied by an activator, the enzyme is stabilized in the active configuration. An inhibitor complexing at the inhibitor site favors the inactive form of the enzyme. There are multiple sites of each type on an enzyme, so they act in concert to promote a given configuration, and when one site of a type is complexed, that configuration is promoted at other sites.

Regulation of Enzyme Synthesis. Besides regulation at the level of enzyme activity, bacterial metabolism may be controlled at the level of enzyme synthesis. Regulation of synthesis generally involves regulation at the genetic level. Some substrates and metabolites can effect enzyme synthesis, while others act to repress the rate of synthesis. Enzymes that are always present whether or not substrate is present are constitutive, while those present only when substrate is available are said to be inducible. The mechanism of enzyme regulation was discovered during Jacob and Monod's investigation of the β-galactosidase system in *E. coli.* A gene product that inhibited synthesis of the enzyme was found; it was called *repressor* and subsequently shown to be a product of a specific gene called a *regulatory gene.* These regulatory, or R, genes were associated with but clearly different from *structural genes* coding for specific enzyme proteins. As shown in Figure 6.9, enzyme repression occurs when the repressor is attached to the operator gene where messenger RNA synthesis is blocked and the proteins specified for by this mRNA cannot be synthesized. Usually the repression depends on an effector molecule (cell metabolite, not shown in the diagram) which binds to the repressor. Transcription occurs if the repressor is not bound to the operator. Enzyme induction occurs when the inducer (another effector

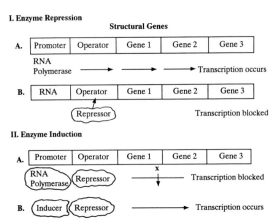

Figure 6.9: Diagrammatic representation of enzyme repression and enzyme induction. In **IA,** transcription occurs because the repressor is unable to bind to the operator. In **IB,** transcription is blocked because repressor binds to operator. In **IIA,** transcription is blocked because the repressor binds to the operator, preventing RNA polymerase action; in **IIB,** transcription occurs because inducer inactivates repressor.

molecule, for example lactose in the β-galactosidase system) binds to the repressor molecule and inactivates it so that it does not bind to the operator. In the absence of the inducer the repressor is free to bind to the operator and transcription is blocked. Thus, inducible enzymes are those for which the cell continually synthesizes repressor. The operator locus controls the expression of adjacent structural genes, and if the repressor does not bind, the structural genes, in this case for the enzymes of lactose metabolism, are expressed and enzymes are produced. An operator together with the genes it controls is called an *operon,* which acts as a unit of coordinated expression. The operon for lactose metabolism contains an operator, the enzyme β-galactosidase, which breaks down lactose, and a permease that transports β-galactoside (lactose) into the cell. The promoter is located next to the operator but distal to the structural genes and is the binding site for RNA polymerase. Its relation to the operator adds to the regulation of transcription by the operator and repressor.

The operon is an efficient control system for metabolic regulation since all enzymes function as a unit. They are present in equivalent amounts and turned on or off at nearly equal rates. Even though enzyme synthesis begins rapidly after induction, several generations must occur before the effects are seen in a culture. This lag occurs because there must be time for the enzyme to reach an adequate level to be effective. In like manner, when repression occurs, the enzyme already present must disappear through dilution and turnover before the effects are seen in the population, or even in the individual organism.

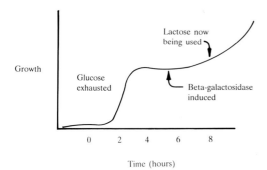

Figure 6.10: Diauxie growth pattern in a mixture of glucose and lactose. The synthesis of β-galactosidase is repressed until glucose is exhausted from the medium. After a brief lag, β-galactosidase is synthesized and growth is resumed with lactose as the growth substrate.

Catabolite Repression. In the examples described above the repressor protein causes the repression of mRNA synthesis. In contrast to this type of negative control there is a positive control in which a regulator protein promotes the binding of RNA polymerase, thereby acting to increase mRNA synthesis. Catabolite repression, one of the best-studied examples of positive control, describes the phenomenon in which the synthesis of several unrelated enzymes is inhibited when cells are grown in the presence of glucose. (Catabolite repression is also called the *glucose effect*). Glucose is utilized more easily than other catabolizable energy sources and its presence inhibits the production of enzymes related to the catabolism of other less readily catabolizable substrates such as lactose. For example, if an organism is grown in the presence of both glucose and lactose, the organism will not utilize the lactose until the glucose has been exhausted. The enzyme β-galactosidase is inducible, and the inducer, lactose, is present, but this enzyme is subject to catabolite repression. This kind of diphasic growth curve is called *diauxie* (Fig. 6.10).

The mechanism for catabolite repression is based on the presence of 1) another allosteric protein, catabolite activator protein (CAP), which must bind first to the promoter site before mRNA, and 2) cyclic adenosine monophosphate (cAMP), another regulatory molecule that must bind to CAP before the CAP can bind to the promoter. cAMP is an activator for the synthesis of many catabolic enzymes. Glucose reduces the cAMP level in the cell and binding of RNA polymerase to the promoter does not occur. If, however, cAMP is added to the medium, catabolite repression does not occur.

Some of these regulatory concepts have been applied to the carbohydrate metabolism of *Streptococcus mutans*. The fermentation of glucose by this organism varies considerably, switches from homolactic to heterolactic according to the availability and concentration of glucose. This variation is based on the regulation of two enzymes, lactic dehydrogenase (LDH) and pyruvate formate lyase (PFL). LDH has an absolute requirement for the activator fructose-1,6-diphosphate (FDP); i.e., FDP is a positive effector. In contrast, PFL is inhibited by galactose-3-phosphate (GA3P). Under conditions of glucose excess the concentrations of both FDP and GA3P are high, leading to a homolactic fermentation as summarized below:

$$\text{High glucose} \longrightarrow \text{allosteric activation of LDH}$$
$$\text{concentration} \quad + \text{ inhibition of PFL}$$
$$\longrightarrow \text{homolactic fermentation.}$$

Under conditions of glucose limitation there are minimal amounts of both FDP and GA3P with negligible turn-on of the LDH system and release the inhibition of PFL with the formation of acetate, formate, and ethanol (heterolactic fermentation):

$$\text{Low glucose} \longrightarrow \text{low FDP,} \longrightarrow$$
$$\text{concentration} \quad \text{low GA3P}$$
$$\text{no LDH activation,} \longrightarrow \text{heterolactic}$$
$$\text{but PFL active} \quad \text{fermentation.}$$

It is now clear why *S. mutans* in plaque produces only lactic acid as the sole fermentation product when given large amounts of glucose or sucrose and produces weaker acids (acetic and formic) and ethanol when these sugars are present in reduced concentrations. This finding has obvious relevance to sugar consumption and caries levels.

Functions of Bacterial Regulatory Mechanisms

Induction, repression, and inhibition are most important mechanisms in bacterial physiology. These mechanisms allow bacteria to control their intracellular activities economically and precisely so that they can adapt to a given environment. *Induction* is important to the economy of bacterial enzyme production in that enzyme production occurs only if the substrate is available. If all the enzymes of a bacterial cell were constitutive, i.e., constantly produced, regardless of their need, then most of the biosynthetic and metabolic machinery of such cells would be so misdirected that the cell could no longer grow because it could not obtain the required energy and metabolites.

Feedback inhibition and *repression* are also important mechanisms that allow bacterial cells to con-

Table 6.1: Cooperative Nutritional Interactions Among Oral Microorganisms

Deficient Organism(s)	"Helper" Organism(s)	Product(s) Provided by "Helper"	Result
Bacteroides melaninogenicus	Facultative diphtheroid	Naphthoquinone	Growth and tissue necrosis
Oral spirochetes, *Treponema*	Fusobacterial species and an anaerobic diphtheroid	Cocarboxylase isobutyrate, putrescine	Growth
Bacteroides asaccharolyticus	*Actinomyces viscosus, Bacteroides melaninogenicus*	Succinate	Growth and infectivity
Fusobacterium fusiforme	*Bacteroides melaninogenicus*	Collagenase	Infectivity
Oral lactobacilli	*Candida albicans*	Vitamins	Growth
Fusobacterium fusiforme	Oral staphylococci, gram-negative cocci	Lowered E_h, growth accessory factors	Chondroitin sulfatase production, gingival destruction
Vibrio sputorum	*Veillonella* species	H_2 from lactate metabolism	In vivo growth
Veillonella sp.	Oral streptococci	Lactate	Growth

trol their endogenous metabolic and biosynthetic activities in relation to the availability of exogenous metabolites. Repression is concerned mostly with control of the synthesis of cell macromolecules that serve as metabolic building blocks. End-product inhibition is related to the control of the economy of metabolite synthesis. The loss of only feedback inhibition by mutation (not by repression) results in the cell producing excessive amounts of the end product and excreting it. Feedback inhibition allows bacteria to produce their metabolic building blocks in such amounts that their excretion does not occur, even under widely varying temperature or pH.

Catabolite repression is another example of physiological economy since the cell does not waste energy producing enzymes to catabolize substrates more difficult to catabolize than glucose. Similarly, if required products (small molecules) are present in the external environment, the cell will no longer produce them internally, since such molecules may be obtained more easily from the environment. This action also allows the cell to manage its metabolic machinery with minimal energy expenditure.

Microbial Interactions

An aspect of bacterial physiology that is often overlooked is that mixed cultures of bacteria, not pure cultures, are the rule in nature. Thus, the interactions of bacteria are essential components of their physiology. This ecological approach is critical to understanding the natural regulation of microbial population levels and activities. Metabolic antagonisms as well as microbial synergisms are as old as the discipline of microbiology and provide the basis for many industrial and ecological applications. Heterotrophic free-living protozoa in soil are estimated to consume between 150 and 900 g of bacteria/m^2/yr and, depending on what kinds of bacteria are present, the soil can be converted to an area capable of supporting a given vegetable flora and fauna. In the rumen of cattle and sheep there are critical microbial interactions among the over 200 different bacterial species known to exist there. These interactions determine whether the animals survive or die. The *Streptococcus bovis/ Megasphera elsdeni* ratios control the rate of acid buildup and consequently the development of lactic acidosis and ulceration; ultimately this microbial interaction determines the amount of useful work the animal can perform.

In the oral cavity numerous possibilities for such interactions exist among the hundreds of bacterial species known to exist there. Some of the cooperative nutritional interactions among oral microorganisms are listed in Table 6.1. For example, fusobacteria and anaerobic diphtheroids ("helper" organisms) reduce the oxidation–reduction potential of plaque to a level that will support spirochete growth (E_h of -200 mV); these two organisms also provide a series of growth factors (isobutyrate, cocarboxylase, and putrescine) for the spirochetes (deficient organisms).

On the negative side of antagonistic interactions are numerous examples of bacterial products that are inhibitory for the growth and metabolism of other oral bacteria, or *bacteriocins*. Bacteriocins are bactericidal proteins, usually heat-labile, that bind to the surfaces of other cells and produce some type of metabolic perturbation (cellular leakage, cessation of respiration, or cessation of DNA, RNA, or protein synthesis). Several oral bacteria produce these proteins, which are thought to destroy other plaque/salivary bacteria, even though many of these proteins are susceptible to the lytic action of proteolytic enzymes that exist in various ecological niches. Another interesting approach has been to utilize these antagonistic relationships to prevent the establishment and growth of pathogens. One of the early goals of microbial ecologists was to prevent and control certain microbial infections by introducing antagonistic, nonvirulent counterparts of disease-producing microorganisms into susceptible host tissues. Ideally, these innocuous counterparts could competitively colonize and establish themselves in an ecosystem, ultimately replacing the virulent strain. The various mechanisms of this "bacterial interference" have not been studied systematically, but some investigators have shown that cariogenic bacteria can be replaced by such counterparts, e.g., lactic dehydrogenase negative mutants of *S. mutans* or noncariogenic strains of *S. salivarius* replace *S. mutans*.

ADDITIONAL READING

Alexander, M. 1971. *Microbial Ecology.* Wiley, New York.

Atkinson, D. E. 1969. Regulation of Enzyme Function. Annu Rev Microbiol, **23,** 47.

Brock, T. T. and Magian, M. T. 1988. *Biology of Microorganisms,* Ed. 5. Prentice Hall, Englewood Cliffs, N.J.

Guirard, B. M., and Snell, E. E. 1962. Nutritional Requirements of Microorganisms. In *The Bacteria,* Vol. IV, edited by E. C. Gunsalus and R. Y. Stanier. Academic Press, New York.

Hammond, B. F. 1986. Ecology—State of the Science Review. In *Dental Plaque Control Measures and Oral Hygiene Practices,* edited by H. Loe and D. Kleinman. IRL Press Ltd., Oxford, England pp. 197–212.

Helmstetter, C. E. 1969. Methods for Studying Microbial Division Cycle. In *Methods in Microbiology,* Vol. 1, edited by J. R. Norris and D. W. Ribbons. Academic Press, New York.

Joklik, W. K., Willett, H. P., and Amos, D. B. (Eds.). 1984. *Zinsser Microbiology,* Ed. 18. Appleton–Century–Crofts, New York.

Koshland, D. E. 1970. The Molecular Basis for Enzyme Regulation. In *The Enzymes,* Ed. 3. Vol. 1, p. 342, edited by P. D. Boyer. Academic Press, New York.

Mallette, M. F. 1969. Evaluation of Growth by Physical and Chemical Means. In *Methods in Microbiology,* Vol. I, edited by J. R. Norris and D. W. Ribbons. Academic Press, New York.

Paigen, K., and Williams, B. 1970. Catabolic Repression and Other Control Mechanisms in Carbohydrate Utilization, Adv Microb Physiol, **4,** 252.

Rogers, J. J. 1970. Bacterial Growth and the Cell Envelope. Bacteriol Rev, **34,** 194.

Yamada, T., and Carlsson, J. C. 1976. The role of pyruvate formate lyase in glucose metabolism of *Strep. mutans.* In *Microbial Aspects of Dental Caries.* Microbiol Abstr./Spec. Suppl. **3,** 809–819.

Part III

Infection and
Resistance

7

Host-Parasite Interactions and Innate Resistance Mechanisms

Keith R. Volkmann

Parasitism

The association of a microorganism with another living entity is called parasitism. This is a natural outcome of the struggle for existence by living organisms. From the constant interactions of microbes with other life and with the physical and chemical environment, the microbial world has developed into life forms with differing requirements for growth, reproduction, and survival. As a result, microorganisms demonstrate varying degrees of dependency on parasitism, and when free-living or parasitic microbes associate with a potential host, there are several possible outcomes (Table 7.1).

Host–Parasite Associations

The human body is constantly bombarded with microorganisms from the environment, with one of several reactions occurring. The intruder may be immediately removed in host secretions or excretions, or destroyed by nonspecific host defense activities after a brief residence. This is the fate of most free-living microorganisms that find themselves translocated from the general environment to the human body because they are unsuited for parasitic life in that host.

Other species find specific sites on or within the host suitable for growth and multiplication. The most successful of these parasites are those which exist in harmony with the host and cause no damage. Such associations result in establishment of the indigenous or normal body flora. With some other parasites the growth and multiplication accidentally cause damage to the host, resulting in a violent reaction called infectious disease. These types of parasites are called pathogens.

In the most unfavorable relationship between host and pathogen, the host is unable to limit the destructive activities of the pathogen and dies. Alternatively, in encounters between a host and pathogen, the host

Table 7.1: Possible Stages in the Development of Parasitism

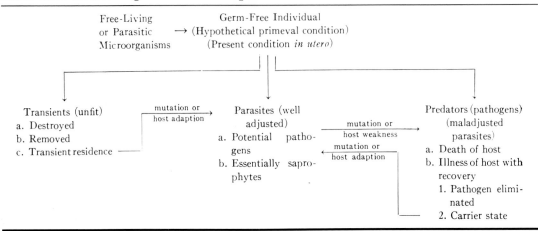

becomes ill and recovers, whereupon the pathogen may be eliminated by the host's adaptive reactions or may persist in the state of truce that we call the carrier state.

Host Adaptations

In an individual, the state of pathogenicity has evolved into a host–parasite complex owing to adaptations of the host. Generally, pathogens are not maintained solely by transfer from diseased to healthy individuals. It is also a great principle that health prevails only so long as the host adaptations can keep the parasite in check. If host adaptations become community-wide over a number of generations, as by hereditary selection, immune responses, and cultural changes, the severity of the disease declines, the carrier state becomes more general, and the parasite may disappear.

Parasite Mutations

A parasite may adjust to an environment by mutation, losing some of its undesirable characteristics. It is not certain how significant this factor has been under natural conditions, although it has been demonstrated experimentally very often.

Facultative Parasites

A number of microorganisms find themselves equally well adapted to existence when they are free in the general environment or as harmless parasites within a host. For example, certain species of *Clostridium* are primarily inhabitants of soil or animal and human intestinal tracts and cause no harm as long as

they remain there. However, under appropriate conditions they can be potent pathogens, producing tetanus or gas gangrene.

Indigenous Parasites

Few of the indigenous parasites of man are found elsewhere except as parasites of other animals and possibly a few plants. This situation appears to have come about through progressive loss (possibly by mutations of the parasites) of functions that could be carried out by the host, and by elimination of nutritionally facultative parasites from the general environment by the antibiotic activities of other microorganisms. The first of the above-mentioned mechanisms is the most likely for the development of viruses and of such transitional forms as the rickettsiae, which are special types of parasitic bacteria. Similarly, it would be difficult for bacteria such as streptococci and lactobacilli to meet their exceedingly complex nutritional requirements in many environments outside their natural hosts. For example, extensive surveys have shown that *Streptococcus mutans* is worldwide in distribution but is found only in the dentulous mouths of man and some lower animals or on saliva-contaminated environmental surfaces. The meningococcus has relatively simple nutritional requirements, but it can carry on its vital functions only within a narrow range of temperature approximating that of the animal body, and it has a very limited ability to survive in an inactive state. On the other hand, *Escherichia coli,* which constitutes a large fraction of animal feces, can synthesize everything it needs from simple media. Its pH and temperature requirements are not critical within a broad range, and it can grow anaerobically as well as aerobically. These needs can

Table 7.2: The Biological Steady State and Infectious Disease

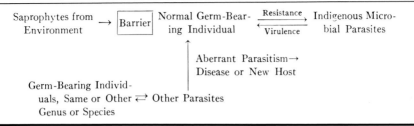

be met in a variety of environments. However, the colonic bacillus is not found in soils and waters not recently contaminated with animal feces; it actually disappears quickly from farm soil, presumably owing to the antibiotic activities of the other microbial residents, for it survives and grows if the soil is autoclaved. It is likely that the colonic bacillus cannot compete successfully in the open and, as an evolutionary adjustment, has taken refuge in the protected environment of the animal gut.

Microbial Steady State

An individual normally harbors an indigenous parasitic flora characteristic for his species and environment (Table 7.2). Environmental saprophytes (free-living organisms) rarely get a foothold. By inherent and adaptive mechanisms, summarized as "resistance," the host holds in check the pathogenic potentialities (virulence) of the parasites. Infectious disease, then, is a combination of the damage to the host's tissues plus the host's adaptive reactions that occur when a parasite gets out of control, either because of an increase in microbial virulence or because of a decrease in the host's resistance.

Probably no microorganisms can be considered nonpathogenic. Under appropriate conditions (e.g., with a compromised host or with excessive contamination) essentially any species may cause varying degrees of damage to the host. In addition, animals reared in a germ-free environment are surprisingly susceptible to generalized invasion by some of the common "nonpathogens," such as lactobacilli and enterococci, in doses that are entirely innocuous for normal germ-bearing animals of the same species, which evidently have built up a tolerance. Dosage, then, is another important determinant. All of these relationships between parasite and host may be summarized in an equation that symbolizes the relative nature of health and disease:

$$\text{Disease or health} = \frac{\text{Virulence of parasite} \times \text{dosage}}{\text{Resistance of host}}.$$

Aberrant Parasitism

If a parasite wanders from its usual habitat into one it is not accustomed to, it may behave as a predator. This is termed aberrant parasitism. The parasite may simply stray from one part of its host to another to produce disease (such as a bacterial endocarditis caused from a bacteremia with an oral organism), or the parasite may be transferred from a symptomless carrier to an uninfected individual of the same species. The result is most dramatic when a virgin population has been infected. Thus, the introduction of measles into the South Sea Islands decimated the native populations. Of epidemiological interest, because of the possible development of new host species, is the transfer of a parasite from its regular host species to a new one, commonly with the production of severe disease. Representative examples can be found among all forms of microorganisms. For example, the rickettsiae are primarily harmless parasites of the intestinal cells of various arthropods, but many of them cause serious disease when transferred to man by the bites of these insects. The initial wandering of a parasite from a well-adjusted association to a foreign host tends to be a biological dead end, since effective mechanisms for transmission within the new host group usually do not exist.

Host Benefits

The universal occurrence of parasitism has raised the question of whether the parasitic biota has become indispensable to its host. Although many instances of useful function by parasites appear possible, it is difficult actually to demonstrate the beneficial aspects of the indigenous flora. Man probably derives most of his vitamin K from his intestinal bacteria, and some individuals can supplement the supply of B vitamins by absorption from the same source. The successful rearing of germ-free animals provided a proper diet demonstrates, however, that the microbial functions are dispensable even though they may play a useful role under natural conditions. It also is possible that small numbers of organisms that enter the bloodstream through small breaks in the mucous membranes of the body openings could induce an immunogenic response. If the antigens from such organisms are closely related to those of given pathogens (e.g., common antigens among *Streptococcus mitis, Streptococcus sanguis,* and the pathogen *Streptococcus pneumoniae*), cross-reacting antibodies may provide some degree of protection against the invading pathogen. This may prevent potential pathogens from establishing in the oral cavity in significant numbers if there are cross-reacting antigens. Secretory IgA also is produced against some indigenous species. Indigenous species also may antagonize the colonization or growth of some invading pathogens, expressing the "first come, first served" adage. For example, it is very difficult to establish a new strain of *S. mutans* in the mouth that is already colonized with an indigenous strain of that organism. The indigenous strain has a selective advantage for specific colonization sites. In addition, suppression of indigenous bacterial flora with antibiotics can result in the proliferation of potentially harmful organisms resistant to the antibiotics, as sometimes occurs in candidiasis or colitis. Thus, the normal indigenous flora apparently assists in keeping some potentially dangerous organisms in check. Since it is not appropriate to rear normal humans in a germ-free state, the potential benefits to man of his indigenous flora will have to be inferred from indirect evidence.

Health Versus Disease

Health and disease are reciprocal concepts. Each is conventionally defined by the absence of the other. However, no independent absolute standard of either health or disease is possible. Therefore, we can only evaluate the degree to which the individual adapts to and functions effectively in relation to his natural environment. The degree to which these adaptations are effective is a measure of the well-being of the individual. The average behavior of a species in a given environment describes the reference standard of its normal health. However, such "average" or "normal" is not necessarily optimal.

When microorganisms first associate with a host, the host is said to be *contaminated.* If the microorganisms establish themselves and grow and multiply for a period of time, the host is said to be *infected.* If the infection causes damage, the host is said to have an *infectious disease.* Thus, an infectious disease is an impairment of host function by an infecting microorganism. With few exceptions, infectious diseases are caused by obligate parasites. Yet only a small fraction of the obligate parasites carried by every form of life are involved in the production of overt disease. Con-

Table 7.3: The Individual in Relation to the Determinants of Internal (Constitutional) and External Environments

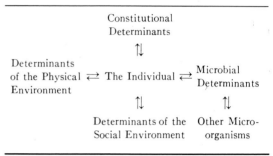

versely, a variety of potentially pathogenic microorganisms can be isolated at any time from healthy individuals. Generally, infectious disease is an infrequent byproduct of parasitization. The fact that parasitization is universal, whereas overt disease is exceptional, means that the host–parasite relationship tends to an equilibrium. Thus, consideration of those factors which maintain or disturb this equilibrium is important to an understanding of health versus disease.

Determinants of Health and Disease

We can group determinants that set the status of the individual into those of the physical environment, social environment (including psychological determinants), the individual's constitution, and the biological, particularly the microbiological, environment (Table 7.3). The arrows in Table 7.3 imply multiple determinants in each case. The use of double arrows pointing in opposite directions symbolizes the fact that not only do the determinants operate on the individual but also that he can alter the nature or effects of the determinants by his adaptive mechanisms. Man especially has brought adaptation to the point that he adjusts the environment to his advantage, rather than merely adjusting himself to it.

Determinants

Physical Determinants. The physical environment comprises such features as geography, climate, season of the year, and such derived factors as the availability and composition of food and water. Geography, for example, determines the availability of minerals. The relationships of fluoride to dental caries and of iodine to thyroid dysfunction are familiar. The seasonal associations of respiratory diseases with winter and poliomyelitis with summer are well known. Streptococcal infections and their rheumatic sequelae seem to be more serious in the semiarid mountain regions of the western United States than in the low-lying humid areas of the south. Mycotic diseases, on the other hand, are more prevalent in the south.

Cultural Determinants. Under natural conditions, adaptations to the physical environment usually take the form of evolution by selection. We are more concerned here with adaptations of a cultural nature, such as housing, clothing, diet, public sanitation, and personal hygiene, occupational conditions, degree of exposure to disease or carriers, and exposure to deleterious chemical and physical agents. The profound possibilities of psychological factors for both benefit and detriment are recognized but are beyond the scope of the present discussion. Cultural habits can be very important. A diet high in marine fish appears to provide beneficial amounts of fluoride and possibly other trace elements. On the other hand, modern preference for diets high in refined sucrose conduces to dental caries. Undoubtedly, the worldwide trend away from agrarian society to urban industrial society has epidemiological consequences that we do not yet suspect.

Constitutional Determinants. Constitutional determinants generally refer to the character of the basic biological equipment with which the individual is born. Specifically, one refers to the factors associated with race, sex, inherent immunity, familial tendencies, mental endowment, and anatomical anomalies. The constitution, however, changes as the individual develops. Human physiology changes with age, and so does the susceptibility to various infections. The common childhood diseases are generally more severe in the adult who escaped them earlier. However, in some instances increasing resistance occurs with age, probably as a result of immunization by previous subclinical experience with the given organism or with an organism conferring cross-immunity. Previous experience with disease also may weaken the general resistance by imposing too great a strain. Man can exercise some control over his constitution. Immunity can be built up by artificial immunization (vaccination). Anatomical anomalies and the effects of some diseases can be corrected surgically. Deficiencies such as diabetes and thyroid dysfunction can be met medically. The general well-being can be fostered by knowledge of diet and personal hygiene and undermined by neglect of this knowledge.

Biological Determinants. The biological environment includes the macroflora and fauna of the external environment as reservoirs and vectors of potentially pathogenic microorganisms. The external and internal microbiota also are important biological determinants. The external microbiota varies quantita- tively and qualitatively from region to region. It is sparse in arid regions, at high altitudes, and in frigid climates. It is more abundant and active in humid tropical areas. It probably differs markedly between actively cultivated agricultural regions and a modern industrial city. The internal (parasitic) microbiota, however, is basically characteristic of the host species, with regional differences superimposed. Both external and internal microbiota are subject to alterations imposed by the level of public and personal hygiene, by changing agricultural practices (e.g., the substitution of chemical fertilizers for animal and human excreta), and by changing customs (the replacement of the horse by the automobile as a means of transportation lowers the incidence of tetanus spores in an urban environment). A thoroughly applied program of active immunization reduces the incidence of the homologous parasite in the community. Another important determinant of the microbial flora is interaction with other microorganisms, which may take the form of indifference (commensalism), antagonism (antibiosis), mutual benefit (symbiosis), or cooperation (synergism) to produce results that are not brought about by any one of them alone.

Human Microbiota

In what is considered to be a state of health, the human host normally exists in some reasonable equilibrium with the bacteria, fungi, viruses and protozoa that compose its normal resident microbiota. Under such conditions the resident microorganisms are parasites and they establish either a commensal, symbiotic, or synergistic relationship with each other and with the host. These parasites may establish an antagonistic or antibiotic relationship with other members of the microbiota, which helps to establish an equilibrium within the microbiota and between the host microbiota and the microorganisms introduced into it.

However, as long as the resident microbial flora maintains a reasonable equilibrium with the human host, it is parasitic and the host is considered to be healthy (i.e., there is absence of clinical disease).

If host resistance decreases, the equilibrium between host and members of the resident microbiota may be upset and a clinically discernible infection (disease) develops in the host. The parasite causing the disease is then a pathogen. Such an infection is termed endogenous, for it is caused by microorganisms that are components of the normal human microbiota. The principal infectious diseases of the oral cavity, such as dental caries and periodontal disease, are endogenous infections in that the microorganisms causing them are normal residents of this region. Many infectious diseases are exogenous in origin, however, for they are introduced into the normal human microbiota at some point, where they invade the host and interfere with his normal functions. In a human infectious disease it must be emphasized that the infection usually takes place among mixed microbiota present on or in the area of the human body where the pathogen was introduced. This, as well as the actions of the causative agent, influences the course of the disease. An understanding of the normal microbiota of the body areas of the host is required for an understanding of the complex situation that exists in health or disease. In the following sections the indigenous microbiota of the human is discussed, as well as factors that affect the growth of microorganisms in the different body areas.

Skin

The skin sustains a relatively abundant and somewhat constant microbial flora that is limited to a relatively few species when compared to the microbiota of other body areas. The outer surface or stratum corneum is a rough surface whose scales are constantly being shed into the environment, carrying some of the resident microorganisms with them. The deeper layers contain sebaceous glands and sweat glands, whose ducts pierce the skin, and hair follicles, which also pass through the skin. The sweat glands secrete a saline solution that contains such nutrients as amino acids, carbohydrates, and vitamins for bacteria and fungi. An adequate but saline water source is available over most of the skin areas. The average temperature of the skin is maintained at 90 to 93°F (32 to 34°C), near the optimum for most pathogenic microorganisms.

Maintenance of the skin microbiota is interfered with by several factors. Sebum, secreted by the sebaceous glands, is composed mostly of lipids, which are broken down into fatty acids that are antibacterial to many microorganisms that might otherwise find the skin a suitable habitat. Another factor is the antibiotic activity of the predominantly gram-positive flora, especially against gram-negative bacteria. The slight acidity (pH 5.2 to 5.8) of the skin also may inhibit prospective microbial residents.

The skin is quite selective in which microorganisms establish temporary or permanent residence. Some fungi and yeast are common residents of the surface of the skin. These include the dermatophytes, which are principally species of *Microsporum, Trichophyton,* and *Epidermophyton*. The two principal bacterial inhabitants are *Propionibacterium acnes (Corynebacterium acnes)* and *Staphylococcus epidermidis*. Although *Mima* species and gram-negative bacilli are considered to be skin residents, the skin microbiota is predominantly gram-positive and is antagonistic to prospective gram-negative residents.

The density of the skin microbiota varies from one region of the integument to another. For example, growth is sparse on the trunk and upper arms and heavy in the axilla, scalp, face, and neck. The average density of microorganisms on the back is about 300/cm^2, while on the scalp it is about 1.5 million/cm^2, and as much as 2.5 million/cm^2 on the skin of the axilla in the male. On a weight basis, it has been estimated that the microbial population is about 530 million/g of skin scurf.

Mouth

The oral cavity is the residence of a wider variety of microorganisms than any other body area. This complex ecosystem is influenced by the morphology of the mouth, the state of oral hygiene, the nature of saliva and its rate of flow, the abrasiveness and nature of the diet, and the physiological state and health of the individual. While all these factors influence the nature and extent of the oral microbiota, saliva is the major mediating factor. Important salivary factors include rate of flow, viscosity, mineral content, ionic strength, buffering capacity, E_h, pH, essential metabolites, presence or absence of salivary gases, the organic content, and antibacterial properties (lysozyme, secretory antibodies, leukocytes).

The oral microbiota is composed of four primary ecosystems on the tongue, the tooth crown, in the gingival crevice, and in saliva. Organisms also colonize the buccal and gingival mucosa. Since each of these ecosystems provides a unique environment, the relative numbers and types of certain species can vary from site to site within the same mouth. Some microbes preferentially colonize only certain sites while other species are widely distributed in the mouth. For example, *Streptococcus sanguis* is commonly found within coronal and gingival crevice plaque, on the tongue and buccal mucosa, and in saliva, whereas *Streptococcus mutans* is most commonly associated with only the tooth surface.

Approximately 200 billion microbial cells are present in a gram of wet coronal dental plaque. This is an incomprehensible number. In fact, it takes about 6,342 years to count to 200 billion at the rate of one numeral every second. Gingival crevice plaque contains a similar concentration of microbes, while each epithelial cell on the surface of the tongue and buccal mucosa contains about 110 and 20 microbial cells, respectively. Since whole saliva bathes all of the microbe-laden oral surfaces and is constantly swallowed and replenished with bacteria-free saliva from the various salivary glands, its microbial concentration varies greatly, with an average of a few hundred million per milliliter.

Over 100 different microbial species have been recovered from the human mouth. On the average, about 35 to 40 species are normal oral residents. While the predominant organisms in the mouth are *Streptococcus, Actinomyces,* and *Veillonella,* other types include lactobacilli and other gram-positive rods or filaments, *Fusobacterium, Bacteroides,* and other gram-negative rods, *Neisseria* and *Branhamella,* micrococci, spirochetes, and occasionally yeasts, other fungi, protozoa, viruses, and mycoplasmas.

Gastrointestinal Tract

The gastrointestinal tract sustains variable numbers of microorganisms that are consistent with the various regions. Depending on the time of the sampling, the esophagus might contain few bacteria or an abundant flora similar to that of saliva or the contaminants of food and drink. At best, however, most, if not all, esophageal bacteria are transients, and the microbial flora fluctuates widely.

The stomach is not a very suitable environment for the growth of most microorganisms due to the high acidity of stomach fluids and the motility of the stomach, which empties itself rather rapidly at periodic intervals following a meal. With the intake of a meal, the microbial flora consists mostly of the salivary bacteria and the contaminants in food and drink. At other times the empty stomach contains a reduced salivary microbiota derived mostly from the swallowing of saliva. It is estimated that about 1 to 2 g of salivary bacteria is swallowed daily.

In the duodenum and the upper jejunum, the intestinal content is also acidic (pH 5 to 6), restricting the microbial population. Below the upper levels of the intestinal tract, the microbiota increases in numbers and complexity, reaching a maximum in the large intestine. Here the intestinal microbiota is predominantly gram-negative. Obligate anaerobic bacteria find the lower bowel suitable for growth, and counts average more than 10^{10}/g of feces. Facultative and aerobic organisms are also present but in lesser numbers. In the final stages of digestion in the lower bowel, the feces is comprised of about 30% bacteria. Over 90% of the fecal flora consists of *Bacteroides* and *Bifidobacterium.* Other principal residents are *Fusobacterium, Eubacterium,* and *Peptostreptococcus,* with lesser numbers of *Propionibacterium, Escherichia coli, Clostridium, Lactobacillus,* enterococci, streptococci, and others.

Upper Respiratory Tract

Many microbes are filtered from the air as it passes through the upper respiratory tract. Since most of these transient species are trapped on the mucous membranes and swallowed, the sinuses, bronchi, and lungs remain free of bacteria under normal conditions. Normal residents in the nose include various gram-positive rods and filamentous forms and staphylococci. Occasional residents are species of *Haemophilus, Neisseria,* and *Branhamella,* as well as pneumococci and moraxellae. The microbiota of the nasopharynx resembles that of the nose, consisting chiefly of staphylococci, streptococci, diphtheroids, and neisseriae, whereas that of the lower pharynx resembles the salivary flora. Here are found most of the microorganisms of the oral cavity, although anaerobic forms are not abundant.

Eye

The eye is remarkably free of a complex resident microbiota, probably owing to the washing action and high lysozyme content of tears. Residents consist of staphylococci and one or more types of gram-positive pleomorphic rods sometimes referred to as diphtheroids. Streptococci, neisseriae, and others may be present as transients.

Genitourinary Tract

The microbiota of the male external genitalia includes yeast, gram-positive bacilli, gram-negative bacilli, cocci, fusiforms, spirochetes, and *Mycobacterium smegmatis.* The microbiota of the vagina varies with age and the physiological conditions. For a month or so after birth, the vaginal epithelium accumulates glycogen as a result of transferred maternal estrogen. This glycogen provides a readily available fermentable substrate for the acidogenic and aciduric flora (principally lactobacilli). Proliferation of these organisms results in a low pH that inhibits growth of many microbial types. As the estrogen is excreted, the utilized glycogen is not replaced and the acidogenic flora decreases. This yields a more alkaline environment and a shift in the types of microbes that can flourish. After puberty, when glycogen is again present, the acidogenic and aciduric flora returns. Microorganisms found in the adult vagina are lactobacilli, diphtheroids, micrococci, staphylococci, streptococci, yeast, and an occasional gram-negative coccus or rod.

Innate Host Resistance

Man's defense against infectious diseases is a combination of innate and acquired mechanisms. Innate resistance is the sum of the defense mechanisms that are the genetic endowment of the individual, regardless of his past experience. Acquired resistance is the sum of specific adaptive reactions to previous contact with microorganisms. Innate resistance depends on the integument as a mechanical barrier, on the inhibition or destruction of microorganisms and their products that find their way onto or into tissues, on inflammation and phagocytosis, and on a vaguely defined quality of insusceptibility, due to the unresponsiveness of an individual to the microorganism or its products.

First Line of Defense—Physical and Chemical Barriers

Skin.   The first line of the body's defense is the skin and mucous membranes, which are not impenetrable mechanical barriers. Hair follicles, sweat glands, and sebaceous glands provide potential sites for microbial localization and growth. The ability of some bacteria to produce infection through the apparently intact skin suggests that they can pass through the interstices between the keratinized cells of the epidermis. However, the skin is never entirely free from microscopic breaks owing to normal wear and tear, allowing microorganisms to penetrate and enter the deeper tissues.

The skin also exerts an important bactericidal action. When millions of cells of *Proteus vulgaris,* for example, or *Staphylococcus aureus* are placed on the skin, nearly all die within 10 minutes to 2 hours. When placed on sterile glass they survive during the same periods. The bactericidal action of the skin relates to the secretion of the sweat glands, which maintain an average dermal pH from 5.2 to 5.8, and to free higher fatty acids, which are bactericidal and fungicidal. A secretion of the apocrine glands that is peculiar to the axillary and inguinal regions of the postpubertal male promotes the growth of fungi. Also contributory to bacterial control in skin is lysozyme, which hydrolyzes the cell walls of many "nonpathogenic" bacteria and kills them. Finally, the indigenous *Propionibacterium acnes (Corynebacterium acnes)* and micrococci are antibiotic to the gram-negative bacteria. The bactericidal action of the skin is greatly reduced within 15 minutes after death, indicating that unidentified mechanisms are also at work.

Alimentary Tract.   When particles such as bacteria are caught in the mucous coating of the mouth, they are washed backward and eventually swallowed. Saliva is inhibitory for nonindigenous organisms. Salivary lysozyme definitely lyses many nonpathogenic, nonindigenous bacteria, but it may injure rather than lyse "pathogenic bacteria." It does not affect any of the species indigenous to the mouth. Since the antibacterial activity of saliva is mostly due to antibiotic activities of the indigenous oral flora, it is an adaptive phenomenon rather than an innate defense. In the stomach, microorganisms are exposed to lethal acidity. A small fraction escape by lodging in particles of food or because of the diluting and buffering action of food and drink. Conditions also are not favorable for bacterial survival in the intestines above the lower half of the jejunum. The full normal intestinal flora is not encountered above the ileum, due to inhibition by the washing and bactericidal action of mucus, a low pH, pancreatic secretions, bile, and possibly lysozyme. It is not certain that living bacteria may not be susceptible to the digestive enzymes of the alimentary tract. In the large intestines, as in the mouth, antagonisms of the normal flora assist in the disposal of nonindigenous forms, especially by their production of antibiotics and bacteriocins.

Respiratory Tract.   Except under heavy exposure, less than 1% of inhaled bacteria ever reach the terminal bronchioles. They are trapped by the hairs and mucus of the nasal passages and on the pharyngeal surfaces. Movement of the ciliated epithelium lining the respiratory tract ("ciliary escalator") keeps the mucous coating in constant motion, from the upper respiratory tract backward and downward and from the trachea and bronchi upward, and the entrapped microorganisms are finally swallowed. Also, as at other sites, the chemical nature of mucous secretion may inhibit many microorganisms, and phagocytosis also contributes to the defenses of the nasal mucosa. Microorganisms that find their way into the terminal bronchioles and alveoli are removed by phagocytosis and lymphatic drainage. Therefore, the trachea, bronchi, and lungs are normally free of microbes.

Urogenital Tract.   The urethra is normally sterile in both sexes, owing in part to the flushing action and slight acidity of the urine. The cellular response to infection of the urogenital tract indicates that phagocytes are readily mobilized in this area. Also, the prostatic secretion is bactericidal. Between puberty and menopause, estrogen causes a marked thickening of the vaginal epithelium and deposition of glycogen, which is fermented by indigenous lactobacilli to lactic acid, so that the pH is too low for most other bacteria. During childhood and after the menopause, the vagina is neutral or slightly alkaline and more susceptible to infection.

Conjunctivae.   Except for a few diphtheroid bacilli, the conjunctivae are normally sterile. Much of their resistance must be due to the flushing action of the lachrymal secretion and to the high lysozyme content.

Second Line of Defense—Inflammation and Phagocytosis

General Description.   Microorganisms penetrate the skin and mucous membranes of the host through abrasions and wounds. Such microorganisms and their toxic agents injure the cells and tissues, eliciting an inflammatory response. This response involves blood vessels, cells, and organized tissues in a series of complex biochemical and morphological events that result in the homeostatic control and repair of the injury. The inflammatory events are manifested clinically by the typical signs of inflammation: heat, redness, swelling, and pain. The constitutional signs and symptoms induced by the local response relate to its severity but usually include fever, weakness, lassitude, headache, and generalized pain. In spite of these reactions, inflammation is essential for the host to combat infection and to contain and dispose of the offending pathogen so that repair can take place. If the inflammatory process loses its homeostatic controls, it becomes destructive, as in glomerulonephritis, rheumatoid arthritis, systemic hypersensitivity inflammatory reactions, and periodontal disease.

Inflammation is innate in that a similar series of events occurs in all normal human beings. The reactions do not require previous exposure to the eliciting agent, and the same reactions occur regardless of the pathogenic microbial species involved or the nature of the microbial toxic agent. However, the final outcome of the reaction may vary considerably, ranging from relatively rapid control and repair of the injury, to mutilation of tissues and to the loss of homeostasis, profound constitutional signs and symptoms, and even death.

Leukocytic Transmigration and Chemotaxis. One of the early events in acute inflammation is the migration of leukocytes across vascular barriers into the infected tissue. The total population of blood polymorphonuclear leukocytes (neutrophils, PMNs) is composed of two readily interchangeable subpopulations. One subpopulation, representing about half of all circulating neutrophils, is found in the central, axial stream within blood vessels. Cells in the marginal pool represent the remainder of the circulating neutrophils; they move out of the axial flow and move slowly along the vascular endothelium. Under normal physiological conditions, the PMNs in the marginal pool adhere to endothelial cells rarely and then only momentarily. However, during inflammation, PMNs in the marginal pool adhere closely to endothelial cells and pass between the junctions of these cells into the extravesicular space, a process known as *diapedisis*. At the same time neutrophils in the axial, central blood flow also begin migrating along endothelial surfaces.

The movement of PMNs from capillary endothelial surfaces to the site of inflammation is directed by chemotactic substances generated at the site of inflammation that diffuse toward local capillaries. In general they are mostly small short-range signaling molecules that are relatively labile. A large number of molecules are chemotactic for leukocytes. Some are normal tissue constituents or components thereof, such as fibronectin or peptides of fibrin and thrombin. One of the most potent chemotactic substances for human neutrophils is C5a, a cleavage product of the C5 component of complement (see Chap. 11). C5a can be generated by either the classic or alternate complement pathway. It has been estimated that human neutrophils have between 100,000 and 300,000 C5a receptors on their cell surface membranes. Neutrophils, monocytes, and macrophages can also respond to very low concentrations of formyl-methionyl peptides released by bacteria. Leukotriene B_4 (LTB_4) is chemotactic for human monocytes, neutrophils, and eosinophils and its activity is greatly enhanced by prostaglandin E_2.

During tissue injury caused by microbial invasion and the subsequent inflammatory response, neutrophils are the first cells to be attracted to the site. Monocytes and macrophages are not as responsive to chemotactic substances as are neutrophils. This is why neutrophils are the predominant cellular infiltrate during acute inflammation. PMNs, particularly when they are lysed, secrete a chemotactic substance to which monocytes and macrophages are responsive. Therefore, macrophages and monocytes accumulate during the subacute and chronic phases of inflammation.

Mononuclear Phagocyte System. The control of a circumscribed infection in deeper tissues is accomplished chiefly by neutrophils and macrophages. However, if an infection is not self-contained in the deeper tissues, pathogenic microorganisms, their soluble toxic products, and other proteins enter the lymphatics and eventually reach the bloodstream. The cells of the mononuclear phagocyte system (MPS) operate as a clearing mechanism. *Mononuclear phagocyte* is a general term applied to populations of phagocytic cells commonly referred to as histiocytes. Cells of the MPS are derived from monoblasts and promonocytes in bone marrow. They enter circulation as monocytes, constituting from 3% to 7% of the circulating white blood cells, then migrate into extravascular tissues as large actively phagocytic macrophages. In the lung, liver, and spleen, large numbers of macrophages populate sinuses and capillaries to form an effective filtering system that removes effete cells and foreign particulate matter from the blood. The MPS (formerly known as the reticuloendothelial system) is involved in almost any significantly severe inflammatory response in the body. When pathogenic microorganisms elicit a severe localized inflammatory response, the area is drained by lymphatics that carry off the cellular and fluid exudates. As the infection intensifies, the pathogenic bacteria enter the lymphatics, which dilate and often become inflamed (lymphangitis). Bacteria and inflammatory detritus are carried toward the closest regional lymph nodes, which attempt to filter them out of lymphatic circulation. The cells of the lymph nodes undergo hypertrophy and hyperplasia (lymphadenitis). If containment is not successful, the affected lymph node barrier breaks down and the infection spreads to other lymph nodes. If an infection is sufficiently severe, the reticuloendothelial system may be overwhelmed and the entire body may become involved in a generalized inflammatory reaction.

Exudate.   Accumulation of an exudate in the affected tissues is a characteristic feature of inflammation. Serous exudates are watery with a low protein content, and fibrinous if they are rich in protein, particularly fibrin. Purulent or suppurative exudates occur if there is much tissue destruction concomitant with pus formation. The exudate is an indicator of the reactions occurring in the inflammatory response. It is also related to the continued presence of a pathogen in the infection. In acute inflammation, removal of the pathogen results in a reversal of the inflammatory reactions, disappearance of the leukocytes, reduced permeability of the blood vessels, removal of fibrin, protein, and water, and return of the tissue to a normal state. If the pathogen and acute inflammation persist, the lysis of neutrophils releases hydrolytic enzymes that lyse tissue and cause an abscess. Such a reaction in the skin is not serious, but a similar reaction in the central nervous system, for example, is most serious.

An inflammatory reaction that becomes chronic is characterized by proliferation and the presence of monocytes and lymphocytes. Healing is characterized by a fibroblastic response that induces the formation of dense, collagenous connective tissue and scars.

The persistence of an exudate may result in a chronic inflammatory focus. This focus is characterized by the accumulation of neutrophils, fibrin, and granulation tissue that walls off the affected tissue, producing a persistent lesion.

Healing and Regeneration.   When the infection and its inflammatory reaction subside, healing and regeneration occur, with either restoration of the tissue to a normal state or its replacement by scar tissue. The regenerative capacity of tissues varies considerably. Most dental structures, endocrine glands, retinal tissue, sense organs, neurons of the central nervous system, renal glomeruli, lung parenchyma, and muscle have limited regenerative capacity. Tissues with considerable or unlimited regenerative capacity include cutaneous and mucosal epithelium, formed cells of the bone marrow, renal tubular epithelium, ductal epithelium of exocrine glands, liver parenchyma, lymphoid tissue, endothelium, and bone.

Granulomatous Inflammation.   Granulomatous inflammation occurs in response to infections such as tuberculosis, some fungal infections, syphilis, and actinomycosis. Lymphocytes, monocytes, and plasma cells are characteristically present in such a response, as are large epitheloid cells (or transformed macrophages) which unite to form multinucleated, giant cells. Also characteristic of the reaction is the peculiar clustering of the tissue macrophages (or histiocytes) about the causative microorganisms or, if the infection has persisted for some time, about a central necrotic area. Granulomatous inflammation ordinarily requires the development of a delayed-type hypersensitivity or at least an intact immunocompetence.

Suppression of Inflammatory Response.   A number of factors may suppress the inflammatory response. Any activity that interferes with bone marrow functions and formation of the short-lived neutrophils (e.g., drugs or radiation) will prevent the initiation or interfere with the continuation of the inflammatory response. The inability to form neutrophils renders an individual highly susceptible to uncontrolled infections. Factors that interfere with the formation of lymphocytes or that produce immunologically incompetent lymphocytes (e.g., chronic granulocytic leukemia) also increase susceptibility to infection.

Disorders of Leukocyte Functions and Their Consequences.   There are several disorders associated with PMNs that alter the individual's ability to successfully defend against infectious diseases. In "lazy leukocyte syndrome," a rare condition, there is a disturbance in the normal mobilization of PMNs and diminished chemotactic responsiveness. Recurrent oral infections are associated with this condition. The bone marrow shows normal numbers and maturation. PMN chemotaxis can be inhibited, usually secondary to another disease, for instance Hodgkin's disease, rheumatoid arthritis, leprosy, and infections with periopathogenic *Capnocytophaga*. Chronic granulomatous disease results in recurrent infections of and granuloma formation in lungs, lymph nodes, skin, liver, spleen, and bone. This condition is inherited and is caused by the functional absence of cytochrome b-245, which disrupts the respiratory burst and halts intracellular bacterial killing. Similar disorders are also found in the cells of the monocyte phagocytic system. In addition, many effector functions of mononuclear cells are dependent on appropriate signals received from a functional immune response. Therefore, any impairment of the immune response that decreases the activity of monocytes and macrophages will adversely affect nonspecific defenses.

Phagocytosis.   One of the principal benefits of inflammation induced by an infection is the activities of phagocytes which help to control the infection. Regardless of which phagocytic cell type is at the site of microbial invasion, the intent is to phagocytose and destroy the offending organism (Fig. 7.1). For

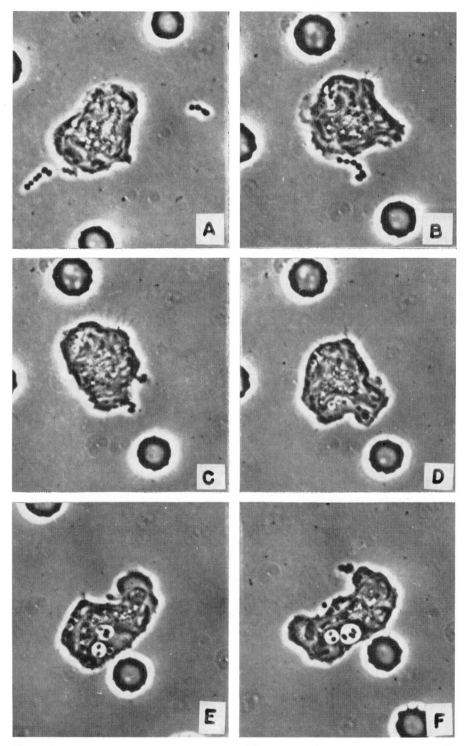

Figure 7.1: Phagocytosis and egestion of streptococci by a mouse polymorphonuclear neutrophil. **(A)** The leukocyte is near two chains of streptococci. **(B)** The shorter chain of streptococci has been phagocytized and is seen in vacuoles in the upper part of the leukocyte. **(C)** The larger chain of streptococci, which has been reproducing by cell division, is being phagocytized. **(D–F)** A streptococcal cell from the small chain is egested from the upper left-hand portion of the leukocyte; streptococci from the longer chain are in vacuoles. (Reproduced with permission from A. T. Wilson: The Egestion of Phagocytized Particles by Leukocytes. *J Exper Med,* **98,** 305, 1953.)

phagocytosis to proceed efficiently, the particle to be internalized must first be coated with opsonin. For instance, cleavage products of the C3 component of complement, a potent opsonin, attach to the surfaces of microorganisms. Some bacteria can activate the alternate complement pathway in the absence of any immune response and thereby generate C3 cleavage products. The classical complement pathway, which does require an immune response, will also generate large quantities of C3 products. Specific antibody molecules that bind to the surface of microorganisms also act as excellent opsonins. Both neutrophils and macrophages have specific receptors on their cell membranes for both C3 cleavage products and the portion of IgG molecules not bound to a microbial surface. In addition, macrophages have receptors for some carbohydrate ligands. If bacteria display these ligands on their surfaces, macrophages can bind to the bacteria directly without an opsonin intermediary. In the absence of microorganisms, the carbohydrate receptors may be important in the clearance of glycoproteins and senescent cells.

After the invading microorganism has been coated with opsonins, phagocytosis can begin, first with the attachment to a phagocytic cell and then with internalization of the microbe. The process occurs in similar fashion in both macrophages and neutrophils. Specific interaction between opsonin-coated microbe and receptors centered over clatharin pits occurs on the phagocytic cell plasma membrane. The bound microbes are then internalized within a phagosome, a phagocytic vesicle derived from the plasma membrane.

Before an internalized microorganism can be enzymatically degraded it must be killed. Phagocytic cells can kill ingested microorganisms by oxygen-dependent and oxygen-independent mechanisms. The oxygen-dependent process begins during the internalization of microorganisms when enzymes located in the phagosomal membrane are activated. There is a sharp increase in the activity of the hexose monophosphate shunt, which provides reduced nicotinamide adenine dinucleotide phosphate (NADPH). NADPH oxidase then acts on oxygen to produce the highly reactive oxygen products superoxide (O_2^-), the OH radical, and singlet oxygen O. The OH radical and singlet oxygen may by themselves be bactericidal. In addition, two superoxide anion radicals may combine in a reaction catalyzed by superoxide dismutase to form hydrogen peroxide. Hydrogen peroxide in the presence of myeloperoxidase and halides such as Cl^- or I^- forms toxic hypohalites. Hypochlorite is particularly lethal to a wide range of microorganisms. Because this process causes a sudden increase in respiratory activity, it is known as the respiratory burst.

The next step in the process involves fusion of the phagosome with preformed lysosomes also present in the cytoplasm of the phagocytic cell. Macrophages contain just one type of lysosome, neutrophils contain two distinct forms. Primary (azurophilic) granules contain a number of lytic enzymes, including acid hydrolases, lysozyme, and myeloperoxidase. The second type of preformed granule found in PMNs is called the secondary (specific) granule and contains lysozyme, lactoferrin and a vitamin B_{12} transport protein, among others. Again, in the case of PMNs, the secondary granule fuses first with the lysosome, followed by fusion with the primary granule. After fusion of the phagosome with lysosome or granules, the lysosomal contents are discharged into the newly formed composite vesicle termed a phagolysosome. When phagolysosome formation occurs, the content of the structure is acidified, typically to a pH of 3.5 to 4.0. This enhances the activity of myeloperoxidase and is the pH optimum of the majority of lysosomal enzymes. If microorganisms are killed by oxygen-independent mechanisms, this too occurs after phagolysosome formation. Lysosomal enzymes that may be important in microbial killing include lysozyme, phospholipase A_2, serine esterases, lipases, and acid phosphatase. The relative microbicidal importance of oxygen-dependent and oxygen-independent mechanisms appears to depend on the type of microorganism ingested. Regardless of the mechanism, once the microorganisms have been killed, they are degraded by lysosomal and granule enzymes.

Some leukocytes have a specialized activity in innate resistance. The eosinophils, for instance, are attracted to the usually extensive exudate of allergic reactions, and they ingest and dispose of the antigen-antibody complexes that form under such conditions. While doing so they lose their granules, as do the neutrophils. They also seem to produce substances that counteract histamine, serotonin, and bradykinin and thereby decrease the amount of the exudate that occurs in such allergic reactions.

The structure of the involved tissues may play a role in phagocytosis. Microorganisms such as *Streptococcus pneumoniae* and *Haemophilus influenzae* are not significantly phagocytized unless homologous antibodies are present. In an infection with such microorganisms, at least 5 or 6 days must elapse before homologous antibodies are detectable in the serum. The question arises as to how a host can survive the first few days of an infection with microorganisms that require homologous antibodies for phagocytosis. Both PMNs and monocytes phagocytize the resistant bacteria before the appearance of homologous antibodies by trapping them against rough tissue surfaces, between phagocytes if the tissue fluid is viscous, or by trapping them in the interstices of fibrin clots. It becomes evident, then, that tissue architecture greatly influences the efficiency of preantibody phagocytosis. This may partially account for the variances in survival rates of infections in tissues with different architecture. Formation of a walled-off necrotic abscess, either acute or chronic, greatly interferes with phagocytosis, and the infecting microorganisms survive quite well in such an environment. Such infections are very resistant to resolution and usually require a drainage procedure to remove the barrier and exudate that interferes with phagocytosis.

Other Innate Defenses

The complement system and the related properdin system, described in detail in a later chapter, are considered innate defense mechanisms. Even though they are frequently effectors of the immune system they are preexisting normal body components that may become active during many types of infectious diseases. Activation of complement directly or through the alternate system by certain bacterial cells, microbial products, or antigen–antibody complexes may result in lysis of gram-negative bacteria or enhancement of the inflammatory responses by increasing leukocyte chemotaxis and facilitating phagocytosis.

Many cells in the body, after infection with a virus, have an innate capacity to synthesize *interferon,* a substance that prevents viral replication in other cells. This is an important nonspecific defense mechanism in man, for many different viruses and other substances can induce the formation of interferon, which is then protective against replication of many different types of viruses.

Modification of Resistance

Nutrition

Malnutrition adds a stress that contributes to the likelihood of infection. Hypoproteinemia and deficiencies in the B vitamins generally increase the susceptibility of experimental animals to bacterial and rickettsial infections. Deficiency of vitamin C, possibly coupled with other nutritional disturbances resulting from alcoholism and fad dieting, for example, may enhance the development of gingivitis. The true relation of other vitamins to resistance is undetermined. There is widespread suspicion that minerals, particularly those ordinarily present in trace amounts, influence innate resistance; except for the protective effect of fluoride against dental caries, unequivocal data for man are scant.

Hormones

The adrenocortical hormones can cause a decrease in host resistance by depressing the inflammatory response. Also, diabetics, unless their disease is adequately controlled by insulin, are unusually susceptible to pyogenic infections of the extremities. The relation of estrogen to vaginal glycogen synthesis and resistance of the vagina to bacteria was discussed earlier.

Miscellaneous

Innate resistance to specific infections varies with race, age, sex, fatigue, and climate, but the specific mechanisms in each case are not well understood.

ADDITIONAL READING

Bartels, H. A. 1961. Host-Parasite Relationships in the Oral Cavity and Their Clinical Significance. NY State Dent J, **27,** 221.

Burnet, F. M. 1962. *Natural History of Infectious Disease,* Ed. 3. Cambridge University Press, Cambridge, England.

Cockburn, A. 1963. *The Evolution and Eradication of Infectious Diseases.* The Johns Hopkins Press, Baltimore.

deLouvois, J., Stanley, V. C., Leask, B. G. S., and Hurley, R. 1975. Ecological Studies of the Microbial Flora of the Female Lower Genital Tract. Proc R Soc Med, **68,** 269.

Dubos, R. J. 1965. *Biochemical Determinants of Microbial Diseases.* Harvard University Press, Cambridge, Mass.

Guba, A. M., Jr., Mulliken, J. B., and Hoopes, J. E. 1975. The Selection of Antibiotics for Human Bites of the Hand. Plast Reconstr Surg, **56,** 538.

Kloos, W. E., Zimmerman, R. J., and Smith, R. F. 1976. Preliminary Studies on the Characterization and Distribution of *Staphylococcus* and *Micrococcus* Species on Animal Skin. Appl Environ Microbiol, **31,** 53.

Lapage, G. 1958. *Parasitic Animals,* Ed. 3. W. Heffer and Sons, Cambridge, England.

Lieberman, J. (Ed.) 1958. Animal Disease and Human Health. Ann NY Acad Sci, **70,** 279.

Noble, W. C. 1975. Skin as a Microhabitat. Postgrad Med J, **51,** 151.

Rosebury, T. 1962. *Microorganisms Indigenous to Man.* McGraw-Hill, New York.

Rutgers University, Bureau of Biological Research. 1960. *Host Influence on Parasite Physiology.* Rutgers University Press, New Brunswick, N.J.

Simon, H. J. 1960. *Attenuated Infection. The Germ Theory in Contemporary Perspective.* J. B. Lippincott, Philadelphia.

Skinner, F. A., and Carr, J. G. 1974. *The Normal Microbial Flora of Man.* Academic Press, New York.

Smith, T. 1934. *Parasitism and Disease.* Princeton University Press, Princeton, N.J.

Society for General Microbiology. 1964. Symposium: *Microbial Behaviour, "In Vivo" and "In Vitro."* Cambridge University Press, New York.

8

Immunity

John A. Molinari

Immune Defense Mechanisms

Immunity is a state of increased reactivity and protection against a substance that comes in contact with a host. To appreciate the importance of immunity to life itself, one must consider the course of infectious disease as a dynamic process, whereby microbial pathogenic factors first trigger nonspecific (innate) host defense mechanisms (see Chap. 7). These innate defense mechanisms may subsequently lead to development of the second component of the immune system, the specific immune response. The intended aim of both the innate and the specific response is to eliminate harmful agents from the body, returning it to a state of homeostasis. However, significant differences exist between these two kinds of defense mechanisms, particularly in their activation or induction, the specificity of response, and manifestations of immunological memory.

Induction

Nonspecific immune defenses are always ready to function and act as the body's first line of protection. The effects of most exposures to infectious agents are limited by these innate mechanisms. They often eliminate the offending microorganisms before clinical or subclinical infection develops. Specific immunity, on the other hand, requires time and a heterogenic, intercellular collaboration to become fully responsive. In addition, specific immune responses usually require the prolonged or continued presence of a stimulus before induction occurs, while innate reactions do not require previous exposure. Thus, foreign microorganisms or toxic substances that are rapidly cleared from the body often elicit only a nonspecific immune response.

Specificity and memory

The nonspecific defense system is effective against many different agents, attempting to rid the body of any substance or infectious organism that is not a component of the normal flora or fauna. In contrast, specific immune defenses respond selectively to a triggering stimulus. The major distinguishing characteristic of this protective reaction is its specificity. On repeated exposure to the same infectious agent, the nonspecific defense system responds in exactly the same fashion to each encounter, but the specific immune system's response is usually faster, more intense, longer lasting, and provides immunological memory on subsequent challenges from the same infectious agent. These features of the specific immune system response are extremely important in the immunological control of infectious diseases. Reexposure of a host to the same infecting microorganism after an immune response has been elicited can result in either a less severe disease process or the prevention of disease entirely. This principle provides the basis for vaccination, or the deliberate immunization against a specific disease before a natural encounter with the infectious agent occurs.

Classification of Forms of Immunity

The classification of the different forms of immunity, as described above, is shown in Table 8.1. Innate defense mechanisms are protective factors concerned with species, race, and certain genetically controlled biochemical and biological reactions that are not acquired during the lifetime of the individual. In contrast to nonspecific defenses, specific or acquired immunity must be developed by the host. Both the natural and artificial components of this form of resistance are summarized in Table 8.1. Aspects of these responses are discussed in later chapters.

General Description of the Immune System

Immunity typically develops against substances that are foreign to the body, including microorganisms, many chemicals, transplanted tissues or cells, and altered components of the host's system. Foreign sub-

Table 8.1: Forms of Immunity

Natural (Innate, Nonspecific)

1. Mechanical barriers
2. Temperature
3. Oxygen concentration
4. Bactericidal activity of tissue fluids
5. Properdin system
6. Phagocytic system
7. Destruction and indifference to toxin
8. Role of normal flora
9. Genetic differences
10. Hormonal activity

Acquired (Specific)

1. Natural
   a) Active: developed by individual during recovery from clinical or subclinical disease.
   b) Passive: neonatal or newborn acquisition of immunity from maternal system, via 1) placental transmission or antibodies, or 2) colostrum during breast-feeding.
2. Artificial
   a) Active: vaccination of nonimmune individual with specific antigen preparation to stimulate active production of host immune factors.
   b) Passive: injection of antiserum into nonimmune individual.

stances capable of inducing an immune response are collectively termed *antigens*. Small- to medium-sized lymphocytes constitute the afferent limb of the immune response and act as a recognition network for antigens. A complex interaction of lymphocyte subclasses and macrophages ensues in secondary lymphoid tissues after antigen recognition has occurred. This ultimately leads to the development of the efferent or effector limb (mediators) of the immune response, which interacts specifically with antigenic chemical groups. These mediators include immunoglobulins (antibodies) and effector lymphocytes. The secondary lymphoid tissues in which the immune mediators develop include lymph nodes, the spleen, gut-associated lymphoid tissue (GALT), and lymphoepithelial tissues such as tonsils and the appendix.

Table 8.2: Properties of Humoral and Cell-Mediated Immune Responses

	Humoral Immunity	Cellular Immunity
Microbial pathogens	Pyogenic and encapsulated bacteria (staphylococci, streptococci, gonococci, pneumococci)	Intracellular parasites; chronic infections (*Mycobacterium tuberculosis,* most viruses, protozoa, and fungi)
Microbial toxins:		
Exotoxins	+	−
Endotoxins	+	−
Active components	Antibody	Specifically sensitized lymphocytes (secretion of lymphokines)
Hypersensitivity reactions	Immediate	Delayed
Transplantation rejection reactions	Hyperacute and chronic rejection phenomena	Major mechanism for rejection of transplanted organs and tissues

The source of cellular components for the immune system in an adult is the bone marrow. Bone marrow-derived lymphocytes require a complex maturation process before they become immunocompetent (i.e., able to respond to antigenic stimuli). This maturation function is provided in humans by primary lymphoid organs such as the thymus and a tissue equivalent of the bursa of Fabricius found in birds.

Immune reactions have been classically divided into humoral immunity, in which protection involves the synthesis of immunoglobulins, and cell-mediated (cellular) immunity, which requires the production of specifically sensitized lymphocytes (Table 8.2). In general, most extracellular parasitic organisms, such as staphylococci, streptococci, and gram-negative bacteria, are recognized and regulated by humoral immune mechanisms, while intracellular parasites, such as viruses, preferentially stimulate cellular immunity. These somewhat artificial separations may be misleading when one views host immunity as a dynamic biological process. A number of infectious microorganisms may actually stimulate both types of responses, owing to the presence of multiple antigens. Both responses also share some common cellular elements and regulatory mechanisms.

ADDITIONAL READING

For additional reading, see Chapter 12, pages 147–149.

9

Antigens (Immunogens) and Immunoglobulins

John A. Molinari

Antigens and the Nature of Immunogenicity

An antigen, more recently called an immunogen, is any substance that is capable, under appropriate conditions, of inducing an immune response and of reacting specifically in some demonstrable manner with the products of the response. There are two distinct parts to the definition, and both are important in determining the potential of natural and synthetic substances to elicit specific responses. A substance that fulfills both criteria—i.e., that has the property of immunogenicity and that can react with specific immunoglobulins or sensitized lymphocytes—is classified as a complete antigen. Many microbial components and products, such as cell wall peptidoglycans, enzymes, exotoxins, and endotoxins, act as complete antigens in exposed hosts.

A large number of substances fall into the category of incomplete antigens, or *haptens*. Haptens are not immunogenic by themselves but can react with the products of a specific response. Numerous examples of haptens are found in dental medicine and medicine. These include antibiotics, local anesthetic preparations, ointments, disinfectants, and antiseptics. Landsteiner demonstrated that when small chemical compounds (molecular weight [MW] <1,000 daltons) were coupled to a larger molecule (i.e., a carrier), they could stimulate the synthesis of immunoglobulins specific for the small molecule. Once bound to the carrier, the hapten–carrier complex formed a complete antigen, and the immunoglobulins which were synthesized were shown to react with the small chemical compound alone. Landsteiner's pioneering work and subsequent studies have allowed for better understanding of the nature of antigenic determinants, as well as the nature of the antigenic binding site on immunoglobulins.

It is important to understand the relationship between structure of an antigenic molecule and its in-

Table 9.1: Classification of Antigens

Foreign (i.e., outside the host)
   Microbial components or products
      (cell walls, pili, enzymes,
      toxins, etc.)
   Drugs
   Environmental antigens
Autoantigens
   Thyroglobulin
   Cellular nucleic acids
   Corneal components
Isoantigens
   Histocompatibility tissue antigens
   Blood group antigens
Heteroantigens
   Heterophile antigens
   Cross-reacting microbial antigens
      (streptococcal cell wall components that share
      immunogenicity with human cardiac and
      glomerular tissues)

teraction with elements of the immune system. The portions of a macromolecule that bind with the recognition elements of the lymphoid system and that also can combine with immunoglobulin are called antigenic determinants. These sites may represent a very small fraction of the entire mass or size of the molecule. Further, multiple types of antigenic determinants are present on or within viable microorganisms. Thus, the body's response to many infections often includes the development of more than one specific immune component.

Characteristics of Antigens

Although an extensive variety of substances can function as antigens, certain minimal properties are required in determining their immunogenicity. These include foreignness, type of molecule (i.e., chemical complexity), molecular weight, and solubility.

Foreignness.   Ordinarily, a substance must be recognized by the immune system of the responding host as foreign, or "not self," in order to stimulate an immune response. This is the single most important property of an antigen. In general, an individual does not respond immunologically to a substance that is part of its own body ("self"). Breakdown in the immune recognition system can occasionally occur, with the subsequent development of autoimmunity, or immunity against self. The degree of foreignness to an individual's tolerated, genetically controlled tissue antigens also provides a basis for the clinical distinction of certain antigens (Table 9.1). Important terms to note here include the following:

Autoantigens: host tissue components that normally are not antigenic in the host but are capa-

ble of inducing a self-destructive autoimmune response when tolerance is broken down.

Alloantigens (isoantigens): genetically controlled antigens that distinguish one individual of a species from another genetically nonidentical member of the same species.

Xenoantigens (heteroantigens): cross-reacting antigens found in a variety of unrelated species. The term **heterophile antigen** is also applicable.

Type of Molecule.   It is generally accepted that the greater the chemical complexity of a substance, the more likely it is to be antigenic. This correlation is illustrated by the different classes of macromolecules listed in Table 9.2. Proteins often serve as the best complete antigens. The heterogeneity of amino acids in the primary structure and their defined secondary and tertiary characteristics are important factors in delineating a protein's immunogenicity. In contrast, homopolymeric polypeptides tend to be poorer antigens. Aromatic amino acids such as tyrosine are more likely to confer antigenicity than are nonaromatic amino acids. Protective immunity against numerous bacterial and viral infections such as tetanus, tuberculosis, and hepatitis B virus infection is directed against specific microbial proteins.

Polysaccharides and carbohydrate-containing molecules may also act as complete antigens. For example, immunity against pneumococcal and meningococcal pneumonia and *Haemophilus influenzae* meningitis is directed at the capsular polysaccharides produced by virulent bacterial strains. Additionally, the immunologic basis of the ABO blood group system is related to the presence of genetically determined amino sugars on erythrocyte plasma membranes.

Table 9.2: Macromolecules as Antigens

Proteins
   Exotoxins
   Enzymes
   Flagella
   Viral capsids
Carbohydrates
   Bacterial capsules
   Blood group antigens
   Lipopolysaccharides (endotoxins)—O-antigen
      portion
Nucleic acids
   DNA
   RNA
Fatty acids and lipids
   Bovine antigen
   Lipopolysaccharides—
      lipid moiety
   Forssman antigens

Nucleic acids are not usually immunogenic; however, in some autoimmune diseases (i.e., systemic lupus erythematosus) antibodies develop to host DNA. Both DNA and RNA have been shown to function primarily as haptens. The least antigenic classes of natural substances are lipids and fatty acids. Lipid portions of complex molecules, such as the lipopolysaccharides from gram-negative bacteria, appear to have more of a potential for tissue toxicity than for immunogenicity.

Molecular Weight. A substance must have a sufficiently high molecular weight in order to function as a complete antigen. Although some synthetic substances with molecular weights of around 2,000 daltons are able to stimulate humoral or cellular immune responses, as a general rule, substances with molecular weights below 10,000 daltons are either weakly antigenic or nonantigenic. Some of the most immunogenic antigens, such as microbial enzymes and exotoxins, are proteins with molecular weights of 100,000 daltons or greater.

Solubility and Position of Antigenic Determinants. In general, the more insoluble an antigenic molecule once it enters the individual's system, the greater is its immunogenicity. Although there are exceptions to this general finding, a host's immune system will more efficiently respond to specific determinants which are present in molecules that are insoluble in tissues. In addition, antigenic determinants must also be available to recognition units on small lymphocytes. Usually this means that the determinants are located on the exterior of a complete antigen.

Immunoglobulin Structure and Function

Immunoglobulins are complex protein molecules produced by plasma cells and some lymphocytes in response to antigenic stimuli. The key concept for their function is *specificity,* as they are able to react in a specific manner with the antigen that triggered the response. Although it is now customary to use the general term immunoglobulin, commonly employed synonyms have been *antibody* and γ-*globulin.* The association of antibody activity with the γ-globulin fraction of electrophoresed serum was first demonstrated by Tiselius and Kabat in 1939. Although most immunoglobulins migrate to this zone, later studies also showed substantial immunoglobulin activity in the β-globulin serum portion.

The immunoglobulins represent a heterogeneous group of glycoproteins found throughout the body. Immunoglobulin molecules of each species are subdivided into different classes on the basis of their backbone structure rather than according to their specificity for distinct antigens. As a consequence of their structure, immunoglobulins exhibit two characteristic functional areas. One area has the ability to physically combine with the antigenic determinants of immunogens. The second area determines the biological activity of immunoglobulin before and after it has complexed with antigen. The basic unit of each immunoglobulin is composed of four polypeptide chains: two identical 25,000-dalton molecular weight chains, termed light (L) chains, and two identical chains, each of 50,000-dalton molecular weight, called heavy (H) chains. These four polypeptide chains are held together by a variable number of interchain disulfide hydrogen bonds (Fig. 9.1).

Our understanding of the basic structure and amino acid sequence of light chains was greatly enhanced by studying patients with certain forms of lymphoid neoplasia. These individuals were found to be suffering from multiple myeloma. A myeloma is a neoplasm composed of a highly uniform population (clone) of malignant plasma cells that can synthesize large amounts of homogeneous immunoglobulin molecules. The concentrations of the plasma cell products may become so high that in many myeloma patients excreted urine contains large quantities of free, identical light chains. These free light chains are called *Bence Jones proteins,* after the physician who discovered them. In addition to serving in light chain structural studies, three-dimensional isolated Bence Jones proteins provided a source of abundant homogeneous material for amino acid sequence analysis.

Light Chains

There are two classes of immunoglobulin light chains in man. About 60% of complete immunoglobulin molecules contain kappa (κ) chains and about 40% have lambda (λ) chains. Although both types are approximately 214 amino acids long, they differ considerably in amino acid sequences. Close examination of the amino acid sequences of light chains has revealed the presence of two domains. The first 110 to 112 amino acids beginning from the amino-terminal end of the light chain show a high degree of sequence variability when the sequences of many light chains of the same class are compared. For this reason, the area composed of the amino-terminal half of the light chain has been called the variable domain (V_L). On the other hand, the amino acid sequences of the carboxy-terminal half of the light chains (approximately 110 to 112 amino acids) show a high degree of homology when light chains of the same class are compared. Therefore, the carboxy-terminal half of the molecule is called the constant domain (C_L). Amino acid sequence differences in light chain constant domains

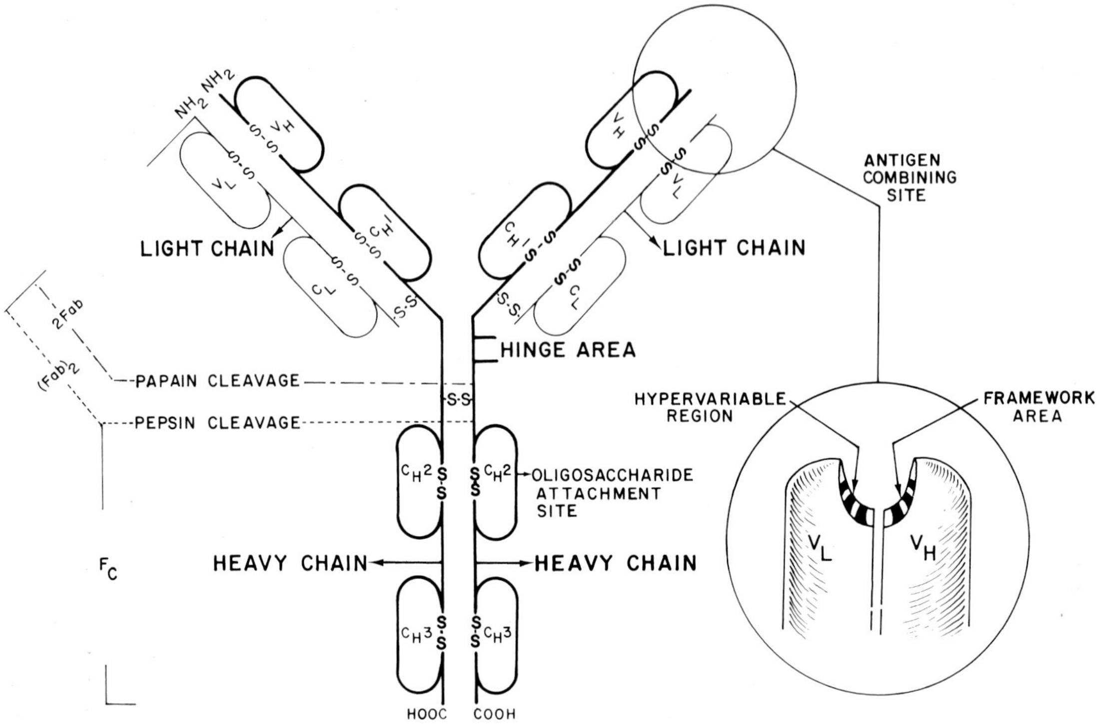

Figure 9.1: Schematic representation of structural features of an IgG molecule. The amino acid sequence of heavy and light chains is arranged in domains, either variable (V_H and V_L) or constant (C_L and C_H1, C_H2, and C_H3). Disulfide bonds (—S—S—) are located within each domain, covalently link light chain to heavy chain, and covalently link heavy chain to heavy chain. Proteolytic enzyme cleavage of the molecule by papain results in three fragments: two identical fragments (2 Fab) and approximately one half of both heavy chains, including the inter-heavy chain disulfide bond (Fc). Proteolytic enzyme cleavage of the molecule by pepsin leaves one large fragment; both light chains and approximately the amino one-half of both heavy chains extending to the interheavy chain disulfide bond (Fab)$_2$. *Inset,* detail of the antigen combining site. *Darkened areas* represent hypervariable regions that actually form the combining site. *White areas* represent framework areas that maintain the overall structure of the variable domains.

specify the light chain class. Each light chain is bound to a heavy chain via a single disulfide bond near the carboxy-terminus of the light chain. Functionally, the light chain variable domain, when paired with the variable domain of a heavy chain, constitutes the antigen-binding site of the complete immunoglobulin molecule. The amino acid sequences of both light chains on a single immunoglobulin molecule are identical.

Heavy Chains and the Three-Dimensional Structure of Immunoglobulins

There are five different classes of heavy chains found in human immunoglobulins, designated α, γ, μ, δ, ϵ. Subclasses of heavy chains have been distinguished within the γ, μ, and α classes. Heavy chain classes have been identified on the basis of both differences in amino acid sequences and qualitative and quantitative differences in oligosaccharide side chains

that are attached to heavy chain constant domains. Whereas the total polypeptide chain length of light chains can be divided into two domains, variable and constant, both of approximately equal length, the full heavy polypeptide chain is composed of one variable domain and an additional three or four constant domains (C_H1 to C_H4), also of approximately equal length. In the completed immunoglobulin molecule, two identical heavy chains are joined together by a minimum of one disulfide bond, located in a linear stretch of amino acids near the midpoint of the polypeptide length.

When the four chains have been joined by disulfide bonds to form an immunoglobulin unit, the variable domains of both light chain (V_L) and heavy chain (V_H) are arranged in a parallel fashion to form the antigen-combining site. The length of heavy chains that extends beyond the attached light chains has been designated the Fc portion. Biological functions that are apparent before and after the immunoglobulin has combined with specific antigenic determinants on antigens are due to properties of the Fc portion of the immunoglobulin. Certain cells—macrophages, for example—contain receptors for the carboxy-terminus of the Fc portion of immunoglobulins on their surface membranes. When antigen–immunoglobulin complexes are formed, macrophages can bind the immunoglobulin at the receptor to enhance phagocytosis. Also, the Fc portion determines whether or not an immunoglobulin will cross the placenta from maternal to fetal circulation. In addition, after an immunoglobulin has combined with antigen to form an immune complex, the Fc portion determines whether or not complement will be fixed.

Based on evidence obtained from a variety of techniques, the typical monomeric immunoglobulin molecule is thought to be T- or Y-shaped. Midway along the length of the H chains near the inter-H chain disulfide bonds is a "hinge" area that allows the arms of the T or Y to flex (see Fig. 9.1). This structure is biologically significant. The monomeric immunoglobulin molecule is symmetric, possessing two antigen-combining sites, and for this reason is termed bivalent. The hinge area allows the antigen-combining sites some degree of mobility, meaning that the immunoglobulin molecule can accommodate to minor variations in the distance between two identical antigenic determinants on the surface of an antigen and still combine in a bivalent fashion.

Proteolytic Enzyme Fragmentation

During early attempts to determine the structure of immunoglobulin molecules, proteolytic enzyme cleavage was employed to assist in analyzing biological function and shape. Knowledge of the resulting fragment names is also helpful because it allows one to identify specific areas of the immunoglobulin molecule that are responsible for individual activities.

Papain Cleavage. When papain is added to IgG, three fragments are produced, two of which are essentially identical and a third that is unique. The identical fragments each contain a portion of the immunoglobulin, which can combine with antigenic determinants in a univalent manner. These fragments are designated Fab (antigen-binding fragments) and correspond to the entire light chain and approximately the amino-terminal half of the heavy chain. The third fragment does not combine with antigen but is so homogeneous that it crystallizes under appropriate conditions and therefore is designated Fc (crystallizable fragment). The Fc portion is located on the carboxy-terminal half of the heavy chains, including the inter-H chain disulfide bonds. This site is important as the portion of the molecule responsible for immunoglobulin attachment to certain cell surfaces.

Pepsin Cleavage. Analysis of the IgG fragments that result from pepsin cleavage reveals one rather large fragment with bivalent antigen-binding activity (designated (Fab)$_2$) but no Fc fragment. The (Fab)$_2$ fragment is composed of the entire length of both light chains and the amino-terminal half of both H chains, including the inter-H chain disulfide bonds and the hinge region. If the inter-H chain disulfide bonds are cleaved, then univalent fragments result that are about 10% heavier (due to increased H chain length) than the corresponding papain fragment (Fab). Therefore, the cleaved pepsin fragment is designated Fab'C instead of Fab.

Immunoglobulin Classes

All immunoglobulin molecules share many structural and some functional features (Table 9.3). In the following section, pertinent differences in structure and biological functioning of human immunoglobulins will be emphasized. The nomenclature of complete immunoglobulins is derived from the designation of their component heavy chains. Thus, an immunoglobulin composed of γ heavy chains becomes immunoglobulin G (IgG); immunoglobulins with μ heavy chains become IgM; with α heavy chains, IgA; with δ heavy chains, IgD; and with ϵ heavy chains, IgE.

IgG

IgG may be divided into four subclasses (IgG1 through IgG4) based on distinctive differences on the Fc segments of their respective heavy chain domains (γ_1 through γ_4). IgG as a class represents about 85% of the total immunoglobulin found in blood. IgG1 is by far the most prevalent IgG, followed in descending order of blood concentration by IgG2, IgG3, and IgG4. Complement-fixing ability is assessed in terms of IgG subclasses: IgG1 and IgG3 fix complement rather efficiently, IgG2 fixes complement less efficiently, and the ability of IgG4 to fix complement is questionable.

IgG molecules are the only class of antibodies that are bound to and actively transported across the placenta. Therefore, maternal IgG provides the source of antibody protection for the developing fetus (i.e., natural passive immunity). After birth, maternal IgG levels gradually diminish and virtually disappear by the time the infant reaches a few months of age.

For protective functions within the body, IgG antibodies are perhaps most useful because of their opsonic capacity (ability to enhance phagocytosis). IgG mainly enhances this function in macrophages, one of the cell types that possess receptors for the Fc portion of IgG molecules on their cell surface membranes.

Table 9.3: Properties of Human Immunoglobulin Classes

Property	IgG	IgM	IgA	IgE	IgD
Molecular weight (x10⁵)	150	800–950	Serum—160 Secretory—400	190	180
Normal serum concentration (mg/100 mL)	1,240	120	Serum—280	0.003	3
Half-life (days)	23	5	6	1–5	3
Heavy chain	$\gamma1, \gamma2, \gamma3, \gamma4$	$\mu1, \mu2$	$\alpha1, \alpha2$	ϵ	δ
Light chain	κ and λ	κ and λ	κ and λ	κ and λ	κ and λ
Extra chains/components		J chains	Serum—J chain Secretory—J chain SC		
Carbohydrate (%)	2.9	11.8	7.5	10.7	12
Biological properties	1. Major Ig in serum 2. Antibacterial, antiviral, antitoxin 3. Ig that crosses placenta 4. Fixes complement 5. Cytophilic for macrophages and PMNs	1. First Ig in response to antigen 2. Blood group antibodies 3. Antibacterial, antiviral 4. Fixes complement	1. Major activity in secretions 2. Antibacterial, antiviral 3. Prevents microbial attachment onto epithelial surfaces	1. Reaginic fixation onto skin 2. Anaphylactic allergies 3. Antiparasitic 4. Homocytotrophic for mast cells, basophils, platelets	1. Major Ig on B-lymphocytes 2. Certain allergic reactions 3. Other functions unknown

Therefore, any antigen to which IgG is bound can be rather efficiently phagocytized by macrophages due to the presence of the IgG Fc receptor. This phenomenon is particularly important in infectious diseases caused by etiological agents that by themselves are not easily phagocytized by macrophages, e.g., encapsulated *Streptococcus pneumoniae*. Specific IgG antibodies also play an important role in viral and toxin neutralization as well. When a sufficient number of IgG antibodies bind to intact virus particles, the virion cannot attach to or penetrate through the cytoplasmic membrane of a susceptible cell. In a similar manner, IgG molecules bound to a bacterial exotoxin inhibit the biological activity of that exotoxin. Of interest, the antigenic determinant on the exotoxin that elicits protective immunoglobulin responses is probably different from the biologically active site of the toxin.

IgG is thought to be the most important immunoglobulin class involved in elimination of extracellular infectious agents, under conditions where circulatory patterns allow the IgG access to body compartments that might harbor such agents. Furthermore, most immunization procedures primarily induce an IgG response, and therefore this Ig is extremely important in vaccination against infectious diseases.

IgM

IgM was originally named macroglobulin because of its high molecular weight (about 900,000 daltons). This large size is due to the fact that IgM is present in blood as a pentamer ($\mu_{10}L_{10}$) composed of five monomeric subunits, each of which is composed of two light chains (either κ or λ) and two heavy chains (μ). Structural studies on IgM were aided by the isolation of high concentrations of IgM from the urine of patients with a particular type of plasma cell myeloma, Waldenström's macroglobulinemia. IgM monomeric subunits are held together with two disulfide bonds linking Fc portions of the μ chains. One disulfide bond is located in the C_H3 domain, the second is located between penultimate amino acids in the C_H4 domain. In addition to amino acid sequence differences and oligosaccharide differences, μ chains differ structurally from γ heavy chains. The former lack a hinge area and have an additional segment of 130 amino acids between the C_H1 and C_H2 domains. In essence, the additional amino acids amount to another domain. Therefore, μ chains are said to have five domains: one variable domain and four constant domains.

Multimeric forms of immunoglobulins such as IgM possess an additional structure not found on IgG or other monomeric forms of immunoglobulin. This is a 15,000-dalton polypeptide that is structurally different from all classes of Ig and is termed the J chain (joining chain). It is synthesized in the same cell in which IgM is synthesized. There is a single J chain for every multimeric immunoglobulin and it is attached to the Fc segment of heavy chains near the carboxy-terminus by two disulfide bonds. Because J chains are seen only in association with multimeric immunoglobulins, it is believed that the J chain is necessary to stabilize these multimeric forms.

IgM accounts for about 10% of the immunoglobulin in normal human blood. It fixes complement very efficiently. Biologically, IgM functions in a manner similar to IgG, with opsonization being one of its most important functions. IgM and IgG can both be produced in response to the same antigenic stimulus. When this occurs, IgM is detected first but is not synthesized for as long or in as large a quantity as is IgG. Monomeric subunits of IgM can be found on the surfaces of B-lymphocytes and probably function as antigen receptors. Finally, IgM acts as an isohemagglutinin that can bind to the specific blood group antigens on the surface of erythrocytes; it is a normal constituent of blood.

IgA

IgA can be present in a monomeric as well as various polymeric forms. In human serum, where it represents approximately 15% of the total serum immunoglobulin, it is present in a typical monomeric form (α_2L_2). IgA is also present in exocrine secretions such as saliva, lacrimal secretions, mucus of the gut and respiratory tree, colostrum, and urogenital mucosa. When present in exocrine secretions, IgA is usually present as a dimer (α_4L_4) and, like the polymeric form of IgM, possesses one J chain per dimer. In addition to the J chain, secretory IgA (sIgA) has a glycoprotein (9% carbohydrate, MW-71,000) attached to the Fc component of α chains via noncovalent bonds and disulfide bonds. This additional glycoprotein is called either secretory component (SC), secretory piece (SP), or transport piece (TP).

Secretory Piece. Secretory piece is attached to the IgA dimer via the approximating Fc portions of the two IgA monomer units. It is not synthesized by the plasma cell that synthesizes IgA but rather is produced by epithelial cells lining the ducts of exocrine glands, termed acinar cells. SP appears to play two important roles in the maturation and function of biologically active sIgA. First, secretory piece may act as a transport molecule, binding dimeric IgA on the tissue side of the epithelial lining and then transporting the dimeric IgA across the epithelial cell to be released on the luminal side of the epithelial lining. After release from the epithelial cell, SP remains attached to the IgA. Second, SP appears to increase the resistance of sIgA to proteolytic enzyme degradation and low pH found in areas such as the gut and oral cavity.

There are two subclasses of α heavy chains, designated α1 and α2. Both α1 and α2 polypeptides have four domains (one variable and three constant). However, α1 has a much larger hinge area that is not present in α2 chains. The hinge area of α1 chains is particularly susceptible to cleavage by proteolytic enzymes released from specific strains of streptococci and neisseria. On the other hand, the foreshortened α2 polypeptides seem to be remarkably resistant to this bacterial proteolytic attack. Therefore, the heavy chain composition of sIgA has definite implications in the ability of sIgA to function extracorporeally, such as in the oral cavity where these organisms are common. Interestingly, approximately 90% of serum IgA is composed of α1 heavy chains, whereas the composition of sIgA seems to be at least equally distributed between α1 and α2 polypeptides, or perhaps a predominance of α2 polypeptides.

Biologically, sIgA acts by interfering with the attachment of bacteria to mucosal surfaces. It may also interfere with the ability of viruses such as influenza virus, which is trophic for mucosal epithelium, to attach to and then penetrate these cells. Finally, sIgA may prevent the absorption of nonliving antigens by the mucosa of the lungs and the gut, and later may prevent the transport of antigens across the mucosa. sIgA is of great importance to dental medicine because it is functionally present in saliva and is a major resistance factor against infections by oral microorganisms and in maintaining the balance of the oral microflora.

IgE

IgE is a very minor component of serum. Because of its low serum concentration (approximately 0.03 μg/mL), its discovery was delayed until the 1960s. Structurally, IgE is composed of two identical ε heavy chains and two identical light chains of either the κ or λ class ($\epsilon_2 L_2$). Like μ heavy chains, ε heavy chains have one variable domain and four constant domains. In addition, ε heavy chains have a high carbohydrate content (approximately 11.5%). IgE is similar to IgG in that it does not tend to form multimeric units.

In terms of biological function, IgE represents a bit of an enigma. The most familiar function of IgE involves its role as a mediator of acute immediate hypersensitivity reactions such as seen in insect venom allergy or hay fever and asthma. It would be difficult to convince a hay fever sufferer that this condition was related to a protective mechanism against some life-threatening infection. However, IgE also plays a role in protection against percutaneous infections of some parasites. In either event, one very important property of IgE is its ability to bind via its Fc portion (C_H4 and perhaps C_H3) to specific receptors located on the surface of mast cells and basophilic leukocytes. These cells contain vasoactive amines that can be released when surface-bound IgE is cross-linked by specific antigen. IgE does not fix complement in the manner that IgG and IgM do. However, aggregated IgE can activate complement via the alternate pathway.

IgD

Although IgD levels vary somewhat in human sera, on average they represent about 2% of the total serum immunoglobulin present. Their overall structure is similar to that of IgG except they do not appear to be as compact as IgG or other immunoglobulins. This may account for their increased sensitivity to proteolysis. IgD is also quite heat labile.

No functional role has been assigned to serum IgD, although this immunoglobulin has been detected in abundance on the surface of B-lymphocytes linked via its Fc portion. IgD may therefore play a role as a specific antigen-binding site on B-lymphocytes, which are the precursor cells of immunoglobulin-producing cells. Furthermore, IgD appears on the B-lymphocyte surface after the appearance of monomeric IgM and may be a step in the normal maturation of immunocompetent B-lymphocytes.

Variable Domains and Antigen-Combining Sites

Variable Domains

Comparison of the amino acid sequences of polypeptide chains from the same class of immunoglobulin molecules shows that they differ from each other at many positions in the 110 to 112 residues at the amino-terminal end. For this reason, this amino-terminal stretch of amino acids has been designated the variable region or domain. Closer examination of this sequence has revealed that these differences are more pronounced at certain areas within the variable domain. These highly variable regions consist of 5 to 10 residues located at positions 30 to 35, 50 to 55, and 95 to 100 on both H chains and L chains, and are termed hypervariable regions. Hypervariable regions comprise the antigen-combining site of the immunoglobulin molecule. Considering the vast array of antigenic determinants present in nature, it is not surprising that extreme amino acid variability in hypervariable regions would be necessary to form a three-dimensional, complementary site to physically accommodate many different antigenic determinants.

The amino acid sequences on either side of the hypervariable regions of many immunoglobulins are far less variable; these are called framework regions. Each variable domain on both the heavy and light chains consists of four relatively constant framework regions and three hypervariable regions. Because of the invariance found in certain framework sequences, variable domains have been divided into three types: one associated with heavy chains, one associated with κ light chains, and one associated with λ light chains. Whereas the hypervariable regions determine the antigenic specificity of the immunoglobulin molecule, the framework regions are extremely important in maintaining a consistent overall shape of the entire variable domain.

Antigen Combining Sites—Light Chain and Heavy Chain Interaction

H chains that have been separated and isolated from a functional immunoglobulin will bind to the antigen, although not as strongly as the original, complete immunoglobulin. Isolated light chains do not bind well with antigen. It thus appears certain that the hypervariable regions of both heavy and light chains contribute to the overall binding properties of the intact immunoglobulin. The variable domains of heavy and light chains are arranged in such a way that the hypervariable regions from both chains form a cleft or pocket that will accommodate all or a portion of the corresponding antigenic determinant.

Three-Dimensional Structure

Each domain, variable or constant, and consisting of a stretch of amino acids approximately 110 to 112 residues long, is arranged in a compact globular shape. The polypeptide chain of each domain is folded in such a way that there are three relatively straight stretches in one plane and four relatively straight stretches in a second, antiparallel plane. In addition, each domain has one intrachain disulfide bond that apparently stabilizes the structure. This conformation gives rise to a sandwich-like or barrel-like structure. Domains residing on the same chain are linked to one another by short, linear interdomain polypeptides. The hinge region, located between C_H1 and C_H2 of heavy chains, also is composed of a linear polypeptide. The length of the hinge region varies according to the class of heavy chain. The hinge region also contains a variable number of cysteine residues that provide the locations for inter-heavy chain disulfide bonds. The fact that this region consists of single linear stretches of amino acids may explain why the hinge region is so susceptible to proteolytic enzyme cleavage.

Bound Carbohydrates

Although immunoglobulin molecules contain distinct carbohydrate side chains, the molecular and clinical functions of the latter are not as yet clearly delineated. Most of these oligosaccharide moieties are linked to asparagine heavy chain polypeptides; however, serine residues have also been found to form glycosidic bonds. In addition to their presence on the Fc portions of heavy chains, carbohydrates have been generally detected attached to J chains and secretory component, but not to light chains. A definitive function for immunoglobulin carbohydrates has not been elucidated. They may play a role in the secretion of the immunoglobulin molecule from plasma cells and may assist in the specific biological activities of the immunoglobulin Fc regions.

ADDITIONAL READING

For additional reading, see Chapter 12, pages 147–149.

10

Tissue and Cellular Basis for the Immune Response

John A. Molinari

Chapter 8 considered innate and acquired immune responses and introduced the concept of intercellular collaboration during the induction of humoral and cellular immunity. Cooperative interaction among a variety of phagocytic and lymphoid cells normally occurs in a series of highly regulated steps aimed at the destruction and elimination of invading microorganisms and foreign antigens. The origins of the defender cells and their individual and combined functions provide the basis for a network of defenses.

Lymphoid Organs and Tissues

The lymphoid system may be divided into three main units, or compartments, each of which plays an important role in the elaboration of end effector cells and immune products. The three compartments are stem cells, primary or central lymphoid tissues, and secondary or peripheral lymphoid tissues.

Stem Cells

Lymphocytes and other formed blood elements are derived from multipotent hematopoietic stem cells. During fetal development the stem cells are initially found in the yolk sac and later in the fetal liver. After birth, stem cells are found in bone marrow. Progenitor cells arising from stem cells develop into immature erythroid cells (which terminally differentiate into erythrocytes), myeloid cells (which ultimately differentiate into granulocytes), and lymphocytes. In the case of early or immature lymphocytes, terminal differentiation into either B- or T-lymphocytes occurs in other primary lymphoid organs—the bursa of Fabricius or its equivalent in humans, and the thymus, respectively.

Primary Lymphoid Tissues

Thymus. The thymus is often referred to as the master organ of the immune system. It is derived from the third and possibly the fourth pharyngeal pouches in the developing embryo as epithelium migrates from these pouches to the midline of the upper thorax. The rudimentary thymus is eventually populated with identifiable cells, termed thymocytes, derived from hematopoietic stem lymphocytes in the fetal liver. These thymocytes are one of the most active sources of lymphocyte proliferation. Only 5% to 10% of the resulting lymphocytes actually mature into long-lived immunocompetent cells, designated T- or thymus-derived lymphocytes. The remainder are short-lived and die within the thymus. Although the maturation process is not completely understood, it is known that only those lymphocytes that emerge from the thymus can carry out T-cell functions.

Abundant data indicate that one or more thymic hormones synthesized by epithelial cells of the thymus trigger the differentiation of less mature thymocytes into immunocompetent T-lymphocytes. After maturation, T-lymphocytes leave the thymus and enter the peripheral blood and lymphatic circulation. In addition, they populate secondary lymphoid tissues such as lymph nodes, the spleen, and gut-associated lymphoid tissue.

The mature thymus consists of a reticular network containing numerous lymphocytes. Thus, this organ contains both lymphoid and epithelial components. It is largest at birth and remains very active until puberty, at which time it begins to involute. The adult thymus is considerably smaller than a prepubescent thymus but continues to be an important source of lymphocytes and humoral immune factors. This information has clinical relevance: thymectomy in an adult does not result in the life-threatening consequences of neonatal thymectomy. When neonatal thymectomy is performed in animals a drastically altered immune response results. The number of circulating lymphocytes is substantially reduced. Additionally, cellular immune manifestations of the acquired immune system, including the ability to reject foreign tissues, the ability to recover from many infectious diseases, and the ability to produce immunoglobulins other than IgM, are greatly reduced or completely eradicated. A similar situation can be seen in human infants if the thymus fails to form embryonically (thymic dysplasia) or does not function properly.

Bursa of Fabricius (Bursal Equivalent). Birds possess a lymphoepithelial organ that anatomically resembles the thymus. It begins as epithelial tissue derived from the intestine and is later populated by migratory immature lymphocytes. When these cells mature in the bursa and become immunocompetent, the resulting lymphocytes are very distinct from mature T-lymphocytes. Cells leaving the bursa have immunoglobulins attached to the surface of the plasma membranes and will produce specific antibodies when stimulated under the appropriate conditions with antigens. These cells are called B-lymphocytes (bursa derived). Mammals do not have a bursa as a discrete organ. The presumption of a bursal equivalent in mammalian species, however, remains a conceptual rationale for the development and differentiation of B-lymphocytes.

Bone Marrow. Substantial data indicate that hematopoietic B-lymphocytes are produced initially by the fetal liver, with the bone marrow assuming this function in the adult. Approximately half of the marrow tissue is devoted to hematopoiesis. Lines of primitive, undifferentiated stem cells mature in bone marrow and are ultimately released as either erythrocytes, granulocytes, platelets, monocytes, or lymphocytes.

Secondary Lymphoid Tissues

Lymph Nodes. Lymphatic vessels begin in peripheral tissues at the capillary level and are structurally similar to venous circulation. Smaller vessels merge to form larger ones until lymphatic flow enters the venous circulation via the thoracic and right lymphatic ducts. Interspersed in this network of lymph vessels are lymph nodes, small lymphoid tissues that function primarily as filtering sites. Representative lymph node activities are phagocytosis of particulate material, concentration of immunogens, and lymphoid cellular activity, by which numerous foreign substances are routinely trapped and eliminated.

Lymph nodes have many structural features in common with primary lymphoid tissues and are similarly involved in the maturation of lymphocytes at the terminal stages of differentiation. There is one striking difference, however, between primary lymphoid tissue and secondary tissue. Primary lymphoid tissue is devoid of any known immunogen, and maturation of precursor lymphocytes appears to be hormonally driven in the thymus. By contrast, secondary lymphoid tissue is very efficient at trapping immunogens, and the final stage of lymphocyte differentiation is triggered by the presence of immunogens.

Architecturally, lymph nodes are small ovoid structures surrounded by a surface capsule. The lymph node is divided into a cortex, including a paracortical region, and a medulla (Fig. 10.1). Many afferent lymph channels join the capsule of the node and empty into a subcapsular sinus located directly under the capsule. The cortex, which is located immediately beneath the subcapsular sinus, is the major site of B-lymphocyte localization. Small B-lymphocytes are clustered into areas termed lymphoid nodules or follicles. Also located within lymphoid follicles are dendritic reticulum cells that have a unique capacity to retain antigens on their surface membranes. The follicles give rise to germinal centers during antigenic stimulation.

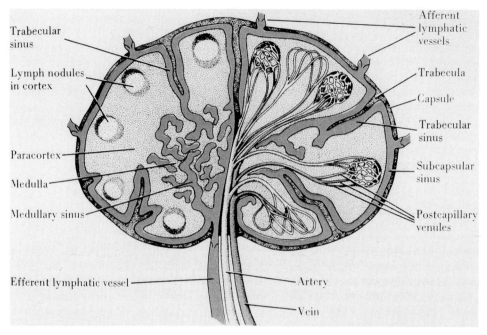

Trabecular sinus

Lymph nodules in cortex

Paracortex

Medulla

Medullary sinus

Efferent lymphatic vessel

Afferent lymphatic vessels

Trabecula

Capsule

Trabecular sinus

Subcapsular sinus

Postcapillary venules

Artery

Vein

Figure 10.1: Schematic diagram of a lymph node. The left side of the figure depicts the general features of a lymph node as seen in section. The substance of the lymph node is divided into a cortex, including a paracortical region, and a medulla. The cortex is the outermost portion; it contains spherical or oval aggregates of lymphocytes called lymph nodules. In an active lymph node, these contain a lighter center called the germinal center. The medulla is the innermost region of the lymph node and extends as far as the hilus of the node. It consists of regions of lymphatic tissue, appearing as irregular cords in section, separated by lymph sinuses, which because of their location in the medulla are referred to as medullary sinuses. The dense population of lymphocytes between the cortex and the medulla constitutes the paracortex. This is the region of the node that contains the postcapillary venules. Surrounding the lymph node is a capsule of dense connective tissue from which trabeculae extend into the substance of the node. Under the capsule and adjacent to the trabeculae are lymph sinuses designated respectively as subcapsular or cortical, and trabecular. Afferent lymphatic vessels penetrate the capsule and empty into the subcapsular sinus. The subcapsular sinus and trabecular sinuses communicate with the medullary sinuses. The right side of the lymph node also shows an artery and vein and the location of the postcapillary venules of the lymph node. (Reproduced with permission from M. Ross and L. Romrell, *Histology. A Text and Atlas,* Ed. 2. Williams & Wilkins, Baltimore, 1989. © 1989 Williams & Wilkins, Baltimore.)

Germinal centers are foci of intense cellular proliferation and hypertrophy, which can result in physical enlargement of the node.

The paracortex, located between the cortex and medulla, is the primary area of T-lymphocyte concentration. Also located within the paracortex are unique postcapillary venules. Recirculating lymphocytes from the bloodstream are able to pass through the specialized endothelial cells of these venules to enter lymph nodes. The medulla of the node is comprised of a network of cords and sinuses. The sinuses link the subcapsular sinus with the origin of a single efferent lymph vessel that drains the entire node. Adhering to the endothelial lining of the medullary sinuses are many macrophages and lymphocytes. After antigenic stimulation, plasma cells producing large quantities of immunoglobulins accumulate within medullary cords. With few exceptions, immunogens in the body tissues will eventually localize in lymph nodes.

Spleen. Immunologically, the spleen functions to filter the blood, much as the lymph nodes monitor lymphatic vessels located in body tissue. Blood-borne immunogens and microorganisms thus tend to be retained within the spleen. The spleen has two anatomical areas, referred to as red pulp and white pulp. Lymphoid follicles (B-lymphocyte areas) and periarteriolar sheaths (T-lymphocyte areas) are found in the white pulp. These two areas are analogous to the lymphoid follicles/germinal centers and the paracortex of lymph nodes, respectively. The red pulp contains cords and sinuses corresponding to similar structures found in the medulla of lymph nodes. The spleen has no afferent lymphatic vessels. Instead, all fluid enters the spleen via arteries. In addition to filtering out blood-borne substances, the spleen may be important in trapping immunogens carried in blood from areas of the body that lack lymphatic drainage, such as the central nervous system.

Table 10.1: Representative Characteristics of T- and B-Lymphocytes

Feature	T-Cells	B-Cells
Origin	Bone marrow	Common stem cells
Maturation	Thymus	Bone marrow
Life span	Both long- and short-lived	Short-lived
Tissue location	Cortex	Germinal centers
Percent lymphocytes		
Peripheral blood	60–70	15–25
Lymph node	75	20
Spleen	35–45	50–60
Bone marrow	<10	<75
Thymus	<75	<10
Recirculation capability	Yes	Little or none

Gut-Associated Lymphoid Tissue. In addition to the centrally located lymphoid tissues described above, other lymphoid tissues are associated with mucosal surfaces. These are arranged in various degrees of organization. The lamina propria of the gastrointestinal (GI) tract possesses lymphocytes and lymphocytic aggregates (gut-associated lymphoid tissue, GALT) within the connective tissue subjacent to epithelial cells. The respiratory tree and urogenital mucosa also have similar accumulations of lymphoid tissue. The immunoglobulins associated with these sites are predominantly of the IgA class. GALT lymphocytes appear to respond to stimulation by substances or infectious agents in the mucous membranes closest to them. The appendix, tonsils, and Peyer's patches represent lymphoepithelial tissue and have a higher degree of organization. These structures are more analogous to lymph nodes than to the small lymphoid aggregates of the lamina propria. The better organized structures have lymphoid follicles and germinal centers populated with B-lymphocytes, as well as diffuse areas of T-lymphocytes.

In summary, lymphoid tissues and organs have two basic functions: 1) Primary lymphoid organs accept precursor lymphocytes and release immunocompetent T- and B-lymphocytes that are capable of responding to immunogenic stimulation. 2) Secondary lymphoid tissues serve as sites for immunocompetent lymphocytes, antigens, and other ancillary cells to localize and then to interact in such a way as to generate the effector responses of the immune system.

Cells of the Immune System

When examined by the light microscope, all small lymphocytes look very much alike. However, the two large groups of lymphocytes, B-lymphocytes and T-lymphocytes, have highly specific immune functions. As immunohistological techniques have become more sensitive and specific, distinct subsets of T- and B-lymphocytes have been further identified and characterized (Tables 10.1 and 10.2). This new information has led to a better understanding of cellular interactions and regulation in acquired immunity.

B-Lymphocytes

B-lymphocytes and their progeny constitute one of the principal cellular components of the immune system. The humoral immune response is mediated by B-lymphocytes. These cells synthesize immunoglobulins against recognized immunogens and differentiate into more specialized cells (immunoblasts and plasma cells). Plasma cells subsequently assume the major

Table 10.2: Characteristics of T-Lymphocyte Subpopulations

Subset	Surface Antigens	Function
T-helper (T_H)	T4	Assist immune activation of B-cells; cooperate with cytotoxic T-cells
T-suppressor (T_S)	T8	Regulate T-cell and B-cell activity
T-cytotoxic (T_C)	T8	Destroy foreign target cells
T-delayed hypersensitivity (T_D)	T4	Responsible for infiltration of macrophages and other inflammatory cells to areas of delayed hypersensitivity reactions

role for production and secretion of antibody molecules.

Precursor B-lymphocytes are first produced in the fetal liver and later in the bone marrow. Approximately 15% of the circulating lymphocytes in the blood are B-cells. The presence of surface immunoglobulins on the cytoplasmic membrane of B-lymphocytes and the lack of a Thy marker (found on more than 95% of T-lymphocytes) formed the initial basis for distinguishing B- from T-lymphocytes. Although early B-cell precursors are unable to produce immunoglobulin, the appearance of IgM is first demonstrable on immature B-lymphocytes, including those that leave the bone marrow. As these cells continue to develop, IgD molecules appear on their surface and eventually become the predominant membrane-bound immunoglobulin. It has been suggested that the presence of IgD on B-cells is an indication of maturation. Other surface immunoglobulins have also been identified on B-lymphocyte surfaces. The Fab portions of surface immunoglobulins are widely regarded as the antigen recognition unit of the B-lymphocyte. Interestingly, if two different immunoglobulin classes occur on the surface of one cell, the variable domains all possess exactly the same receptor specificity for one antigenic determinant. Practically all B-lymphocytes have receptors on their surface membranes for the Fc portions of aggregated immunoglobulins. Aggregation can occur as a result of the binding to immunogens or it can occur in vitro when immunoglobulins are denatured.

In addition to surface immunoglobulins, B-cells express an array of other membrane markers and receptors that are necessary for immune system function. Receptors for certain complement components (C3d and C3b), interferons, a β-stimulating factor (BSF-1), and interleukin-2 are found either before (resting) or after B-cell activation. The interaction of macromolecules or microorganisms with these receptors can have direct clinical significance. For example, the C3d binding site is also the receptor for the Epstein–Barr virus. This is but one example of a microbial structure or product serving to activate B-lymphocytes and trigger immune sequelae.

A variety of antigenic stimuli can activate B-lymphocytes. Out of a pool of approximately 10^{12} cells, only a small percentage are able to bind the antigen onto their surfaces when an immunogen is introduced into a host system. The immunogens most likely to stimulate B-lymphocytes are soluble macromolecules containing multiple antigenic determinants, blood-borne infectious organisms, or structural components of infectious microorganisms.

With the availability of increasingly sophisticated in vitro and in vivo techniques, it has become apparent that antigen interaction with immunocompetent B-lymphocytes alone does not necessarily result in antibody production. In addition to specific binding onto surface immunoglobulins of B-cells, immune processing of most immunogens requires both T-helper lymphocyte and macrophage cooperation (Fig. 10.2). The cellular interactions that occur may be triggered by a number of mechanisms, and both the nature of the immunogen and the genetically controlled surface receptors determine the sequence of activation.

A variety of immunogenic molecules are termed T-cell–dependent antigens. These antigens contain many structurally different antigenic determinants that are available to interact with B-lymphocytes. Such substances constitute the vast majority of immunogens found in nature. A few substances, called T-cell–independent antigens, are able to directly stimulate B-lymphocytes. They usually contain structurally repeating subunits, and they appear to bind with the B-cell surface by cross-linking appropriate surface immunoglobulin receptors. Examples of macromolecules included in this group are lipopolysaccharides of gram-negative bacteria and staphylococcal protein A.

T-Lymphocytes

The demonstration of a second major class of human lymphocytes, the T-lymphocytes, heralded a new era in scientific understanding of how lymphoid tissues and cells function. As with B-lymphocytes, T-cell precursors originate in the bone marrow in late fetal life. The maturation process for T-cells is quite different, however, as they undergo a complex maturation in the thymus, as described earlier. Approximately 60% to 70% of the lymphocytes found in the blood are mature T-cells. Characterization of T-lymphocyte subsets is primarily associated with specific markers detected on the cell surfaces (see Table 10.1).

Analysis of immunological markers on cell surface membranes delineates two major T-lymphocyte subpopulations: T-helper cells (T4 lymphocytes) and T-suppressor cells (T8 lymphocytes). T-helper lymphocytes serve as important antigen recognition and processing cells in the earliest portions of humoral immune responses and substantially facilitate immunoglobulin production. T-suppressor cells exert a regulatory role by controlling and inhibiting immunoglobulin synthesis.

The effector portion of activated T-lymphocyte function is accomplished through the activities of soluble substances called lymphokines. Lymphokines are produced and released after the T-cells have become sensitized to specific immunogens. These molecules are nonspecific and should not be confused with immunoglobulins. Individual lymphokines basically act on lymphoid or mononuclear cells or other target

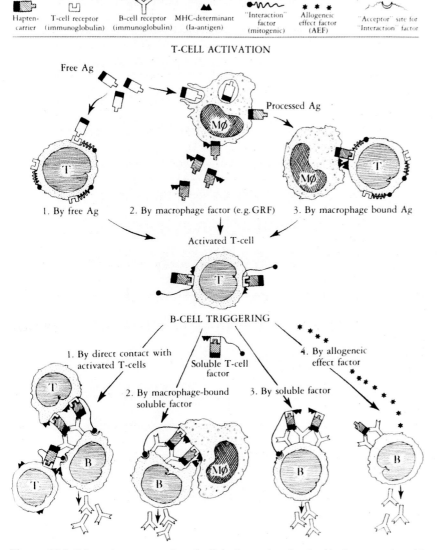

Hapten-carrier	T-cell receptor (immunoglobulin)	B-cell receptor (immunoglobulin)	MHC-determinant (Ia-antigen)	"Interaction" factor (mitogenic)	Allogeneic effect factor (AEF)	"Acceptor" site for "Interaction" factor

T-CELL ACTIVATION

Free Ag

Processed Ag

Mϕ

Mϕ

1. By free Ag   2. By macrophage factor (e.g. GRF)   3. By macrophage bound Ag

Activated T-cell

B-CELL TRIGGERING

1. By direct contact with activated T-cells

Soluble T-cell factor

4. By allogeneic effect factor

2. By macrophage-bound soluble factor

3. By soluble factor

Mϕ

Figure 10.2: Schematic representation of cellular interactions involved in the generation of the humoral immune responses. Note that T-cells can be activated in three ways: 1) by free antigen (*Ag*); 2) by macrophage-processed antigen; or 3) by macrophage-associated antigen. In turn, B-cells may be triggered to produce antibody in four ways: 1) by direct contact with Ag-bearing activated T-cells; 2) by macrophage-bound factor; 3) by a soluble Ag-specific T-cell factor; or 4) by a nonspecific (allogeneic effect) factor produced by T-cells. (Reproduced with permission from J. Bellanti, *Immunology III*. Saunders, Philadelphia, 1985.)

cells and greatly enhance the ability of sensitized T-lymphocytes to respond successfully to foreign antigens. These lymphocyte products are discussed further in Chapter 12.

Null Cells

A class of lymphocyte has been found that lacks surface markers for either T- or B-lymphocytes. These cells, termed null cells, appear to represent a het-erogeneous mixture of immature hematopoietic cells with properties intermediate between those of T-lymphocytes and myelomonocytic cells. Functionally, two subclasses of null cells have been identified. One subset has been designated killer cells (K cells). K cells are monocytes that have surface receptors for the Fc portion of immunoglobulins bound to antigens. If the immunoglobulins are linked to antigens on a cell surface, then the binding of a K cell to this surface-bound immunoglobulin results in lysis of the antibody-coated cell. The second line of null cells consists of natural killer cells (NK cells). NK cells have the ability to destroy virus-infected, transformed, or various tumor cells without prior immunization.

Plasma Cells

Plasma cells are highly specialized, terminally differentiated B-lymphocytes. They function as classic immunoglobulin-producing cells. The pathway leading to their development begins after B-cells are antigenically stimulated in the early stages of immune induction. Intermediate plasmablasts exhibit properties of both parent B-lymphocytes and progeny plasma cells. The latter contain very few surface-bound immunoglobulins, and other typical B-cell surface markers are generally undetectable on mature plasma cells. The cellular structure of plasma cells is directed at promoting the synthesis of large amounts of protein. The presence of ribosomes and an extensive endoplasmic reticulum make the cell well suited for this purpose. Even though the typical plasma cell may live for only a few days, it is capable of producing up to 2,000 antibody molecules per second.

The microscopic appearance of plasma cells is characteristic and makes them readily identifiable. Cells are ovoid, with an eccentric spoke–wheel or cog–wheel nucleus. The cytoplasm stains intensely basophilic. Plasma cells are only infrequently detected in the peripheral circulation, as most are observable in certain areas of lymphoid tissues, such as the medullary cords of lymph nodes, the red pulp of the spleen, and the bone marrow.

Macrophages

The macrophage plays a central role in both nonspecific and acquired host defenses. In addition to their role as nonspecific scavengers, macrophages are intimately involved in the development of specific humoral and cellular immune responses. There is good evidence to suggest that macrophages present antigens, after modifying them, to both T- and B-lymphocytes. This "accessory" antigen-processing role is fundamental to the efficiency of all acquired immune system responses. In vitro experiments have shown that when macrophages are added to a cell system designed to produce immunoglobulins after antigenic stimulation, significantly less antigen is required to drive the system. There is evidence to indicate that macrophages in close physical proximity to antigen-sensitive B- and T-lymphocytes secrete a polypeptide hormone, interleukin-1 (IL-1), which triggers activation of these lymphocytes. Finally, macrophages can act as effector cells in an immune response. In certain cell-mediated responses, activated macrophages become more aggressive phagocytic cells

with an enhanced capacity to kill ingested microorganisms. Because macrophages have Fc receptors on their surfaces, antigens with immunoglobulin bound to them are easily phagocytosed (opsonization). Thus, in the body's attempt to rid itself of noxious agents, the macrophage appears to play prominent roles at several stages.

Humoral Immune Response in the Immunocompetent Host

Stimulation of an immunocompetent host with immunogens capable of inducing a humoral (antibody) response triggers a series of interrelated molecular and cellular events. Under appropriate conditions, these result in a measurable synthesis of immunoglobulins capable of specifically binding to their corresponding antigenic determinant sites. The route of antigen entrance often determines which lymphoid tissues will respond to an immunologic stimulus. For example, if the immunogen is located in tissue (with the exception of the CNS), antibody production will most likely occur in the regional lymph node responsible for clearance of the area where the immunogen is located. Primary deposition of an immunogen in the bloodstream or CNS, on the other hand, will usually result in activation of lymphoid cells that reside in the spleen.

Secondary lymphoid tissues such as the spleen and lymph nodes are architecturally organized in such a way as to 1) provide an interaction between antigen-bearing macrophages, T_h-cells, and antigen-sensitive B-lymphocytes; 2) provide a location for development of plasma cells; and 3) provide a mechanism for distributing secreted antibody. The latter uses efferent lymphatic channels leading to the thoracic duct in the release from lymph nodes, and the venous circulation in the case of antibody synthesis in the spleen. Secretory IgA synthesis and secretion, however, varies from this pattern of central processing and distribution. Secretory IgA is typically produced locally near the site of immunogen entry through the affected mucosa, and later in all exocrine glands.

The increase in concentration of specific antibody with respect to time after antigenic stimulation may be measured by sampling the host's serum at various intervals. In this manner the patterns of IgM and IgG synthesis (most notably for systemic immunity) and IgA (primarily for secretory immune responses) can be observed as indications of immune reactivity.

Primary Humoral Immune Response

When an immunologically intact host is exposed for the first time with a T-cell–dependent immunogen, a lag period of several days ensues before any specific immunoglobulin is detected in the serum. The sequence of events that occurs in this instance is called the primary immune response. The first immunoglobulin class to appear is IgM. Its production peaks in 3 to 4 days, after which the concentration diminishes, with the IgM gradually replaced by IgG of the same antigenic specificity. This change corresponds to the observation that the same sensitized plasma cell switches from IgM to IgG synthesis, without producing two immunoglobulin classes at the same time. In many instances IgG production peaks 14 to 21 days after antigenic stimulation, and then gradually declines to a level where residual concentrations in serum are slightly above the preimmunization level. The biological half-life of IgG in serum is about 23 days, whereas that for IgM is about 5 days. As antibody production increases during the primary response, the affinity of the antibodies for antigenic determinants also increases.

The pattern described above represents a typical sequence for the initial appearance of immunoglobulins. The route of immunogen administration, the type of antigenic molecule, and the presence of immunostimulators all can substantially alter the course of the response. Aspects of these factors will be considered in a later section.

Secondary Humoral Immune Response

When an immunized host has a second exposure to the same or a cross-reacting antigen, the resulting specific response is different from the initial encounter. The lag time between stimulation and the appearance of free antibody in the circulation is shorter than for the primary response. Immunoglobulin production occurs at a more rapid rate and persists longer. This results in a significantly higher antibody concentration than seen in the primary humoral response. IgM levels are basically the same in both responses. The major difference occurs with IgG synthesis. The levels of this antibody class rapidly increase over a long period of time and constitute the most demonstrable characteristic of the secondary immune response. The host responds as if it remembered the initial immunogenic exposure; in fact, this response is due to the production and persistence of specific "memory cells," which develop at the same time that antigen-sensitive B-lymphocytes are differentiating into plasmablasts and mature plasma cells. It is through the activities of memory cells that the immune system can respond faster and to a greater degree on rechallenge; hence the synonyms *anamnestic, memory,* or *recall response.*

The biological advantage of such a system is of great significance when one considers the host's response to infectious agents. During primary exposure the immunoglobulins produced are often essential for eliminating the invading microorganisms from the body. In addition, later reinfection by the same microbe would induce a secondary immune response. Because of the shortened lag time and increased immunoglobulin synthesis, this recall reaction can prevent clinical manifestations of the disease in many cases or at least substantially diminish the severity of the symptoms.

T-Lymphocyte–Independent Immunogens

Immunogens that do not require T-helper cell cooperation in order to stimulate B-lymphocytes appear to have two important properties. 1) They tend to be high molecular weight polymers, particularly polysaccharides, that have repeating, identical antigenic determinants. They are thus capable of binding to many surface immunoglobulin receptors on B-lymphocytes. This satisfies the antigen-specific signal necessary for B-cell activation. 2) These immunogens also have the intrinsic ability to provide the mitogenic signal required for B-cell proliferation. In fact, lipopolysaccharides are such potent B-lymphocyte mitogens (substances that activate cells and induce them to divide) that they can nonspecifically induce proliferation and antibody secretion of many B-lymphocyte clones.

In contrast to T-cell–dependent antigens, however, no IgM–IgG switch is noted after sensitization with T-cell–independent immunogens. Plasma cells derived from those B-cells stimulated by the latter produce only IgM. In addition, immunological memory fails to develop or is of short duration. The time course and degree of immunoglobulin synthesis after second and subsequent challenges with T-cell–independent immunogens are virtually the same as after the initial encounter.

Principles of Immunization

By manipulating the immune response, medical science has been able to protect individuals from numerous pathogenic microorganisms. The list of public health immunizations includes many highly communicable viral diseases (e.g., measles, mumps), diseases produced by potent bacterial exotoxins (e.g., tetanus, diphtheria), and many infections produced by virulent bacteria themselves (e.g., bacterial pneumonia) (Table 10.3). Health care professionals are now also able to receive a highly effective vaccine to protect against infection with hepatitis B virus, one of the major occupational infectious diseases. The vaccine preparations are classified into four categories: 1) killed or inactivated microorganisms, 2) attenuated microorganisms, 3) microbial products, and 4) microbial components.

Table 10.3: Vaccines Available in the United States, by Type and Recommended Routes of Administration*

Vaccine	Type	Route
BCG (bacillus Calmette–Guérin)	Live bacteria	Intradermal or subcutaneous
Cholera	Inactivated bacteria	Subcutaneous or intradermal†
DTP (D = diphtheria) (T = tetanus) (P = pertussis)	Toxoids and inactivated bacteria	Intramuscular
HB (Hepatitis B)	Inactive viral antigen	Intramuscular
Haemophilus influenzae b Polysaccharide (HbPV) or conjugate (HbCV)	Bacterial polysaccharide Polysaccharide conjugated to protein	Subcutaneous or intramuscular‡ Intramuscular
Influenza	Inactivated virus or viral components	Intramuscular
IPV (inactivated polio-virus vaccine)	Inactivated viruses of all 3 serotypes	Subcutaneous
Measles	Live virus	Subcutaneous
Meningococcal	Bacterial polysaccharides of serotypes A/C/Y/W-135	Subcutaneous
MMR (M = measles) (M = mumps) (R = rubella)	Live viruses	Subcutaneous
Mumps	Live virus	Subcutaneous
OPV (oral poliovirus vaccine)	Live viruses of all 3 sero-types	Oral
Plague	Inactivated bacteria	Intramuscular
Pneumococcal	Bacterial polysaccharides of 23 pneumococcal types	Intramuscular or subcutaneous
Rabies	Inactivated virus	Subcutaneous or intradermal§
Rubella	Live virus	Subcutaneous
Tetanus	Inactivated toxin (toxoid)	Intramuscular‖
Td or DT** (T = tetanus) (D or d = diphtheria)	Inactivated toxins (toxoids)	Intramuscular‖
Typhoid	Inactivated bacteria	Subcutaneous††
Yellow fever	Live virus	Subcutaneous

*From Centers for Disease Control, Immunization Practices Advisory Committee: General Recommendations on Immunization. *MMWR*, **38**, 205–227, 1989.

†The intradermal dose is lower.

‡Route depends on the manufacturer; consult package insert for recommendation for specific product used.

§Intradermal dose is lower and used only for preexposure vaccination.

‖Preparations with adjuvants should be given intramuscularly.

**DT = tetanus and diphtheria toxoids for use in children aged <7 years. Td = tetanus and diphtheria toxoids for use in persons aged ≥7 years. Td contains the same amount of tetanus toxoid as DTP or DT but a reduced dose of diphtheria toxoid.

††Boosters may be given intradermally unless acetone-killed and dried vaccine is used.

Active Immunization

Active immunization attempts to stimulate an individual's immune system with a particular antigen in order to produce a primary immune response. The immune response is accompanied by an increase in antigen-sensitive B-lymphocytes (humoral immunity) or T-lymphocytes (cellular immunity) capable of responding to the antigen. A critical factor in primary immunization is to use an immunogen that does not cause illness yet is antigenically similar or identical to the disease-causing agent. For example, in the case of bacterial exotoxins, the biologically active sites are altered but the antigenicity of the molecule remains essentially the same (toxoids). In many viral vaccines, the virus may be "killed" so that it cannot replicate in tissue, but the viral surface immunogenicity is not altered. Alternatively, the virus may be attenuated (i.e., its virulence is weakened while the virus retains its viability) in the laboratory. When the resulting vaccine is administered to humans, the microorganism will replicate in tissue but not cause disease. An attenuated vaccine contains the same surface antigenicity as the wild-type organism.

Once a primary response has been mounted against the relatively innocuous vaccine agent, the hope is that little or no clinical disease will develop when the virulent microbial form is encountered in nature. Active immunization has effectively controlled many serious infectious diseases. It should also be stressed that active immunization is most effective when instituted before an individual is exposed to the natural disease agent or substance. The advantage of active immunization is that the probability of ensuing protection is high and may last for years.

Passive Immunization

Passive immunization, unlike active immunization, does not stimulate the individual's own immune system. In fact, in many instances the host's immune apparatus may actually be inhibited by passive immunization. What is this technique and what is its rationale?

Immunotherapy classically denotes artificial passive immunization—the use of whole serum or serum γ-globulins to treat or prevent certain infectious diseases. The basic premise involves the injection of antibodies from an immune person into a nonimmune host. The antibody preparation, which is predominantly of the IgG class, is obtained from donors who have developed antibodies either through immunization by vaccine or through exposure to and recovery from a microbial disease. The rationale is that the transferred antibody will help clear the infectious agent or toxin from the recipient before symptomatic or asymptomatic disease results. Passive immunization is almost always performed after a nonimmune individual has been exposed to a specific disease (e.g., after exposure to tetanus or hepatitis A virus). Exogenously administered immunoglobulins are immediately available to the recipient, thereby filling the gap between exposure to antigen and the appearance of a protective immune response. However, because the injected antibody can be rapidly cleared from the system, the recipient's own immune tissues may not have time to respond.

The advantage of passive immunization is that it may prevent or lessen the severity of disease in the nonimmune host. The disadvantages are that immunity is of short duration, owing to the biological half-life of the administered immunoglobulins; and the recipient's own immune system may not be stimulated. Under some circumstances, active and passive immunization may be utilized concurrently to prevent disease (e.g., after rabies exposure, and to prevent perinatal transmission of HBV). Historically, the hyperimmune serum used for passive immunization was prepared in animal species, most notably the horse. This practice has largely been abandoned, however, because of the development of serious hypersensitivity reactions.

Passive immunization also occurs in nature. Examples of this natural passive immunity occur both when maternal IgG is transferred across the placenta to the fetal circulation and when secretory IgA, found in colostrum and breast milk, is transferred to nursing infants.

Antigen Administration

Deliberate immunization of humans and animals has yielded important clinical information about effective antigen administration. Determination of the best site for antigen administration should consider such factors as the irritancy and volume of the substance being injected. Antigenic substances have been administered into the skin (intradermally), subcutaneously, or intramuscularly. They have been successfully injected intravenously and intraperitoneally in animal experiments. Inhalation has also been utilized as a route of antigen administration, particularly when preferential synthesis of secretory IgA is desired. One must be cautioned, however, that inhalation of immunogen is associated with an increased risk of IgE synthesis, leading to subsequent hypersensitivity sequelae. Ingestion of immunogens is usually not particularly successful, in part because antigens are easily degraded in the digestive tract.

Adjuvants

For immunization to occur the antigen must persist for a period of time after it has entered the body. A portion of immunogen is initially catabolized, phagocytized, or otherwise degraded after it enters the body and is thus unavailable to stimulate the immune system. Some crucial minimal threshold amount must therefore persist for an unknown but essential period of time in order to trigger the development of a host response.

One way to enhance the persistence of immunogens, particularly soluble ones, is to inject a mixture of immunogen and adjuvant. An adjuvant is defined as a nonspecific potentiator of immune responses. These immunostimulators initially form an insoluble complex with antigen. This bolus of material acts as a depot, slowly releasing antigen over a relatively long time period; in effect, providing multiple immune challenges. Because an inflammatory reaction is stimulated at the site of antigen–adjuvant localization in tissue, concentrations of macrophages and lymphocytes are greatly increased. Thus, retention of immunogen leads to the enhanced recruitment of immune processing cells, making the ultimate response more efficient.

Substances capable of nonspecific immunopotentiation include a variety of macromolecules that can augment either humoral or cellular immune responses, or both. Commonly used adjuvants include the following: 1) intact microorganisms such as human and animal strains of mycobacteria (i.e., bacillus Calmette-Guèrin) and gram-positive bacilli (i.e., *Corynebacterium parvum*); 2) structural components of bacteria such as lipopolysaccharides from gram-negative bacteria; 3) synthetic macromolecules (i.e., nucleic acids, polyinosinic acid); 4) lymphokines; and 5) small molecules such as alum and silica. Classic experimental adjuvants were first developed by Freund. These were water-in-oil emulsions, which were primarily allowed only in certain animal investigations. Freund's "complete" adjuvant consists of a water-in-oil emulsion in which living or dead mycobacteria are suspended. This complete adjuvant causes an intense chronic inflammatory response at the site of deposit, thereby precluding its use in humans. Freund's "incomplete" adjuvant (without mycobacteria) is not as effective as the complete adjuvant but has been successful when used clinically.

Immunological Tolerance

It has long been recognized that individuals normally do not respond to their own antigens. Recognition of self antigens, and the lack of immune response against them, is termed tolerance. Experimentally, it is possible to take a substance that is usually immunogenic and present it to an immunocompetent host in such a way that the host fails to respond to the antigen. Once induced, this type of tolerance is antigen-specific, meaning that the host is immunologically unresponsive only to the antigen used to induce the tolerant state. Immunity or tolerance may then be viewed as alternative outcomes in response to the same substance.

Factors That Favor Induction of Tolerance. It is easier to induce tolerance in fetal and newborn members of a species than in mature adults. This may be due to the fact that immature B-cells in the neonate are more readily made tolerant than B-cells from the adult. The antigen dose appears to be another important factor. Every immunogen has an optimum dose range needed to elicit an immune response. Doses that greatly exceed the optimal dose tend to result in high-dose tolerance. This effect may involve a B-cell or T-cell tolerance. In contrast, tolerance can also be produced with quantities of antigen substantially below the optimal dose. This so-called low-dose tolerance appears to affect mainly T-cells. A third factor is the physical state of the immunogen. The more soluble or less aggregated an immunogen, the more likely it is to induce tolerance. On the other hand, particu-

late immunogens such as bacteria and viruses are almost always immunogenic and can be made tolerogenic only with great difficulty. Finally, the route of antigen administration can be a factor, especially in the case of soluble antigens.

Maturation of the Humoral Immune Response

The immune system begins to develop and mature during the early stages of fetal life. However, not all elements of the humoral immune response begin to function until 9 to 10 years after birth. B-lymphocytes bearing IgM or IgG surface markers can be detected in the fetus by the 10th week of gestation. When a fetal spleen is examined at the 15th week of gestation, the proportion of lymphocytes containing surface immunoglobulins of all classes is essentially similar to the distribution in adults. However, secretion of immunoglobulins is not observed until the 20th week, and then IgM is the predominant antibody secreted, with only sparse concentrations of IgG. IgA secretion is first observed some time after birth.

Even though secreted immunoglobulins may be detected in a relatively young fetus, it should not be inferred that the fetus can respond to a wide variety of immunogenic challenges. Protective levels of immunoglobulins are not reached until after birth. In addition, although fetal B-lymphocytes can respond to antigens in vitro, the limited responsiveness in vivo may be due to the maturational state of macrophages. This is in contrast to the vigorous plasma cell development and concomitant IgM secretion in the fetus in response to congenital infections such as syphilis.

The highest concentration of serum immunoglobulin at birth is IgG. The majority of this antibody is of maternal origin, since IgG is the only immunoglobulin that is selectively transported across the placenta. At birth the infant therefore possesses an IgG repertoire equivalent to that of its mother. During the first 8 to 10 weeks of neonatal life there is continuous loss of maternal IgG as antibody molecules are catabolized. Total IgG levels then begin to rise again as the infant produces greater quantities of IgG. Adult concentrations of serum IgM are found in the infant within the first year after birth, followed by IgG at 3 to 4 years, by IgA at 9 to 10 years, and finally by IgE at about 10 to 15 years. Because of the sequential secretion of immunoglobulins, coupled with the rapid loss of maternal IgG, the infant is particularly vulnerable to infectious diseases from approximately the second to the fifth month of life.

ADDITIONAL READING

For additional reading, see Chapter 12, pages 147–149.

11

Complement, Serology, and Antibody-Mediated Disease

John A. Molinari

Complement

It has been long recognized that a normal, nonimmunoglobulin group of serum proteins plays a critical role in host defenses against many bacteria and other pathogens. These macromolecules most often exert their biological effects in the presence of antigen–antibody complexes. Historically, it was observed in the early 1900s that cholera vibrios were lysed within a short time when added to serum from an immunized animal. It was also noted that the nonimmune serum constituent was heat labile, because the lytic activity was destroyed after the immune serum was heated to 56°C for a few minutes. Lytic activity was restored to the immune serum after heat treatment by adding fresh serum from a normal animal. Therefore, lysis appeared to be dependent on two factors: 1) specific antigen–antibody complex formation, and 2) the presence of a normal constituent of serum, now termed complement.

The complement system consists not of a single entity but of 15 proteins that act in an ordered, prescribed sequence. These heterogeneous proteins circulate in blood in an inactive form and account for about 10% of the globulins in normal human serum. Activated complement proteins that function early in the sequence are cleaved so that one cleavage product becomes a proteolytic enzyme to react specifically with only the next complement component in the sequence. Later cleavage products may have nonenzymatic biological activity, such as causing inflammatory tissue changes. Such changes include increased vascular permeability and attraction of high concentrations of polymorphonuclear leukocytes (PMNs, neutrophils). This chemotaxis recruits phagocytic cells to the affected area of tissue, resulting in ingestion and destruction of the foreign microorganisms. Complement proteins that function late in the cascade do not behave as enzymes, but rather aggregate to form complexes that alter the permeability characteristics of cytoplasmic membranes. This frequently triggers the lysis of target cells coated with the products of the reactions. Such destruction is protective against numerous bacterial and viral infections. When complement is initiated by antigen–antibody complexes, the resulting sequence is known as the classical complement pathway. When the complement system is activated by substances other than antigen–antibody complexes, the sequence is called the alternate complement pathway.

Early Steps of Complement Sequence

Initiation of Classical Complement Pathway. The classical complement pathway can be initiated by antigen–antibody complexes formed by IgM, IgG1, IgG2, or IgG3. The classic example of pathway induction assumes that the antigen is a gram-negative bacterial cell wall component. In the case of IgG complexes, individual IgG molecules must aggregate in sufficient numbers and compactness to ensure that two adjacent antibody molecules are close enough for the first complement protein to physically bridge the distance between adjacent Fc (crystallizable fragment) regions. Because IgM is a pentamer with five closely apposed Fc regions, the interaction of a single IgM molecule with an antigen is sufficient to bind the first complement protein (C1). A conformational change occurs within the antibody molecule after the appropriate immunoglobulin complexes with antigen. This opens up a C1 receptor located on the C_H2 domain of immunoglobulin heavy chains.

C1 is actually a complex of three separate proteins, designated C1q, C1r, and C1s, that are held together in the presence of calcium ions (Fig. 11.1). C1q is the portion of the molecule that binds with the antibody in the immune complex initiating the complement activation sequence by binding to exposed receptors on the C_H2 domains of immunoglobulins (no prior activation step is necessary other than formation of the requisite antigen–antibody complex). Binding of C1q causes a conformational change in the molecule that results in the activation of C1r and then C1s. First, C1r is cleaved and becomes a proteolytic enzyme ($\overline{C1r}$), which in turn cleaves C1s, whose active form is also a proteolytic enzyme ($\overline{C1s}$). (A complement component or complex with a line over it denotes the enzymatically active form, e.g., $\overline{C1s,C4b,2a}$.) One additional requirement for the proper functioning of C1 is Ca^{2+}, which is necessary to stabilize the complex.

The next component to react in the sequence is C4. Complement proteins are numbered in the order in which they were discovered, not in the sequence in which they react. C1s cleaves C4 into two fragments: a small fragment, C4a, and a larger fragment, C4b. A single C1s activates hundreds of C4 molecules, with

the result that some C4b remains attached to the Ag-Ab$\overline{C1}$ complex and some C4b becomes bound to the nearby bacterial cell membrane. Membrane-bound C4b enhances the cleavage of, and acts as a receptor for, the split product of the next protein in the sequence, C2. C2, like C4, is a natural substrate for C1s. When C2 is cleaved, two fragments result. C2a, the major fragment, binds to membrane-bound C4b in the presence of Mg^{2+}. C2b, the minor fragment, is biologically inactive and diffuses away.

The membrane-bound, bimolecular $\overline{C4b,2a}$ complex is also called C3 convertase. It is physically separated from the Ag-Ab$\overline{C1}$ complex and acts as a proteolytic enzyme that is specific for C3, the next protein to be activated in the sequence. The enzymatically active site of C3 convertase is the C2a moiety, which cleaves C3 into a small C3a fragment and a larger C3b fragment that joins the membrane-bound $\overline{C4b,2a}$ complex to form the larger $\overline{C4b,2a,3b}$ complex, which in turn will activate the next component, C5.

There is another sequence of events that culminates in the cleavage of C3 and that does not require specific antigen–antibody complex formation to initiate the complement cascade. This alternate complement pathway does not utilize C1, C2, or C4. It does, however, depend on other normal constituents of serum that also react in sequence before C3 is cleaved. This pathway will be discussed before we return to the common remaining late steps in the complete complement sequence.

Initiation of the Alternate Complete Pathway. Complex polysaccharides of bacterial and fungal origin, lipopolysaccharides from gram-negative bacteria, IgG4, and aggregated IgA all can initiate the alternate complement pathway. The early proteins of the alternate pathway are normal serum constituents that are always active and depend on the activity of normal inhibitors to keep the system in check. It is only when these inhibitors can be bypassed that significant quantities of C3 are cleaved and the complement sequence can go to completion. The continuously active serum proteins in the alternate pathway are factor B, factor D, properdin (P), and trace amounts of C3b. These are also normally found in serum. Factor B binds to C3b to form the complex C3b,B. Factor D, an active protease, cleaves factor b in the complex into Ba, which is inactive, and Bb. The $\overline{C3b,Bb}$ complex in turn cleaves C3 into C3a and C3b, perhaps accounting for the ever-present small quantities of C3b in serum. In addition, the $\overline{C3b,Bb}$ complex is rather unstable and readily dissociates into its inactive components. However, if the complex binds to properdin, the resulting new complex, $P,\overline{C3b,Bb}$, becomes a relatively stable C3-splitting enzyme. Left unchecked, this enzyme could trigger the remaining

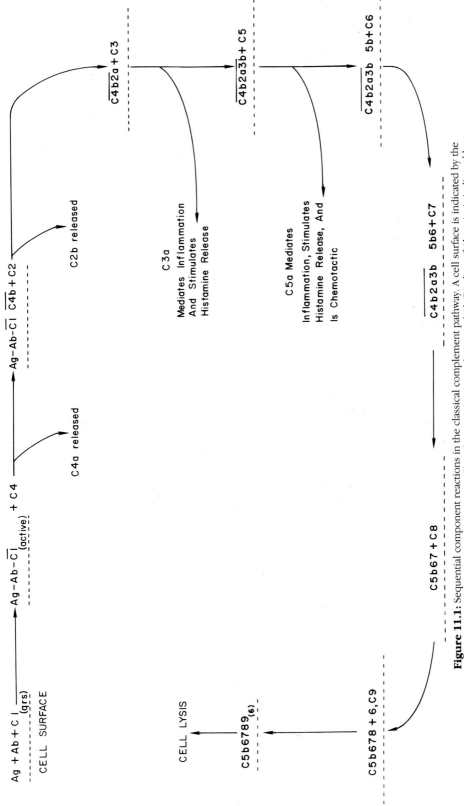

Figure 11.1: Sequential component reactions in the classical complement pathway: A cell surface is indicated by the dashed line (- -). Antibody specific for a cell surface component is designated *Ab*. Binding of Ab to Ag is indicated by a single dash (—), and binding of subsequent complement components is indicated by consecutive numbered components. Enzymatically active complement components and complexes are indicated by a bar drawn over the component.

components of the complement sequence. Under normal circumstances, however, there are two regulatory proteins that, working in concert, first inactivate C3b and then dissociate the P,$\overline{C3b,Bb}$ complex.

Returning to the bacterial cell used as an example of the triggering antigen in the classical pathway, the P,$\overline{C3b,Bb}$ complex can bind to complex polysaccharides or lipopolysaccharides. Binding of the complex under these conditions apparently protects C3b from the regulatory proteins, and now C3 can be cleaved in sufficient quantities to trigger the rest of the complement sequence, owing to the formation of a new enzymatically active complex, P,$\overline{C3b_2,Bb}$.

Late Steps of Complement Sequence

Up to this point, we recognize that there exist two enzyme complexes, both of which can activate C5, the next complement protein in the sequence—the $\overline{C4b,2a,3b}$ complex from the antigen–antibody complex–driven classical pathway and the P,$\overline{C3b_2,Bb}$ complex from the alternate pathway. Recall also that in the examples given, both of these complexes are located near a bacterial cytoplasmic membrane.

Regardless of which enzymatic complex is involved, C5 is cleaved into two fragments, C5a and C5b. If C5 is split by the membrane-bound $\overline{C4b,2a,3b}$ enzyme, then C5b binds to the bacterial cell membrane at a topographical site independent of the enzyme site (see Fig. 11.1). If, on the other hand, C5 is split by the P,$\overline{C3b_2,Bb}$ complex, C5b also adheres to the bacterial cell membrane even though the enzyme complex may not be in direct contact with the membrane.

The sequence that follows C5 cleavage is quite different from what preceded it. Instead of enzymatic cleavage to activate succeeding components, there is an aggregation of succeeding components, one to another. After C5b has become membrane-bound, one molecule of C6 joins each C5b molecule, followed by one molecule of C7 joining to C6. The C5b,6,7 aggregate provides a binding site for one molecule of C8, to which up to six molecules of C9 attach by adsorption.

Membrane Injury. Permeability changes are first seen in the affected cell membrane when component C8 is bound to the C5b,6,7 complex and intracellular constituents slowly begin to leak out of the cell. When C9s are added, the flow rate increases 10-fold. With regard to the target bacterial cell example, lysis occurs with the passage of water into the cell. Complement-mediated lysis of red blood cells occurs in the same fashion. However, complement attachment to nucleated cells results first in the slow release of small intracellular substances, followed by release of larger substances such as nucleotides and finally proteins. The suggestion has been made that, as the complex assembles, hydrophobic regions of the proteins are exposed that interact with lipids of the cell membrane, creating a transmembrane channel that enlarges with addition of C9s.

C3a and C5a. It was mentioned previously that the two small split fragments, C3a and C5a, although not a part of the continuing complement sequence, do possess biological activity. Originally called anaphylatoxins because they caused inflammatory tissue changes, C3a and C5a stimulate mast cells to secrete histamine, resulting in a marked increase in capillary permeability. In addition, C5a along with the C5b,6,7 complex is chemotactic for PMNs and eosinophils. Furthermore, C3a has been shown to cause smooth muscle contraction in vitro independently of histamine.

Summary

Any cell within the body to which an appropriate antigen–antibody complex may attach or to which a complex polysaccharide may attach is a potential target cell for complement-mediated lysis. The medical importance of this will become more apparent in the following section. In addition, it should be kept in mind that just one $\overline{C4a,2b,3b}$ complex or just one P,$\overline{C3B_2,Bb}$ complex on a cell surface can result in the formation of many C5b,6,7,8,9 lytic complexes on a single cell. This amplification of the system is based on the fact that many C5s can be split by just one of the aforementioned complexes. Finally, macrophages and neutrophils have specific receptors on their cell surfaces for C3b, perhaps accounting for the opsonic properties of complement.

Serology

The specificity with which immunoglobulins can discriminate between immunogens of similar structure and selectively bind to the single antigenic site that induces antibody formation should be clear at this point. In addition to a high degree of specificity, immunoglobulins possess an extraordinary degree of sensitivity in vitro. The term *serology* denotes the study of antigen–antibody reactions; the term is derived from the primary use of serum to measure these reactions. Over the years, a wide range of serologic procedures have been developed to assist in the diagnosis of infections and the determination of host immunity. These assays make use of functional properties of different immunoglobulin classes and have greatly expanded the immunologic armamentarium of those responsible for patient care (Table 11.1). In general, the type of antigen–antibody reaction detected depends primarily on the physical nature of the antigen—that is, on whether it is soluble,

Table 11.1: Immunologic Procedures Used in Diagnosis and/or Microbial Identification*

Procedure	Principle Involved	Positive Test Results	Applications Include:
Agglutination	Antibody clumps cells or other particulate antigen preparations	Aggregates (clumps) of antigens	1. Diagnosis of typhus and Rocky Mountain spotted fever (Weil–Felix test) 2. Diagnosis of typhoid fever (Widal test)
Complement fixation	Antigen–antibody complex of test system binds complement, which is thereby unavailable for binding by sheep RBCs and hemolysin of the indicator system	Cloudy red suspension	Diagnosis of various bacterial, mycotic, protozoan, viral, and helminthic (worm) diseases
Ferritin-conjugated antibodies	Antibody, to which ferritin (iron-containing) particles are attached, binds various types of antigens	Presence of localized dark spheres in electron micrographs	Locating bacterial, fungal, viral, and other biological antigens by electron microscopy
Hemagglutination	Homologous antibody (hemagglutinin) aggregates of RBCs†	Aggregates of RBCs	Blood typing
Hemagglutination inhibition (viral)	Antibody inhibits the agglutination of RBCs by coating hemagglutinating virus	Formation of a circle of unagglutinated cells	1. Determining the immune status toward German measles 2. Virus identification
Immunodiffusion	Antibody and soluble antigen diffuse toward one another through an agar gel and react where homologous antibody is in proper proportion to homologous antigen	Lines of precipitate form within the agar	Antigen and/or antibody identification
Immunofluorescent microscopy	Antibody (usually) or antigen is labeled with a fluorescent dye, which fluoresces on exposure to ultraviolet or blue light	Glowing on exposure to ultraviolet light	1. Detection of antigen or antibody 2. Identification of microbial pathogens, such as rabies, syphilis, etc.
Precipitation	Antibody and soluble antigen react where they are in proper proportion to one another	Lines of precipitate form	1. Diagnosis of microbial diseases 2. Detection of antigens
Radioimmunoassay	Antibody or antigen can be labeled with radioactive element, and the resulting complex precipitated and monitored for radioactivity	Radioactivity counts	1. Detection of antigen and/or antibody 2. Detection of hepatitis antigen
Virus neutralization	Antibody neutralizes infectivity	Absence of virus destructive effects	1. Determining neutralizing effects of antibody 2. Virus identification and diagnosis

*Adapted with permission of Macmillan Publishing Company from G. A. Wistreich and M. D. Lechtman: *Microbiology*, Ed. 3. Glencoe Publishing Co., Calif, 1988. Copyright © 1988 by Macmillan Publishing Company.
†Hemagglutination reactions caused by certain viruses and bacteria generally do not involve antibody.

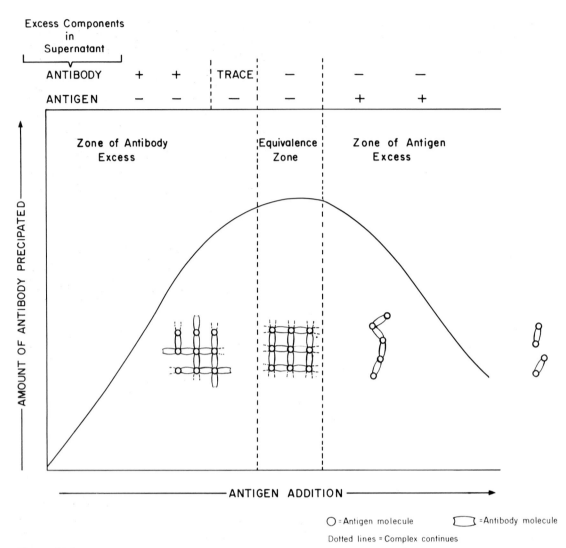

Excess Components
in
Supernatant

ANTIBODY	+	+	TRACE	−	−	−
ANTIGEN	−	−	−	−	+	+

Zone of Antibody
Excess

Equivalence
Zone

Zone of Antigen
Excess

AMOUNT OF ANTIBODY PRECIPITATED

ANTIGEN ADDITION

◯ = Antigen molecule   ⬭ = Antibody molecule

Dotted lines = Complex continues

Figure 11.2: Quantitative precipitin curve for a single antigen and its homologous antibody. The curve rises sharply as more antigen is added in the zone of antibody excess, reaching a maximum level with a plateau in the equivalence zone and then declining in the zone of antigen excess. The presumed antigen–antibody lattice configuration for each zone is depicted under the precipitin curve.

particulate, and so forth. Many important medical diagnostic tests also take advantage of different immunoglobulin biochemical properties to detect minute quantities of antigens or antibodies in biological specimens. The sensitivity of these assays has increased over the years as sophisticated indicator systems have been developed that detect the presence of extremely small quantities of antigen–antibody complexes. Representative tests will be discussed to illustrate the diverse nature of the procedures available.

Quantitative Precipitin Curve

The first visual demonstration of specific antigen–antibody interaction occurred when it was found that antigen and antibody mixed in correct proportions in a test tube yielded a stable, white flocculent precipitate. This observation led to the development of the quantitative precipitin curve. The curve is experimentally developed by starting with a series of tubes, each containing a known, constant amount of antibody. To each tube in this series is added an incrementally greater amount of a single antigen so that the first tube in the series contains the least amount of antigen and the last tube contains the greatest amount. Reaction mixtures are incubated to allow precipitates to form. If one then quantitatively measures the amount of precipitate formed in each tube, a curve is generated, as shown in Figure 11.2. This curve shows that the maximum amount of precipitate is formed in tubes where the concentration of antigen is roughly equivalent to the concentration of antibody, termed the *equivalence zone*. To either side of the equivalence zone on the curve (antibody excess or antigen excess), progressively less precipitate is detected. To account for the observed precipitation, it is assumed that as equivalence is approached, each antigen molecule is linked to more than one antibody molecule and each antibody molecule is linked to more than one antigen molecule. When the growing aggregate reaches a critical size it becomes insoluble and falls out of solution. In both antibody and antigen excess zones, aggregates of this critical size cannot develop.

Precipitin Reactions in Gels

A modification of the precipitin reaction that allows the analysis of multiple antigen systems involves diffusion of antigens through a semisolid agar gel rather than a liquid medium. Depending on the procedure employed, the antigen or antibody can diffuse in a single dimension or in two dimensions. Regardless of the procedure, the principle is the same. Multiple antigens diffuse at different rates, depending on their diffusion coefficients. These are partially determined by the substances' molecular weights and three-dimensional shapes. The same is true for the diffusion of immunoglobulins. At some point during diffusion, antigen and specific antibody will meet at concentrations corresponding to the equivalence zone of the quantitative precipitin curve, and a precipitate will be formed. This reaction is manifested as an opaque, opalescent line. Each antigen in the original mixture for which there is a specific immunoglobulin will appear as a separate line.

Oudin developed a technique whereby antiserum is mixed with agar in the liquid state and poured into a small tube. When the agar has solidified, a solution of antigen is poured over the antiserum containing agar. Precipitin lines develop as the antigen diffuses into the gel. A modification of this technique was developed in which antiserum is first added to a tube, then a column of agar is added, and finally antigen is layered over the top of the agar gel. Antiserum diffuses upward into the gel and antigens diffuse downward into the gel. Again, precipitin bands develop in the gel where antigen and antibody meet in a zone of relative equivalence.

Ouchterlony developed one of the most useful agar diffusion techniques which allows one to determine the degree of identity existing between antigens from different sources (Fig. 11.3). Agar is poured to a uniform thickness on a glass plate and when the gel has solidified, small cylinders of agar are removed, which creates wells in the remaining agar. Antigens and antibodies are then added to the wells and both con-

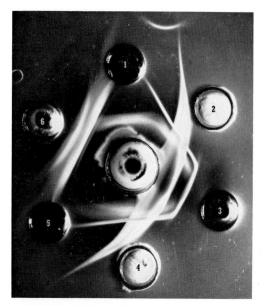

Figure 11.3: Double diffusion test (Ouchterlony technique) between antisaliva serum from a rabbit (*center well*) and six antigen solutions, showing the presence of amylase and several serum proteins in saliva. (*1*) Cohn fraction V, human serum. (*2*) Whole human serum. (*3*) Human parotid saliva. (*4*) Whole human serum. (*5*) Cohn fraction II-1, 2, human serum. (*6*) Whole human saliva. The heavy arc from well *3* is due to amylase + antiamylase (Courtesy of S. A. Ellison.)

stituents diffuse out from the wells in all directions. Precipitin lines are formed at a point where the advancing fronts meet.

Immunoelectrophoresis is another variation of agar diffusion. This assay is particularly useful for analyzing complicated mixtures of antigens such as those present in serum. Serum is first placed in a well cut in an agar slab, then a potential difference is applied across the agar. Serum proteins are separated according to their net electrical charges, molecular weights, and diffusion constants. After separation has been accomplished, a long trough is cut in the agar, parallel to the applied potential difference. The trough is subsequently filled with antiserum (serum-containing antibodies raised against the test serum proteins). The electrically separated proteins and the antiserum diffuse toward each other and precipitin lines are formed (Fig. 11.4). Though not very sensitive, this technique is useful for detecting deficiencies in, or absences of, normal serum constituents. In fact, all of the gel methods described so far can be viewed as qualitative tests. They measure the presence or absence of an antigen rather than how much antigen is present.

In contrast, radial immunodiffusion can be used to quantify antigen concentration. In this technique,

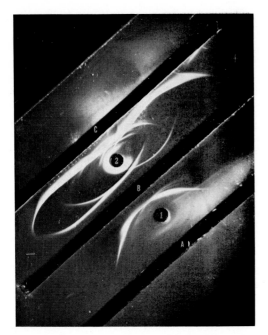

Figure 11.4: Immunoelectrophoretic test with human saliva, human serum, and respective rabbit antisera. A layer of buffered agar about 1 mm thick was formed on a glass plate. Wells 1 and 2 and troughs A, B, and C were cut from the agar. Saliva in well 1 and whole serum in well 2 were subjected to electrophoresis along the strips of agar by electrodes applied across the plate at + and −. The current was interrupted and rabbit antiserum against human saliva was placed in trough B, rabbit antiserum against human serum in troughs A and C. Between trough B and well 1 is the amylase band and two minor bands. Serum proteins in the saliva were too dilute to give bands between trough A and well 1. However, antibodies against several serum proteins were present in the antisaliva serum, as shown by the three bands between trough B and well 2. (Courtesy of S. A. Ellison.)

monospecific antibody is incorporated into an agar gel. Again, wells are cut in the agar and antigen is added. If the antiserum is specific for the antigen, a precipitin ring will develop around and at some distance from the antigen well. The diameter of the precipitin ring can be correlated with antigen concentration by comparing the diameters of unknown antigen concentrations with the diameters of rings developed from known antigen concentrations.

Agglutination Reactions

Under the appropriate conditions, bacteria, fungi, and red blood cells (RBCs) can be agglutinated (clumped) in the presence of immunoglobulins specific for some surface antigen on these cells. Furthermore, the presence or absence of agglutination is quite visible either microscopically or macroscopically. Agglutination thus provides an easily observed indicator of the presence or absence of immune com-

plex formation. In principle, agglutination is very similar to observable precipitation, i.e., at the appropriate concentrations one immunoglobulin is attached to more than one cell and each cell is bound by more than one immunoglobulin so that a large aggregate is formed.

Agglutination forms the basis for some of the most clinically useful diagnostic tests available. Not only do these tests indicate the presence or absence of a specific immune complex, but they also can reveal relative concentrations of either antigen or antibody. Usually agglutination tests are employed to determine whether or not an individual has been exposed to a specific infectious agent. This can be determined by measuring an increase in specific antibody to a particular agent over background levels. In many cases this provides a retrospective diagnosis because significant increases in unbound immunoglobulins may only be present in serum after the acute phase of clinical illness. In order to determine the relative concentration of specific immunoglobulins present in an individual's serum, the serum may be serially diluted in 2-fold fashion. The last dilution of the serum that yields a "positive reaction" with a constant amount of antigen is taken as the end point. The relative concentration of immunoglobulins is expressed as a titer, which is the reciprocal of the highest dilution that caused agglutination of the antigen. For example, if a dilution of 1:256 causes agglutination but a dilution of 1:512 does not, then the titer is expressed as 256.

Passive Agglutination

Although the direct agglutination of some bacteria and fungi by serum can be used in the diagnosis of some diseases, the majority of agglutination tests take advantage of the fact that a wide variety of antigens can be passively coupled to the surfaces of RBCs or latex spheres to produce an easily observable agglutination or lack thereof. Many antigens, including some viruses, bacterial antigens, endotoxins, and proteins, will spontaneously adsorb to the surface of RBCs. In addition, the repertoire of antigens can be expanded by using coupling agents such as tannic acid, glutaraldehyde, and carbodiimides to passively bind antigens to RBC surfaces.

Regardless of the antigen used, the mechanics of the test are the same. A constant amount of antigen-covered erythrocytes is placed in a series of small test tubes or the wells of microtiter plates. Increasing dilutions of a patient's serum are added to the tubes or wells and the mixture is incubated to allow agglutination to occur. In some cases, sera with high specific titers fail to agglutinate RBCs at low serum dilutions. This seemingly false negative reaction is termed the *prozone phenomenon* and is analogous to the lack of precipitation found in the antibody excess zone of the precipitin curve. In essence, there is such an abundance of antibody that significant cross-linking of RBCs does not occur. At higher serum dilutions, however, agglutination does occur.

Hemagglutination Inhibition

Many viruses, such as the influenza and parainfluenza viruses, have the ability to spontaneously agglutinate RBCs. One method of determining the specific antiviral serum titers to these viruses is the hemagglutination inhibition test, which involves two steps. In the first step, a constant number of erythrocytes is added to each reaction mixture. If specific antibody is present, it will bind with the viral capsid surface, thereby interfering with the ability of the virus to agglutinate the RBCs. The titer of the serum is thus determined by the highest dilution at which no agglutination is observed. Small quantities of antigen can also be detected by this method. In this case the first step involves mixing the test antigen with a known amount of specific antibody. In the second step, a known number of RBCs coated with the same antigen is added to the test mixtures. If antigen was indeed present in the test solution, it will bind the available antibody, and hemagglutination of the antigen-coated erythrocytes will not occur. The degree to which antigen in the test solution successfully competes for the available antibody gives a measure of the amount of antigen present.

Antiglobulin Test (Coombs Test)

During the development and testing of many hemagglutinating systems, it was found that many specific antibody preparations failed to agglutinate antigen-coated RBCs. Either the antibody concentration was too low to cause large aggregate formation or, for some reason, the immunoglobulin molecules did not form a bridge between antigen-coated erythrocytes. A typical example of such a nonagglutinating antibody is the antibody specific for the Rh determinants on human RBCs. Coombs discovered that RBCs coated with antibodies specific for a surface antigen could be agglutinated if antibody specific for the cell-bound immunoglobulin was added to the mixture. Furthermore, one can determine the immunoglobulin class of bound antibody by adding antiglobulin specific for each heavy chain class.

Complement Fixation

Because many antigen–antibody complexes fix complement, the consumption of complement in vitro can be used to detect and measure antigens, antibodies, or both. This test also is a two-stage procedure. In the first stage, antigen, antibody, and a known amount of complement (often of guinea pig origin) are mixed. If antigen–antibody complexes form, then complement will be consumed. In the second stage, antibody-coated sheep erythrocytes are added to the test mixtures. If complement has been consumed in the test mixture, it will be unavailable to lyse the antibody-coated RBCs. Therefore, absence of RBC lysis is a positive test result. On the other hand, if antigen and antibody did not complex in the test mixture, then complement will be available to lyse the RBCs in the indicator system. Lysis of RBCs in this instance constitutes a negative result.

Fluorescent Antibody Techniques

Fluorescent antibody tests are particularly useful for detecting the presence of cell-bound antigens or antibodies. The cells can be of bacterial, fungal, or human origin. Regardless of the cell origin, the first step involves fixing the cells to a microscope slide. In the direct fluorescent antibody technique, a fluorescent dye, either fluorescein isothyocyanate, which appears green under ultraviolet light, or tetramethylrodamine isothiocyanate, which appears red when excited by ultraviolet light, is covalently coupled to specific antibody. The resulting conjugated antibody is allowed to react with the cell preparation and then the slide is thoroughly washed to remove any unbound antibody. The specimen is then examined microscopically with ultraviolet illumination. Bound antibody is detected from the presence of the characteristic dye color which is seen against a dark background (Fig. 11.5).

A modification of this technique that enhances the sensitivity of the test and reduces the number of different conjugated antibodies necessary is the indirect immunofluorescent test. In the first stage of this test, specific antibody is added that does not have a fluorescent dye conjugated to it. After thorough washing, an antibody preparation that reacts specifically with human immunoglobulins is added. This second antibody is conjugated with a fluorescent dye and then the slide is observed for specific dye color. The advantage of the indirect method is that one conjugated anti-human serum preparation can be used for all test systems that use specific human immunoglobulins (see Fig. 11.5). Both of these methods are very useful. However, careful attention must be paid to technical details and appropriate positive and negative controls.

Radioimmunoassays

Radioimmunoassays (RIAs) are among the most sensitive immunological tests now available. If properly used, RIAs can detect less than 1.0 pg of material. They have been employed to detect hepatitis B virus surface antigen and serum IgE for specific allergens.

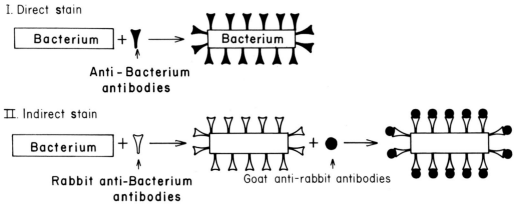

Figure 11.5: Direct and indirect immunofluorescence assays. In the direct procedure, the antigens on the bacterial cell react with specific antibodies that are labeled with a fluorescent dye (*black*). In the indirect staining procedure, the antigens on the bacterial cell react with unlabeled antibodies (*white*) produced, in this case, in a rabbit. Antibodies against rabbit immunoglobulins, produced in a goat, are labeled with a fluorescent dye (*black*) and react with the rabbit anti-bacterial cell antibodies, resulting in a visible complex. Thus, one labeled antibody preparation can be used as a stain for a variety of serologically specific reactions.

There are many variations of this technique, but one of the most popular methods is based on the observation that almost all antibodies and some antigens can be adsorbed to the surface of plastic, usually polystyrene spheres or tubes. After antibody is bound to the plastic, a solution of unknown antigen is added. If that antigen is bound to the solid-phase antibody, two methods can be used to detect the presence of the antigen–antibody complexes. In one scheme, a second antibody is added that is radioactively labeled and also is specific for the test antigen. If antigen is bound to the solid-phase antibody, then the radioactively labeled antibody will bind to the antigen as well. Thus, the antigen is sandwiched between two layers of antibody, and antigen–antibody complex is detected in a radiodetector. In the second scheme, a mixture of antigens is added to the solid-phase antibody that consists of a known quantity of radiolabeled antigen and an unknown quantity of the test antigen. In this case, labeled and unlabeled antigen compete for a limited number of antibodies. The amount of labeled antigen bound is dependent on the concentration of antigen in the unknown solution; i.e., the higher the concentration of unlabeled antigen present, the less labeled antigen will be bound by antibody.

Antibody-Mediated Disease

Up to this point, the immune response, particularly the humoral immune response, has been presented as a beneficial component of the body's defense against invading microorganisms and other noxious substances. However, the immunological sword can cut in two directions. For example, the injection of a small amount of bee venom into the skin of a person hardly seems to constitute a serious problem, yet an adverse immune response to that venom can kill within minutes. Similarly, it is difficult to understand why a protective system should produce acute glomerulonephritis in the process of ridding the body of an infectious agent. In the following sections, these unfavorable phenomena will be discussed and an attempt made to explain these phenomena in terms of an inappropriate, overly vigorous immune response or an insufficient immune response.

These types of reactions may be grouped under the general heading of allergy or hypersensitivity. Although some semantic differences exist, the terms are often used synonymously. Hypersensitive or allergic reactions are defined as altered immune responses that cause harm or tissue damage and do not occur in all members of the same species. Such adverse reactions may develop to a wide variety of plants, foods, drugs and many other substances and have been known for centuries. Manifestations may range from mild to life-threatening and are potential hazards during patient treatment. Although there are a number of reasons why allergic responses are of importance to dental professionals, three major ones are: 1) Many chemicals, drugs, and dental materials used in patient care may evoke hypersensitivities. 2) Certain allergic reactions may directly affect the oral cavity. 3) Practitioners will be treating patients who suffer from various allergies, and who may present problems during certain procedures by responding adversely.

Two general classification systems have been devised for hypersensitivity reactions, in addition to the major categories of immediate and delayed responses (Table 11.2). In general, types I, II, and III would

Table 11.2: Hypersensitivity Reactions*

	Type I: Anaphylactic	Type II: Cytotoxic (Antibody-Mediated)	Type III: Immune Complex (Arthus, Serum Sickness)	Type IV: Cell-Mediated (Delayed)
Indicator Etiology and mechanism	IgE, rarely IgG4 Reagin with antigen causes release of pharmacologic mediators of anaphylaxis	IgG, IgM, rarely IgA Antibody combining with tissue antigens causes activation of complement system, which causes cytolysis	IgG (usually) Antibody and soluble antigen form insoluble complexes that 1) deposit at various sites, causing inflammation, etc., and 2) cause activation of complement system	Cellular Immune lymphoid cell reaction with antigenic cells or proteins causes 1) direct killing of antigenic cells, 2) production of mediators of cell-mediated immune response, causing accumulation of PMNs, monocytes, etc., the liberation of lysosomal enzymes, and inflammation
Examples	Penicillin allergy, insect sting hypersensitivity, many food and drug allergies	RBC destruction in transfusion reactions, systemic lupus erythematosus, poststreptococcal glomerulonephritis, rheumatic fever	Allergic granulomatous angiitis, serum sickness, lupus nephritis, chronic glomerulonephritis	Contact dermatitis, poison ivy allergy

*Adapted with permission from the publisher and R. D. Guttmann et al.: *Immunology*. The Upjohn Co, Kalamazoo, Mich., 1987.

be considered immediate hypersensitivity reactions, since each involves immunoglobulin activity. The following discussion will be limited to types I and III, as these are considered by many immunologists to be classic forms of immediate-type allergic responses. An earlier section of this chapter discussed some of the sequelae of complement fixation in tissues.

Immediate-type Hypersensitivity— Anaphylaxis

Most immune responses categorized as immediate allergic or hypersensitivity responses are mediated by IgE. There appear to be at least two groups of antigens that tend to elicit an IgE response. One group consists of haptens. Examples of this group are penicillin and its metabolic products, which efficiently bind to the circulating carriers necessary to make the hapten immunogenic. The second group consists of environmental immunogens and includes various plant pollens, spores, and animal danders that are unusually resistant to enzymatic degradation after entering the body. Those immunogens that usually elicit an IgE rather than an IgG response are called sensitizers, reagins, or allergens. Usually, very low antigen doses are required to stimulate an IgE response.

IgE-producing plasma cells have routinely been found in the intestinal mucosa, respiratory mucosa, and mesenteric lymph nodes. Even in these locations, however, IgE-bearing B-lymphocytes are outnumbered by IgA-bearing lymphocytes. IgE-producing plasma cells or IgE-bearing B-lymphocytes are rarely found in other regional lymph nodes or in the spleen, accounting for the extremely low serum levels of IgE. The paucity of IgE production and the relatively few incidents of IgE-mediated disease both suggest that IgE production is under stringent regulation. In the compass of all immunoglobulin production, IgE production is the most dependent on T-helper cell activity. Furthermore, IgE production is considerably more susceptible to T-suppressor cell activity than is IgG production. When IgE is produced, a series of events is set into motion that is quite different from any of the humoral responses discussed previously.

Cytotropic Nature of IgE

IgE has the ability to bind to mast cells and basophilic polymorphonuclear leukocytes (basophils). Mast cells are nonmotile connective tissue cells found peripheral to capillaries. They are especially prevalent in skin, lungs, and the gastrointestinal and genitourinary tracts. Basophils are derived from hematopoietic stem cells of the white blood cell series and are motile. IgE is bound via specific IgE (Fc) receptors on the surface of mast cells and basophils via the Fc portion of its heavy chains. The high affinity of IgE for these receptors accounts for the long-term sensitivity to IgE-eliciting antigens.

Mast Cell/Basophil Activation

In order for mast cells or basophils to be activated, two conditions must be met. 1) IgE must be bound to mast cell or basophil surface receptors. This implies that the individual has had at least one previous exposure to the antigen to induce initial synthesis of IgE (i.e., a sensitizing dose). 2) Antigen during a second or subsequent exposure (i.e., challenge dose) must specifically cross-link a minimum of two surface-bound IgE molecules. This causes the aggregation of surface Fc receptors. When receptor aggregation has occurred, mast cells are said to degranulate. During degranulation, preformed granules residing within the cytoplasm of these cells and containing histamine, heparin, and other substances fuse with the cytoplasmic membrane, emptying their contents to the exterior of the cell. Degranulation does not involve destruction of the cell. The substances released from granules are pharmacologically active, and because they are preformed they are classified as primary mediators of immediate hypersensitivity. In addition, after degranulation begins, other pharmacologically active mediators are rapidly synthesized by the cell and secreted into the surrounding environment. These latter substances are called secondary mediators. The released mediators, whether primary or secondary, actually cause the physical manifestations observed in immediate-type hypersensitivity. Representative examples of each type of mediator are described below.

Primary Mediators

Histamine. Histamine is formed from L-histidine and is found throughout the body but is present in high concentrations in the granules of mast cells and basophils in addition to platelets. Mast cells are the major source of histamine in host tissues.

Physiologically, the action of histamine is exerted by its interaction with two distinct cell surface receptors, H_1 and H_2. The H_1-receptor controls the inflammatory responses, including increased capillary permeability, the smooth muscle contraction of bronchi that results in a profound increase in airway resistance, and the smooth muscle contraction of the intestines. Histamine effects mediated through H_1-receptors can be reversed by antihistamines. The noninflammatory effects of histamine are mediated through H_2-receptors. These effects include increased gastric secretion of HCl and cardiac stimulation. These actions cannot be blocked by antihistamines but rather require thiourea derivatives.

Species vary in their sensitivity to histamine, and man is exquisitely sensitive to its actions. Therefore, histamine release is a major contributor to the manifestations of anaphylactic hypersensitivity.

Serotonin (5-hydroxytryptamine, 5-HT). Serotonin is a vasoactive amine formed from L-tryptophan. Its body distribution varies in different species. In some rodent species it is found preformed in the granules of mast cells and basophils and is released during typical IgE–antigen complex formation. In humans, serotonin is not found in mast cells or basophils but in platelets, the brain, and the enterochromaffin cells of the gastrointestinal tract. In humans, serotonin can be released from platelets during an IgE-mediated response by a secondary mediator (see below) produced in mast cells and basophils after degranulation. The pharmacological effects of serotonin are very similar to those of histamine, i.e., smooth muscle contraction and venule leakiness. Many rodents are quite sensitive to this substance but humans are rather resistant to serotonin. Therefore, its role as an active mediator in human anaphylaxis is believed to be a minor one at best.

Eosinophil Chemotactic Factors of Anaphylaxis (ECF-A). ECF-As are highly selective chemoattractants for eosinophils that are found preformed in human mast cells and basophils. The association of eosinophils with allergic reactions is classic, and eosinophilia in the circulation of localized tissues is an important clinical indicator of hypersensitivity or parasitic infestation.

The best characterized ECF-As consist of two acidic tetrapeptides, but a much larger polypeptide with the same function also is known to exist in granules. ECF-A is important because eosinophils exhibit multiple functions during these immediate allergic reactions. They serve as scavenger cells, ingesting and degrading antigen–antibody complexes, and they also release a substance that inhibits the actions of slow-reacting substance of anaphylaxis, a secondary mediator of type I hypersensitivity reactions.

Heparin. Heparin is a proteoglycan that is located in the granules of human mast cells. Heparin has the ability to block complement activity and inhibits both coagulation and fibrinolysis.

Secondary Mediators

Slow-Reacting Substance of Anaphylaxis (SRS-A). SRS-A is comprised of a mixture of arachidonic acid metabolites, collectively termed leukotrienes. SRS-A appears in an immediate-type hypersensitivity response after mast cell and basophil degranulation is complete (approximately 5 minutes).

Because SRS-A is not preformed prior to IgE–antigen complex formation on the surface of mast cells and basophils, it is classified as a secondary mediator. Nonetheless, degranulation must in some way trigger its synthesis. The most notable pharmacological effect of SRS-A in humans is a profound ability to cause bronchiolar constriction and vascular permeability. The smooth muscle contraction is greater and of longer duration than that produced by histamine. For this reason, SRS-A is considered to be the most important cause of asthma. Furthermore, the action of SRS-A is not blocked by antihistamines, and exogenously administered epinephrine may be required to reduce bronchiole constriction. However, the body does have substances that will block the action of SRS-A, namely the arylsulfatases released by eosinophils. It now becomes clear why ECF-A release is important: this substance and the subsequent release of arylsulfatases provide a mechanism for returning the system to homeostasis.

Platelet-Activating Factor (PAF). Platelet-activating factors also are synthesized and released from mast cells and basophils after these cells have been degranulated. The major PAFs are phospholipids which, when released, both aggregate platelets and stimulate the release of serotonin from platelets.

Physical Manifestations of Immediate-type Hypersensitivity

The degree and the severity of physical manifestations of an IgE-mediated response depend on several factors: the total number of mast cells and/or basophils that are coated with surface IgE specific for a particular antigen (usually a function of the number of exposures a responding individual has had to the sensitizing antigen); the site of antigen administration (topical via skin, inhalation into the lung, ingestion, or systemically administered); and to some extent the amount of antigen administered. In individuals who are mildly sensitized, local cutaneous administration of the sensitizing antigen typically produces localized symptoms as soon as 2 to 3 minutes after antigen administration. The first symptom usually experienced is itching at the site of penetration, followed quickly by a pale edematous raised zone surrounded by a halo of erythema, termed a wheal-and-flare reaction. The response reaches maximal intensity by about 10 minutes, persists for another 10 to 20 minutes, and then gradually subsides. This phenomenon is referred to as cutaneous anaphylaxis, wheal-and-erythema, wheal-and-flare, or a hive (Fig. 11.6). At the other end of the spectrum, injection, deliberate or otherwise, of the same amount of antigen in a hypersensitive individual can result in a dramatic increase in the speed of onset, distribution, and intensity of the anaphylactic

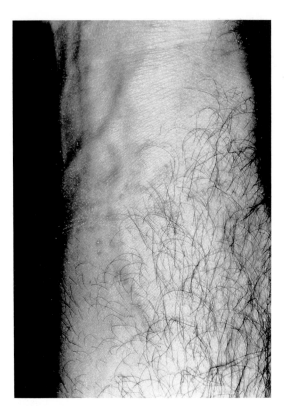

Figure 11.6: Cutaneous anaphylaxis on arm in an individual allergic to animal (mouse) dander.

response. In generalized or systemic anaphylaxis, massive edema can develop around the site of antigen injection. Difficulty in breathing and swallowing is encountered, owing to bronchial and laryngeal constriction and edema, and there may be profound hypovolemic shock, owing to peripheral capillary permeability and vasodilation. Anaphylactic death in humans can occur very rapidly and is primarily related to asphyxia. After a response of this intensity, if the individual does not die, recovery is usually complete within an hour. The important points for clinicians to keep in mind are 1) demonstration on the part of patients of any of these symptoms is cause for concern, and 2) demonstration of difficulty in breathing demands rapid and decisive intervention.

Atopy.   There appears to be a heritable predisposition for some individuals to easily become hypersensitive to a few or many environmental allergens. Hypersensitivity develops spontaneously when these allergens are inhaled or ingested. Airborne plant pollens, particularly ragweed pollen, are the most common and well-studied allergens in the United States. In addition, tree and grass pollens, microbial spores, house dust (which is composed of epidermal products of man and animals, bacteria, molds, and insect parts), bovine milk constituents, and egg albumin all can be potent allergens. The two most common physi-

cal manifestations of inhalation allergy are hay fever, more properly termed allergic rhinitis, and asthma. Allergic rhinitis is characterized by sneezing, nasal congestion, and watery discharge, increased lacrimation, periorbital edema, and conjunctival itching. On the other hand, symptoms of bronchial asthma are paroxysmal seizures of dyspnea associated with coughing and wheezing. Chest tightness is an early symptom and in some cases is preceded by allergic rhinitis. Unlike emphysema, asthma is episodic, leaves no permanent tissue damage, and usually is not brought on by exertion.

Desensitization.   One way of preventing allergic responses is avoidance of the allergen. Since avoidance may not be a practical solution, a common strategy involves active treatment of an individual with the hope of preventing IgE-mediated responses. This involves induction of noncytotropic-blocking antibodies by repeated injections of small and increasing amounts of the allergen to induce the production of IgG. The rationale for this procedure is predicated on the concept that in the presence of high concentrations of IgG, the allergen would be bound by the IgG before it had the opportunity to bind either to mast cell and basophil-bound IgE, or the opportunity to elicit more IgE production. IgG thus serves as a competitive inhibitor for IgE binding and sequelae. The clinical results of this procedure are somewhat unpredictable and by no means universally successful. As a very rough estimate, approximately 50% of atopic individuals who have been through a desensitization series demonstrate some clinical improvement. Interestingly, many individuals who do not show improvement do have high levels of allergen-specific serum IgG.

Passive Transfer of IgE

Because immediate-type hypersensitivity is mediated by an immunoglobulin, it would seem reasonable to expect that sensitivity to a particular allergen could be transferred by serum from a sensitized to a nonsensitized individual. Indeed this is the case. The guinea pig has been a consistently reliable model for human anaphylactic responses, and passive transfer of hypersensitivity has been studied in great detail in this animal species.

Passive Cutaneous Anaphylaxis (PCA).   If a small quantity of dilute serum from a previously sensitized guinea pig is injected into the skin of a normal guinea pig, and if this transfer is followed the next day by an injection of the sensitizing allergen at the same site, then a typical wheal-and-flare reaction will be observed within minutes of injection of the allergen. A minimal latent period of 3 to 6 hours between serum injection and allergen injection is required, however, presumably to allow time for the transferred

Table 11.3: Immunological Characteristics of Human Immediate Hypersensitivity Reactions

Feature	Anaphylaxis	Arthus Reaction	Serum Sickness
Time	Minutes	2–4 hr	7–10 days
Histology	Edema, few cells	Infiltration by neutrophils	Infiltration by neutrophils
Tissue effects	Localized or systemic	Localized	Systemic
Ig involved	IgE	IgG, IgM	IgG, IgM
Complement	−	+	+
Pathogenesis	IgE, mast cells, basophils, platelets	Ag-Ab complexes and $C \rightarrow$ PMNs	Ag-Ab complexes and $C \rightarrow$ PMNs

IgE to bind to the surfaces of mast cells and basophils in the immediate vicinity of the injection site. The PCA phenomenon can be made more visible if a dye such as Evans blue is injected intravenously just prior to the injection of antigen. Because of the mediator-induced increase in capillary permeability, the blood-borne dye leaks into the tissue surrounding the antigen injection site. In fact, measurement of the diameter of the blue-stained area has been used as a semiquantitative measure of IgE concentration.

Prausnitz–Küstner Reaction. Passive cutaneous anaphylaxis can be demonstrated in humans by following essentially the same procedure used to demonstrate PCA in guinea pigs. PCA in humans is termed the Prausnitz–Küstner reaction after those who first described it in 1921. Again, a small amount of diluted serum from an atopic individual is injected into the skin of a nonsensitized person. In humans, the latent period required between serum injection and allergen injection is 10 to 20 hours. As in PCA in the guinea pig, if the donor's serum contains IgE specific for the allergen, a typical wheal-and-flare reaction will develop very quickly at the injection site. The Prausnitz–Küstner reaction was used in humans as a safe alternative to direct skin testing of atopic individuals.

Schultz–Dale Reaction. Returning to the guinea pig model, there is one additional method used for demonstrating immediate-type hypersensitivity induced either actively or passively. The Schultz–Dale reaction occurs when isolated uterine or intestinal strips from a sensitized animal contract in vitro with the addition of antigen to the bathing solution.

Immune Complex Diseases

After the discovery of anaphylaxis, other types of antibody-dependent tissue reactions were described that differed from anaphylaxis in the time of onset, were not mediated by IgE, and produced different histopathologic findings at the tissue reaction sites (Table 11.3). Although tissue injury caused by immune complexes can manifest in many parts of the body, the principles of the reaction can be initially illustrated by the cutaneous Arthus reaction, named after the French physiologist who first described the response.

Arthus Reaction (Passive Cutaneous Form)

To demonstrate an Arthus reaction, immune serum from one individual is injected intravenously into a nonimmune recipient, then the specific antigen used to induce the immune serum is injected into the recipient's skin. One to two hours later the skin injection site appears edematous and erythematous. This is followed by punctate hemorrhages that reach a maximum 6 to 12 hours after injection; then the reaction slowly subsides. During severe cutaneous Arthus reactions, one finds evidence of tissue necrosis at the injection site.

Three essential elements must be present simultaneously in order to produce this lesion: soluble antigen–antibody complexes, complement, and PMNs. The appropriate soluble antigen–antibody complexes are produced when the concentration of antigen is greater than the concentration of corresponding antibody (slight antigen excess) and they are small so that they can remain suspended in circulating blood. These small complexes are of the configuration Ag_3Ab_2 or Ag_5Ab_3 and easily settle out of circulation along the walls of small blood vessels between endothelial cells and in contact with the elastic lamina. The final condition that these complexes must satisfy is that the complexed antibodies must be able to fix complement, e.g., IgG1, IgG3, or IgM.

After the antigen–antibody complexes have settled along vessel walls, complement is fixed via the classical pathway and the attendant release of C5a and perhaps C3a attracts and localizes PMNs. In the cells' attempt to phagocytize immune complexes, the lysosomal contents of the PMNs—acid phosphatases, neutral and acid proteases, collagenase, elastase, and acid lipases—are released and cause focal necrosis of the vessel wall. This accounts for the hemorrhage seen at the injection site. Necrotic PMNs are gradually replaced by macrophages and eosinophils and because the latter two cell types are able to phagocytize and degrade the immune complexes the inflammation disappears. Even though histamine is probably released from mast cells because of the action of C5a and C3a, the administration of antihistamines does not block the Arthus reaction.

Serum Sickness and Serum Sickness-like Syndromes

During the early days of clinical passive immunity procedures, it was common to induce the production of immunoglobulins specific for many infectious disease agents in rabbits and horses. Subsequently these animal sera were passively administered to humans. After repeated injections, or in some cases after a single injection, some of the human recipients developed a syndrome after 7 to 10 days that was characterized by enlarged lymph nodes and spleen, fever, erythematous and urticarial rashes, arthritis, and fever. In most cases the disease subsided in a few days, but in some cases the affected individuals died. Autopsy revealed disseminated vascular inflammatory lesions very similar to those observed in an Arthus reaction.

Because of subtle differences in the structure of animal serum proteins, they are recognized as foreign antigens by the immune systems of the human hosts. However, and again because they are serum proteins, they enjoy a normal biological half-life and remain in circulation for a relatively long period of time. As complement-fixing antibodies begin to appear in the host, the foreign serum proteins are present in antigen excess and therefore the necessary conditions prevail for the formation of soluble antigen–antibody complexes. It is important to understand that, even though the clinical manifestations of the accumulated reactions may take longer than a week to develop, serum sickness syndrome is still classified as an immediate hypersensitivity, because of the presence and activity of antibodies.

Unlike the localized Arthus reaction, in serum sickness any small vessel in the body is a potential target for antigen–antibody complex deposition, complement fixation, and localized vascular necrosis. The mechanisms for both reactions are very similar, and often serum sickness is described as a "systemic Arthus response." The systemic scope of immune complex deposition provides some explanation for the symptoms. Vessel damage near skin surfaces explains the rash. Systemic release of endogenous pyrogen from PMNs explains the fever, and systemic production of immunoglobulins is the basis for lymph node and spleen enlargement. Finally, synovial joints appear to be a preferred location for complex deposition, accounting for arthritic symptoms. In addition to synovial joints, other tissues that are primarily involved include the heart, which may reveal endocardial proliferation, valvular vegetations, myocarditis, and pericarditis; the arteries, which reveal necrosis involving all layers of the arterial wall; and the kidneys.

Because of the obvious potential danger of administering foreign serum proteins, the use of animal serum preparations is reserved for certain rare instances. Even though serum sickness was first recognized as a sequel to injection of foreign serum proteins, it is important to realize that any antigen that can, for one reason or another, remain in circulation for relatively long periods of time can also cause a serum sickness-like syndrome. As examples, chronic viral and bacterial diseases provide a continuous source of antigenic material capable of forming soluble complexes.

Glomerulonephritis

For reasons that are poorly understood, the basement membrane of glomerular capillaries of the kidney are particularly susceptible to localization of soluble immune complexes, regardless of the antigen. Furthermore, because glomerulonephritis is a common sequel of untreated streptococcal disease caused especially by a nephritogenic strain, it deserves separate attention. During immune complex disease in the kidney, the glomerular basement membrane is the primary site of injury. Microscopic examination reveals necrotic lesions in the basement membrane, while urinalysis reveals proteinuria followed by hematuria. If the damage is severe enough, the afflicted individual may experience renal failure. As the degenerative inflammatory process continues, endothelial proliferation occurs, along with slight basement membrane thickening. In the case of poststreptococcal glomerulonephritis, streptococcal antigens have been demonstrated in basement membrane immune complexes. In addition, antigens from the malarial strain *Plasmodium malariae* and hepatitis B viral antigens both commonly form soluble complexes with antibodies that localize in the kidney. In the case of chronic hepatitis B infection, the suggestion has been made that long-standing immune complex disease, including glomerulonephritis, occurs in individuals who are unable to mount a massive immunoglobulin response that would clear circulating antigens. Instead, these individuals appear to mount an intermediate response that, coupled with constant antigen production, leaves them in chronic antigen excess without antigen clearance.

ADDITIONAL READING

For additional reading, see Chapter 12, pages 147–149.

12

Cell-Mediated Immunity, Tumor Immunology, Transplantation, and Immunodeficiency Disorders

John A. Molinari

Up to this point the discussion of the immune system has been limited to specific humoral responses and the sequelae mediated by immunoglobulin molecules. In this chapter the functional role played by T-cells will be more fully developed. Several immune system responses, such as delayed-type hypersensitivity, rejection of transplanted tissue, and tumor immunology, appear to be mediated primarily by T-lymphocytes and their secreted products. Each of these responses is necessary for continued optimal function of specific host defenses. In addition, the rapidly expanding area of immunodeficiency disorders will be considered using information presented in this and earlier chapters.

Major Histocompatibility Antigens

All nucleated cells of the body have surface antigens coded for by genes associated with immune response functions. These antigens as a group are referred to as the major histocompatibility complex (MHC). In humans, the MHC is divided into two classes. Class I comprises the human leukocyte antigens (HLA). Although all nucleated cells have these antigens, their density varies greatly from one cell type to another. In a given individual, all HLA antigens are identical, and it is probable that the HLA antigens form the basis of self-recognition by the immune system. T-lymphocytes are particularly sensitive in recognizing subtle differences in or alterations to self-HLA antigens. Immunologically, T-cells are activated to become effector cells when they encounter foreign HLA antigens or when they encounter small cell-bound antigens that alter the character of self-HLA antigens.

Genetics of Human MHC

HLA-A to HLA-C Loci. Human population studies have revealed that HLA antigens can be arranged into three groups, HLA-A, B, and C. Allelic polymorphism among these HLA groups is considerable. The gene products of these alleles can be identified by specific antisera developed against human leukocytes and by newer assays that measure T-lymphocyte recognition. Individuals within the population are heterozygous for two alleles specified by each of the three loci. Each parent contributes one allele from each locus to the offspring at fertilization. The point to be stressed is that in an outbred human population tremendous diversity exists in HLA antigens due to the combinations of alleles possible at each locus. Conversely, the chances of finding phenotypic identity at each of these three loci in two nonrelated individuals are indeed remote.

HLA-D and HLA-DR. In addition to HLA-A, B, and C antigens, a second class of MHC antigens (class II) exists. Within this group HLA-D, DR, and DQ (D-related) loci are known. They are more limited than the former group of HLA loci with regard to their tissue distribution. HLA-DR, and DQ are found on the surfaces of B-lymphocytes, activated T-cells, and macrophages. These antigens may also be recognized by specific antisera and are considered important in determining whether or not B- and T-cell interactions will occur.

Structure of MHC Products

HLA-A to HLA-C. The A, B, and C loci each code for a polypeptide chain of approximately 45,000 daltons molecular weight (MW). In addition, there is an oligosaccharide component attached to the polypeptide, accounting for about 10% of the total molecular weight. The oligosaccharide can be enzymatically removed without altering the antigenicity of the molecule. This finding implies that the varied antigenicity of these polypeptides resides exclusively in the amino acid sequence. The carboxy end of the heavy chain has a hydrophobic segment that apparently interacts in a stable manner with cell membrane lipids.

Each heavy chain on the cell membrane is associated noncovalently with a lighter chain, β_2-microglobulin (MW = 12,000 daltons). The light chain also shares properties with immunoglobulin molecules in that portions of its amino acid sequence are homologous with those of C_H domains. Unlike the amino acid sequence heterogeneity seen in HLA heavy chains, the light chains associated with all heavy chains are identical within a species; furthermore, they do not extend into the cell membrane.

HLA-D. The HLA-D gene product is also a glycoprotein composed of two chains (α and β) per molecule that are of about equal molecular weight. Both chains extend into the cell membrane. Some chain pairs have interchain disulfide bonds, others do not.

The manner in which T-lymphocytes recognize MHC gene products—self, nonself, or altered self—has great significance in terms of how or if they will respond. The most familiar example involves T-cell–mediated destruction of transplanted tissue bearing foreign histocompatibility antigens.

Cell-Mediated Immunity and Infectious Disease

Antigens that primarily elicit a cell-mediated response have one important common feature. Unlike the rather large, particulate, macromolecular antigens of extracellular parasites, which tend to stimulate B-cells, antigens that stimulate antigen-reactive T-cells are often small and cell-bound. In contrast to B-cell activation, T-lymphocytes are not triggered by free antigen. Instead, surface receptors recognize antigenic moieties, which are bound to larger protein components on accessory cells. For example, small antigens derived from parasites capable of intracellular life, such as the tubercle bacillus, easily become bound to infected cell surfaces. In addition, virally infected cells have virus-coded antigens inserted in their surface membranes. When a circulating, antigen-sensitive T-cell comes in contact with an antigen-bearing cell, it recognizes the altered surface of the infected cell. It may recognize the new surface antigen in addition to the "self" HLA antigens, or, if the new antigen is on or near the "self" HLA antigens, it may recognize an alteration to the HLA antigens themselves.

Generation of Effector T-Lymphocytes

Once stimulated, antigen-reactive T-cells migrate to either a regional lymph node or the spleen, where cellular proliferation occurs in predominantly T-cell areas. The result of proliferation is an expanded pool of two subsets of effector cells. One effector subset, termed T_D (for delayed-type hypersensitivity), secretes biologically active substances termed lymphokines when it comes in contact with its specific antigen-bearing cell. This lymphocyte subclass is found within the group of T-cells exhibiting T4 surface antigens. Both the T_D and T-helper cells carry the T4 alloantigen (see Chap. 10), but from a functional standpoint they appear to be quite different cells. A second effector subset is termed cytotoxic T-lymphocyte (Tc) or T-killer cells (T_K), which specifically lyse target cells carrying the appropriate surface antigen. After proliferation, effector cells return to the site or sites or target antigens. These activated or sensitized T-lymphocytes are capable of synthesizing and releasing a vast array of substances called lymphokines. These soluble products of ac-

Table 12.1: Prominent Biological Properties of Human Lymphokines*

Lymphokine	Biological Properties
Interleukin-1 (α and β)	Activates resting T-cells; cofactor for hematopoietic growth factors; induces fever, sleep, ACTH release, neutrophilia, and other systemic acute-phase responses; stimulates synthesis of lymphokines, collagen, and collagenases; activates endothelial and macrophagic cells; mediates inflammation, catabolic processes, and nonspecific resistance to infection
Interleukin-2	Growth factor for activated T-cells; induces the synthesis of other lymphokines; activates cytotoxic lymphocytes
Interleukin-3	Supports the growth of pluripotent (multilineage) bone marrow stem cells; growth factor for mast cells
Colony-stimulating factor (CSF):	
Granulocyte-macrophage CSF	Promotes neutrophilic, eosinophilic, and macrophagic bone marrow colonies; activates mature granulocytes
Granulocyte CSF	Promotes neutrophilic colonies
Macrophage CSF	Promotes macrophagic colonies
Interleukin-4 (B-cell–stimulating factor-1)	Growth factor for activated B-cells; induces DR expression on B-cells; growth factor for resting T-cells; enhances cytolytic activity of cytotoxic T-cells; mast cell growth factor
B-cell–stimulating factor-2 (B-cell–differentiating factor)	Induces the differentiation of activated B-cells into immunoglobulin-secreting plasma cells; identical with β-interferon, plasmacytoma growth factor, and hepatocyte-stimulating factor
γ-Interferon	Induces class I, class II (DR), and other surface antigens on a variety of cells; activates macrophages and endothelial cells; augments or inhibits other lymphokine activities; augments natural killer cell activity; exerts antiviral activity
Interferon (α and β)	Exerts antiviral activity; induces class I antigen expression; augments natural killer cell activity; has fever-inducing and antiproliferative properties
Tumor necrosis factor (α and β)	Direct cytotoxin for some tumor cells; induces fever, sleep, and other systemic acute-phase responses; stimulates the synthesis of lymphokines, collagen, and collagenases; activates endothelial and macrophagic cells; mediates inflammation, catabolic processes, and septic shock

*Reproduced by permission of *The New England Journal of Medicine* from C. A. Dinarello and J. W. Mier. Lymphokines. *N Engl J Med,* **317,** 940–945, 1987.

tivated lymphocytes are primarily responsible for the manifestations of cellular immune responses. Although originally thought to be released only by T-cells, lymphokines have been found as products of other cells, including macrophages and B-lymphocytes. For this reason the more general term cytokine is often applied in place of lymphokine. The latter designation will be used in the present discussion, as the secreted products of lymphoid cells will be emphasized.

Many different lymphokines have been described (Table 12.1). An interesting property of lymphokines is that a specific T-cell–antigen interaction is necessary for their release but, once released, the actions of lymphokines are immunologically nonspecific. Representative examples of a few well-characterized lymphokine functions are described below.

Migration Inhibitory Factor (MIF). MIF was the first lymphokine to be described. Biochemically it is a heat-stable, nondialyzable protein. When MIF is released at the site of T_D-cell–target cell interaction, it inhibits the random migration of macrophages in vitro and presumably in vivo as well. Migrating macrophages therefore remain localized at the antigen site. This appears to have an important functional application for macrophage activity. Affected macrophages will tend to accumulate in those tissue sites where the immunologic stimulus or injury has occurred; thus, they have the overall effect of enhancing the immune system's capacity to eradicate foreign microorganisms.

Macrophage Activation Factor (MAF). Macrophages that have been incubated with MAF in vitro exhibit a number of morphological, metabolic, and functional changes. They are then termed activated macrophages. Activated macrophages are more aggressive and efficient phagocytes and possess an enhanced ability to kill phagocytosed microorganisms compared to nonactivated macrophages. In addition, activated macrophages exhibit the interesting property of enhanced ability to kill certain tumor cells but not their normal counterparts.

Leukocyte Inhibition Factor (LIF). LIF inhibits the migration of polymorphonuclear leukocytes (PMNs) in much the same manner that MIF inhibits macrophage motility. However, LIF is specific only for PMNs. It also may enhance the phagocytic ability of PMNs.

Lymphocyte Mitogenic Factor (LMF). T_D cells release a factor or factors that nonspecifically stimulate other noncommitted T-lymphocytes to undergo blast transformation and proliferation at the local peripheral site of antigen-bearing target cell. The result is a local expansion of the number of specific T_D-cells. The proliferation may be quite similar to the proliferation that takes place in regional lymph nodes.

The three aforementioned lymphokines—MIF/MAF, LIF, and LMF—all illustrate the remarkable efficiency and economy of cell-mediated responses. A very small number of T-cells migrating from a lymph node or spleen and localizing at some distant antigen site can locally recruit and activate a large number of uncommitted phagocytic cells and lymphocytes that attempt to clear the infectious agent from the area. Histologically, an intense inflammatory response occurs that causes a considerable amount of nonspecific tissue destruction, owing to the release of cytolytic enzymes from the accumulated phagocytic cells. In the case of intracellular bacterial and fungal pathogens, and considering the entire local cellular infiltrate, perhaps the most important defensive cells are the activated macrophages, because these cells have an enhanced ability to kill phagocytosed organisms. Recall that these same pathogens grow with impunity in nonactivated phagocytic cells.

Osteoclast Activating Factor (OAF).   Osteoclast activating factor is an interesting lymphokine whose presence and functional capacities have been described in vitro but whose in vivo significance remains to be determined. OAF is of particular interest to the dental community because its in vitro production stimulates the differentiation of osteoclasts, which in turn resorb bone. OAF can be elicited by specific antigen stimulation of T-cells or by nonspecific polyclonal T-cell mitogens such as phytohemagglutinin. OAF release by stimulated T-cells requires intimate interaction of the T-cell with a macrophage. This cellular interaction is not seen in the release of other lymphokines. It would be interesting to know whether or not T-cell stimulation by subgingival bacterial antigens with subsequent release of OAF plays a role in the pathogenic bone resorption seen in aggressive periodontal disease.

Tissue Response Mediated by CTLs

Cytotoxic lymphocytes or killer T-cells carry the T8 antigens, as do suppressor T-cells, but again, these cells appear to be functionally different. These effector T-cells have the ability to specifically lyse target cells with foreign antigens, such as those with virus-specific glycoproteins on their surfaces. Contact between CTL and target cell is required for lysis, but interaction with accessory cells such as macrophages is not required. With regard to the protective properties of cell-mediated responses against intracellular

parasites, CTLs appear to be particularly advantageous in viral disease. Cells in which viruses are replicating can be specifically killed and any infectious virus that is released during lysis may then be cleared by specific antibodies.

Cell-mediated immunity directed against infectious agents is very similar to the humoral response in terms of time course and memory. Effector cells in a primary response are first seen experimentally 5 to 7 days after exposure to the antigen. If reexposure to the same antigen occurs, a secondary (anamnestic) response occurs faster, with greater intensity and longer duration than the primary response. As for the secondary humoral response, this is presumably due to an expanded pool of specific antigen-reactive T-lymphocytes. Finally, as for the humoral immune response, tissue damage can be directly linked to the cellular immune response itself. For example, the large inflammatory lesions in response to infection by *Mycobacterium tuberculosis* causing the destruction of large areas of lung parenchyma are probably due to T_D-cells and the sequence of events following their release of lymphokines.

Cutaneous Delayed-Type Hypersensitivity (Type IV)

A host immunized with partially purified proteins extracted from an organism such as *M. tuberculosis* will develop a skin lesion on subsequent challenge with the same antigens (Fig. 12.1). Usually no reaction is seen for at least 10 hours after the protein preparation has been injected. Then erythema, swelling, and induration gradually appear, reaching maximal size and intensity at 24 to 72 hours. The lesion slowly resolves over the next several days. In a highly sensitive human, injection of this substance can cause local necrosis, ulceration, and scarring. Historically, the time course of this response distinguished it from immediate-type hypersensitivity and the cutaneous Arthus response, hence the term delayed-type hypersensitivity (DTH) or type IV hypersensitivity (see Table 11.2).

Histologically, DTH is readily distinguished from both immediate-type hypersensitivity and the Arthus response. In a mild to moderate DTH reaction, the earliest cellular infiltrate consists of small to medium-sized lymphocytes, neutrophils, monocytes, and macrophages that accumulate around postcapillary venules. At the time of maximal tissue response, the entire dermis is involved and mononuclear cells may be found in the epidermis. Necrosis of blood vessels, muscle, connective tissue, and epidermis may occur to varying degrees, depending on the sensitivity of the individual.

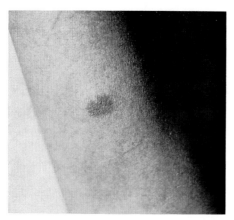

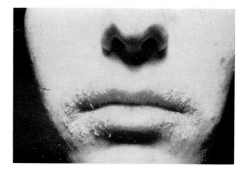

Figure 12.2: Contact dermatitis, an acute allergic reaction about the lips, cause unknown. (AFIP 57–7757–1.)

Figure 12.1: Positive reaction for tuberculin test. (AFIP 53–1280.)

Presumably the injected proteins become bound to cells in the dermis and are recognized by antigen-reactive T-cells, which became sensitized during the first exposure to *M. tuberculosis*. The resulting inflammatory lesion is a secondary cellular immune response and represents a localized cutaneous counterpart to the T_D-cell–mediated response mentioned previously. Similar responses may be induced by other antigens to which an individual has been sensitized.

Contact Skin Sensitivity

A variety of small molecular weight chemicals (<1,000 daltons) are capable of causing an allergic skin reaction in man simply by coming in contact with skin. The catechols of the poison ivy plant, soaps and detergents, drugs, many dental materials, and cosmetics all commonly cause allergic contact dermatitis. The initial exposure to a potential sensitizing substance usually does not elicit any visible skin response. In some individuals, however, if reexposure to the same substance occurs anywhere on the skin surface just 4 to 5 days after initial exposure, a localized DTH response is elicited. In other individuals, several exposures to the substance may be necessary before any visible manifestation is observed.

The time course of contact dermatitis is the same as that for a cutaneous DTH reaction of the tuberculin type. Erythema and swelling appear at 10 to 12 hours and reach a maximum between 27 and 72 hours. Usually intense reactions can produce necrosis, but even in the absence of necrosis, complete recovery can take several weeks. The dermis at the site of contact is invaded by macrophages, lymphocytes, and basophils, resembling the DTH response to tuberculin. The superficial epidermis, however, looks different. It becomes hyperplastic, invaded by macrophages and lymphocytes, and in man, intraepidermal vesicles or blisters form that are filled with serous fluid and a variety of cell types. Histologically, these lesions develop slowly, reaching a peak 3 to 6 days after contact (Figs. 12.2 and 12.3).

According to the general properties of antigens (see Chap. 9), it would seem that these substances are too small to act as complete antigens, but instead act as haptens which covalently bind to skin cell proteins. The covalent skin protein derivatives then behave as the complete antigen. As for other cell-mediated responses, antigen-reactive T-cells recognize both the antigen and MHC gene products, and as with all immune responses, reactions become more intense and last longer with each succeeding exposure. Once established, contact sensitivity can last for several years and then slowly diminish.

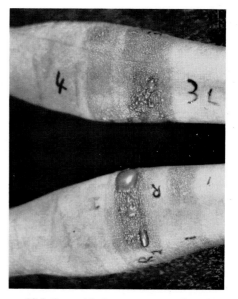

Figure 12.3: Dermatitis due to reaction to drugs. (AFIP 54–1548; 1st MFL–104.)

Transplantation

The study of tissue transplantation began as an unwelcome consequence of early cancer studies. It was found that when some tumors were transplanted to recipients in an outbred animal population, the tumor cells were killed. This observation led many investigators to believe that the immune control of cancer was a rather easily attainable goal. However, more rigorous experiments demonstrated that transplanted normal tissue was rejected as fast as or faster than tumor tissue. Although a cellular immune phenomenon caused tissue destruction in both cases, it was quickly appreciated that the critical antigens were not specific tumor antigens but rather normal cell surface antigens. Experimental work in transplantation immunology has increased our understanding of histocompatibility antigens, the role they play in cell-mediated responses in general, and their function in tissue rejection in particular. When the cellular immune response is viewed in broad perspective, tissue rejection is a minor consequence of the much broader protective functions of immune surveillance against deleterious nonself antigens, including infectious agents.

Types of Tissue Grafts

Autografts are transplants of tissue from one site to another on the same individual. If the surgical procedure employed is sound, autographs usually survive.

Isografts are transplants of tissue from one individual to a genetically identical individual. In humans, isografts are possible only between monozygotic twins. In animal populations, inbred strains can be produced by a series of brother–sister matings that result in an entire population of genetically identical individuals. Again, isografts, if performed correctly, usually survive in the recipient.

Allografts or homografts are transplants of tissue from one individual of the same species to a genetically nonidentical member of the same species. These transplants represent the bulk of human transplant procedures. Their success or failure is based on the degree of similarity between the MHC antigens as well as minor antigens of donor and recipient.

Heterografts or xenografts are transplants of tissue from one species to another species. They usually do not survive unless extraordinary measures are taken to eliminate cell surface antigens.

Responses to Transplantation

Typical rejection phenomena are well illustrated when skin is transplanted from a mouse of one strain to another mouse of a different strain. Technically, skin is relatively easy to transplant; its macroscopic fate is easy to observe; and tissue specimens are easily obtained for microscopic examination. The median survival time of the grafted tissue gives an indication of the intensity of the recipient's immune response. However, the same principles are involved in grafts of other tissues in other species, including man.

When a skin allograft is placed on a surgically prepared bed on the recipient animal, the graft is vascularized and cells within the graft proliferate. Host and graft tissue also attempt to heal the surgical site. However, 10 to 14 days later an intense inflammatory reaction can be observed in the allograft that results in death of the transplanted tissue, and finally the entire allograft is sloughed. If a second allograft is performed between the same donor and recipient, the rejection process is accelerated, beginning as early as 5 to 6 days after transplantation, and is more intense, meaning that once the rejection is started it is completed faster than the first rejection. This second-set rejection is histocompatibility antigen-specific, because an allograft from a second donor does not result in an accelerated rejection reaction. Second-set rejection also can be elicited by prior injection of virtually any donor cells other than red blood cells (RBCs). The cellular nature of this response may be demonstrated by two techniques. Transplantation immunity can be passively transferred by giving the prospective recipient presensitized, genetically identical lymphocytes, but not by transferring serum or immunoglobulins. Secondly, if a semipermeable membrane that inhibits cell migration but not fluid flow is placed between the grafted tissue and the recipient, the graft survives.

During rejection the histological picture resembles a typical DTM response with its massive accumulation of inflammatory cells and is, in all likelihood, directly mediated by both T_D-cells and CTLs, as well as their product lymphokines.

Graft-Versus-Host Reactions

In newborn animals that are immunologically unresponsive, or in humans who lack T-cell function, transplanted lymphocytes from immunocompetent adult donors often are not rejected. However, the donor lymphocytes can and do respond to the recipient's histocompatibility antigens. In the ensuing graft-versus-host reaction, the recipient animal fails to gain weight normally, develops skin lesions and diarrhea, and usually dies within a few weeks. In this situation the transplanted tissue literally has destroyed the recipient. This same phenomenon can occur in humans who are given bone marrow transplants in an attempt to repopulate their immune system to remedy congenital immunological defects or after sublethal whole body irradiation or cytotoxic drugs given during antineoplastic chemotherapy.

A similar response can be demonstrated in vitro when peripheral lymphocytes from two genetically different individuals are present in the same culture. The mixed lymphocyte reaction (MLR) occurs when each set of lymphocytes recognizes different MHC antigens on the other, and both sets of lymphocytes undergo blast formation, incorporate radioactively labeled thymidine, and begin proliferating. In humans, this response appears to be particularly dependent on differences in HLA-D and HLA-DR antigens. The reaction can be made unidirectional (just one set of lymphocytes proliferate) by pretreating the lymphocytes of one donor with inhibitors of DNA synthesis or mitosis. This technique has been used as a method for checking the immune compatibility of potential tissue donors and recipients in humans.

Human Transplantation

As in any transplantation situation, the long-term survival of transplanted tissue in humans depends on the degree to which HLA-A, B, C, D, and DR gene products are matched between donor and recipient. An extensive bank of specific antisera against most of the known HLA alleles is available; these antisera, in addition to MLR tests, can accurately identify histocompatibility markers. These procedures have greatly enhanced our ability to find reasonably compatible tissue and organ donors, but, except for homozygotic twins, exact matches are difficult to achieve. The best matches are usually found within the immediate family, either between parents and children or between siblings.

Increased allograft survival in humans can also be achieved by modifying the immune system of the recipient. It is not unusual to administer antilymphocyte serum (antibodies that destroy T-lymphocytes) either directly after transplantation or at the earliest signs of graft rejection. In addition, immunosuppressive drugs usually are administered. The timing of drug therapy appears to be crucial to maximum effectiveness. At present, a great deal of controversy surrounds the clinical indicators of the best time to intervene with certain drugs.

Tumor Immunology

Neoantigens Expressed by Tumor Cells

Despite the observation made long ago that rejection of a transplanted tumor was more dependent on histoincompatibility of normal cell antigens than on the immune system's recognition of tumor-specific antigens, experimental tumors in animal systems have revealed the presence of neoantigens on the surfaces of tumor cells. For instance, chemical carcinogens randomly induce the appearance of tumor-specific antigens. The same chemical carcinogen does not result in the appearance of the same antigen when given to different members of the same animal species. On the other hand, oncogenic animal viruses are also capable of inducing neoantigens on the surface of tumor cells; in this case, the tumor antigens are of the same specificity from individual to individual and unique to each virus. It has been definitively established that oncogenic viruses for man exist (see Chap. 47), and even though it is difficult to demonstrate tumor-specific antigens on tumors induced by chemical carcinogens in man, neoantigens have been found on human tumor cells.

Two of the demonstrable neoantigens are expressed in fetal development but are rarely if ever normally produced after birth. α-Fetoprotein (AFP) is synthesized at maximum levels between the third and sixth month of gestation and then gradually disappears. However, high serum levels of AFP are seen in humans with primary liver cancer, teratomas, and in some individuals with cancer of the stomach and pancreas. AFP is not immunogenic in the species of origin, but rabbits experimentally immunized with human AFP develop antibodies that cross-react with their own AFP. For some reason, the cross-reacting antibodies do not seem to influence the growth of the tumor. Serum levels of carcinoembryonic antigen (CEA) are elevated in individuals with primary cancers of the colon and pancreas, and CEA can be isolated from metastases to the liver. Specific isolated antibodies produced by injecting human CEA into rabbits will bind to human tumor cells. Perhaps because of the heterogeneity of CEA antibodies, they seem to have little effect on tumor growth. The continued decrease in serum CEA levels is used as a measure of the success of surgical extirpation of primary tumors, however.

A variety of immune mechanisms can lead to the destruction of tumor cells. T_D-cells, CTLs, and activated macrophages, under the appropriate conditions, all can kill tumor cells. In addition, complement-fixing antibodies specific for animal cell tumor-specific antigens can lyse tumor cells via the classical complement pathway. Another antibody-dependent cytolytic process involves null or killer (K) cells. These cells do not express the alloantigens of typical T-cells and they do not have surface immunoglobulins of typical B-cells (see Chap. 10). However, null cells have surface receptors for the Fc portions of immunoglobulins. If antibody is bound to tumor-specific antigens on tumor cells, null cells then can bind to the immunoglobulin, and the result of this interaction is tumor

Table 12.2: The Major Human Blood Groups

Group	Antigen in Erythrocyte	Isoagglutinin in Serum	Erythrocytes Agglutinated by Serum of Group	Serum Agglutinates Erythrocytes of Group
A	A	Anti-B (β)	B and O	B and AB
B	B	Anti-A (α)	A and O	A and AB
AB	AB	None	A, B, and O	None
O	O*	Anti-A, anti-B (α and β)	None	A, B, and AB

*Group O erythrocytes possess a specific antigen (H) but the homologous isoagglutinin rarely appears in human sera.

cell lysis. This process, termed antibody-dependent, cell-mediated cytotoxicity, is not dependent on complement. Finally, a population of lymphocytes has been found that does not resemble B-cells, T-cells, killer cells, or macrophages in surface antigens. These cells, termed natural killer cells (NK cells), were described in Chapter 10.

Even though tumor-specific antigens can be found on tumor cells and tumoricidal immune mechanisms can be demonstrated, in most cases tumors appear to grow in an uninterrupted manner, eventually killing the host. How do tumors escape immune surveillance? There is good evidence that tumor-specific antigens (TSA) readily elicit T-suppressor cells that would block any further response. It is also possible that the more aggressive tumors have TSAs that are only weakly immunogenic. Blocking antibodies may appear in the absence of null cells that effectively interfere with recognition by T-cells. This situation would be similar to the enhancing antibodies discussed under Transplantation. Finally, successful tumors may escape immune recognition until they reach some critical mass, at which point the immune system is overwhelmed in its attempt to destroy the tumor.

Blood Groups and Transfusion

Human red blood cells (RBCs) do not express HLA antigens or minor histocompatibility antigens on their surfaces but they do express blood group antigens that are capable of inducing an immune response in an incompatible host. Major blood group antigens belong to the ABO system, and currently 16 additional minor blood group systems have been identified. Familial studies revealed that the ABO gene has three alleles, A, B, and O, with A and B being codominant over O. An individual receives one allele from each parent. Furthermore, individuals naturally possess agglutinating antibodies of the IgM class in their serum for ABO antigens that they do not possess. Thus, type

A individuals have isoagglutinins for B, type B individuals have isoagglutinins for A, type AB individuals have no isoagglutinins, and type O individuals have isoagglutinins for A and B (Table 12.2). There are no isoagglutinins for the O marker, as it is not routinely immunogenic in man.

Chemically, the blood group substances are derived from a single large glycopeptide onto which various sugars that correspond to the A and B specificities are sequentially added. The backbone glycoprotein corresponding to the group O substance is termed H. The name *H substance* was derived from the observation that this membrane component is found in many unrelated (heterogeneic) species. It is thought that a genetic locus separate from the ABO group is responsible for controlling H substance in humans. A simplified chemical chart for each is shown in Figure 12.4. As each sugar is added it introduces a new antigenic specificity masking the previous one. The question of why specific IgM isoagglutinins appear for A and B substances not present in the body has been the subject of extensive study. Accumulated data suggest that the immunogenicity of the A and B substances may be shared by antigenic determinants on polysaccharides of common gastrointestinal bacteria. These macromolecules in turn provide the necessary antigenic stimulation. Exposed infants begin producing anti-A or anti-B antibodies within the first few months of life. In addition, A and B substances are found on other cells of the body and are secreted in saliva. Approximately 80% of the population secrete these blood group antigens in saliva and other body fluids.

Transfusion of mismatched A, B, and O blood types can lead to hemolytic destruction of the transfused RBCs. Type A blood will by lysed in a type B or a type O recipient. Type B blood will be lysed in a type A or a type O recipient. An individual with type AB blood will not respond adversely to any ABO group and therefore is known as a *universal recipient*. In contrast, a type O individual can donate blood to both A

Gene	Terminal End	(Ag)
O	β—GAL (1→3 or 1→4) GNAc $\quad$ ↑ α-1,2 $\quad$ Fucose	(H)
A	α—GAL NAc—(1→3) β—GAL (1→3 or 1→4) GNAc $\quad$ ↑ α-1,2 $\quad$ Fucose	(A)
B	α—GAL (1→3) β—GAL (1→3 or 1→4) GNAc $\quad$ ↑ α-1,2 $\quad$ Fucose	(B)

Figure 12.4: Chemistry of ABO blood groups. H substance for type O is present in a variety of other species and so is called heterogenetic.

and B individuals, since each recipient can accept type O erythrocytes. The term *universal donor* is therefore given to individuals with type O blood. Furthermore, after transfusion of ABO-incompatible blood, IgG immunoglobulins are elicited, in addition to the preexisting IgM. Because normal isoagglutinins are IgM that cannot cross the placenta, a developing fetus with a blood type differing from the maternal type will be relatively safe from hemolytic disease.

Rh Antigen

In addition to the ABO substances, approximately 85% of the population express an Rh antigen (Rh$^+$) and 15% do not (Rh$^-$). This was discovered serendipitously when rabbit antiserum prepared against rhesus monkey RBCs agglutinated 85% of the samples of human RBCs. Rhesus monkeys and humans thus share a common RBC surface antigen. The Rh factor also must be matched for transfusion because it is more immunogenic than A and B antigens. Parental couples in which the mother is Rh$^-$ and the father is Rh$^+$ run the major risk of serious hemolytic disease in their newborn. Some fetal RBCs cross the placenta during normal development. Since in this instance the fetal blood would be Rh$^+$ and the maternal blood would be Rh$^-$, the mother would respond to the immunogenic stimulus with IgG directed against the Rh factor. During a first pregnancy, the degree of anti-Rh stimulation is usually not great enough to cause the fetus serious, if any, harm. However, at the time of birth, when the placenta separates from the uterine wall, a significant "shower" of fetal RBCs occurs, and these RBCs are absorbed into the maternal circulation. This many result in a significant antigenic challenge. The risk of serious fetal hemolytic disease called erythroblastosis fetalis, or hemolytic disease of the newborn, during succeeding pregnancies is therefore greatly increased. In its most severe manifestation, hemolytic disease of the newborn can result in the infant's death.

Prevention of Rh Disease

The incidence of Rh disease is less when the Rh$^-$ mother and the Rh$^+$ baby also differ in ABO type. Rapid removal of fetal cells from maternal circulation by anti-A or anti-B antibodies apparently reduces the likelihood of anti-Rh stimulation. This observation has led to an effective method of reducing the incidence of erythroblastosis fetalis. After each delivery, the mother is injected with anti-Rh antibodies, causing rapid elimination of Rh$^+$ cells from maternal circulation.

Immunodeficiency

Although a variety of immunodeficiency disease and conditions have been described in the past four decades, the acquired immunodeficiency syndrome (AIDS) has become overwhelmingly important. The present discussion will consider some underlying principles of immunodeficiency, and representative immune deficiency states that result in defects in the functional capacities of B- and T-lymphocytes, phagocytic cells, and complement. Basically, if the condition is due to a B-cell defect, one can expect impaired function of all or part of the humoral response, but T-cell–mediated responses should remain intact. On the other hand, if the defect impairs the ability of T-lymphocytes to function properly, one would expect not only T-cell responses to be diminished, but also T-cell–dependent humoral responses would be adversely affected.

Classification of Immunodeficiency Conditions

Immune deficiencies may be broadly divided into two major groups, primary or congenital, and secondary or acquired. Congenital immune deficiencies are often detected in young children as they experience

---

Table 12.3: Classification of Selected Immunodeficiency Disorders

---

Primary

B-lymphocyte (immunoglobulin) deficiency:
    Infantile X-linked agammaglobulinemia
    Congenital hypogammaglobulinemia
    Common variable immunodeficiency
    Selective IgA deficiency
    Selective IgM deficiency
    Immunodeficiency with hyper-IgM

T-lymphocyte (cellular) deficiency:
    DiGeorge syndrome (congenital thymic aplasia)
    Chronic mucocutaneous candidiasis

Combined B- and T-lymphocyte deficiency:
    Severe combined immunodeficiency
    Nezelof's syndrome (cellular immunodeficiency with abnormal immunoglobulin)
    Ataxia–telangiectasia
    Wiskott–Aldrich syndrome
    Acquired immunodeficiency syndrome (AIDS)

Phagocytic cell dysfunction:
    Chediak–Higashi syndrome
    Chronic granulomatous disease
    Myeloperoxidase deficiency
    Hyper-IgE syndrome

Complement component deficiencies:
    C1q, C1n, C1s deficiency
    C4, C2, C3, C5 (deficiency; dysfunction), C6, C7, C8, C9

Secondary

Condition	Immunodeficiencies
Tuberculosis	Decreased T-cell responses; decreased MIF
Hodgkin's disease	Reduced delayed hypersensitivity (DTH); some increased Ig; decreased phagocyte chemotaxis
Systemic lupus erythematosus (SLE)	Elevated Ig levels; some complement deficiencies; decreased T-cell and DTH
AIDS	Reduced T^4/T^8 cell ratios; elevated Ig levels
Diabetes	Impaired phagocytic activity
Aging	Decreased T-cell responses; increased B-cell responses (often autoantibodies)

---

numerous bacterial, viral, or mycotic infections. Table 12.3 lists some immune deficiency conditions in each of the four groupings. Review of this information also indicates that the diagnosis of specific conditions can be aided by noting the types of infections associated with different immune system deficiencies.

A large number of conditions are associated with acquired or secondary immune deficiency disorders. Many of these occur most frequently in adults and range in severity from transient and mild to life-threatening. Often more than one factor is responsible for the onset of an immune deficiency disorder, and therefore treatment, where possible, may involve multiple therapeutic strategies.

B-Lymphocyte Immunodeficiencies

Infantile X-Linked Agammaglobulinemia. This X-linked genetic condition occurs overtly in males and is carried symptom-free by heterozygous females. Male infants with congenital agammaglobulinemia usually remain in general good health for the first 9 months of life and then, depending on their environment and exposure to various infectious agents, become ill. The most frequent infecting pathogens are staphylococci, pneumococci, streptococci, and *Haemophilus influenzae.* The disease conditions can be controlled with appropriate antibiotic therapy, but persistent recurrences are common. Interestingly enough, these children do not seem to have any unusual difficulty with common childhood viral diseases and are not overly susceptible to protozoal or mycotic infections.

The sera of children with X-linked agammaglobulinemia show a profound reduction in immunoglobulin levels of all classes compared to the normal child. Even more striking, these children have few or no lymphocytes with surface immunoglobulins. Therefore, their B-cells are unable to respond to immunogenic stimuli. There appears to be either a stem cell defect or a defect in the process leading to mature, functional B-lymphocytes. Diagnosis of this condition may involve lymph node biopsy after deliberate attempts at immunizing the patient. The histological picture reveals a highly disorganized cellular arrangement and a striking lack of plasma cells. The purely cellular immune responses are intact, although at reduced levels in some individuals. Other serum constituents involved in resistance to infection, such as complement, lysozyme, and properdin levels, are normal. The most effective treatment for these individuals is monthly injection of commercially available γ-globulin preparations (i.e., artificial passive immunity).

Selective IgA Deficiency. Selective IgA deficiency is the most common immunoglobulin deficiency, occurring in 0.1% of the population. The more appropriate term for this type of disorder is dysgammaglobulinemia. In patients with selective IgA deficiency the serum IgA levels are below 5 mg/mL, with the other antibody levels being either normal or elevated. Cellular immune functions remain normal. The condition is heritable and can be transmitted as either an autosomal recessive trait or an autosomal dominant trait. In addition, there is evidence that selective IgA deficiency can be acquired, as it has been associated with congenital infections, including rubella. Patients with this condition have relatively normal concentrations of IgA-bearing B-lymphocytes, and in vitro assays indicate that these cells can be induced to proliferate when exposed to immunologically nonspecific mitogens. The accumulated data to date suggest that this deficiency may be in large part due to a decreased synthesis or secretion of IgA.

Most individuals with selective IgA deficiency suffer from recurrent sinopulmonary infections, multiple allergies, an increased incidence of abnormal gastrointestinal conditions, and a variety of autoimmune diseases. Treatment is mostly aimed at eliminating microbial infections and controlling the secondary immune dysfunctions such as systemic lupus erythematosus, rheumatoid arthritis, and celiac disease. Administration of pooled human γ-globulin is not indicated, since the host is capable of developing anti-IgA antibodies against injected foreign IgA.

T-Cell Deficiency States

In addition to immunodeficiency states that primarily affect B-cells, leading to immunoglobulin deficiencies, there are also deficiency states that primarily affect T-cell functions.

Thymic Aplasia. Thymic aplasia, also called DiGeorge syndrome, is caused by a defect in the development of the third and fourth pharyngeal pouches, which give rise to the thymus, parathyroid, and thyroid glands. In addition to hormonal disorders, affected children suffer from a severely compromised immune system. Their blood lymphocytes are virtually all immunoglobulin-bearing B-cells. They lack practically all T-cell–mediated functions and suffer from severe recurring infections; they show no DTH responses to common bacterial antigens and do not develop contact sensitivity to potent sensitizers. If these infants live beyond their first 2 years, they show a surprisingly sound IgG response, even to antigens considered to be T-cell dependent. The probable explanation is that these individuals do in fact have some thymus function.

Acquired Immunodeficiency Syndrome (AIDS). The definition of AIDS has been modified three times by the U.S. Centers for Disease Control (CDC) since the first cases were reported in 1981. The definition now includes an extensive list of opportunistic infections and immunological abnormalities resulting from human immunodeficiency virus (HIV) infection. A detailed discussion of HIV, AIDS, and infectious sequelae is presented in Chapter 47. A variety of immunological events occur during the course of HIV infection, the most pronounced of which is the reduction of T-helper/suppressor cell ratios. Host cellular immune functions become severely depressed, eventually leading to recurrent infections by microorganisms that are normally kept in check by T-lymphocyte responses. Other immunological manifestations include a pronounced lymphopenia, reduced lymphocyte responses to certain mitogens, elevated immunoglobulin levels, diminished natural killer cell function, and reduced synthesis of lymphokines such as interleukin-2. At present, the treatment of this immunosuppressive disorder is mainly aimed at affecting HIV replication, since attempts at immune reconstitution have not been successful.

Severe Combined Immunodeficiency Disease. Individuals with severe combined immunodeficiency disease have a crippling absence of both T- and B-cell functions, probably due to a profound hematopoietic stem cell defect. Without heroic efforts to protect affected infants from infection, death at an early age is a common fate. Attempts have been made to reconstitute the immune system of these individuals with bone marrow transplants. Success depends on an excellent histocompatibility match between donor and recipient. Because of the vulnerability of the recipient, graft-versus-host disease is a constant problem in bone marrow transplants of this type.

ADDITIONAL READING (CHAPTERS 8–12)

Abbas, A. K. 1979. Hypothesis: Two Distinct Mechanisms of B-Lymphocyte Tolerance. Cell Immunol, **46,** 178.

Amzel, L. M., and Poljak, R. J. 1979. Three-Dimensional Structure of Immunoglobulins. Annu Rev Biochem, **48**, 961.

Bach, F. H., and Sachs, D. H. 1987. Transplantation Immunology. N Engl J Med, **317**, 489.

Barnett, E. V., Knutson, D. W., Abrass, C. K., Chia, D. S., Young, L. S., and Liebling, M. R. 1979. Circulating Immune Complexes: Their Immunochemistry, Detection, and Importance. Ann Intern Med, **91**, 430.

Bellanti, J. A. 1985. *Immunology III.* Saunders, Philadelphia.

Bienenstock, J., and Befus, A. D. 1980. Review—Mucosal Immunology. Immunology, **41**, 249.

Brandtzaeg, P. 1981. Transport Models for Secretory IgA and Secretory IgM. Clin Exp Immunol, **44**, 221.

Carpenter, C. B. 1981. The Cellular Basis of Allograft Rejection. Immunol Today, **2**, 50.

Centers for Disease Control, Immunization Practices Advisory Committee. 1989. General Recommendations on Immunization. MMWR, **38**, 205.

Conger, J. D., Lewis, G. K., and Goodman, J. W. 1981. Idiotype Profile of an Immune Response: I. Contrasts in Idiotype Dominance between Primary and Secondary Responses and between IgM and IgG Plaque-Forming Cells. J Exp Med, **153**, 1173.

Cooper, M. D. 1987. B Lymphocytes: Normal Development and Function. N Engl J Med, **317**, 1452.

Cosimi, A. B. 1981. The Clinical Value of Antilymphocyte Antibodies. Transplant Proc, **13**, 462.

Cotner, T., Mashimo, H., Kung, P. C., Goldstein, G., and Strominger, J. L. 1981. Human T Cell Surface Antigens Bearing a Structural Relationship to HLA Antigens. Proc Natl Acad Sci, **78**, 3858.

Edelman, R. 1980. Vaccine Adjuvants. Rev Infect Dis, **2**, 370.

Fey, G., and Colten, H. R. 1981. Biosynthesis of Complement Components. Fed Proc, **40**, 2099.

Fitch, F. W. 1986. T-Cell Clones and T-Cell Receptors. Microbiol Rev, **50**, 50.

Fitchen, J. H., Foon, K. A., and Cline, M. J. 1981. The Antigenic Characteristics of Hematopoietic Stem Cells. N Engl J Med, **305**, 17.

Frank, M. M. 1979. The Complement System in Host Defense and Inflammation. Rev Infect Dis, **1**, 483.

Golding, H., and Singer, A. 1984. Role of Accessory Cell Processing and Presentation of Shed H-2 Alloantigens in Allospecific Cytotoxic T Lymphocyte Responses. J Immunol, **133**, 597.

Gottlieb, M. S., Schroff, R., Schanker, H. M., et al. 1981. *Pneumocystis carinii* Pneumonia and Mucosal Candidiasis in Previously Healthy Homosexual Men: Evidence For a New Acquired Cellular Immunodeficiency. N Engl J Med, **305**, 1425.

Hall, B. M., Gurley, K., and Dorsch, S. E. 1985. Do T Helper-Inducer Cells Mediate Rejection Without T Cytotoxic-Suppressor Cells? Transplant Proc, **17**, 233.

Hasek, M., and Chutna, J. 1979. Complexity of the State of Immunological Tolerance. Immunol Rev, **46**, 3.

Heddle, R. J., Kwitko, A. O., and Shearman, D. J. C. 1980. Specific IgM and IgG Antibodies in IgA Deficiency. Clin Exp Immunol, **41**, 453.

Herberman, R. B., Djeu, J. Y., Kay, H. D., Ortaldo, J. R., Riccardi, C., Bonnard, G. D., Holden, H. T., Fagnani, R., and Puccetti, S. and P. 1979. Natural Killer Cells: Characteristics and Regulation of Activity. Immunol Rev, **44**, 43.

Horton, J. E., Koopman, W. J., Farrar, J. J., Fuller-Bonar, J., and Mergenhagen, S. E. 1979. Partial Purification of a Bone-Resorbing Factor Elaborated from Human Allogeneic Cultures. Cell Immunol, **43**, 1.

Horton, J. E., Oppenheim, J. J., Mergenhagen, S. E., and Raisz, L. G. 1974. Macrophage-Lymphocyte Synergy in the Production of Osteoclast Activating Factor. J Immunol, **113**, 1278.

Ishizaka, K., and Ishizaka, T. 1978. Mechanisms of Reaginic Hypersensitivity and IgE Antibody Response. Immunol Rev, **44**, 109.

Johnsen, H. E., and Madsen, M. 1979. Lymphocyte Subpopulations in Man: Characterization of Human Killer Cells Against Allogeneic Targets Sensitized with HLA Antibodies. Scand J Immunol, **9**, 429.

Johnstone, D. E. 1981. Immunotherapy in Children: Past, Present and Future (Parts I and II). Ann Allergy, **46**, 1, 59.

Koshland, M. E. 1975. Structure and Function of J Chain. Adv Immunol, **20**, 41.

Kulczycki, A. 1981. Role of Immunoglobulin E and Immunoglobulin E Receptors in Bronchial Asthma. J Allergy Clin Immunol, **68**, 5.

Levy, J. A. 1989. Human Immunodeficiency Viruses and the Pathogenesis of AIDS. JAMA, **261**, 2997.

Lewis, R. A., and Austen, K. F. 1984. The Biologically Active Leukotrienes: Biosynthesis, Metabolism, Receptors, Functions, and Pharmacology. J Clin Invest, **73**, 889.

Lin, L. C., and Putnam, F. W. 1981. Primary Structure of the F_c Region of Human Immunoglobulin D: Implications for Evolutionary Origin and Biological Function. Proc Natl Acad Sci, **78**, 504.

Lu, C. Y., Calamai, E. G., and Unanue, E. R. 1979. A Defect in the Antigen-Presenting Function of Macrophages from Neonatal Mice. Nature, **282**, 327.

Male, D. 1986. *Immunology: An Illustrated Outline.* C. V. Mosby, St. Louis.

Mandel, T. E., Phipps, R. P., Abbot, A., and Tew, J. G. 1980. The Follicular Dendritic Cell: Long Term Antigen Retention During Immunity. Immunol Rev, **53**, 29.

Marsh, D. G., Hsu, S. H., Hussain, R., Meyers, D. A., Freidhoff, L. R., and Bias, W. B. 1980. Genetics of Human Immune Response to Allergens. J Allergy Clin Immunol, **65**, 322.

Masur, H., Michelis, M. A., Greene, J. B., et al. 1981. An Outbreak of Community-Acquired *Pneumocystis carinii* pneumonia: Initial Manifestation of Cellular Immune Dysfunction. N Engl J Med, **305**, 1431-8.

Melchers, F., and Andersson, J. 1986. Factors Controlling the B-Cell Cycle. Annu Rev Immunol, **4**, 13.

Miyawaki, T., Moriya, N., Nagaoki, T., and Taniguchi, N. 1981. Maturation of B-Cell Differentiation Ability and T-Cell Regulatory Function in Infancy and Childhood. Immunol Rev, **57**, 61.

Moen, T., Albrechtsen, D., Flatmark, A., Jakobsen, A., Jervell, J., Halvorsen, S., Solheim, B. G., and Thorsby, E. 1980. Importance of HLA-DR Matching in Cadaveric Renal Transplantation—A Prospective One-Center Study of 170 Transplants. N Engl J Med, **303**, 850.

Moore, S. B. 1979. HLA. Mayo Clin Proc, **54**, 385.

Nossal, G. J. V. 1987. The Basic Components of the Immune System. N Engl J Med, **316**, 1320.

O'Reilly, R. J., Kapoor, N., Pollack, M., Sorell, M., Chaganti, R. S. K., Blaese, R. M., Wank, R., Good, R. A., and Dupont, B. 1979. Reconstitution of Immunologic Function in a Patient with Severe Combined Immunodeficiency Following Transplantation of Bone Marrow from an HLA-A, B, C Nonidentical but MLC-Compatible Paternal Donor. Transplant Proc, **11**, 1934.

Osmond, D. G. 1986. Population Dynamics of Bone Marrow B Lymphocytes. Immunol Rev, **93**, 103.

Plaut, A. G., Gilbert, J. V., and Wistar, R., Jr. 1977. Loss of Antibody Activity in Human Immunoglobulin A Exposed to Extracellular Immunoglobulin A Proteases of *Neisseria gonorrhoeae* and *Streptococcus sanguis.* Infect Immun, **17**, 130.

Quesenberry, P., and Levitt, L. 1979. Hematopoietic Stem Cells. N Engl J Med, **301,** 755, 819, 868.

Rocklin, R. E., Sheffer, A. L., Greineder, D. K., and Melmon, K. L. 1980. Generation of Antigen-Specific Suppressor Cells During Allergy Desensitization. N Engl J Med, **302,** 1213.

Roitt, I. M., and Lehner, T. 1980. *Immunology of Oral Diseases.* Blackwell Scientific Publications, Oxford.

Ross, M. H., and Romrell, L. J. 1989. *Histology: A Text and Atlas,* Ed. 2. Williams & Wilkins, Baltimore.

Russell, J. H., Masakowski, V. R., and Dobos, C. B. 1980. Mechanisms of Immune Lysis: I. Physiological Distinction between Target Cell Death Mediated by Cytotoxic T Lymphocytes and Antibody Plus Complement. J Immunol, **124,** 1100.

Sabin, A. B. 1981. Immunization: Evaluation of Some Currently Available and Prospective Vaccines. JAMA, **246,** 236.

Sakano, H., Maki, R., Kurosawa, Y., Roeder, W., and Tonegawa, S. 1980. Two Types of Somatic Recombination Are Necessary for the Generation of Complete Immunoglobulin Heavy-Chain Genes. Nature, **286,** 676.

Salaman, J. R. 1981. Pharmacologic Immunosuppression. Transplant Proc, **13,** 311.

Schreiber, R. D., Morrison, D. C., Podack, E. R., and Muller-Ekerhard, H. J. 1979. Bactericidal Activity of the Alternative Complement Pathway Generated from 11 Isolated Plasma Proteins. J Exp Med, **149,** 870.

Serafin, W. E., and Austen, K. F. 1987. Mediators of Immediate Hypersensitivity Reactions. N Engl J Med, **317,** 30.

Shillitoe, E. J., and Rapp, F. 1979. Virus-Induced Cell Surface Antigens and Cell-Mediated Immune Responses. Springer Semin Immunopathol, **2,** 237.

Siegal, F. P., Lopez, C., Hammer, G. S., et al. 1981. Severe Acquired Immunodeficiency in Male Homosexuals Manifested by Chronic Perianal Ulcerative Herpes Simplex Lesions. N Engl J Med, **305,** 1439.

Silverstein, A. M., and Bialasiewicz, A. A. 1980. History of Immunology: A History of Theories of Acquired Immunity. Cell Immunol, **51,** 151.

Smith, P. L., Kagey-Sabotka, A., Bleecker, E. R., et al. 1980. Physiologic Manifestations of Human Anaphylaxis. J Clin Invest, **66,** 1072.

Steinmuller, D. 1985. Which T Cells Mediate Allograft Rejection? Transplantation, **40,** 229.

Stiles, D. P., Stobo, J. D., and Wells, J. V. 1987. *Basic and Clinical Immunology,* Ed. 6. Lange Medical Publications, Los Altos, Calif.

Stuart, F. P., McKearn, T. J., Weiss, A., and Fitch, F. W. 1980. Suppression of Rat Renal Allograft Rejection by Antigen and Antibody. Immunol Rev, **49,** 127.

Taubman, M. A., Smith, D. J., and Murray, R. 1978. Immunoglobulin Susceptibility to Proteolytic Effects of Human Dental Plaque Extracts. Arch Oral Biol, **23,** 949.

Ting, C. C., and Rodrigues, D. 1980. Switching on the Macrophage-Mediated Suppressor Mechanism by Tumor Cells to Evade Host Immune Surveillance. Proc Natl Acad Sci, **77,** 4265.

Unanue, E. R., and Allen, P. M. 1987. The Basis for the Immunoregulatory Role of Macrophages and Other Accessory Cells. Science, **236,** 551.

Van Es, A., Persign, G. G., Van Hoff-Eijkenboom, Y. E. A., Kalff, M. W., and Van Hoff, J. P. 1981. Blood Transfusions, HLA-A, and B,DR Matching, Graft Survival, and Clinical Course After Cadaveric Kidney Transplantation. Transplant Proc, **13,** 172.

Weigert, M., and Riblet, R. 1978. The Genetic Control of Antibody Variable Regions in the Mouse. Springer Semin Immunopathol, **1,** 133.

Weissman, G., Smolen, J. E., and Korchak, H. M. 1980. Release of Inflammatory Mediators from Stimulated Neutrophils. N Engl J Med, **303,** 27.

Williams, R. C. 1981. Immune Complexes in Human Diseases. Annu Rev Med, **32,** 13.

Part IV

**Microbial Control
and Mechanisms
of Pathogenicity**

13

Sterilization and Disinfection

John A. Molinari

Accumulated information indicates that the individuals who are at greatest occupational risk from cross-infection in dental practice are the health professionals themselves. Because the oral cavity normally contains a diversity of potentially pathogenic microorganisms, the routine use of effective infection control procedures is an important aspect of clinical dentistry. A few of the varied "occupational" infections are listed in Table 13.1. Many of the agents find favorable growth environments in various areas of the mouth and may be spread by direct contact with a lesion or microorganisms, by indirect contact via contaminated instruments or office equipment, by inhalation of aerosols induced by handpieces and ultrasonic cleaners, and by the routine scrubbing of instruments (Fig. 13.1).

A part of the problem with cross-infection in the dental setting is that most persons with an increased potential for transmitting infection are asymptomatic. For example, undetected hepatitis B carriers and persons secreting herpes simplex viruses in saliva often are treated in dental offices and clinics. In addition,

many treatment providers fail to appreciate the infection potential presented by saliva and blood. By neglecting to implement effective precautions and procedures, health professionals place innocent bystanders at risk, including their own family members and other patients in the practice. The potential dangers are often missed, since much of the spatter coming from the patient's mouth is not readily noticed. Organic debris may be transparent or translucent and dries as a clear film on skin, clothing, and other tissues. Since diseases such as hepatitis B and tuberculosis may also have long incubation periods, it is difficult to trace the source of suspected outbreaks. For these reasons, dental professionals must be certain they are doing their utmost to provide "safe" oral procedures for their patients.

The above considerations constitute some of the major infection control concerns. Recognition of the potential for cross-contamination should lead to the implementation of infection control precautions based on the following principles: 1) reduction of the concentration of pathogens to allow normal host re-

Table 13.1: Representative Infectious Disease Risks in Dentistry

Disease	Etiologic Agent	Incubation Period
Bacterial		
Staphylococcal infections	*Staphylococcus aureus*	4–10 days
Tuberculosis	*Mycobacterium tuberculosis*	Up to 6 mo
Streptococcal infections	*Streptococcus pyogenes*	1–3 days
Gonorrhea	*Neisseria gonorrhoeae*	1–7 days
Syphilis	*Treponema pallidum*	2–12 wk
Tetanus	*Clostridium tetani*	1–10 days
Viral		
Recurrent herpetic lesion	Herpes simplex, types 1 and 2	Up to 2 wk
Rubella	Rubella virus	9–11 days
Hepatitis A	Hepatitis A virus	2–7 wk
Hepatitis B	Hepatitis B virus	6 wk to 6 mo
Delta hepatitis (Hepatitis D)	Hepatitis D virus	Weeks to months
Infectious mononucleosis	Epstein–Barr virus	4–7 wk
Hand-foot-and-mouth disease	Primarily coxsackievirus A16	2 days to >3 wk
Herpangina	Coxsackieviruses group A	5 days
Acquired immunodeficiency syndrome (AIDS)	Human immunodeficiency virus	Months to years
Fungal		
Dermatomycoses (superficial skin infections)	*Trichophyton, Microsporum, Epidermophyton* and *Candida*	Days to weeks
Candidiasis	*Candida albicans*	Days to weeks
Miscellaneous		
Infections of fingers, hands and eyes from dental plaque and calculus	Variety of microorganisms	1–8 days

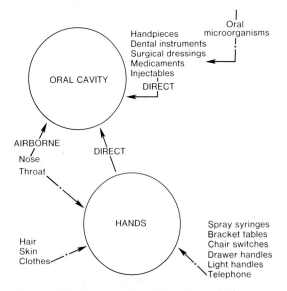

Figure 13.1: Representative vehicles of microbial cross-contamination in dental practice. (Adapted with permission from J. J. Crawford: Sterilization, Disinfection and Asepsis in Dentistry. In *Disinfection, Sterilization and Preservation,* edited by S. S. Block. Lea & Febiger, Philadelphia, 1977.)

sistance mechanisms to prevent infections; 2) break the cycle of infection and eliminate cross-infection; 3) treat every patient and instrument as potentially infectious (i.e., employ universal precautions); and 4) protect patients and personnel from occupational infection.

The utilization of proper sterilization, disinfection, and clinical aseptic procedures minimizes the infectious risk of treating certain patients. This chapter considers 1) aseptic technique, 2) patient screening, 3) personal protection, 4) instrument sterilization, 5) disinfection procedures, 6) equipment asepsis, and 7) dental laboratory asepsis.

Terminology

Sterilization is defined as the destruction or removal of all forms of life, with particular reference to microorganisms. The practical criterion of sterility is the absence of microbial growth in suitable media. Other criteria are loss of motility and inhibition of metabolism and particular enzymes. The ultimate requirement for sterilization is the destruction of bacterial and fungal spores. Agents capable of sterilizing are 1) steam under pressure, 2) high temperature, including an open flame, 3) filters, 4) ethylene oxide, 5) radiation, and 6) certain chemical sterilants.

Germicide literally means "a killer of germs"; the term is not ambiguous. *Antiseptic* indicates an agent that inhibits growth as long as there is contact between agent and microorganism. By custom, the term antiseptic is reserved for agents that can be applied to living tissues and that destroy or inhibit microorganisms.

Disinfection properly refers only to the inhibition or destruction of pathogens. By custom, the term *disinfectant* is reserved for agents applied to inanimate objects. *Bacteriostatic agents* act by inhibiting the growth of microorganisms without killing them, and their effects are reversible. Conversely, *bactericidal agents* kill microorganisms by an action that is not reversible.

In another group of substances are the *sanitizers,* which includes the detergents. These are agents or processes involving agents that are used to maintain the microbial flora of drinking water and food-handling equipment, for example, at safe public health levels.

Asepsis, in contrast to antisepsis, denotes the avoidance of pathogenic microorganisms. In practice, it refers to techniques that aim to exclude all microorganisms. Modern surgery is antiseptic in its attempts to chemically destroy microbes at the site of the operation and on the hands of the surgeon. It is aseptic in the use of sterile instruments, sutures, and dressings and the wearing of sterile masks, caps, gowns, and rubber gloves. Bacteriological laboratory techniques are likewise aseptic. They minimize contamination by flaming wire transfer loops and other instruments, flaming the mouths of containers when opened, exposing open Petri plates and other containers for the shortest time possible, and working under as dust-free conditions as possible.

While each of the above defined terms may be distinguished on the basis of clinical and antimicrobial application, the expression *cold sterilization* represents an often abused aspect of office asepsis. This concept refers to disinfection of instruments at room temperature by immersion in a chemical solution. Since the solutions routinely used often cannot guarantee destruction of all microbial forms, cold sterilization is actually a misnomer, and the practice should not be confused with acceptable methods of sterilization.

The goal of antimicrobial sterilization and disinfection is to reduce the spread of infectious agents. This necessitates an understanding of *cross-infection,* that is, the passage of microorganisms from one person to another. The potential for cross-infection in the dental office exists for direct or indirect transmission, as well as via aerosols routinely created during clinical procedures.

Aseptic Technique

Aseptic technique refers to the use of procedures that break the circle of infection and, ideally, eliminate cross-contamination. The idea of surgical cleanliness was first advocated by Joseph Lister in 1867. His concerns and approaches for resolution of cross-infection risks were fundamental to all that has occurred since. Concern for effective, logical aseptic techniques runs as a thread through other areas of infection control. Practical applications of this concept include integrating each area into an organized, efficient program, minimizing surface exposure and contact during treatment, minimizing the number of items that are contaminated during treatment procedures, and preventing interruptions in patient treatment. The routine use of a pretreatment mouth rinse for patients also lowers the microbial load at a primary source for infection, the patient's mouth.

Patient Screening

It is important to develop an informative patient history profile before providing routine care. An appropriate medical history can help identify factors that assist in the diagnosis of oral and systemic disorders. The presence of certain conditions may alter or modify the routine delivery of care and may alert dental professionals to prepare for medical emergencies (i.e., allergic episodes). Since potentially infectious patients often fail to relate this information, each patient should be treated as potentially infectious for hepatitis B virus (HBV), human immunodeficiency virus (HIV), or other blood-borne pathogens. This important, fundamental application of infection control is referred to as "universal precautions." It is not only a major professional standard of care, but also makes good sense. The routine use of blood and body fluid precautions substantially reduces the clinical guesswork previously employed in the determination of a patient's infection status.

Personal Protection

Repeated exposure to saliva and blood during intraoral, often invasive procedures can challenge the health professional's immune defenses with a wide range of microbial agents. Personal protection in this context involves two basic considerations: immunological protection and barrier protection. The former requires that treatment providers receive available vaccines of proven efficacy to prevent the onset of clinical or subclinical infection. The occupational risk of contracting hepatitis B, measles, rubella, influenza, and certain other microbial infections can be minimized considerably by stimulating artificial active immunity. Approved vaccines are available for each of these diseases and should be used by individuals providing patient care.

While vaccination and the subsequent development of protective immunity are effective in minimizing the transmission of certain infections, they are not sufficient for protection against the range of potential pathogens encountered during patient treatment. Physical barriers make up an essential component of an infection control program. The routine use of disposable gloves, face masks, and protective eyewear during treatment procedures minimizes the infectious exposure.

Gloves. Properly fitting gloves protect the dental care provider from exposure through cuts and abrasions often found on hands. The latter serve as routes of microbial entry into the system when ungloved hands are placed in patients' mouths ("wet-fingered dentistry"). Even scrupulous hand washing cannot serve as a replacement for the use of gloves. Glove reuse is not recommended, since washing of gloves with handwash antiseptics increases both the size and number of pinholes in the gloves and compromises the integrity of commercial gloves. The latex examination gloves employed during routine nonsurgical treatment were not formulated to withstand prolonged exposure to secretions or chemical agents. Glove integrity may also be compromised during long procedures. Because of these kinds of factors, gloves may have to be changed during a treatment session. Continued advances in the quality and manufacture of gloves can only expand the protection afforded by this fundamentally important barrier.

A current alternative for latex gloves is to use medical grade vinyl gloves. This action may be necessitated when a treatment provider develops a documented allergy to latex or to glove powder. Individuals who wear vinyl gloves often immediately note the difference from latex gloves. Tactile sensation with vinyl gloves may be altered, and they may tear more easily because they are more rigid. Newer generation gloves of this type have attempted to correct these inherent differences in the original polyvinyl products.

Protective Eyewear. The eyes are particularly susceptible to physical and microbial injury by virtue of their limited vascularity and diminished immune capacities. Aerosolized droplets containing microbial contaminants can lead to the development of conjunctivitis in dental personnel. This may keep the individual away from work for a minimum of 1 to 2 weeks. Protective eyewear or an appropriate face shield should therefore be worn during treatment procedures, in the dental laboratory, and in the sterilization/disinfection area when chemicals are mixed and poured.

Masks. The use of an approved face mask will protect the dentist, hygienist, assistant, and laboratory technician from microbe-laden aerosolized droplets. According to current technology and recommendations, the best masks are those that filter at least 95% of droplet particles 3.0 to 3.2 μm in diameter.

The mask should fit properly for both wearer comfort and barrier efficiency. Masks should be changed for each patient, since a mask's efficiency decreases as it traps moisture during dental procedures. The wet fabric serves as a vehicle for microbial transfer through the mask.

Operatory Attire. Appropriate uniforms or gowns must be worn for all dental treatment. Debate regarding the appropriateness of either long- or short-sleeved uniforms or clinic jackets is continuing, as positive and negative features are inherent with each type.

Changing the gown or uniform or wearing a protective cover over the uniform when an aerosol spray is being generated is recommended. All clinical attire should be of synthetic material so that contaminants are not easily absorbed into the material. Seams, buttons, and buckles should be kept to a minimum for the same reason.

Other Barriers. Most dental students learn to use a rubber dam when performing restorative or endodontic procedures. A rubber dam is helpful when water-spray handpieces are used. A combination of a high-speed suction device and rubber dam can sharply reduce the microbial load in the aerosols produced. The use of disposable covers or drapes on operatory surfaces will also diminish the collection of splatter on equipment that can only be disinfected.

Factors Affecting the Death Rate of Microorganisms

Time and Concentration of Organisms. The concentration of microorganisms affects the rate at which they are killed. Microorganisms exposed to a sterilizing agent die at a progressively decreasing rate that is proportional to the number of survivors. Whatever the agent, the graph of logarithms of number of survivors against time falls in a straight line over most of its course (Fig. 13.2). The greater the size of inoculum at the outset, the longer it takes to reach complete sterility.

Time and Concentration of Agent. The con-

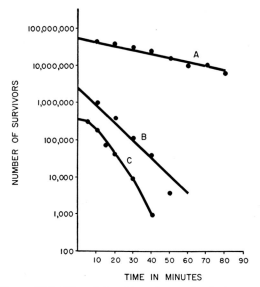

Figure 13.2: Effect of size of inoculum on the death rate of bacteria. Three experiments with *Escherichia coli* in 0.005 N sodium hydroxide at 30°C. In all cases, the death rate was logarithmic over most of the course. Starting with 55,000,000 cells per mL (*A*), however, only 2.5% of survivors died per minute, whereas starting with 2,500,000 (*B*) or 350,000 (*C*), the rate was 10% per minute. A similar although less pronounced effect of numbers was observed with heat at 55°C at neutrality. Even though the death rate is approximately the same in *B* and *C,* 70 minutes would have been required to reduce the survivors in *B* to 1,000, whereas *C* reached this figure in 40 minutes. Theoretically, *A* would have required 7 hours. *C* illustrates also the lag that often occurs at the beginning and the acceleration of killing at the end, when the numbers are very small. Frequently, however, the death rate at the end is much slower, owing to a fraction of more resistant cells in the original population. (Data for compilation of graph from I. H. Watkins and C. E. A. Winslow: Factors Determining the Rate of Mortality of Bacteria Exposed to Alkalinity and Heat. *J Bacteriol,* **24,** 243, 1932.)

centration of the agent also affects the rate at which microorganisms are killed. The time necessary for sterilization by a chemical decreases as the agent's concentration increases, and vice versa. For many chemicals, doubling the concentration halves the time required. For some chemicals, such as phenols and alcohol, the efficacy changes extremely rapidly with changes in concentration (Fig. 13.3).

Time and Temperature. Temperature affects the rate at which microorganisms are killed. Two effects of temperature must be distinguished: the increase in activity of a chemical with rising temperature, and killing by heat alone. The rate of sterilization behaves like a chemical reaction; that is, it doubles or trebles for every 10°C rise in temperature.

The susceptibility of microorganisms to heat has been expressed as thermal death time or thermal death point (more accurately, thermal death tempera-

ture). Thermal death time is defined as the time it takes to kill microorganisms at a given temperature. The thermal death point of bacteria is defined as the lowest temperature that sterilizes a 24-hour culture in broth at pH 7 in 10 minutes.

Effect of Organic Matter. The chemicals considered in this chapter act for the most part by chemical combination with microbial protoplasm. They also combine with the constituents of tissue, especially proteins and glycoproteins. This usually reduces the efficacy of the chemicals and thus diminishes their effectiveness. The effects of bioburden (i.e., blood, saliva, exudate, etc.) on disinfectants will be discussed in a later section.

Hydrogen ion concentration affects the killing of microorganisms. Acids and acidic substances are generally more easily sterilized than are neutral or alkaline substances. Organic acids produced in fermentations often protect fluids and solid food and the gastrointestinal tract from the activities of undesirable contaminating microorganisms.

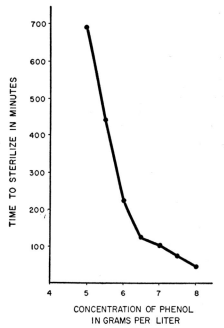

Figure 13.3: Effect of changing concentration of phenol on time required to sterilize paratyphoid bacilli in a concentration of 6,000,000 per mL in aqueous phenol at 20°C. The data fit closely the curve, $C_5 t = 6.65$, which means that doubling the concentration reduces the time required 45-fold ($= 2^{55}$) and vice versa. By extrapolation, a concentration of 1% (10 g/L) would have sterilized in 14 minutes, and 2%, in 20 seconds. Note, however, that concentrations of phenol as low as 0.25% may be used to protect solutions from contamination. (Reproduced with permission from H. E. Watson: A Note on the Variation of the Rate of Disinfection with Change in the Concentration of the Disinfectant. *J Hygiene (Cambridge),* **8,** 536, 1908.)

Evaluation of Sterilizing Agents

Laboratory Measurement of Antimicrobial Action. Sterilization in vitro is determined either by exposure of organisms to an agent in liquid medium with subsequent tests for viability, or by direct application of the agent to cultures on solid culture media. The former is exemplified by the determination of the *phenol coefficient*. A standard inoculum of a standard strain of *Staphylococcus aureus* or *Salmonella typhi* is added to a series of dilutions of phenol in a standard broth at 20°C and to a series of dilutions of the substance under comparison. After 5, 10, and 15 minutes, a standard sample of each mixture is transferred to fresh broth containing, if necessary, a neutralizer of the agent being tested. After incubation, the subcultures in which growth occurred are noted, and which dilutions of the substances killed all organisms in 10 minutes but not in 5.

Microbial testing for viability by animal inoculation can be applied to organisms that are difficult to culture. This procedure has been used for the assay of antibiotics, with known amounts of the pure substance used instead of phenol in the reference series. When done in this way, the test resembles the agar plate method, in which a test organism is seeded in a pour plate or streaked uniformly on the surface and a sample of the agent is applied directly, or in hollow cylinders, or in impregnated thick disks of filter paper. After incubation, growth develops as a lawn culture except in the vicinity of the agent (Fig. 13.4). The area of the clear zones is proportional to the amount of the agent applied.

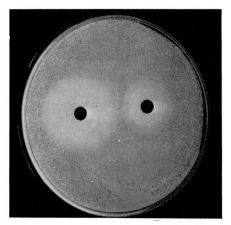

Figure 13.4: The plate method for determining sensitivity of microorganisms to antibiotics. A poured plate is prepared on the test organism(s), the disks impregnated with a given concentration of antibiotic(s) are placed on the surface, and the plate is incubated. The area of clear zone about the disks is proportional to the amount of agent applied and to the sensitivity of the microorganism.

Evaluation in Use. Some physical and chemical methods have been found useful in general sanitation and for the sterilization of inanimate objects. The success of a chemical against a defined infection can be measured satisfactorily, as for example with the use of silver nitrate to prevent gonococcal ophthalmia neonatorum.

Physical Methods of Sterilization

Certain routine procedures must be employed to sterilize all instruments, mirrors, burs, metal bands, and other intraoral materials that can withstand effective procedures. The following section considers the most appropriate physical methods of sterilization— steam autoclaving, dry heat, and chemical vapor—and other physical modes useful in microbiology as sterilizing systems. Effective conditions and wrapping requirements for the major physical modes are given in Table 13.2.

Moist Heat

Boiling. Moist heat is the most widely utilized means of sterilizing heat-stable items. The application of this method may occur in several forms: boiling, steam at atmospheric pressure, and steam under pressure. When applied at 100°C or higher, heat is effective by denaturation of proteins. Microbial destruction can be achieved by immersing articles in boiling water for 10 to 20 minutes. All vegetative cells and most spores are destroyed in this way, but a fraction of tetanus, gas gangrene, and botulinum spores are likely to survive. In addition, because of the unrealistically prolonged time necessary for ultimate destruction of all spores, immersion in 100°C water is not considered a sterilizing process. Nevertheless, this method has certain advantages as a disinfection mode: it is rapid, economical, does not require any elaborate equipment, has effective penetration capability, and is harmless to a wide range of dental materials. A serious disadvantage is that it dulls the edges of cutting instruments. The use of stainless steel instruments can alleviate this problem, while the dulling effects can be reduced somewhat by the addition of sodium carbonate to the water.

Steam Sterilization. Complete sterilization is achieved by the use of moist heat at higher temperatures in the form of saturated steam under pressure in air-tight vessels such as an autoclave. Under the appropriate conditions, autoclaving is a very efficient sterilization process. Steam may also be employed as free-flowing at atmospheric conditions, although at 1 atmosphere pressure its efficacy is only analogous to that of boiling water.

Most commonly, a temperature of 121°C (250°F) is

Table 13.2: Major Methods of Sterilization*

Method	Temperature	Pressure	Cycle Time	Packaging Material Requirements	Acceptable Materials	Unacceptable Materials
Steam autoclave	121°C 134°C	15 psi 30 psi	15–20 min 3–5 min	Must allow steam to penetrate	Paper, plastic, surgical muslin	Closed metal and glass containers
Dry heat oven	160°C 170°C		2 hr 1 hr	Must not insulate items from heat; must not be destroyed by temperature used	Paper bags, muslin, aluminum foil, aluminum trays, pans	Plastic bags
Unsaturated chemical vapor	131°C	20 psi	30 min	Vapors must be allowed to precipitate on contents; vapors must not react with packaging material; plastics should not contact sides of sterilizer	Perforated metal trays, paper	Metal trays, sealed glass jars
Ethylene oxide	Room temperature (25°C)		10–16 hr (depends on material)	Gas must be allowed to penetrate	Paper, plastic bags	Sealed metal or glass containers

*Adapted with permission from J. A. Molinari and J. York: *Detroit Dental Bull*, **49**, 5, 1980; and R. J. Whitacre, et al.: *Dental Asepsis*. Stoma Press, Seattle, 1979.

applied for 15 to 20 minutes. These conditions yield 15 pounds pressure of steam at sea level. Direct exposure to saturated steam at 121°C for 10 minutes normally destroys all forms of life. In practice, an additional "safety factor" interval must be allowed for the temperature to reach this point in the center of thick packages of dressings or large containers of liquids. In most instances, a maximal sterilization period of 30 minutes suffices. Higher temperatures and pressures for shorter periods of time are employed in newer equipment used in many dental facilities.

As efficient as autoclaving can be in instrument sterilization, this procedure is effective only when suitable conditions are present in the pressured chamber. Problems arise with steam sterilization if the materials have not been adequately prepared for sterilization (the packaging does not allow penetration of steam), the instrument chamber has been improperly loaded, the sterilizer is not functioning properly (failure to reach requisite temperature or pressure), air is in the chamber (may delay microbial destruction up to 10 times longer), and the steam holds excess water (can serve as passageway for microorganisms to get through wet instrument packages).

Unsaturated Chemical Vapor. Chemical vapor sterilization in dental practices and clinics is considered an acceptable method of sterilization by the ADA Council on Dental Therapeutics and its use has increased substantially in recent years. This system depends on heat, water, and chemical synergism for its efficacy; a mixture of alcohols, formaldehyde, ketone, acetone, and water is employed. As shown in Table 13.2, higher temperatures and pressures are necessary for chemical vapor sterilization than for autoclaving. The principle of operation has similarities to steam sterilization, but also some important distinctions. The solution of premixed chemicals added to the jacket reservoir must be purchased from the manufacturer, since the ratio of each component in the preparation is critical. The apparatus is preheated and clean, dry, loosely wrapped instruments are placed in the chamber. The package wraps must be loose enough to allow the chemical vapors to condense on the instrument surfaces during the cycle. Thick, tightly wrapped items will require longer exposure because unsaturated chemical vapors cannot penetrate as well as saturated steam under pressure. Metal instruments must be dry before sterilization or the chemicals will accumulate in the wet surfaces and corrosion will occur.

The major advantages of chemical vapor sterilization are a short cycle time, analogous to that for the autoclave; no rusting of instruments and burs, in contrast to steam sterilization; the removal of dry instruments at the end of the cycle; and automatic, preset cycle timing. The 8% to 9% water vapor in the chemical solution is significantly below the 15% minimum for rusting and dulling and prevents destruction of dental items such as endodontic files, orthodontic pliers, wires and bands, burs, and carbon steel instruments. A wide range of items can therefore be routinely sterilized. The requirement for adequate ventilation can be a problem for practitioners who use this apparatus, however. Chemical vapors, particularly formaldehyde, may be released when the chamber door is opened at the end of the cycle; these vapors leave a temporary unpleasant odor in the area. Although numerous toxicity studies by the manufacturer indicate little chance of eye irritation from these residual vapors, dental personnel may occasionally report some discomfort if the sterilizer is in an area with poor air circulation. To counteract this detrimental aspect, later models were equipped with a special filtration device that further reduces the amount of vapor left in the chamber at the end of the cycle.

Dry Heat

The destruction of all forms of microbial life in the absence of moisture requires very different conditions from those discussed previously. As proteins dry, their resistance to denaturation increases. Thus, at a given temperature, dry heat sterilizes much less efficiently than moist heat, and, as shown in Table 13.2, higher temperatures are necessary for a properly functioning hot air oven.

Destruction of microorganisms by dry heat is accomplished either by incineration or by placing items in a hot air oven. Direct flaming, the most dramatic application of dry heat, is also one of the simplest procedures. No special apparatus is necessary and 100% effectiveness is guaranteed. Disposal of infectious materials and organic wastes is safely accomplished using large incinerators. The practical application of this method in clinical areas, however, is limited at best. Other than wire loops, which are flamed in the microbiology laboratory before the sterile inoculation of cultures, other metallic items do not maintain their integrity with repeated flaming.

The proper use of a dry heat oven is recognized as an effective means of sterilization in dental practices. Since dry air does not conduct heat as efficiently as moist air at the same temperature, a much higher temperature is necessary for sterilization. The usual recommendation is to hold the temperature at 160°C for 2 hours. A 1-hour exposure at 170°C will also be effective. These conditions are suitable for sterilizing glassware and metal instruments that rust or dull in the presence of water vapor. Many dental practitioners prefer the use of dry heat sterilizers in their offices because of the preservation of sharp, cutting edges on their surgical instruments. In addition, many types of oils and powders with high heat resistance may be

Table 13.3: Features of Sterilization Methods

Method	Advantages	Disadvantages
Autoclaving	1. Short cycle time 2. Good penetration 3. Wide range of materials can be processed without destruction	1. Corrosion of unprotected carbon steel instruments 2. Dulling of unprotected cutting edges 3. Packages may remain wet at end of cycle 4. May destroy heat-sensitive materials
Dry heat	1. Effective and safe for sterilization of metal instruments and mirrors 2. Does not dull cutting edges 3. Does not rust or corrode	1. Long cycle required for sterilization 2. Poor penetration 3. May discolor and char fabric 4. Destroys heat-labile items
Unsaturated chemical vapor	1. Short cycle time 2. Does not rust or corrode metal instruments, including carbon steel 3. Does not dull cutting edges 4. Suitable for orthodontic stainless wires	1. Instruments must be completely dried before processing 2. Will destroy heat-sensitive plastics 3. Chemical odor in poorly ventilated areas
Ethylene oxide	1. High capacity for penetration 2. Does not damage heat-labile materials (including rubber & handpieces) 3. Evaporates without leaving a residue 4. Suitable for materials that cannot be exposed to moisture	1. Slow—requires very long cycle times 2. Retained in liquids and rubber material for prolonged intervals 3. Causes tissue irritation if not well aerated 4. Requires special "spark-shield"—explosive in presence of flame or sparks

sterilized at 160 to 170°C. However, these high temperatures will destroy many rubber and plastic-based materials, melt the solder of most impression trays, and weaken some fabrics, as well as discolor other fabrics and paper materials. As with the design of newer generations of autoclaves, advances in the technology for dry heat sterilization are continuing. Dry heat convection units are currently available that use higher temperatures and require substantially shorter sterilization times.

A common problem with using a dry heat sterilizer is the failure of clinic personnel to time the sterilization interval. Since dry heat penetrates slowly into the center of the pack, depending on the size of packages and the type of wrapping material, one must be certain that a proper temperature is achieved in the chamber (by preheating) before setting the timer. Thick wraps and larger than normal packages can significantly increase the interval required for assured sterility. Some individuals also view the prolonged exposure times for dry heat as a disadvantage. The argument is made that if only one sterilizer is available, the 1- to 2-hour period plus cooling time disrupts the smooth flow of instrument recirculation. These problems may be compared with those inherent in autoclaving and use of chemical vapor (Table 13.3).

Pasteurization

Pasteurization is principally used in the food-processing industries (milk and other dairy products, fruit juices, wine and beer). Its purpose is to disinfect and to postpone spoilage. As defined for the treatment of milk, pasteurization consists of holding the fluid at 143°F (61.7°C) for 30 minutes in tanks or at 160°F (71.1°C) for 15 seconds for continuous flow through heat exchangers. The infectious agents that cause milk-borne diseases, such as tuberculosis, brucellosis, salmonellosis, Q fever, and diphtheria, are destroyed under these conditions; in fact, the killing of *Mycobacterium tuberculosis* and *Mycobacterium bovis* was classically used to test the efficiency of the pasteurization process. Microbial spores are not inactivated, however, and some nonpathogens like *Streptococcus lactis* can also survive.

Radiant Energy

Lethal levels of energy may be transmitted to microorganisms by ultraviolet light, which is absorbed in their DNA over a considerable range of wavelengths from 220 to 290 nm. Bactericidal efficacy is proportional to adsorption. Killing of microorganisms by ultraviolet light involves inducing lethal mutations or sufficient chemical modification of DNA so as to interfere with subsequent replication. Ultraviolet light may act indirectly on DNA, by production of H_2O_2 or organic peroxides in fluids that contain oxygen and organic compounds. Modern germicidal lamps are usually of the mercury vapor type, because they can be designed to have most of their output at 254 nm, the resonance radiation of mercury. Unfortunately, the poor penetration capability of the energy rays seriously limits their use. Ultraviolet light is so readily absorbed by glass, liquids, and a variety of organic substances that it is effective only on surfaces or thin layers of material.

High-energy electromagnetic waves (x-rays and γ-rays) and particulate radiations (cathode, α-, and β-rays; fast protons, neutrons, and deuterons; heavy atomic particles from nuclear fission) have been tested extensively as sterilizing agents. They are called ionizing radiations because they ionize molecules in their path which absorb them. Their lethal action may occur directly on such vital molecules as enzymes and nucleic acids, particularly DNA. For the most part they act indirectly by splitting water into hydroxyl radicals and hydrogen atoms, both of which are highly reactive and interfere with vital cellular activities.

The practical effectiveness of ionizing radiation in sterilization is limited because it depends on random hits of molecules; therefore, complete killing of bacterial cells requires many times the dosage that reduces the population partially. The sensitivity of bacteria to ionizing radiation varies with the growth phase, being least during the lag phase, greatest during the logarithmic phase, and gradually decreasing in the latter to the sensitivity of "resting" bacteria. Freezing decreases sensitivity, as does drying.

The vegetative forms of bacteria are most susceptible to ionizing radiation, but there is little difference between gram-positive and gram-negative species. Bacterial spores are quite resistant, those of *Clostridium botulinum* most of all. A major medical industrial application of electromagnetic waves is found in the sterilization of heat-sensitive plastic hypodermic syringes and sutures.

Ionizing radiation has also been studied as a means of sterilization, pasteurization, disinfection, or disinfestation, or all four, particularly with regard to food preservation. Studies have been made of the preservation of foods by ionizing radiation, and irradiated bacon was the first food so treated found acceptable for human consumption by the Food and Drug Administration, in 1963. In general, the sterilization of foods with ionizing radiation has not proved acceptable to the Food and Drug Administration. The high level of irradiation required to achieve sterility in foods also causes sufficient changes to make them unacceptable or potentially dangerous as foods.

Ultrasonic Vibration

Cells of all kinds can be disrupted by intense sonic and ultrasonic vibrations generated by magnetostriction oscillators or piezoelectric crystals. This technique is widely used as a laboratory tool for the release of cell contents with minimal damage, such as nuclei, mitochondria, antigens, and enzymes, but it is not a practical means of sterilization. Bacteria and viruses are more resistant to it than are mammalian cells. Ultrasonic vibration is often successfully used to clean, but not to sterilize, dental instruments. The apparatus efficiently removes blood, pus, and other tissue debris from grooves and other areas that are difficult to clean. The effective scrubbing capabilities of ultrasonic cleaners make them a valuable piece of equipment in dental offices as a preparatory step to instrument sterilization.

Filtration

In microbiology, filtration is used to free liquids and gases from suspended particles, either inanimate or animate. The Seitz, sintered glass, and membrane filters are in common use in microbiology.

Seitz filter pads are made of a mixture of asbestos and cellulose, supported by a woven base and held in place by a suitable holder. Numerous types of filter pad holders are available for either pressure or vacuum filtration, but such filters should not be subjected to a change in pressure of more than 5 pounds per square inch. Seitz filters and holders may be sterilized by autoclaving.

Sintered glass filters are available in several grades. The pores of such filters are not uniform, however, necessitating the determination and certification of the average pore diameter of each filter. Sintered glass disks are either fused into glass funnels or fitted into funnels by means of rubber cones.

Membrane filters are composed mostly of cellulose esters, usually cellulose acetate or triacetate, but not cellulose nitrate. Common pore sizes range from 0.22 to 10 μm, but filters can be produced with a pore size as small as 0.05 μm. Each square centimeter of a membrane filter with an average pore size of 0.45 ± 0.02 μm contains millions of pores, the volume of the open spaces being about 80% and the solid material about 20% of the total volume. A membrane filter with a 0.45 μm pore size will prevent the passage of almost all nonviral microorganisms. Membrane filters have a flow rate at least 40 times greater than that of other types of filters with similar pore size. Clogging occurs with stable gels and with liquid-borne particles that are approximately pore size. Liquid-borne particles larger than pore size and airborne particles cause negligible clogging because they do not penetrate into the pore structure.

Membrane filters are widely used to prepare cell-free solutions, particularly those that will not withstand heat. They are also used for the separation of bacteria and viruses; for the clarification of solutions by removing cells; for microbial isolation and cultivation—bacteria collected on a membrane filter can be cultivated by placing the filter in contact with nutrients; for analysis of airborne microorganisms and biological specimens; for contamination control and microbial analysis of food, meats, soft drinks, and dairy products; for investigation of antibiotics, antiseptics, and disinfectants; for water and sewage control; and for soil microbiology.

Freezing

Depending on the species, the composition of the suspending fluid, the rate of temperature reduction or increase, and the temperature at which microorganisms are stored, freezing both kills and preserves viable microorganisms. Freezing of bacterial cells usually does not occur until they are supercooled to -10 to $-15°C$. Water either freezes inside the cells or moves out of the cells, dehydrating them in either instance. When a microbial suspension is cooled, considerable ice crystal formation occurs inside the cell. The formation and the movements of internal ice crystals disrupt the cell by cytoplasmic and membrane damage. The rate of thawing also affects the survival of frozen microbial cells. Slow thawing is more harmful than rapid thawing.

As the microbial cells become dehydrated during cooling, their salts tend to concentrate in pockets sufficiently to crystallize when the temperature is lowered to their eutectic point, about $-20°C$ for NaCl. Local concentration and crystallization of intracellular salts damages the cytoplasm, cell wall, and membrane.

When present in the suspending medium, nonelectrolytes such as glycerol, sucrose, or dimethyl sulfoxide partially protect bacteria from damage during freezing by preventing electrolytes from concentrating locally in cells. While most metabolic activities of bacteria cease below the freezing point of water, microorganisms are best preserved at the lowest temperature possible. Untoward reactions occur at a temperature as low as $-130°C$, but the temperatures commonly used are those of solid carbon dioxide ($-78°C$) and liquid nitrogen ($-180°C$).

Drying

The preservation of microorganisms by drying from the frozen state was discussed earlier. The spontaneous drying of water or saline suspensions of bacteria on glass usually kills them, while viruses are more resistant. The smaller particles of salivary spray expelled during coughing, sneezing, many dental procedures, or simply talking dry within seconds, encasing their bacterial contents in a protective mucinous coat. In this way, viable hemolytic streptococci can survive indoors for at least several weeks. Staphylococci in dried exudate may survive for several months. On the other hand, pneumococci, meningococci, and *Haemophilus influenzae* do not survive for more than a few days under such conditions. Air-dried spores may remain viable for years.

Monitoring of Sterilization

An integral component of offfice sterilization procedures is monitoring the efficiency of the system. A multitude of factors may diminish the effectiveness of an autoclave, dry heat sterilizer, or unsaturated chemical vapor apparatus. Frequent problems encountered are improper wrapping of instruments, which prevents adequate penetration to the instrument surface; human error in timing the cycle; defective control gauges that do not reflect actual conditions inside the sterilizer; and sterilizer malfunction.

One may employ chemically treated tapes that change color or biological controls to check for the proper functioning of an office sterilizer. Materials that change color generally inform the practitioner that sterilizing conditions have been reached but do not necessarily indicate that sterilization of the chamber contents has been achieved. In addition, certain indicators change color long before sterilization occurs and before appropriate conditions are met. Autoclave tape is probably the worst offender in this regard, as it will change to show the striped markings following very brief exposure to steam. It appears that the major use of specific chemical indicators to monitor sterilization is as a routine check for each load of items processed through the sterilizer. Gross malfunctions can usually be detected very quickly by using indicator labels, strips, and steam pattern cards.

The use of calibrated biological controls remains the main guarantee of sterilization. These preparations contain bacterial spores, which are more resistant to heat than viruses and vegetative bacteria. Since a spore vehicle designed for one sterilization method is not necessarily appropriate to use for other procedures, manufacturers produce both glass vials containing spores and biological test strips. The organisms most often used are calibrated concentrations of either *Bacillus stearothermophilus* or *Bacillus subtilis* spores. These are either suspended in a nutrient medium (ampule form) or impregnated onto a paper strip. A pH indicator in the growth medium changes color when spores germinate, thereby providing a visual key to sterilization failure. Since the spore preparations are relatively heat resistant, the proof of their destruction after exposure to the sterilization cycle is used to infer that all microorganisms exposed to the same conditions have been destroyed. The demonstration of sporicidal activity by an office sterilizer thus represents the most sensitive check for efficiency.

Chemical Agents

Antiseptics and disinfectants are the most widely used of all drugs in public health practice, in hospital practice, in sanitation, and in the household. These agents are used extensively in dental practices and hospitals despite the demonstrably limited effectiveness of certain substances. Many are applied to the skin of the patient, to the hands of the health professional, and

---

Table 13.4: Properties of an Ideal Disinfectant*

1. Broad spectrum: Should always have the widest possible antimicrobial spectrum.
2. Fast-acting: Should have a rapidly lethal action on all vegetative forms and spores of bacteria and fungi, protozoa, and viruses.
3. Not affected by physical factors:
   a) Active in the presence of organic matter such as blood, sputum, and feces (i.e., cleaning capability).
   b) Should be compatible with soaps, detergents and other chemicals encountered in use.
4. Nontoxic
5. Surface compatibility:
   a) Should not corrode instruments and other metallic surfaces.
   b) Should not cause the disintegration of cloth, rubber, plastics, or other materials.
6. Residual effect on treated surfaces
7. Easy to use
8. Odorless: An inoffensive odor would facilitate its routine use.
9. Economical: Cost should not be prohibitively high.

---

*Adapted with permission from J. A. Molinari, M. D. Campbell, and J. York: Minimizing Potential Infections in Dental Practice. *J Mich Dent Assoc,* **64,** 411, 1982.

---

to environmental surfaces for use in controlling microbial contamination.

Ideal Properties

A variety of chemical disinfectants and antiseptics may be employed. The antimicrobial spectrum of these agents ranges from limited to very broad. The most appropriate agent may be difficult to determine, since exaggerated claims may cloud actual performance capabilities. It is therefore advisable to compare the qualities of any product with the desirable properties of an ideal agent. The latter are summarized in Table 13.4.

Modes of Action and Adverse Features

Most chemicals that act as antiseptics or disinfectants function as cytoplasmic poisons. This lack of specificity generally limits the application of the agents to inanimate objects and the outer surfaces of the body. Any or all of the three major portions of cells may be affected: the cell wall, cytoplasm (particularly enzymes), and nuclear material. The resultant microbial destruction is accomplished by one of a limited number of reactions or by a combination of them; these effects with representative chemical substances are summarized in Table 13.5.

All available disinfectants also have undesirable effects on tissues or inanimate surfaces. Corrosiveness and epithelial toxicity are factors that are often overlooked when chemical disinfectants are used. For example, epithelial hypersensitivity and nonspecific dermatitis are common problems noted with repeated exposure to certain disinfectant preparations (Table 13.6). These adverse reactions can be avoided by wearing heavy duty gloves during clean-up and disinfection procedures.

Surface-Active Substances (Detergents)

Surface-active substances are those that alter the nature of interfaces to lower surface tension and increase detergency. At the cell membrane, the effect is to alter the osmotic barrier and increase permeability so that the cell cannot maintain its integrity. Surface denaturation of enzymes in the cell membrane may also occur.

The surface-active substances are classified as nonionic, anionic, cationic, or amphoteric. Nonionic

---

Table 13.5: Antimicrobial Mechanisms of Chemical Agents

Mechanism of Action	Representative Substances
Protein denaturation	Alcohols
	Phenols
	Detergents
	Acids
	Organic solvents
Hydrolysis	Acids
	Alkalis
Formation of insoluble or poorly dissociable salts of proteins	Mercuric, cupric, and silver ions
Oxidation	Hypochlorite
	Hydrogen peroxide
Halogenation	Iodine
	Iodophors
	Chlorine
Disruptive, increased membrane permeability	Detergents
	Alcohols
	Phenols
Poisoning active groups of enzymes	Mercurials
	Detergents
	Acid dyes
Production of an unfavorable oxidation–reduction potential	Dyes
Inhibition of enzymes containing iron or copper	Cyanide
	Azide
	Hydroxylamine

Table 13.6: Chemical Disinfectants

Disinfectant	Activity	Adverse Features
Alcohol	Bactericidal and tuberculocidal; not sporicidal; limited virucidal activity	Denatures proteins, making it difficult to remove them from surfaces. Denatured proteins protect bacteria from the effects of alcohol. Rapid evaporation from treated surfaces.
Chlorine dioxide*	Rapid disinfection activity; can be used for sterilization with 6 hr exposure.	Corrosive; activity greatly reduced in the presence of protein and organic debris; requires good ventilation.
Glutaraldehyde*	As 2.0%–3.2% immersion preparation, broad-spectrum antimicrobial activity; sporicidal after 10 hours' exposure; long use life. Surface disinfectant product available at 0.25% concentration.	Very corrosive to skin and mucous membranes; allergenic with repeated exposures.
Hypochlorite*	Rapid-acting, broad-spectrum bactericidal, sporicidal, virucidal agent.	Irritating to skin; corrosive; can degrade plastics.
Iodophors*	Rapid-acting, broad-spectrum disinfectant; residual antimicrobial activity remains on surface after drying.	Corrosive to some metals; may discolor some surfaces; inactivated by hard water.
Phenols*	Broad-spectrum antimicrobial activity; effective in the presence of detergents.	Can degrade plastics; irritating to skin and eyes; inactivated by hard water and organic debris.
Quaternary amines	Effective against gram-positive bacteria.	Not tuberculocidal nor virucidal; inactivated by soaps and hard water; inactivated by organic debris.

Note: Protective gloves should be worn when using disinfectant preparations.

*Approved for surface disinfection in the dental office by the American Dental Association, the Centers for Disease Control, and the Environmental Protection Agency.

agents have essentially no antibacterial effect. Anionic substances are soaps and synthetic anionic detergents. Soaps are the salts of the long-chain aliphatic carboxylic acids of animal and plant fats. Most synthetic anionic detergents are alkyl, aryl, or alkyl–aryl sulfates or sulfonates. The alkali content and sodium salt are responsible for the cidal effect of soaps on treponemes, streptococci, pneumococci, gonococci, meningococci, and influenza viruses. They are not very active against most gram-negative bacilli and quite ineffective against staphylococci. Overall, the value of anionic detergents seems to depend as much on their mechanical cleansing power as on their germicidal action.

Cationic surface-active substances (also termed quaternary ammonium salts) are modifications of a basic formula in which the four hydrogen atoms of the ammonium ion have been replaced with alkyl and alkyl–aryl groups. Cationic surface-active agents are germicidal in a much lower concentration than anionic detergents and are bacteriostatic in surprisingly high dilutions. They persist when they are applied to inanimate objects and form a film on the skin, the inner surface of which is not antibacterial. They likely act on the cell membrane, releasing essential enzymes and metabolites of both gram-positive and gram-negative bacteria; however, the cationic detergents are much more effective against gram-positive bacteria. They have little or no action on bacterial spores, viruses, or fungi. The use of cationic detergents is severely limited by their inability to penetrate organic debris on instrument surfaces and by their incompatibility with anionic agents or soaps, calcium, magnesium, and iron of hard waters, and organic matter. They are also readily absorbed by porous material (cotton, rubber, and other materials). Quaternary ammonium solutions are easily contaminated by gram-negative bacteria.

Substantial scientific evidence has proved the ineffectiveness of quaternary ammonium compounds against many pathogenic microorganisms that are transmitted in dental practice, including the causative agents for hepatitis B and tuberculosis. Since dental personnel are at significant occupational risk of infection by these agents, it is unfortunate that some practitioners continue to use aqueous quaternary ammonium preparations for the disinfection of environmental surfaces and instruments. In 1978 the ADA Council on Dental Therapeutics eliminated quaternary ammonium preparations from the Acceptance Program as disinfecting agents, thereby removing any doubt concerning the effectiveness of these preparations. Thus, benzalkonium chloride, dibenzalkonium chloride, and cetyldimethylethylammonium bromide are no longer recommended for routine use in dentistry.

Heavy Metals

All metallic ions inhibit microorganisms if applied in sufficient concentration, but only a few are useful antiseptics or disinfectants. None is of practical use in killing bacterial spores. Metals inhibit nonsporulating bacteria in very low concentration (1:1,000,000 or less) by what is termed oligodynamic action. This potency in small concentrations means simply that the ions of these elements have an exceptionally strong affinity for proteins, and especially for sulfhydryl groups. Bacterial cells or other organic matter readily absorb them out of solution. As with many other chemical antiseptics and disinfectants, the antimicrobial activity of metallic ion substances is sharply reduced by the presence of organic matter.

Mercury Compounds.   The mercuric ion, far from being an ideal antiseptic, is both an indiscriminate protein precipitant and an inactivator of sulfhydryl enzymes, the latter action being easily reversible.

Mercury Bichloride. Mercuric chloride, N.F., the oldest of the mercury antiseptics, is used for skin antisepsis and, previously, for disinfecting inanimate objects, including some surgical instruments, but it is ineffective against spores. Water-insoluble mercury compounds are used principally for treatment of skin infections. The organic mercurial antiseptics are, in general, less irritating, less toxic, and more antiseptic than the inorganic mercurial salts.

Merbromin, N.F. (Mercurochrome), used widely for application to skin, wounds, and mucous membranes, is not an effective germicide. Some other organic mercurials (*thimerosal,* N.F., *phenylmercuric nitrate,* N.F., and *nitromersol,* N.F.) are used in solutions, ointments, tinctures, jellies, and suppositories. They are not effective against spores, cannot be depended on to disinfect instruments, and are prone to cause allergic sensitization.

Mercury-containing compounds, particularly the soluble salts of mercury, are a common cause of poisoning. In acute poisoning mercury is extremely toxic to the alimentary tract and causes irreversible kidney damage. In chronic poisoning it causes gastric irritation and gingivitis, in addition to nephritis and hepatitis.

Silver Compounds.   Simple silver salts (silver nitrate, silver lactate, silver picrate) are used as antiseptics. Silver nitrate is used as a caustic and in lesser concentrations for local application as an antiseptic or astringent. The routine application of 1% or 2% silver nitrate to the eyes of newborn infants has practically eliminated gonococcal ophthalmia.

Zinc Compounds.   *Zinc sulfate,* U.S.P., *zinc chloride,* U.S.P., and *zinc oxide,* U.S.P., are mild antiseptics, mostly noted for their astringent action. They are used in the treatment of conjunctivitis, skin infections, and as a nasal spray.

Copper Compounds.   Although many copper salts act as astringents, germicides, and fungicides, the concentration required for bacterial activity is usually too great to be useful.

Alcohols

Ethyl alcohol and isopropyl alcohol have been used as surface disinfectants and antiseptics. Both of these agents effectively denature proteins and act as lipid solvents. This latter property probably enhances their range of activity because of the destructive effect on many enveloped viruses. Alcohols exhibit a fairly broad antimicrobial spectrum of activity under certain conditions. They are not recommended for use as surface disinfectants, however, because of a number of serious problems inherent with their use. They are not very effective in the presence of tissue proteins, such as those found in saliva and blood (i.e., they are poor cleaning agents in the presence of bioburden). Alcohol denatures these proteins to make them insoluble and adherent to most surfaces, including the surfaces of contaminant microorganisms. A coating of denatured bioburden may then protect microorganisms from the antimicrobial effects of the alcohols for prolonged intervals. Rapid evaporation of alcohol from environmental surfaces also inhibits their activity on protein-coated bacteria and viruses, which are commonly found in the spatter generated during dental procedures. Other problems include the corrosiveness of alcohols on metal surfaces, lack of sporicidal activity, and destruction of certain construction materials, such as plastic items and vinyl coverings.

Vegetative bacteria are killed by exposure to high concentrations of alcohol (70% optimum), the most notable pathogen being *M. tuberculosis.* The concentration of an alcohol preparation is critical to its antimicrobial effectiveness. When the concentration exceeds 70%, the initial dehydration of microbial proteins allows these cell components to resist the subsequent detrimental denaturation effects. Thus, the exposed microorganisms can remain viable for longer periods of time.

Ethyl alcohol is relatively nontoxic, colorless, nearly odorless and tasteless, and readily evaporates without residue. Isopropanol is less corrosive than ethanol, since it is not oxidized as rapidly to acetic acid and acetaldehyde. As a general consideration, neither is regarded as a very effective cleaning agent, required as a first step in preparation for disinfection and sterilization procedures. For these reasons neither the ADA nor the CDC currently recommends alcohol as a surface disinfectant for dental practice.

Halogens

Iodine. Iodine is one of the oldest antiseptics for application to skin, mucous membranes, abrasions, and other wounds. The high reactivity of this halogen with its substrate provides iodine with potent germicidal effects. It acts by iodination of proteins and subsequent formation of protein salts. Since iodine is insoluble in water, it has been routinely prepared as a tincture by dissolving an iodide salt in alcohol. Iodine in this form continues to be an effective antiseptic, as shown by the fact that at different concentrations, tinctures of iodine are toxic to both gram-positive and gram-negative bacteria, *M. tuberculosis,* spores, fungi, and most viruses. However, this chemical suffers from some serious drawbacks: it is irritating, allergenic, corrodes metals, and stains skin and clothing. Hypersensitivity reactions to iodine are not uncommon and may range from very mild to severe.

Iodophors. Attempts to utilize the powerful germicidal action of iodine while reducing its caustic and staining effects have led to the synthesis of later generation iodine compounds by formulating preparations in which the iodine is held in dissociable complexes. These compounds, called iodophors, retain a similar broad-spectrum antimicrobial range as that of iodine tinctures but have the following added features: less irritation to tissues, significantly less allergic, do not stain skin or clothing, and have a prolonged activity after application. Iodophors are prepared by combining iodine with a solubilizing agent or carrier. One of the most common carriers for iodophors is polyvinylpyrrolidine (PVP). This agent stabilizes the iodine, minimizes its toxicity, and slowly releases the halogen to the tissues. The carriers themselves are surface-acting substances (usually nonionic) that are water soluble and react with epithelial areas to increase tissue permeability. Thus, the active iodine that is released is better absorbed. Iodophor antiseptics are useful in preparing the oral mucosa for local anesthetic injections and surgical procedures. Iodophors have also been found to be effective hand washing antiseptics. In addition to removing microbial populations from the skin in large numbers, these cleansers are not generally washed off completely; therefore, a residual antimicrobial effect may remain in the scrubbed areas. Other iodophor preparations serve as disinfectants in hospitals, clinics, and similar health care facilities. Their surfactant properties make them excellent surface cleaning agents prior to disinfection. It must be noted here that diluting iodophor disinfectants in hard water may cause rapid loss of antimicrobial activity. The general recommendation is therefore to use distilled water, or at least softened water, to dilute the iodophors prior to use.

Chlorine. Chlorine has been used to arrest putrefaction and destroy odors since shortly after its discovery in 1774. Chlorine acts primarily by oxidation, as hypochlorous acid, into which it is quickly converted by water:

$$Cl_2 + H_2O \leftrightarrows HOCl + HCl$$
$$HOCl + NaOH \leftrightarrows NaOCl + H_2O$$

Chlorine is therefore more active in acid solutions. Elemental chlorine is a very potent germicide, killing most bacteria in 15 to 30 seconds at concentrations of 0.10 to 0.25 ppm. Accepted chlorine-containing compounds in common use are hypochlorite solutions and chlorine dioxide preparations. Diluted bleach (1:10 to 1:100) in water is very useful as a disinfectant, especially in areas considered to have been contaminated with hepatitis viruses. The CDC has recommended the use of 500 to 5,000 ppm (0.05% to 0.5%) sodium hypochlorite as an effective agent in destroying hepatitis B viruses. Since this chemical is unstable, fresh solutions must be prepared daily. Despite its effectiveness as a disinfectant, this chlorine-releasing preparation has some obvious disadvantages. It is corrosive to metals and very irritating to skin and other tissues, and destroys many fabrics.

Phenols and Derivatives

The classic antiseptic for surgical procedures was carbolic acid. It was first thought that postoperative infections would be virtually eradicated with the widespread use of this phenol. However, due to the severe toxicity reported in individuals exposed to carbolic acid, its application was curtailed. Other phenolic compounds have filled roles as effective disinfectants or antiseptics. These agents act as cytoplasmic poisons by penetrating and disrupting microbial cell walls, leading to denaturation of intracellular proteins. The intense penetration capability of phenols is probably the major factor in their antimicrobial activity. Unfortunately, they can also penetrate intact skin, causing local tissue damage and possible systemic complications. Thus, with the exception of the bisphenols, most phenolic derivatives are used primarily as disinfectants.

Phenol. Phenol is bacteriostatic at about 0.2%, lethal to most bacteria at 1.0%, and fungicidal at about 1.3%. Its penetrating power on epithelial surfaces can cause necrosis and gangrene. Phenol is now seldom used as a disinfectant or germicide but has slight value as a fungicide. It remains as the in vitro standard against which other antimicrobial chemicals are compared.

Hexylresorcinol. This phenolic derivative is widely used as an antiseptic, specifically as an anthelminthic. In addition, some commercial mouth rinses also contain hexylresorcinol in very low concentrations.

Cresols. Cresols, which are alkyl derivatives of phenol, are composed of mixtures of *ortho*-cresol, *meta*-cresol, and *para*-cresol. Cresols are widely used and are superior to phenol as disinfectants. This latter property is illustrated by the greater tuberculocidal activity of cresols. The primary disinfection of many inanimate areas such as floors and walls is accomplished through routine use of these agents. Because they retain the capacity to irritate superficial tissues, cresols are not applicable as antiseptics. Concentrations that are nonirritating are ineffective against most bacteria.

Halogenated Phenols. Chlorinated phenols are active germicides, Camphorated *p*-chlorophenol (1 part *p*-chlorophenol and 2 parts camphor; also, 1 part *p*-chlorophenol and 7 parts camphor) has been used in dentistry as a root canal antiseptic. Its spectrum of activity and toxicity are similar to those of phenol; however, the antimicrobial efficacy of the chlorinated phenols appears to be greater due to halogen substitution.

Parachlorometaxylenol (PCMX) is a halogen-substituted phenol that is currently employed as the active agent in a class of hand wash antiseptics. PCMX is bactericidal for gram-positive and gram-negative bacteria and is fungicidal.

Bisphenols. This group of phenolic compounds contains agents possessing properties which make them effective hand wash antiseptics. Hexachlorophene and chlorhexidine, by virtue of their dual phenolic ring structure, have a relatively low toxicity and a high bacteriostatic action at low concentrations. Although they are somewhat insoluble in water, they are soluble in dilute alkali. Thus, both antiseptics remain effective even when mixed wih soaps. Bisphenols possess properties that make them suitable as routine hand washing agents. Although hexachlorophene and chlorhexidine significantly diminish the concentration of resident skin microorganisms after a single application, repeated washings throughout the day are necessary for maximal effectiveness. Both preparations can accumulate and remain on the skin in an active form for prolonged periods, thereby leaving a residual antibacterial effect after each wash. This property, called *substantivity,* fosters the buildup of an "antimicrobial layer" against many common skin contaminants. Since neither hexachloraphene nor chlorhexidine is effective against tubercle bacilli and spores, present formulations are not functional as disinfectants.

Complex (Synthetic) Phenols. In the mid-1980s a new class of phenolic compounds was approved by the EPA as surface disinfectants. These contain more than one phenolic agent. Currently most products contain two, but newer formulations have three phenols as the active compounds. After appropriate dilution in water, these phenolics act in a synergistic manner to offer a broad antimicrobial spectrum, including tuberculocidal activity. They also serve as good surface cleaners and are effective in the presence of detergents. Unfortunately, the penetration properties of phenols tend to cause epithelial toxicity in exposed tissues.

Oxidants

Oxidizing agents are toxic to microorganisms. The most common oxidants used as antiseptic drugs are hydrogen and metallic peroxides. Hydrogen peroxide is still frequently employed as an oxygenating agent in the treatment of oral anaerobic infections, such as acute gingivitis, necrotizing ulcerative gingivitis, and maxillofacial abscesses.

Hydrogen peroxide in quite small concentrations will inhibit bacteria in culture, but its antiseptic action is brief when applied to tissues, owing to its rapid decomposition by tissue catalase. Zinc peroxide releases its oxygen more slowly than hydrogen peroxide and leaves a residue of zinc oxide, an astringent. The other metallic peroxides, used extensively in the past, are seldom used now.

Dyes

Dyes have been recognized as antiseptics for many years, even though their practical use is very limited. Some are used as antiprotozoal and wound-healing agents. In general, they are more active against gram-positive than gram-negative bacteria. Dyes are used in selective culture media and in some diagnostic procedures. Merbromin (Mercurochrome), a combination of mercury and fluorescein, although widely used, has limited value for the disinfection of skin, mucous membranes, and wounds. The triphenylmethane rosaniline dyes, a group of basic dyes, of which gentian or crystal violet is the most important, are active against bacteria and some pathogenic fungi. Crystal violet is also used as a differential bacterial stain (Gram stain).

Glutaraldehydes

Glutaraldehyde ($C_5H_8O_2$) has two aldehyde units, one at each end of the carbon chain. Different commercial preparations are formulated to have maximal activity at alkaline, acidic, or neutral pH. Those products that are active at alkaline or neutral pH utilize an activator that brings the final 2.0% to 3.2% glutaraldehyde to the desired pH. At these concentrations glutaraldehydes are effective against all vegetative bacteria, including *M. tuberculosis,* fungi, and viruses, and are able to destroy microbial spores in 6 to 10 hours. They therefore offer an alternative as immersion sterilants for those few items that cannot withstand repeated heat sterilization and are not disposable.

In addition to their wide antimicrobial range, glutaraldehydes also offer other important advantages as disinfectants. Their low surface tension permits them to penetrate blood or exudate to reach instrument surfaces, and facilitates rinsing. Rubber and plastic items are not degraded during prolonged immersion, and in fact these chemicals are useful in removing blood from suction hoses. Unfortunately, glutaraldehydes can damage many metallic items if misused. For example, nickel-coated impression trays will often discolor and carbon steel burs will corrode when immersed in a 2.0% to 3.2% glutaraldehyde solution for prolonged periods.

Sterilization of instruments by immersion in glutaraldehyde solutions can be useful in certain circumstances but may also be the most abused aspect of office asepsis. The misleading term "cold sterilization" was derived from such practices. Chemical sterilization techniques and the use of chemical holding solutions are not acceptable substitutes for heat sterilization. Important considerations that directly relate to glutaraldehyde biocidal activity include their shelf life, use life, and reuse life. *Shelf life* is the time that a product may be safely stored. *Use life* is the life expectancy for the solution once it is activated but has not yet been put into use with contaminated items. *Reuse life* is the amount of time a solution can be used and reused as it is challenged with instruments which are wet or coated with bioburden. Reuse life takes into account a dilution factor due to added water from wet instruments, the effects of soap and other detergents, and evaporation. The Environmental Protection Agency started accepting reuse claims from glutaraldehyde manufacturers in 1985. Acceptance allows the manufacturer to include a reuse statement on the product label.

Although glutaraldehydes are highly effective as disinfectants, they are not functional as antiseptics. Irritation of hands is common, so that direct physical contact between glutaraldehyde solutions and tissues should not occur. Heavy duty gloves should always be worn when handling any glutaraldehyde solution. They can rapidly induce hypersensitivity and other dermatological reactions with repeated exposures. For these reasons, immersed items should be thoroughly rinsed with sterile water prior to use.

Vapors and Gases

Glycol Vapors. In 1941 it was demonstrated that glycol vapors readily kill bacteria in air. Aerosols of propylene or trimethylene glycol, hypochlorite, or substituted phenols were widely tested for sterilization of air. Their use is limited because of difficulty in controlling humidity, distribution of the vapors, and the accumulation of glycol films with little or no antibacterial activity on room surfaces.

Formaldehyde. Formaldehyde, a gas at room temperature, was formerly used for fumigation. It is too toxic to apply to body tissues and is allergenic, causing eczematoid dermatitis. It is used in solution (formalin) as a tissue specimen fixative.

β-Propiolactone. β-Propiolactone, in its vapor phase, was previously used to disinfect dental instruments. It is more active than formaldehyde and is a good sporicide, but there was some indication that it may be carcinogenic.

Ethylene Oxide. Ethylene oxide is a highly penetrative, colorless gas at room temperature. This agent is unusually effective against spores, is virucidal, does no damage to materials, and evaporates without a residue. These features have led to the acceptance of ethylene oxide as a recognized method of sterilization (see Table 13.2), especially for items that can be damaged by moisture or heat. Materials such as suction tubing, all handpieces, radiographic film holders, and dental prostheses may be sterilized without adverse effect by this means.

Since pure ethylene oxide is rather toxic, allergenic, slow in action, and forms explosive mixtures with air, commercial preparations are mixed with carbon dioxide or an inert gas to form a more stable combination. This preparation functions as an alkylating agent by irreversibly inactivating cellular nucleic acids and proteins. Susceptible chemical groups of these intracellular molecules are the $-NH_2$, $-COOH$, $-SH$, and $-OH$ sites. Since the toxic effects are not selective for microbial substrates and the potential remains for explosion, materials must be processed in a special container placed in a well-ventilated area.

The slow penetration of gas throughout the container necessitates a protracted sterilization period followed by another prolonged aeration interval. Usually, 10 to 16 hours is sufficient for sterilization of most non-rubber-based items. For items containing rubber, an additional 24 hours may be necessary to allow for complete dissipation of ethylene oxide from the porous material. Trapped gas can cause painful burns when the improperly aerated item comes into contact with epithelial tissues. Liquids to be sterilized may have to aerate even longer and may not be treatable with ethylene oxide.

Asepsis in the Dental Practice

Instrument Recirculation

Processing reusable items includes cleaning, packaging, sterilizing, monitoring, and storage of packaged instruments. Accumulated debris, such as blood and saliva, can lengthen the interval necessary for sterilization or even prevent sterilization under certain conditions.

The initial requirement for instrument recirculation is to remove any collected organic matter. Hand scrubbing can accomplish this cleaning, although caution must always be exercised to prevent skin punctures. Puncture-resistant utility gloves should be worn to prevent this type of accident. An alternative or additional method of cleaning instruments utilizes an ultrasonic bath. This apparatus must be operated with a cover to prevent aerosolization of contaminants. Cleaning solutions are manufactured that are compatible with this type of unit. The metal container within the ultrasonic unit should also be wiped with a suitable cleanser/disinfectant at frequent intervals (i.e., periodically during the day or after each use, depending on instrument load size).

The packaging of items for heat sterilization will depend on the type of sterilizer used and the characteristics of the instruments. Cleaned instruments should be placed in heat-stable wraps, sealed, and dated. Sterilized instruments should remain wrapped until use. Many commercial wraps and sealed plastic pouches will remain sterile for months if unopened. Taking sterilized instruments out of a package and placing them in cabinet drawers for later use is *not* recommended. An updated list formulated by the ADA regarding the application of various sterilization modalities for instruments and other intra-oral items is presented in Table 13.7. Corrosion or rusting of metallic instruments is a major fault of using steam under pressure for sterilization. Even the best autoclaves contain sufficient oxygen to cause corrosion of carbon steel during sterilization. An approach has been made using chemicals that vaporize in the autoclave and protect iron or steel from oxidation by hydrolysis. The utilization of a dry heat oven, chemical vapor sterilizer, or an ethylene oxide unit prevents the above adverse effect.

Handpiece Asepsis

The issue of handpiece sterilization has been addressed in the last few years. Previously, heat sterilization was not feasible for this equipment, as handpieces could not withstand elevated temperatures. As a result, practitioners became used to disinfecting the outer surfaces of the handpiece. Asepsis of internal components that were also exposed to saliva and blood was not accomplished. Advances in technology are resolving many of these problems, with the result being the routine manufacture and sale of heat-sterilization handpieces for dental practice. Current infection control guidelines include a statement for the sterilization of dental handpieces after use with each patient.

The current recommended methods for heat sterilization of handpieces are use of an autoclave or an unsaturated chemical vapor sterilizer, although newer generation, shorter cycle, dry heat units also appear to be feasible. For those handpieces that cannot withstand heat, the CDC has outlined a compromise precleaning/disinfection protocol. It should be noted here that handpieces should never be immersed in a disinfectant solution or treated with 2.0% to 3.0% glutaraldehyde preparations. Such misuse of these chemicals will shorten handpiece life dramatically, as well as increase the chances for glutaraldehyde toxicity reactions during operator handling.

Handpieces should be properly lubricated before they are wrapped for sterilization. Failure to maintain the handpiece properly in this manner can diminish its efficiency. These same procedures and precautions apply to items like air/water syringe tips and ultrasonic scalers.

Surface Disinfection

Although the use of disposable covers is increasing, surfaces that cannot be covered must be cleaned and disinfected. If one considers the large number of operatory surfaces that may become contaminated with saliva, blood, or exudate (bioburden), it is apparent that surface disinfection is a major factor in achieving asepsis in the dental office. Disinfection of environmental surfaces is a two-step procedure. An initial mechanical removal of organic proteinaceous debris (precleaning) is required. This is followed by application of an appropriate disinfectant, with adequate time allowed for the chemical to achieve disinfection. Since proteinaceous debris renders coated microorganisms more resistant to the effect of many disinfectants, surface precleaning is a mandatory first step before chemical disinfection. A product that is unable to penetrate and remove accumulated debris would fail at the first step of surface asepsis. The use of a disinfectant that provides residual antimicrobial effect with repeated use is also desirable.

Manufacturers recommend that their products be used on precleaned surfaces. Although separate surface cleaners and surface disinfectants may be employed, use of a chemical agent that accomplishes both functions during the two-step protocol provides a more efficient approach.

Equipment Asepsis

Dental equipment that is heat resistant should be sterilized. All other equipment must be covered or disinfected. Thus, infection control should be considered when new equipment is to be purchased. Office design, traffic flow, construction materials, and fixtures are all elements that should be taken into account when implementing an asepsis regimen. Design features that minimize contact between hand and contaminated surfaces include sink faucets that are controlled by a foot, forearm, or electrically; soap dispensers that are controlled by a foot or forearm; towel dispensers that dispense disposable paper towels without requiring handling of the release mechanism; waste containers that are plastic lined and recessed under cabinets beneath a countertop opening; an air circulation exchange system or single-room air filtration unit that reduces the amount of "airborne" microbes; and a floor covering such as vinyl that is constructed in a smooth and continuous manner, eliminating crevices that can trap debris.

Disposable barriers should be used whenever possible to avoid the necessity of excessive cleaning of both surfaces and equipment. Aluminum foil, plastic wrap, plastic bags, plastic-lined paper, or any other impervious sheeting can be used as a cover/barrier on equipment and surfaces. Cleaning followed by disinfection is recommended for equipment surfaces that cannot be covered.

Hand Washing

Hands must be washed thoroughly immediately before and after the treatment of each patient. The use of gloves is not a substitute for routine hand washing with an effective liquid antiseptic. The rationale here includes the recognition that gloves may tear or perforate during patient treatment, and that bacteria either remaining on the skin after washing or entering through a compromised glove can multiply rapidly under the glove.

Substituted phenol preparations, such as chlorhexidine gluconate (a bisphenol) and parachlorometaxylenol (PCMX), are the best hand washing agents currently available. With both agents repeated washings are necessary throughout the day for maximal substantivity effectiveness. Hands should be dried with air or disposable paper towels, not with reusable cloth towels.

Disposables

Items manufactured and identified for single use only, such as needles, saliva ejectors, and prophylaxis cups, are not to be reused. The availability of disposables continues to increase as manufacturers, distributors, and office personnel recognize their usefulness. Some recently marketed disposable items include disposable prophylaxis angles, rag wheels, and evacuation line traps. These products present less

cross-contamination risks since they do not undergo recleaning and recycling, but they must be disposed of properly. This is especially important for needles and other sharp instruments, which 1) should not be recapped by hand and 2) should be placed in puncture-resistant containers for disposal.

Laboratory Asepsis

Impressions, prosthetic devices, and the instruments used in their construction generally require handling by multiple individuals both in the dental office and in commercial dental laboratories. These items, contaminated with the patient's saliva, blood, and, in the case of old prostheses, plaque deposits, can serve as sources of infection. The ADA Council on Dental Therapeutics and Prosthetic Services and the Council on Dental Laboratory Relations updated guidelines for infection control in dental laboratories in 1988. The ADA and the CDC have recommended that impressions, appliances, and other items removed from the mouth of a patient be cleaned and disinfected before being sent to the laboratory. Additionally, items received from the laboratory for delivery to a patient must be cleaned and disinfected prior to placement.

Materials and the instrumentation used in the construction of dental prostheses pose special problems in maintaining an aseptic environment and in the delivery of a noncontaminated prosthesis to the patient. Many of these items may be damaged by exposure to heat or the chemicals used for disinfection. The use of barriers to prevent contamination, of separate materials for new devices and those previously inserted in the mouth, and of unit doses of polishing materials will minimize cross-contamination in the dental laboratory setting.

Dental impressions and prostheses must be disinfected carefully to avoid distorting the impressions and damaging the metal, porcelain, or acrylic surfaces of prostheses. Several groups of investigators have evaluated the effects of various disinfectant solutions on these materials. Table 13.8 presents recommendations for disinfection of impressions and prostheses based on the results of a number of research investigations. Immersion is preferred over spraying when possible since this ensures that all surfaces are adequately exposed to the disinfectant. Thorough rinsing under running tap water is essential both before disinfection to remove bioburden and after disinfection to remove any residual disinfectant.

Summary

Effective infection control must be a routine component of professional activity. The use of universal pre-

Table 13.7: Sterilization and Disinfection of Dental Instruments, Materials, and Some Commonly Used Items*

	Steam Autoclave	Dry Heat Oven	Chemical Vapor	Ethylene Oxide	Chemical Disinfection/ Sterilization	Other Methods/ Comments
Angle attachments†	+	+	+	++	+	
Burs						
Carbon steel	−	++	++	+++	−	
Steel	++	+++	+++	+++	+++	
Tungsten–carbide	++	+++	++	+++	+++	
Condensers	++	+	+	+++	+++	
Dapen dishes	++					
Endodontic instruments (broaches, files, reamers)						Hot salt/glass bead sterilizer 10 to 15 sec. 218°C (425°F)
Stainless steel handles	+	++	++	++	+	
Stainless steel with plastic handles	++	++	−	++	−	
Fluoride gel trays						
Heat-resistant plastic	++	− −	−	+++	− −	
Non-heat-resistant plastic	− −	− −	−	+++	−	Discard (+ +)
Glass slabs	++	++	++	+++	+	
Hand instruments						
Carbon steel	− [Steam autoclave with chemical protection (1% sodium nitrite)]	++	++	+++	−	
Stainless steel	++	++	++	++	+	
Handpieces†					+	Sterilizable preferably
Sterilizable†	(+ +)†	−	(+)†	++	− −	
Contra-angles†	−	−	−	+++	+ +	Combination synthetic phenolics or iodophors (−)
Nonsterilizable†	−	−	−	+++	+ +	
Prophylaxis angles†	+	+	+	+	−	
Impression materials‡						
Impression trays						
Aluminum metal	++	++	++	+++	−	
Chrome-plated	++	++	++	+++	+++	
Custom acrylic resin	− −	− −	− −	+++	+++	
Plastic	− −	− −	− −	+++	− −	Discard (+ +) preferred
Instruments in packs	++	+ Small packs	++	++ Small packs	− −	
Instrument tray setups						
Restorative or surgical	Size limit	+	Size limit	++ Size limit	−	

Item	1	2	3	4	5	6	Notes
Mirrors	–		++	++	++	+	
Needles							
Disposable	–	–	–	–	–	–	Discard (++) Do not reuse
Nitrous oxide							
Nose piece	(++)†	–	(++)†	++	++	(+)†	
Hoses	(++)†	–	(++)†	++	++	(+)†	
Orthodontic pliers							
High-quality stainless	++	++	++	++	++	+	
Low-quality stainless	–	++	–	++	++	–	
With plastic parts	++	++	++	++	++	++	
Pluggers	–	–	–	+	++	–	
Polishing wheels and disks							
Garnet and cuttle	–	–	–	+	++	–	
Rag	++	+	+	++	++	– –	
Rubber	–	–	–	+	++	++	
Prostheses, removable				+			
Rubber dam equipment							
Carbon steel clamps	–	++	++	++	++	–	
Metal frames	++	++	++	++	++	++	
Plastic frames	–	–	–	–	++	++	
Punches	–	++	++	++	++	++	
Stainless steel clamps	++	++	++	++	++	++	
Rubber items	–	–	–	–	++	–	
Prophylaxis cups	–		–	++	++	–	Discard (++)
Saliva evacuators, ejectors							
Low-melting plastic	–	–	–	–	++	++	Discard (++)
High-melting plastic	++	+	+	++	++	++	
Stones							
Diamond	++	++	++	++	++	+	
Polishing	++	+	+	++	++	–	
Sharpening	++	++	++	++	–		
Surgical instruments							
Stainless steel	++	++	++	++	++	++	
Ultrasonic scaling tips	+	–	–	–	++	++	
Water–air syringe tips	++	++	++	++	++	++	
X-ray equipment							
Plastic film holders	(++)†	–	(+)†	++	++	++	
Collimating devices	–	–	–	–	++	+	

Note: ++ denotes effective and preferred methods, + denotes effective and acceptable method, – denotes effective method but risk of damage to materials, – – denotes ineffective method with risk of damage to materials.

*Reproduced with permission from the Council on Dental Therapeutics, American Dental Association: Infection control recommendations for the dental office and the dental laboratory. *JADA,* **116,** 241, 1988. The table is adapted from *Accepted Dental Therapeutics* and *Dentists' Desk Reference: Materials, Instruments, and Equipment.*

†As manufacturers use a variety of alloys and materials in these products, confirmation with the equipment manufacturers is recommended, especially for handpieces and their attachments.

‡No standards were available on impression materials when this table was originally printed. Subsequent work has provided information about these materials. (See Table 13.8.)

Table 13.8: Guide for Selecting Disinfectant Solutions

Use	Glutaraldehydes*	Iodophors†	Chlorine Compounds‡	Complex Phenolics*	Phenolic Glutaraldehyde§
Impressions					
Alginate	−	?	+	−	−
Polysulfide rubber base	+	+	+	+	+
Silicone rubber	+	+	+	+	+
Polyether	−	−	+	−	−
ZOE impression paste	+	+	−	?	+
Reversible hydrocolloid	−	+	+	?	+
Compound	−	+	+	−	+
Prostheses‖					
Fixed (metal/porcelain)	+	+/−	−	?	+
Removable (acrylic/porcelain)	−	+	+	−	−
Removable (metal/acrylic)	−	+/−	+/−	−	−

Note: + denotes recommended method, − denotes not recommended, +/− denotes could damage material, ? denotes data inconclusive or not available.

Minimum exposure time should be that recommended for disinfection with the selected product. Thorough rinsing of impressions and prostheses under running tap water to remove any residual disinfectant is essential.

*Prepared according to the manufacturer's instructions.
†1:213 dilution
‡1:10 dilution of commercial bleach
§1:16 dilution
‖May also be ethylene oxide sterilized.

cautions in the management of all patients greatly minimizes occupational exposure to microbial pathogens, by addressing the reality that most potentially infectious individuals are asymptomatic and therefore undiagnosed.

Procedures aimed at preventing the spread of infectious disease during dental treatment are also constantly being evaluated by the profession and an increasingly inquisitive public. The dilemma faced by dental practitioners was concisely summarized by Crawford (1978):

> Discrepancies between "the ideal" and "the real" in dental asepsis provide fertile ground for rash statements of two kinds: "Sterilize everything!" versus "Do nothing, the mouth is a dirty place!" Both are expressions of compulsion, fear or frustration about a seemingly impossible dilemma. They may reflect the sentiment, "Go away; let me alone." Practical reality, of course, dictates that to prevent the possible spread of infectious diseases, dental professionals must be provided with inclusive, up-to-date information that can be utilized to develop an optimal program of asepsis.

When such a program has been implemented by the practitioner and auxiliary staff, the risk of disease transmission is significantly reduced.

ADDITIONAL READING

ADA Council on Dental Materials and Devices, Council on Dental Therapeutics. 1978. Infection Control in the Dental Office. J Am Dent Assoc, **97,** 673.

Allen, A. L., and Organ, R. J. 1982. Occult Blood Accumulation Under the Fingernails: A Mechanism for the Spread of Bloodborne Infection. J Am Dent Assoc, **105,** 455.

American Dental Association Council on Dental Therapeutics. 1978. Quaternary Ammonium Compounds Not Acceptable for Disinfection of Instruments and Environmental Surfaces. J Am Dent Assoc, **97, 855.**

Block, S. S. (Ed.). 1983. *Disinfection, Sterilization and Preservation.* Lea & Febiger, Philadelphia.

Centers for Disease Control. 1980. Viral Hepatitis Type B, Tuberculosis and Dental Care of Indochinese Refugees. MMWR, **29,** 1.

Centers for Disease Control. 1983. Acquired Immunodeficiency Syndrome (AIDS): Precautions for Health Care Workers and Allied Professionals. MMWR, **32,** 450.

Centers for Disease Control. 1986. Recommended Infection Control Practices for Dentistry. MMWR, **35,** 237.

Centers for Disease Control. 1987. Recommendations for Prevention of HIV Transmission in Health Care Settings. MMWR, **36(2S),** 1.

Centers for Disease Control. 1988. Update: Universal Precautions for Prevention of Transmission of Human Immunodeficiency Virus, Hepatitis B Virus and Other Bloodbourne Pathogens in Health-Care Settings. MMWR, **37,** 377.

Cottone, J. A. 1986. Infection Control in Dentistry. In *Proceedings of a National Conference on Infection Control in Dentistry,* Chicago, p. 34, edited by E. W. Mitchell and S. B. Corbin. American Dental Association, Chicago.

Council on Dental Materials, Instruments, and Equipment, Council on Dental Practice, and Council on Dental Therapeutics. 1988. Infection Control Recommendations for the Dental Office and the Dental Laboratory. J Am Dent Assoc, **116,** 241.

Crawford, J. J. 1978. *Clinical Asepsis in Dentistry.* R. A. Kolstad, Dallas.

Crawford, J. J. 1983. Sterilization, Disinfection and Asepsis in Dentistry. In *Disinfection, Sterilization and Preservation,* pp. 505–523, edited by S. S. Block. Lea & Febiger, Philadelphia.

Crawford, J. J. 1985. State-of-the-Art: Practical Infection Control in Dentistry. J Am Dent Assoc, **110,** 629.

Dineen, P. 1978. Handwashing Degerming: A Comparison of Povidone-Iodine and Chlorhexidine. Clin Pharm Ther, **23,** 63.

Ernst, R. R. 1974. Ethylene Oxide Sterilization Kinetics. Biotechnol Bioeng Symp, **4,** 865.

Favero, M. S. 1985. Sterilization, Disinfection and Antisepsis in the Hospital. In *Manual of Clinical Microbiology,* Ed. 4, p. 129. American Society for Microbiology, Washington, D.C.

Hales, R. H. 1970. Ocular Injuries Sustained in the Dental Office. Am J Ophthal **70,** 221.

Kimbrough, R. D. 1973. Review of Recent Evidence of Toxic Effects of Hexachlorophene. Pediatrics, **51,** 391.

Lister, J. 1987. On a New Method of Treating Compound Fracture, Abscess, etc. with Observations on the Condition of Suppuration. Lancet i, **326,** 387.

Merchant, V. A., Herrera, S. P., and Dwan, J. J. 1987. Marginal Fit of Cast Gold MO Inlays from Disinfected Elastomeric Impressions. J Prosthetic Dent, **58,** 276.

Molinari, J. A., Campbell, M. D., and York, J. 1982. Minimizing Potential Infections in Dental Practice. J Mich Dent Assoc, **64,** 411.

Molinari, J. A., Gleason, M. J., and Merchant, V. A. 1988. Infection Control. An Overview for Dentistry. Calif Dent Assoc J, **16,** 14.

Palenik, C. J. 1981. Eye Protection for the Entire Dental Office. J Ind Dent Assoc, **60,** 23.

Peterson, A. F., Rosenberg, A., and Alatary, S. D. 1978. Comparative Evaluation of Surgical Scrub Preparations. Surg Gynecol Obstet, **164,** 63.

Riley, R. L. 1971. Air Disinfection in Corridors by Upper Air Irradiation with Ultraviolet Light. Arch Environ Health, **22,** 551.

Runnells, R. R. 1988. *Dental Infection Control. Update '88.* I.C. Publications, North Salt Lake, Utah.

Soulsby, M. E., Barnett, J. B., and Maddox, S. 1986. The Efficacy of Chlorhexidine Gluconate-Containing Surgical Scrub Preparations. Infect Control, **7,** 223.

Sykes, G. 1969. Methods and Equipment for Sterilization of Laboratory Apparatus and Media. In *Methods in Microbiology,* Vol. 1, p. 77, edited by J. R. Norris and D. W. Ribbons. Academic Press, New York.

Taber, D., Lazaras, J. C., Faucher, O. E., and Calandra, J. C. 1971. The Accumulation and Persistence of Antibacterial Agents in Human Skin. J Soc Cosmet Chem, **22,** 369.

Whitacre, R. J., Robins, S. K., Williams, B. L., and Crawford, J. J. 1979. *Dental Asepsis.* Stoma Press, Seattle.

14

Antimicrobial Chemotherapy

John T. Wilson

The advent of antibiotics for the treatment of infectious diseases began in 1928 with Sir Alexander Fleming's chance observation that staphylococci growing on a culture plate were inhibited by contamination with a species of *Penicillium*. This mold produced an antibiotic that Fleming called penicillin. After much investigation, penicillin was isolated by Ernst Boris Chain and Sir Howard W. Florey as an impure brown powder, and by 1941 an extensive systematic search was under way for molds and bacteria that might produce other antibiotics. The results indicated that many types of penicillin were produced by mutant strains and species of *P. notatum* and *P. chrysogenum* as well as other *Penicillium* species. The search also revealed that many *Streptomyces* species and a few *Bacillus* species produced antibiotics. Some species of *Nocardia* and *Aspergillus* also produce antibiotics. As the search continues, new antibiotics will undoubtedly be discovered, either produced naturally by microorganisms or synthesized by biochemists.

The list of microbial agents causing oral and maxillofacial infections continues to expand as cultural and diagnostic procedures become more sensitive. The dental practitioner is thus required to be familiar with the principles and general approaches to chemotherapy as they relate to the wide range of infections encountered. Many of these infections, such as those involving strict anaerobes, frequently were not diagnosed correctly and often led to long-term complications for both patient and dentist. It is not the purpose of this chapter to present an exhaustive pharmacological discussion of antibiotics. Excellent texts and references (see Additional Readings) have recently been published that provide the student and practitioner with detailed therapeutic information on virtually every chemical agent. Instead, the intent is to present an overview of the principles of antimicrobial chemotherapy with the emphasis on different mechanisms by which antibiotics interfere with infectious microorganisms. Selected drugs of use in dental medicine are discussed in relation to these mechanisms.

Characteristics of Ideal Chemotherapeutic Agents

As the search for useful chemotherapeutic agents progressed it became evident that they must have certain properties. These characteristics of an ideal agent have served as a useful guide in the ongoing search for natural antibiotics and in the development of chemosynthetic agents. However, agents that do not have all of the requisite properties of an ideal agent may still be of considerable practical use, depending on the clinical circumstances.

An ideal chemotherapeutic agent:

1. Should have selective activity. It will have true selectivity if it affects some essential biochemical reaction of the microorganism that is not an essential reaction of the host. The agent may have relative selectivity even if the reaction is essential to both pathogen and host. For instance, such an agent would be useful if the pathogen metabolized or reproduced more rapidly than the host cells, or if the membranes of the pathogen were more permeable to the agent than those of the host cells.

2. Should have a spectrum of activity that includes only the causative pathogen or pathogens involved in a given disease. It should not upset the normal microbiota of the various body areas.

3. Is generally more useful if it is bactericidal rather than bacteriostatic.

4. Should not induce bacterial resistance.

5. Should have no significant toxic effects on the host at its highest useful dose.

6. Should not be allergenic.

7. Should retain its activity in the presence of body fluids and tissues.

8. Should be soluble and stable in water.

9. Rapidly achieves a bactericidal blood level that can be maintained for the time necessary to effect a cure.

10. Can be administered either parenterally or orally.

11. Is easily disposed of by the body at a rate that will maintain a bactericidal blood level.

12. Is reasonable in cost.

Classification of Antibiotics and Chemotherapeutics

Antibiotics and chemotherapeutic agents can be classified by their mode of action on microbial cells (Table 14.1). Thus, the various agents can be divided into groups that 1) interfere with cell wall synthesis, 2) inhibit or interfere with protein synthesis, 3) affect nucleic acid function, 4) damage plasma membranes, or 5) are metabolite antagonists.

As shown in Table 14.1, penicillin, cycloserine, vancomycin, bacitracin, and novobiocin inhibit the synthesis of bacterial cell walls or, more specifically, interfere with some phase of peptidoglycan synthesis. Antibiotics that inhibit protein synthesis can be sub-

Table 14.1: Chemotherapeutic Agents According to Their Mode of Action

Mode of Action	Antibiotic

Inhibitors of cell wall formation	Beta-lactams
	  Penicillin
	  Cephalosporins
	  Monobactams
	  Carbopenems
	Cycloserine
	Vancomycin
	Bacitracin
	Novobiocin (partially)

Inhibitors of protein synthesis: A. At the level of transcription	Actinomycin
B. At the level of translation	Rifampin Streptomycin Neomycin Paromomycin Kanamycin Gentamicin Spectinomycin Chloramphenicol Erythromycin Lincomycin Clindamycin Amikacin Tobramycin Tetracyclines
Inhibitors of nucleic acid function	Mitomycin Nalidixic acid Novobiocin Griseofulvin
Inhibitors causing cytoplasmic membrane damage	Polymyxin Nystatin Amphotericin B
Metabolite antagonists	Sulfonamides Sulfones *p*-Aminosalicylic acid Isoniazid

divided into one group comprising agents that affect protein synthesis at the level of transcription (actinomycin, rifampin) and another group comprising agents that inhibit microbial protein synthesis at the level of translation. The latter group includes streptomycin, neomycin, paromomycin, kanamycin, gentamicin, spectinomycin, chloramphenicol, erythromycin, lincomycin, clindamycin, and the tetracyclines. Although there are a number of inhibitors of nucleic acid function, most are not routinely used because of their deleterious effects on the host. Many nucleic acid inhibitors that are not included in Table 14.1, such as the alkylating agents nitrogen mustard and cyclophosphamide, have an important role in antineoplastic treatment regimens.

The cell or cytoplasmic membrane is also an important regulator of bacterial cell activity, particularly as a selective barrier affecting the transport of compounds into and out of the cell, and in biosynthesis and metabolism. Polymyxin, nystatin, and amphotericin B are examples of antibiotics that attack the cytoplasmic cell membrane directly. These agents are relatively nonspecific, for they usually are not able to distinguish between mammalian and target microbial membranes. This affects their application and will be discussed in a later section.

The sulfonamides and related compounds are classified in a group of antimetabolites that interfere with the enzymes involved in the production and utilization of essential bacterial growth factors (vitamins, amino acids). These essential enzymes combine with antimetabolites that are structurally related to their normal substrate and prevent normal substrate–enzyme reaction.

No classification scheme for antibiotics appears to be appropriate in all instances. While each method is plagued by exceptions and footnoted explanations, a few approaches other than the classification shown in Table 14.1 must be mentioned. First, antibiotics and chemotherapeutic agents can be classified by their antimicrobial spectrum. This classification, quite useful in clinical practice, divides the agents into 1) those that have primarily a gram-positive spectrum, 2) those that have primarily a gram-negative spectrum, 3) those active against a broad spectrum of microbes, 4) antifungal agents, and 5) antiviral agents. Agents with a gram-positive spectrum include penicillin, erythromycin, lincomycin, bacitracin, and vancomycin. Agents with a gram-negative spectrum include gentamicin, tobramycin, and polymyxin B. Broad-spectrum agents, acting on both gram-positive and gram-negative bacteria, include tetracycline, kanamycin, neomycin, cephalosporin, chloramphenicol, and streptomycin. Antifungal agents are nystatin, amphotericin B, and griseofulvin. There are few antiviral agents, but 5-iodo-2'-deoxyuridine, vidarabine, amantadine, and AZT are clinically useful.

Another method of categorizing antimicrobial agents is by their route of administration. Routes of administration are topical or systemic (oral and parenteral). Some agents that are applied topically include bacitracin and nystatin. Some agents that can be applied both topically and systemically are polymyxin and neomycin. Among the numerous agents that are applied systemically, griseofulvin, streptomycin, amphotericin B, the cephalosporins, tetracycline, clindamycin, erythromycin, and the penicillins have found application in dental medicine.

A less useful method of classifying antimicrobial agents, at least clinically, is by their source. Sources are 1) fungi or molds, 2) bacteria, and 3) synthetic compounds. Antibiotics produced by fungi include the penicillins, griseofulvin, and cephalosporins. Major agents derived from bacteria are polymyxin, colis-

tin, and bacitracin. Most antibiotics derived from bacteria are applied locally. The majority of such antibiotics in current use are produced by actinomycetes. They include streptomycin, neomycin, kanamycin, vancomycin, clindamycin, nystatin, amphotericin B, and erythromycin. Another source of antibiotics and chemotherapeutic agents is by synthesis or semisynthesis. The most notable examples of this type of agent are the semisynthetic penicillins.

Inhibitors of Cell Wall Formation

Most bacteria have rugged cell walls composed of a murein backbone and tetrapeptide cross-bridges (see Chap. 3). Beta-lactam antibiotics inhibit cell wall synthesis by disrupting the transpeptidation processes that link the various peptidoglycan components. The mechanism of action of beta-lactam antibiotics has not been fully elucidated. However, it is believed that they bind to specific proteins, penicillin-binding proteins (PBPs). PBPs are enzymes, i.e., carboxypeptidases, transpeptidases, and endopeptidases involved in the assembly and reshaping of the bacterial cell wall.

The various beta-lactam antibiotics are either bactericidal or bacteriostatic, depending on which species of PBP they have inhibited. In contrast, other antibiotics—cycloserine, bacitracin, novobiocin, and vancomycin—do not bind to PBPs but interfere with other processes involved in cell wall synthesis.

Penicillins. The basic structure of penicillins consists of a condensation product of the D-isomers of an alanine and a β-dimethyl-cysteine residue, to which is attached an R-C-group (Fig. 14.1). From strains of *P. notatum* and *P. chrysogenum* grown in ordinary culture media, many useful types of penicillin have been isolated, designated as G, K, X, O, V, F, and dihydro-F. Penicillin G, O, and V are useful therapeutically. Many additional "biosynthetic" penicillins have been isolated by the addition of certain chemical intermediates, as sources of different R-groups, to species and strains of *Penicillium* grown in standard media. For penicillin to have antibacterial activity, the lactam and thiazolidine rings must be intact. Most forms of bacterial penicillinase inactivate penicillins by breaking the lactam ring, resulting in inactive penicilloic acid. The side chain, or R'-group, largely determines the stability of the molecule and is responsible for many of the antibacterial and pharmacological features of different penicillins. In 1959, 6-aminopenicillanic acid was obtained in crystalline form without side chain precursors. Although it has little or no antibacterial activity, it can be acylated to yield strongly antibacterial semisynthetic penicillins, which have become very important in the treatment of certain penicillin-resistant and gram-negative infections. A functional classification of the major penicillins is presented in

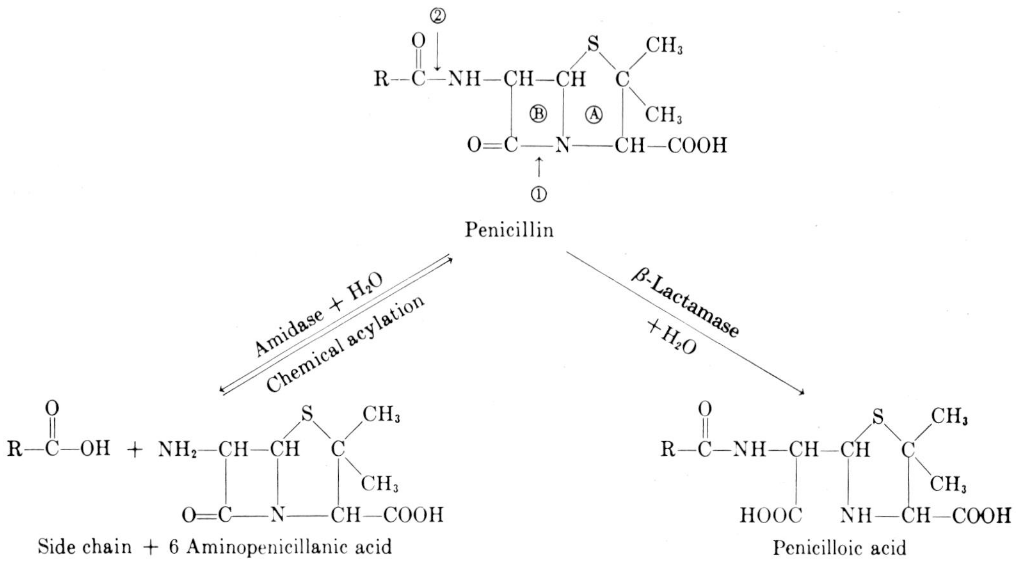

Figure 14.1: Basic structure of penicillins, and some of their important chemical reactions: Ⓐ, thiazolidine ring; Ⓑ, beta-lactam ring; ①, site of action of β-lactamase; ②, site of action of amidase.

Table 14.2. Structural formulas of the principal penicillins in use are diagramed in Figure 14.2.

Penicillin Activity. Penicillins are mainly effective against gram-positive bacteria, spirochetes, and a few gram-negative bacteria (see Table 14.2). However, in high concentrations they are effective against many gram-negative microorganisms.

The semisynthetic penicillins include some with broadened antimicrobial spectra. For example, 6-aminobenzylpenicillin (ampicillin) is much more active than penicillin G against many gram-negative bacteria. This is evidently due to its greater ability to penetrate through the gram-negative cell envelope. Ampicillin, however, is less active than penicillin G against many gram-positive microorganisms.

Penicillin Resistance. Penicillin-resistant microorganisms usually develop by the production of the adaptive enzyme penicillinase. Although pathogenic strains of *Staphylococcus aureus* are the major infectious agents possessing this enzyme, other infections have been traced in recent years to penicillinase-producing strains of *Neisseria gonorrhoeae* and *Haemophilus influenzae*. These strains are becoming increasingly prevalent. In addition, penicillin-resistant strains of *Streptococcus pneumoniae* began appearing in South African outbreaks in 1977, and since that time a number of countries, including the United States and Canada, have reported strains resistant to up to 2 μg/mL penicillin. Multiple drug resistance has also become a characteristic feature of these pneumococci.

Penicillinase synthesized by adaptive mutants can occur in either a beta-lactamase or an amidase form

(see Fig. 14.1). The first is the most common, resulting in cleavage of the beta-lactam ring with subsequent inactivation of the drug. Most *S. aureus* and gram-negative bacteria that produce a penicillinase do so by releasing a beta-lactamase. The amidase type of enzyme destroys the antimicrobial activity of penicillins by cleaving side groups from the parent molecule. The development of semisynthetic penicillins such as methicillin and oxacillin has countered some of the above resistance, as these forms of the drug are penicillinase resistant. They are poor substrates for beta-lactamase and thus are not inactivated in the presence of lactamase-producing strains. Agents such as methicillin, cloxacillin, nafcillin, and oxacillin have found significant use in dental medicine against penicillin G–resistant staphylococcal infections.

Penicillin Toxicity. The penicillins in common use have very little significant toxicity or pharmacological action per se even when used in large dosages. They are toxic when applied directly to the central nervous system in concentrated solution, but not in dilute solution. After parenteral or oral administration, very little penicillin reaches the undiseased central nervous system.

Penicillins, however, seem to be among the worst allergens of the antibiotics in current use. Largely because of the indiscriminate use of penicillins, more than 10% of the population has become seriously hypersensitive to them. Some 25% of all patients treated with penicillins show some form of dermal sensitivity. The less severe symptoms of penicillin sensitivity are epidermal reactions (urticaria, dermatitis), gastrointestinal disturbances (diarrhea is common with

Table 14.2: Penicillins and the Infectious Organisms for Which They Are the Antimicrobial Agents of Choice*

Penicillin G
  Streptococcus pneumoniae†
  Streptococcus pyogenes
  Viridans streptococci
  Anaerobic streptococci
  Staphylococcus aureus (nonpenicillinase-producing)
  Neisseria meningitidis
  Neisseria gonorrhoeae‡
  Bacillus anthracis
  Clostridium
  Leptotrichia buccalis
  Erysipelothrix rhusiopathiae
  Pasteurella multocida
  Streptobacillus moniliformis
  Bacteroides (non-*fragilis* strains)
  Treponema pallidum
  Sprillum minor
  Leptospira
  Fusiform bacteria
  Actinomyces israelii
Methicillin, oxacillin, nafcillin, cloxacillin, dicloxacillin
  Staphylococcus aureus (penicillinase-producing)
Ampicillin
  Streptococcus faecalis§
  Proteus mirabilis
  Haemophilus influenzae†
  Actinomyces muris ratti
  Listeria monocytogenes
  Salmonella other than *S. typhi*
Carbenicillin, piperacillin,§ mezlocillin,§ azlocillin§
  Pseudomonas aeruginosa

---

*Reproduced with permission from C. J. Wilkowske: Special Series on Antimicrobial Agents. *Mayo Clin Proc,* **52**, 616, 1977.
†Penicillin-resistant strains occur in the absence of penicillinase synthesis.
‡Penicillinase-producing resistant strains occur.
§Usually with an aminoglycoside.

ampicillin), pain in muscles or joints, headache, eosinophilia, fever resembling serum sickness, and malaise. Most of these reactions are transient and subside when penicillin is no longer administered. The use of long-lasting or repository types of penicillin complicates the treatment of allergic reactions, for even when the use of such penicillins is discontinued, the drug persists in the tissues. The most serious sensitivity reaction is anaphylactic shock. Its occurrence is infrequent and usually, but not always, follows parenteral administration.

Routes of Administration. Penicillins can be administered orally (PO), intramuscularly (IM), or intravenously (IV). The onset of antibacterial action following various routes of penicillin administration relates to the rate of absorption, the tissue level obtained, the resistance to degradation by gastric acids, and the degree of protein binding. Two of these factors, extent of

absorption after oral administration and acid resistance, are very noteworthy to the practicing dentist and specialist (Table 14.3).

Only about one third of orally administered penicillin G is absorbed, mostly from the duodenum; the remaining two thirds is destroyed in the stomach and colon. Some penicillins are resistant to gastric juices and are well absorbed, particularly from an empty stomach. Oral administration also yields a lower blood serum concentration than is obtained by the other routes. The IM administration of penicillin is more effective than the oral route, but the risk of an untoward reaction is greater. Blood serum concentrations obtained by IM injection are intermediate between oral (lowest) and IV (highest) administration. Finally, the IV injection of penicillins is most dangerous with regard to hypersensitivity, but a high serum concentration can be achieved almost immediately. It is not routinely used except in life-threatening situations.

Metabolism and Excretion. A number of substances in the body act on penicillin. Most penicillins are hydrolyzed to some extent by gastric acids. Amidases convert penicillins into the inactive 6-aminopenicillanic acid. Bacterial penicillinase (beta-lactamase) converts penicillins to penicilloic acid. Absorbed penicillins that are not hydrolyzed in the body are excreted unchanged. Most penicillin (60% to 90%) is excreted in urine; the remainder is excreted in bile, saliva, or other body fluids.

Dosage of Penicillin. The dosage for IM administration is usually from 300,000 to 1 million units/day. Orally, penicillin is generally administered three to four times daily in 400,000 to 500,000 unit doses.

Cephalosporins. The cephalosporins, semisynthetic derivatives of 7-aminocephalosporanic acid, are antibacterial compounds produced by the fungus *Cephalosporium acremonium.* 7-Aminocephalosporanic acid is the active component of the fungal product cephalosporin C. The nucleus of cephalosporin C is closely related to penicillin in structure and mechanism of antibacterial action (Fig. 14.3). The major difference between the structures of the cephalosporins and the penicillins is the presence of a dihydrothiazine ring in place of the penicillins' five-membered thiazolidine ring. The R^1 and R^2 side groups distinguish the various cephalosporins from each other with regard to antimicrobial spectrum, stability, and oral absorption. The available forms of cephalosporins are categorized in Table 14.4.

Various cephalosporins are commonly referred to as either first-, second-, or third-generation drugs. The initial compounds developed (first-generation drugs) have a narrower spectrum of antimicrobial activity than the later second- and third-generation drugs and are primarily useful for certain gram-pos-

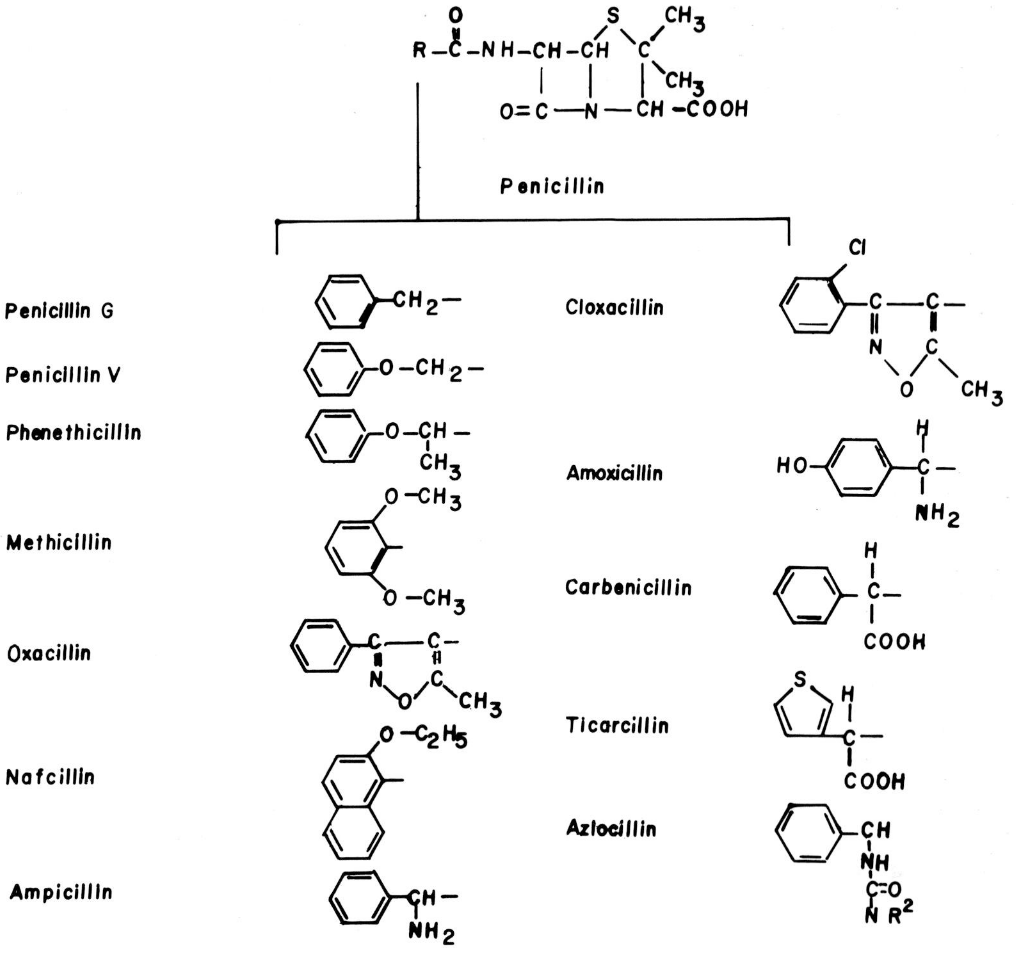

Figure 14.2: Structures of penicillins.

itive microorganisms. However, whereas the second- and third-generation cephalosporins have an increased gram-negative spectrum, they are not as active against gram-positive bacteria as are the first-generation cephalosporins. Third-generation cephalosporins generally have a longer half-life than the first- and second-generation drugs.

Cephalosporin Activity. These drugs usually are reserved for serious infections in hospitalized patients, although in general the cephalosporins are bactericidal against most gram-positive cocci and common gram-negative bacilli such as *Escherichia coli, Klebsiella pneumoniae, Proteus mirabilis, Salmonella* species and *Shigella* species. A notable exception among the gram-positive cocci is the resistance demonstrated by enterococci, specifically *Streptococcus faecalis.* Maxillofacial and periapical abscesses caused by this bacterium are as resistant to cephalosporins as they are to simple penicillins. The above antimicrobial spectrum is remarkably similar for most of the

cephalosporins. The main exceptions are cefamandole and cefoxitin, which have broad spectra.

This group of antibiotics is rarely mentioned as the agent of choice for treatment of dental infections, although cephalosporins are effective against certain orofacial infections that are refractory to penicillins. Serious methacillin-resistant *S. aureus* infections serve as examples for the use of an agent like cephalothin, in conjunction with an aminoglycoside such as gentamicin, as an appropriate replacement for ineffective penicillin regimens.

Patients with a history of minor penicillin hypersensitivity have also been transferred to a cephalosporin, generally without any subsequent incidents. Although there is some immunological cross-reactivity between penicillins and cephalosporins, scientists and clinicians have found that the latter usually are contraindicated only in patients with anaphylactic or other severe immediate hypersensitivities.

The major route of excretion of cephalosporins is

Table 14.3: Classification of Penicillins*

Types/Generic Names	Trade Names	Oral Absorption	Acid Resistance
Natural			
Penicillin G	Many	Variable (poor)	+
Phenoxymethyl penicillin (penicillin V)	Many	Good	+ +
Phenoxymethyl penicillin (phenethicillin)	Many	Good	+ + +
Semisynthetic			
Penicillinase-resistant			
Methicillin	Staphcillin	Poor	0
Oxacillin	Bactocill, Prostaphlin	Good	+ +
Nafcillin	Unipen	Variable	+ +
Cloxacillin	Tegopen	Good	+ + +
Dicloxacillin	Dynapen, Pathocil, Veracillin	Good	
Extended spectrum			
Ampicillin	Many	Good	+ + +
Bacampicillin	Spectrobid	Good	+ + +
Hetacillin	Versapen	Good	+ + +
Amoxicillin	Larotid, Amoxil, Polymox	Excellent	+ + +
Carbenicillin	Geopen, Pyopen	Poor	+ +
Ticarcillin	Ticar	Poor	0
Azlocillin	Azlin	Poor	0
Mezlocillin	Mezlin	Poor	0
Piperacillin	Pipracil	Poor	0

Note: 0 = acid sensitive; + = slightly resistant; + + = moderately resistant; + + + = highly resistant.

*Adapted with permission C. J. Wilkowske: Special Series on Antimicrobial Agents. *Mayo Clin Proc,* **52,** 616, 1977.

via the renal system. A notable exception is the third-generation drug cetoperazone, which is primarily (70%) excreted through the biliary system, and therefore dosage reductions would not be necessary in patients with renal failure.

Cephalosporin Resistance. Induced mechanisms of antimicrobial resistance are similar to those demonstrated against the penicillins. Beta-lactamases, or more specifically cephalosporinases, are capable of inactivating the drugs in a fashion analogous to that for penicillinase. In addition, mutant bacteria can pre-vent the penetration of most cephalosporins to the active site in the cell wall. These two forms of resistance can be overcome by substituting a less susceptible cephalosporin. For example, cefamandole can be used against soft tissue infections caused by beta-lactamase-producing gram-negative bacilli.

Cephalosporin Toxicity. The development of allergic reactions is the major adverse manifestation. These are most commonly maculopapular rashes, with anaphylactic responses occurring only occasionally. A positive Coombs test is a frequent problem in

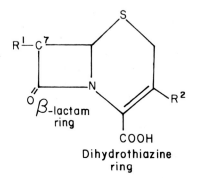

Figure 14.3: General structure of cephalosporins.

Table 14.4: Types of Cephalosporins*

Parenteral Use	Oral Use	Extended Spectrum
Cephalothin†	Cephalexin†	Cefamandole‡
Cephapirin†	Cephradine†	Cefoxitin‡
Cefazolin†	Cefadroxil†	
Cephaloridine		
Cephradine†	Cefalcor‡	

*Adapted with permission from R. L. Thompson: Special Series on Antimicrobial Agents. *Mayo Clin Proc,* **52,** 625, 1977.

†First-generation drugs.

‡Second-generation drugs.

individuals receiving larger doses of cephalosporins; fortunately, hemolysis generally does not occur in this situation. In the main, similar adverse effects are associated with both cephalosporins and penicillins.

Cycloserine. Cycloserine is a broad-spectrum antibiotic that has been isolated from *Streptomyces orchidaceus* as well as synthesized commercially. It is a structural analogue of D-alanine that disrupts cell wall synthesis by inhibiting D-alanyl-D-alanine synthetase and D-alanine racemase. These enzymes are responsible for the incorporation of D-alanine into the murein. Adverse reactions to cycloserine include central nervous system toxicity, which encompasses both neurologic and psychic disturbances, and hypersensitivity. Because of the potential for severe nervous system toxicity, cycloserine is generally restricted to treatment of *Mycobacterium* infections that are refractory to other chemotherapeutic agents.

Vancomycin. Vancomycin, produced by *Streptomyces orientalis,* is active against a few gram-positive bacteria and spirochetes. It has a complex molecular structure composed of amino acids and sugars, and it acts by interfering with the second stage of cell wall formation and preventing the transfer of subunits from the carrier to the growing peptidoglycan component. Vancomycin should only be used if penicillins, cephalosporins, and other classes of antibiotics cannot be employed. An application in dentistry is the prophylactic administration of IV vancomycin to a patient with a history of endocarditis or rheumatic heart disease and who is allergic to penicillin and erythromycin. Vancomycin also is effective in treating endocarditis caused by viridans streptococci in a similar patient. An unexpected use of vancomycin came to light recently during investigations of the etiology of pseudomembranous colitis. The causative organism, *Clostridium difficile,* is an exotoxin-producing bacillus that is susceptible to orally administered vancomycin. Since the antibiotic is poorly absorbed through the intestinal lining, it remains in the lumen and is thus bactericidal to the *C. difficile* present.

Bacteria seldom develop resistance to vancomycin, and it does not exhibit cross-resistance with other antibiotics. However, vancomycin is ototoxic, nephrotoxic, allergenic, and occasionally causes dermatitis and localized phlebitis. It should not be administered to patients with impaired renal function.

Bacitracin. Bacitracin is an antibiotic produced by strains of *Bacillus subtilis.* It is active against many gram-positive bacteria as well as against *Neisseria* species, *Haemophilus influenzae,* and *Treponema pallidum.* Bacitracin functions by interfering with dephosphorylation of the carrier lipid formed in the course of subunit transfer to the growing cell wall. Bacitracin frequently induces nephrotoxicity after parenteral administration, so its use is limited to topical application. The dental practitioner would have little occasion to use this drug.

Novobiocin. Novobiocin, produced by *Streptomyces niveus, Streptomyces griseus,* and *Streptomyces spheroides,* is bactericidal against gram-positive bacteria, with an antibacterial spectrum similar to that of penicillin and erythromycin. Novobiocin interferes with the integrity of the cytoplasmic membrane, DNA replication, and cell wall formation. It does not induce formation of spheroplasts and in fact is quite active against L forms and spheroplasts. Still, novobiocin has serious drawbacks in clinical use. Susceptible bacteria readily develop resistance to it, and the drug is allergenic and toxic. The toxic symptoms, principally anemia, leukopenia, pancytopenia, and gastrointestinal irritation, preclude clinical utilization of this antibiotic.

Inhibitors of Protein Synthesis

Protein Synthesis. Two major processes are essential to protein synthesis. One is transcription, in which a complementary sequence of RNA is formed by RNA polymerase in response to the genetic information present in DNA. In transcription, antibiotics may alter the structure of template DNA or inhibit RNA polymerases. The other process relates to the translation of mRNA, formed in transcription, into protein. Translation of mRNA into the synthesis of a peptide chain occurs in initiation, elongation, and termination stages. This complex activity, resembling an assembly line, occurs in ribosomes that undergo assembly and disassembly while synthesizing protein.

Translation differs between prokaryotes and eukaryotes both in structural features of mRNA and ribosomes and in the specific steps involving initiation and elongation of polypeptides. These differences allow the inhibition of microbial protein synthetic mechanisms with a minimum of concurrent disruption of mammalian intracellular functions.

There are a relatively large number of clinically useful chemotherapeutic agents that inhibit some stage of translation. These antibiotics can be categorized primarily into groups according to their reaction with either 30S or 50S ribosomal subunits of prokaryotes. In addition to their inhibitory activity against certain pathogenic microorganisms in disease, many of the chemotherapeutic agents described below have also been used to delineate individual steps in the process of protein synthesis.

Inhibitors of Transcription

Actinomycin. Actinomycin, produced by several *Streptomyces* species, is an oligopeptide that interferes with protein synthesis in both gram-positive and gram-negative bacteria and mammalian cells. Its clinical usage has been in the form of the derivative, dactinomycin, a potent antineoplastic chemotherapeutic agent.

Rifampin. Rifampin is a semisynthetic derivative of rifamycin B, the latter being produced by *Streptomyces mediteranei*. Rifampin is effective against numerous gram-positive and enteric gram-negative bacteria, *Chlamydia*, and some viruses, but it is best used clinically as a potent antitubercular drug. It has the widest range of activity in vitro of all the major agents against *Mycobacterium* species. Rifampin's bactericidal effect is directed against DNA-dependent RNA polymerase, impairing RNA synthesis. It has little or no effect on mammalian RNA polymerases, owing to their inability to bind the drug. Because of the rapid emergence of bacterial resistance, this antibiotic is not used alone in the treatment of tuberculosis. Instead, rifampin administered concurrently with isoniazid constitutes the most effective drug combination for antitubercular therapy. Oral rifampin has also been successfully used as prophylactic therapy for *Neisseria meningitidis* infection.

Side effects, which vary with use of the drug, include the development of an orange-pink color to saliva, tears, urine, and perspiration. Less frequent adverse reactions include rashes, nausea, vomiting, fever, and jaundice.

Inhibitors of Translation

Streptomycin and Other Aminoglycosides. Streptomycin, an aminoglycoside produced by *Streptomyces griseus*, inhibits many gram-positive and gram-negative bacteria as well as *Mycobacterium tuberculosis*. Although it is toxic to the eighth cranial nerve and vestibular apparatus, it is sometimes used in combination with other drugs to treat tuberculosis, meningitis caused by *Haemophilus influenzae*, plague, tularemia, and *Salmonella* and *Shigella* infections. Orofacial infections and endocarditis caused by enterococci (i.e., *Streptococcus faecalis*) are controlled by IM administration of streptomycin in combination with oral ampicillin. Nevertheless, because of its toxicity and the rapid development of bacterial resistance, streptomycin is not a commonly employed antibiotic in dental medicine.

In vitro, streptomycin binds irreversibly to the 30S ribosomal subunit of a sensitive bacterial cell, inhibiting protein synthesis at the initiation of the cycle and inducing a misreading of mRNA and phenotypic suppression. The net result of the addition of streptomycin to growing bacteria is a reduction in their negative surface charge, resulting in agglutination, a rapid discharge of potassium into the environment, cessation of protein synthesis, depression of DNA and RNA synthesis, RNA dissolution, and death of the cell.

In addition to streptomycin, a number of other aminoglycoside antibiotics mostly produced by *Streptomyces* species prevent protein synthesis by reacting with the 30S ribosomal subunits. All contain amino acids and sugars and either a streptamine (streptomycin) or a deoxystreptamine moiety (kanamycin, neomycin). Of this group, neomycin, gentamicin, kanamycin, tobramycin, and amikacin are used clinically to suppress the growth of gram-negative rods like *Pseudomonas aeruginosa* in burns and wounds and in some types of gastroenteritis. Although a bacterium may develop resistance to one aminoglycoside during such treatment, it will still be sensitive to the other drugs of this group.

Tetracyclines. Tetracyclines, produced by various species of *Streptomyces*, belong to a group of closely related bacteriostatic antibiotics that include tetracycline, chlortetracycline, dimethylchlortetracycline, doxycycline, and oxytetracycline. They are termed broad-spectrum antibiotics since they act against both gram-positive and gram-negative bacteria as well as against microorganisms that are insensitive to other antibiotics. Bacteria that become insensitive to one tetracycline are insensitive to all others. The clinical value of tetracyclines as drugs of first choice and alternative therapy is summarized in Table 14.5. The recognition of appropriate and inappropriate application becomes very important when dental practitioners consider using one of these drugs to treat routine oral infections.

Tetracyclines act by inhibiting protein synthesis. Inhibition is accomplished by preventing the binding of aminoacyl-tRNA to the acceptor site on the 30S ribosome, stopping peptide chain formation. Figure 14.4 shows the basic structure of tetracycline.

Tetracyclines may be administered orally or parenterally and are absorbed into all tissues except the brain. Tetracyclines do enter the cerebrospinal fluid. Due to their chelating activity, tetracyclines are deposited in forming bones and teeth, causing discoloration. They also interfere with the normal growth and development of bones and teeth. Accordingly, their use should be avoided during the last trimester of pregnancy, the neonatal period, and early childhood. Their affinity for calcium may also result in vitamin K deficiency and a prolonged clotting time.

Although tetracyclines have a relatively low systemic toxicity, they can produce untoward effects, and some decomposition products are toxic. In addition, oral administration of tetracyclines can upset the normal microbiota of the mouth, vagina, and intestine. *Candida albicans*, which is not susceptible to the tetracyclines, is ordinarily held in check by the normal bacterial flora. During tetracycline therapy it may

Table 14.5: Major Clinical Applications of Tetracyclines

Acne vulgaris	Pneumonia (*Hemophilus influenzae*
Actinomycosis	and *Klebsiella* spp.)
Conjunctivitis (chlamydial)	Sinusitis
Genitourinary tract infections	Psitticosis
Lymphogranuloma venereum	Rickettsial Pox
Meningococcal carriers	Rocky Mountain Spotted Fever
Necrotizing ulcerative	Skin and soft tissue infections
gingivostomatitis	Syphilis
Otitis media	Urethritis (non-gonococcal)
Pharyngitis	

grow in abundance, causing local and even systemic infection. In addition, staphylococcal enteritis or pseudomembranous colitis may develop when the normal ecological balance is upset during prolonged tetracycline therapy.

Chloramphenicol. Closely related to the tetracyclines in its antibiotic spectrum but not in its chemical structure is chloramphenicol, produced either by *Streptomyces venezuelae* or synthetically. Chloramphenicol, a bacteriostatic antibiotic, is active against gram-positive and gram-negative bacteria, *Rickettsia,* and *Chlamydia*. Because of its toxicity, the use of chloramphenicol is restricted to the treatment of typhoid fever, salmonellosis, staphylococcal infections resistant to other less toxic antibiotics, anaerobic infections such as *Bacteroides fragilis* sepsis, and some other severe, life-threatening infections.

The chief toxic effects are severe blood dyscrasias, optic neuritis, and depression of marrow activity. Less serious symptoms of toxicity are bitter taste, dry mouth, gastritis, diarrhea, and nausea. Although it is toxic, chloramphenicol can be administered with reasonable safety to seriously ill patients if proper precautions are observed.

The mode of antibacterial action of chloramphenicol is to prevent protein synthesis by binding exclusively to 50S ribosomal subunits. The antibiotic does not inhibit the initiation of protein synthesis, but interferes with peptide bond formation (transpeptidation). Chloramphenicol does not react with mammalian ribosomes, owing to the absence of appropriate reacting sites.

Chloramphenicol, erythromycin, lincomycin, and clindamycin compete for the same binding sites on 50S ribosomal subunits. Therefore, the simultaneous use of antibiotics affecting these sites is of no more value than if they are used singly. Resistance to such antibiotics generally develops by the bacteria either becoming impermeable to the drug or acquiring the ability to degrade the antibiotic to an inactive form.

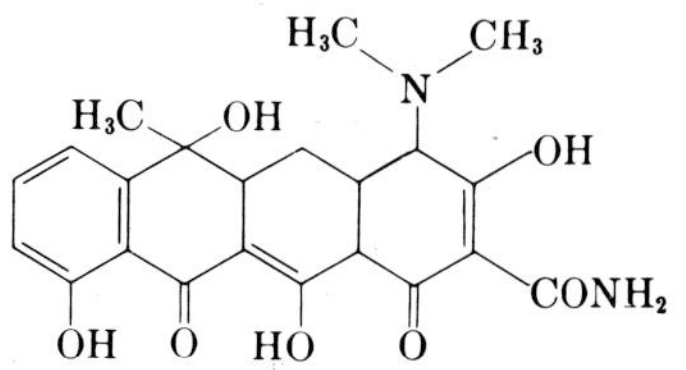

Macrolide Antibiotics. The macrolide group, which includes erythromycin, oleandomycin, and spiramycin, also inhibits bacteria by reacting with 50S ribosomal subunits. These antibiotics have an antibacterial spectrum similar to penicillin and are primarily bacteriostatic.

Erythromycin, produced by *Streptomyces erythraeus,* is frequently employed as a therapeutic drug in dental medicine. Many general practitioners and specialists use this macrolide as an alternative to penicillins for common infections. This complex compound is effective both as a drug of first choice and as an alternative choice for individuals with demonstrated penicillin hypersensitivity (Table 14.6). Erythromycin prevents protein synthesis by reacting with 50S ribosomal subunits near or at the same site as chloramphenicol. The coupling of the peptide bonds is inhibited, but the ribosome cycle continues without protein synthesis. Resistance to erythromycin is generally controlled with bacterial acquisition of a plasmid that can result in alteration of the bacterial RNA. This change, which occurs primarily after exposure to low concentrations of the antibiotic, diminishes the bacteriostatic effectiveness of the macrolide.

Lincomycin and Clindamycin. Lincomycin, produced by *Streptomyces lincolnensis,* is structurally related to other antibiotics but has an antibacterial spectrum similar to that of erythromycin. The 7-deoxy, 7-chloro derivative of lincomycin, termed clindamycin, is better absorbed than the parent molecule and is more active with fewer adverse reactions. Therefore, clindamycin has replaced lincomycin in clinical usage. Clindamycin is used in dental medicine as a substitute for penicillin in patients allergic to the drug and also in cases of anaerobic infection, especially where *Bacteroides fragilis* is involved. The antibiotic binds to 50S ribosomes, interfering with the binding of aminoacyl-tRNA and resulting in the breakdown of polyribosomes. It does not bind to mammalian rRNA,

Figure 14.4: Basic structural formula of tetracycline.

Table 14.6: Uses of Erythromycins

Source
Produced from a strain of *Streptomyces erythraeus*

Chemical Group
Macrolide group

Forms
Erythromycin (oral)
Erythromycin Estolate (oral)
Erythromycin Ethylsuccinate (oral)
Erythromycin Gluceptate (parenteral)
Erythromycin Lactobionate (parenteral)
Erythromycin Stearate (oral)

Major Indications
Actinomycosis
Bacterial endocarditis (prophylaxis in penicillin-allergic
   patients)
Chlamydial infections: conjunctivitis, genitourinary tract
   infections, pneumonia
Gonorrhea
Legionnaires' disease
Lymphogranuloma venereum
Pharyngitis (caused by group A beta-hemolytic
   streptococci)
Pneumonia (mycoplasma)
Rheumatic fever (long-term prophylaxis)
Sinusitis
Skin and soft tissue infections (caused by *Streptococcus
   pyogenes* and *Staphylococcus aureus*
Urethritis (non-gonococcal)

---

thereby furthering its usefulness. However, since diarrhea can occur and can lead to pseudomembranous colitis, clindamycin is advised only when other antimicrobials are contraindicated.

Inhibitors of Nucleic Acid Function

A number of antibiotics interfere with DNA structure and function, but only a few are clinically useful because their toxic action is not very selective. These antibiotics affect DNA by either cross-linking or intercalation.

Mitomycin. Mitomycin, produced by *Streptomyces* species, has been used principally in the study of bacteriophages and as an antineoplastic agent. In vitro it blocks DNA synthesis, causing filamentous forms, cessation of growth, and ultimately death. In vivo it is converted to an active hydroquinone derivative that cross-links with DNA on each of its complementary strands, preventing their separation and halting DNA synthesis. Mitomycin has some selectivity, for it will sometimes halt bacterial cell DNA synthesis but allow the synthesis of bacteriophages.

The Quinolones. A new class of antibiotics that is becoming clinically important comprises the quinolones. These antibiotics are basic molecular modifications of nalidixic acid. Quinolones are believed to inhibit bacterial DNA synthesis by interfering with the bacterial enzyme topoisomerase II (DNA gyrase). This enzyme is necessary for maintaining the bacterial chromosome in a supercoiled state and is involved in repair during DNA replication.

Nalidixic Acid. Nalidixic acid, the "original" quinolone, is a synthetic compound used clinically against urinary tract infections caused by species of *Escherichia, Aerobacter,* and *Proteus.* Because it inhibits DNA synthesis, it also has been used to study the factors regulating bacterial cell division.

Fluorinated Quinolones (Ciprofloxacin, Nonfloxacin, Ofloxacin, Pefloxacin). The new fluorinated quinolones have a wider spectrum of activity than nalidixic acid. They are well absorbed orally and are very active against *E. coli, Salmonella, Shigella, Citrobacter, Enterobacter, Proteus,* and *Neisseria* and moderately active against *Pseudomonas aeruginosa.* The fluorinated quinolones have substantially longer half-lifes than nalidixic acid. The long half-life, coupled with the high degree of antimicrobial activity, allows chemotherapeutic dosing at 12-hour intervals. Currently, no serious adverse reactions have been reported.

Griseofulvin. Griseofulvin is produced by *Penicillium griseofulvum.* It has few toxic effects and does not elicit resistance in clinical use. It is useful in the treatment of superficial mycotic infections by interfering with DNA replication. Griseofulvin is given orally and is assimilated through the intestinal wall into the blood. The drug eventually localizes in the new epithelial tissues of the skin, nails, and hair as the old tissues are sloughed from fungal infection. This antibiotic thus localizes in the specific tissue area infected with dermatophytes.

Inhibitors Causing Cytoplasmic Membrane Damage

Several antibiotics affect one or more essential activities of microbial cytoplasmic membranes. Among those in clinical use are polymyxin, nystatin, and amphotericin B.

Polymyxins. The polymyxins, produced by *Bacillus polymyxa,* are a group of five polypeptides, of which polymyxin B and polymyxin E (colistin) are of clinical value. They act on gram-negative bacteria and are used in urinary tract infections and infections caused by resistant *Pseudomonas aeruginosa* and *Shigella* species. The polymyxins are sufficiently nephrotoxic that their use must be strictly limited. Polymyxins bind specifically to cytoplasmic membranes, break down the osmotic barrier, and cause metabolites to leak out of the cell.

Nystatin. Nystatin, produced by *Streptomyces noursei,* is a relatively nontoxic member of the polyene group of antibiotics. It is active against many fungi, particularly *Candida albicans.* This yeast-like fungus is the most common cause of intraoral mycotic infection. Nystatin binds to a sterol-containing site on the cytoplasmic membranes of fungi, causing leakage. Nystatin is not active against bacteria since the cell membranes of bacteria contain no sterol.

Amphotericin B. Amphotericin B, produced by *Streptomyces nodosus,* is also a member of the polyene group of antibiotics. It is active against many pathogenic fungi but can be nephrotoxic to the patient. Administered IV, amphotericin B reacts with a sterol-containing site on the fungal cytoplasmic membrane, causing it to leak intracellular constituents.

Metabolite Antagonists

Sulfonamides. Even though sulfonamides are rarely used in dental medicine, the history of their discovery and development as therapeutic agents is important. Elucidation of their antimicrobial activity, absorption, and toxicity set the stage for investigation of later antibiotics. The following sections are thus presented in detail, despite the limited application of sulfonamides in dental therapeutics.

In 1932 the German physician and biochemist Gerhard Domagk developed Prontosil, an azo dye containing *p*-aminobenzenesulfonamide, which was inactive in vitro. It was active in vivo, however, for with it he successfully treated experimental streptococcal infection in mice in 1935. In the same year French investigators found that Prontosil owed its antibacterial activity in the mammalian body to the release of its *p*-aminobenzenesulfonamide moiety (sulfanilamide).

Sulfanilamide proved too toxic for general therapy but its discovery stimulated a successful search for variant compounds that were antibacterial and sufficiently nontoxic for systemic human therapy. This effort resulted in the production of thousands of sulfanilamide derivatives, sulfones, and other related compounds, but only a dozen or so are useful therapeutic agents.

Sulfonamides are effective because they competitively inhibit the synthesis of folic acid. As structural analogues of *p*-aminobenzoic acid, an essential metabolite that is a precursor of folic acid, sulfonamides interfere with the synthesis of these compounds. In general, the sulfonamides are administered orally and only in exceptional circumstances, intravenously. Most of the sulfonamides are readily absorbed from the gastrointestinal tract, but a few are poorly absorbed. After absorption they are well distributed to all tissues except the central nervous system.

The sulfonamides are bacteriostatic and their inhibiting activity can be easily reversed by their dilution or removal, or by the addition of *p*-aminobenzoic acid. Their successful use in vivo requires active phagocytosis. In vitro, they have a wide range of antibacterial activity against gram-positive and gram-negative bacteria. Clinically useful sulfonamides include sulfadiazine, used in the treatment of meningitis; sulfisoxazole, sulfamethoxazole, and sulfamethoxydiazine, used in the treatment of urinary tract infections; sulfadimethoxine, used in respiratory tract infections; and phthalylsulfathiazole and succinylsulfathiazole, used preoperatively to control the intestinal flora or to treat bacillary dysentery.

Renal damage is the most common complication of sulfonamide therapy. Hypersensitivity, usually manifested as a dermatitis, may develop, particularly if sulfonamides are administered for long periods of time.

Sulfones. A class of sulfonamide derivatives, the sulfones can be orally administered and are useful in the treatment of leprosy. Such derivatives as sodium sulfoxone, dapsone, and sodium glucosulfone are used. Oral sulfone therapy usually effects clinical improvement if given for months or years, but it is not certain that it has ever eliminated *Mycobacterium leprae* completely. Toxic manifestations include hemolytic anemia, methemoglobinemia, sulfhemoglobinemia, allergy, and the Jarisch-Herxheimer reaction. Another complication is that after extended treatment the resident bacterial flora of the patient becomes resistant to sulfonamides in general.

Further Considerations of Antimicrobial Chemotherapy in Dental Practice

The management of infectious diseases with antibiotic therapy is well established in dental medicine. Dental practitioners routinely use chemotherapeutic drugs for the prevention and treatment of infections. Unfortunately, a tendency has persisted to abuse the therapeutic knowledge accumulated in this area. Much of this casual, uninformed approach stems from the observation that many routine cases of dentally related infections can be controlled with the empirical use of penicillin. The intelligent management of a patient with an infection requires a complete medical history, an understanding of the cause of the infection, and knowledge of the different uses of available antibiotics. These major responsibilities involve some fundamental actions and comprehensions on the part of the practitioner.

Diagnosis and Antibiotic Sensitivity Testing

A dental clinician is familiar with the discomfort, soft tissue edema, erythema, and dysfunction that characterize a localized dentoalveolar infection. A more complete diagnosis is reached by evaluating the onset and sequence of symptoms; the presence of malaise or nausea, suggesting intermittent bacteremia or septicemia; the development of palpable lymphadenopathy; the presence of a skin rash or joint pain; and the presence or absence of fever. The practitioner also should consider the significance of localized disease processes in relation to other factors such as age (very young or old), preexisting cardiac, liver, or kidney disease, the presence of diabetes mellitis, and steroid use.

A definitive diagnosis in any infectious process depends on a microbial culture. Until recently, collection of a specimen for culture was a neglected art not only in dentistry but in other disciplines as well, primarily because "shotgun" therapy with penicillin or broad-spectrum antibiotics seemed effective. The materials necessary for taking a culture are readily available for both aerobic and anaerobic specimens. Materials for sampling aerobic specimens provide an oxygen-free environment for the culture material and must be used if one is to have a complete picture of bacterial growth in many facial infections. Disposable collection devices with appropriate culture media have a prolonged shelf-life and can be obtained, along with the necessary descriptive paperwork for identification, from a commercial microbiology laboratory. The clinician should submit with this specimen a concise description of the site of the infection, the patient's current antibiotic therapy, and the request for aerobic and/or anaerobic bacterial and/or fungal culture with antimicrobial sensitivity patterns. Many hospital and clinical laboratories also request a slide smear preparation from the infection site. The laboratory can then perform a routine stain procedure, such as the gram stain, to assess the kinds of microbial forms present in the lesion at the time of culture. Procedures for obtaining and preparing samples from various types of lesions have been described in Chapter 2. When the laboratory has the specimen and requisite clinical information, microbial identification and determination of antibiotic susceptibility may proceed. The major antibiotic sensitivity procedures employed are summarized in Table 14.7. For many infections, even though antibiotic therapy would have been initiated at the time of sample collection, the practitioner should at least have a tentative identification from the laboratory within 12 to 48 hours. The dentist will then be able to better assess the value of the initial antibiotic prescribed and to modify the regimen if necessary.

Table 14.7: Comparison of Antimicrobial Susceptibility Tests*

Property	Type of Susceptibility Test			
	Dilution			Agar Disc Diffusion (Bauer-Kirby)
	Broth		Agar	
	Tube	Micro†		
Will give minimum inhibitory concentration	+	+	+	−
Can be used to determine lethal action of antimicrobial agent	+	+	−	−
Accurate to within ± 1 dilution	+	+	+	−
Requires relatively little effort (cost)	−	+	+‡	+
Information about a large number of microorganisms easily obtainable	−	+	+	+
Contamination easily recognized	−	−	+	+

*Reproduced with permission from G. Youmans, P. Paterson, and H. Sommers: *The Biologic and Clinical Basis of Infectious Diseases,* Ed. 2, Saunders, Philadelphia, 1980.

†Microdilution performed in microtiter dilution plates.

‡Will depend on number of isolates.

Therapeutic Indication and Use

Once it has been established that continued antibiotic therapy is necessary, the proper agent should be administered in an appropriate dosage for a sufficient period of time to permit destruction and removal of the infectious organisms. The patient should be monitored at frequent intervals to ascertain that the chosen antibiotics are effective in controlling the symptoms and course of the infection.

Prophylactic Indications

Much has been written concerning appropriate indications for antibiotic prophylaxis in dental medicine. The only definitive instances agreed upon by pharmacologists, microbiologists, and clinicians are for those patients with rheumatic heart diseases or other cardiac valvular damage, and individuals with heart prostheses. At present there is substantial disagreement regarding chemotherapeutic coverage for circumstances involving those individuals with hip prostheses and for the prevention of post-dental surgical infection. Detailed discussions dealing with the beneficial and detrimental aspects of dental and medical prophylaxis may be found by consulting specific references cited at the end of this chapter.

Factors Influencing Antibiotic Use

Superinfection. Antibiotics can suppress the normal microbial flora and may result in the development of superinfections, especially when the host's resistance is lowered. Examples of such superinfections are oral or systemic candidiasis and staphylococcal pneumonia. Broad-spectrum agents often allow the greatest opportunities for superinfection. Organisms such as *Candida albicans* that are not affected by routine antibiotics are no longer held in check by the drug-sensitive resident flora and may proliferate in a virtually uncontrolled environment. This situation can lead to microbial replacement in normal ecological niches with potential pathogens, culminating in an abnormally high presence of drug-insensitive organisms with resultant clinical superinfection.

Nature of Antibiotic and Host Factors. The state of activity of the infecting bacteria influences the effectiveness of antibiotics. For instance, penicillin and other antibiotics affecting cell walls require actively growing cells to be effective. The dosage of an antibiotic also is influenced by the extent of the infection and the tissues involved. For an antibiotic to be effective, a minimal concentration of the antibiotic must be achieved in the circulation and in the affected tissues. This concentration is influenced by dosage, absorption, vascularity of the infected tissue, swelling, and the extent of protein binding by the drug.

In choosing an antibiotic the clinician also must consider host factors that may influence the patient's response to treatment. Whether an agent is bactericidal or bacteriostatic must be taken into consideration. Bacteriostatic antibiotics inhibit the replication and growth of the organism but depend on the defenses of the host to actually eradicate the organism; bactericidal antibiotics interfere with the integrity of the microbial cell itself and directly kill the organism. The effectiveness of bacteriostatic antibiotics thus depends on the ability of the patient to overcome the infecting agent with his own defense mechanisms. When host defenses are altered or compromised, as in pregnant women, the elderly, steroid-dependent individuals, diabetics, patients with advanced liver disease or nutritional compromise, or individuals on prolonged steroid therapy, bacteriostatic antibiotics may prove insufficient and should not be prescribed. Toxic reactions to antibiotics also may be increased by allergies, decreased liver or kidney function, and other debilitating diseases.

Development of Microbial Resistance. The induction of resistance to therapeutic drugs remains a constant threat during antibiotic treatment. The most common mechanisms of acquired resistance were mentioned in previous sections describing specific antibiotics. A brief summarization of the induction of drug resistance is presented in Table 14.8.

Complications of Antibiotic Therapy. Local tissue or organ irritation may result from antibiotic therapy. This may occur in the oral cavity in response to oral administration as a stomatitis or glossitis; at the site of absorption in the gastrointestinal tract, resulting in nausea, vomiting, and diarrhea; or at the site of elimination as colitis or a perianal lesion.

Antibiotics of value in dental medicine also may cause irritation of organ systems. The principal irrita-

---

Table 14.8: Mechanisms for Development of Antimicrobial Resistance

Mechanism	Examples of Antibiotics to Which Resistance Is Acquired
Induction of specific drug-inactivating enzymes	Penicillins
	Chloramphenicol
Prevention of drug entrance into cell	Tetracyclines
	Isoniazid
Decreased affinity of drug due to alteration of receptor site	Erythromycin
	Streptomycin
	Sulfonamides
Loss of enzymes responsible for intracellular drug conversion	Flucytosine (antimycotic)
Alteration in concentration of drug receptor	Sulfonamides

tions of this type are neurotoxicity, particularly of the eighth cranial nerve; nephrotoxicity; hepatotoxicity; and depression of the hepatopoietic system.

Allergic reactions have become increasingly frequent complications of dental-related antibiotic therapy. These reactions may occur locally as a stomatitis or dermatitis, or they may occur as systemic reactions ranging in severity from a mild reaction such as hives, itching, and urticaria to anaphylactic shock. Chemotherapeutic agents discussed earlier that are quite allergenic are the sulfonamides, penicillin, and amphotericin. Tetracyclines are moderately allergenic; erythromycin and nystatin are seldom allergenic.

Antibiotic Combinations. Most infections treated by general dentists and specialists are effectively managed by the judicious use of a single appropriate antibiotic. In some instances, however, combinations of agents are appropriate. Multidrug regimens may be necessary in acutely ill hospitalized patients with undiagnosed bacterial infections requiring broad antimicrobial coverage; in cases of orofacial infection with a mixed bacterial etiology and different antibiotic susceptibility patterns; to prevent the development of resistant mutants against a single antibiotic; and to achieve an additive or synergistic antimicrobial effect against very adaptable microorganisms. Specific examples of antibiotic combinations are given in Table 14.9.

Despite their effectiveness in certain clinical infections, the use of multiple antibiotic combinations is recommended only when the therapeutic efficacy of a single drug is deemed unsatisfactory. In addition to possible antagonism between the agents, resulting in minimal activity, the risk of superinfection is usually greater, as is the potential for increased toxicity reactions.

Table 14.9: Representative Therapeutic Antibiotic Combinations

Drug Combination	Clinical Efficacy
Carbenicillin or ticarcillin with tobramycin or gentamicin	Synergistic activity against *Pseudomonas aeruginosa*
Ampicillin with streptomycin	Effective against enterococcal infection (i.e., *Streptococcus faecalis*)
A cephalosporin with an aminoglycoside	Effective against severe *Klebsiella pneumoniae* infections
Isoniazid with rifampin	Therapeutic and prevents development of resistant *Mycobacterium tuberculosis*

ADDITIONAL READING

Athar, M. A., and Winner, H. I. 1971. The Development of Resistance by *Candida* Species to Polyene Antibiotics *In Vitro*. J Med Microbiol, **4**, 505.

Bartlett, J. G., Chang, T. W., Gurwith, M., Gorbach, S. L., and Onderdonk, A. B. 1978. Antibiotic-Associated Pseudomembranous Colitis Due to Toxin-Producing Clostridia. N Engl J Med, **298**, 531.

Bartlett, J. G., Chang, T. W., Taylor, N. S., and Onderdonk, A. B. 1979. Colitis Induced by *Clostridium difficile*. Rev Infect Dis, **1**, 370.

Bennett, J. E. 1974. Chemotherapy of Systemic Mycoses: Parts I and II. N Engl J Med, **290**, 30, 320.

Benveniste, R., and Davies, J. 1973. Mechanism of Antibiotic Resistance in Bacteria. Annu Rev Biochem, **42**, 471.

Cefamandole and Cefoxitin. 1979. Med Lett Drugs Ther, **21**, 13.

Dipiro, J. T., Bowden, T. A., Jr., and Hooks, V. H. III. 1984. Prophylactic Parenteral Cephalosporins in Surgery: Are the Newer Agents Better? JAMA, **252**, 3277–3279.

Donowitz, G. R., and Mandell, G. L. 1988. Beta-Lactam Antibiotics: Parts I and II. N Engl J Med, **318**, 419.

Fried, J. S., and Hinthorn, D. R. 1985. The Cephalosporins. DM, **31**(7), 1–60.

Ginsberg, M., and Tager, I. 1980. *Practical Guide to Antimicrobial Agents*. Williams & Wilkins, Baltimore.

Goldberg, I. H., and Friedman, P. A. 1971. Antibiotics and Nucleic Acids. Annu Rev Biochem, **40**, 775.

Greenwood, D., and O'Grady, F. 1975. Lysis Enhancement: A Novel Form of Interaction Between β-Lactam Antibiotics. J Med Microbiol, **8**, 205.

Handbook of Antimicrobial Therapy. 1980. Medical Letter Inc., New Rochelle, New York.

Hodge, W. R., and Schneider, L. S. 1972. A New Antibacterial Mode of Action for Sulfonamides. J Pharm Sci, **61**, 142.

Hooper, D. C., and Wolfson, J. S. 1985. The Fluoroquinolones: Pharmacology, Clinical Uses, and Toxicities in Humans. Antimicro Agents Chemother, **28**, 716–721.

Jacobs, M. R., Koornhof, H. J., Robins-Browne, R. M., et al. 1978. Emergence of Multiply Resistant Pneumococci. N Engl J Med, **299**, 735.

Koch, A. L. 1981. Evolution of Antibiotic Resistance Gene Function. Microbiol Rev, **45**, 355.

Montes, L. F. 1971. Oral Amphotericin B in Superficial Candidiasis. Clin Med, **78**, 14.

Neu, H. C. 1983. Penicillin-binding Proteins and Role of Amdinocillin in Causing Bacterial Cell Death. Am J Med, **75**, Suppl 2A, 9–20.

Olson, R. E., Morello, J. A., and Kieff, E. D. 1975. Antibiotic Treatment of Oral Anaerobic Infections. J Oral Surg, **33**, 619.

Petz, L. D. 1978. Immunologic Cross-Reactivity Between Penicillins and Cephalosporins: A Review. J Infect Dis, **137**, 574.

Pratt, W. B. 1977. *Chemotherapy of Infection*. Oxford University Press, New York.

Sabiston, C. B., Jr., Grigsby, W. R., and Segerstrom, N. 1976. Bacterial Study of Pyogenic Infections of Dental Origin. Oral Surg, **41**, 430.

Schuen, N. J., Panzer, J. D., and Atkinson, W. H. 1974. A Comparison of Clindamycin and Penicillin V in the Treatment of Oral Infections. J Oral Surg, **32**, 503.

Thompson, R. L. 1977. The Cephalosporins. Mayo Clin Proc, **52**, 625.

Thompson, R. L., and Wright, A. J. 1983. Cephalosporin Antibiotics. Mayo Clin Proc, **58**, 79–87.

Thornsberry, C., Gavan, T. L., and Gerlach, E. H. 1977. *New Developments in Antimicrobial Agent Susceptibility Test-*

ing. Coordinating Ed., J. C. Sherris. American Society for Microbiology, Washington, D.C.

Tipper, D. J. 1986. Mode of Action of Beta-Lactam Antibiotics. In *Beta-Lactam Antibiotics for Clinical Use,* edited by S. F. Queener et al., New York, Marcel Dekker, pp. 17–47.

Tomasz, A. 1979. The Mechanism of the Irreversible Antimicrobial Effects of Penicillins: How the Beta-lactam Antibiotics Kill and Lyse Bacteria. Annu Rev Microbiol, **33,** 113–137.

Tomasz, A. 1986. Penicillin-binding Proteins and the Antibacterial Effectiveness of β-lactam Antibiotics. Rev Infect Dis, **8,** Suppl 3, S260–S278.

Turner, J. E., Moore, D. W., and Shaw, B. S. 1975. Prevalence and Antibiotic Susceptibility of Organisms Isolated from Acute Soft-Tissue Abscesses Secondary to Dental Caries. Oral Surg, **39,** 848.

Waxman, D. J., and Strominger, J. L. 1983. Penicillin-binding Proteins and the Mechanism of Action of β-lactam Antibiotics. Annu Rev Biochem, **52,** 825–869.

Wilkowske, C. J. 1977. The Penicillins. Mayo Clin Proc, **52,** 616.

Yocum, R. R., Rasmussin, J. R., and Strominger, S. L. 1980. The Mechanism of Action of Penicillin: Penicillin Activates the Active Site of *Bacillus stearothermophilus* D-Alanine Carboxypeptidase. J Biol Chem, **255,** 3977–3986.

15

Microbial Pathogenicity

Keith R. Volkmann

Pathogenicity is the ability of a microorganism to cause disease. Within the realm of pathogenicity, microbes express degrees of disease-producing ability referred to as virulence. For example, a highly virulent microorganism may cause damage to the host at low dosages while another pathogenic microorganism of low virulence may damage the host only at high dosages. In addition, a single pathogenic species may contain strains that are highly virulent, of intermediate virulence, or avirulent, depending on changes in specific disease-producing properties.

The pathogenicity of even a highly virulent microorganism may not be expressed as clinically detectable damage in a host if the host's resistance is sufficient. Thus, health and disease are functions of the virulence and dosage of the infecting organism versus the resistance of the host.

Development of an Infectious Disease

The infectious disease process is very complex and many events must take place before the virulence of

an infecting microorganism is expressed as clinically detectable damage in the host. This becomes evident on examination of the stages in the development of an infectious disease (Fig. 15.1). Of particular importance, the control of infectious diseases can be approached by interrupting or preventing any one of these stages.

Causative Agent

The requirement for a causative agent in the development of an infectious disease is obvious. The factors listed in Table 15.1 in general apply to all types of potentially pathogenic microorganisms—bacteria, viruses, fungi, and protozoa. The sources of the causative agents are most often previously infected hosts who are obviously ill or who are natural or asymptomatic, transient or chronic carriers of the agent. The inanimate environment may also serve as a source of infectious disease agents.

Transmissibility

Although the microbial properties related to the transmission of pathogens between suitable hosts are

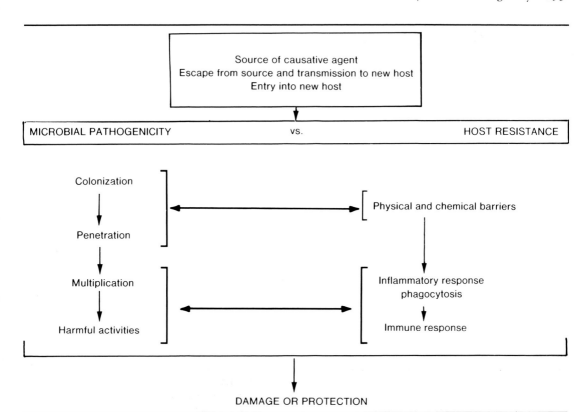

Figure 15.1: Stages in the development of an infectious disease.

not necessarily pathogenic properties, transmission is a vital function of most human disease agents. Transmission is important not only to the parasite, which must occasionally find a new host, but also to the human host in relation to the communicability or spread of infectious diseases. Since many human pathogens are obligate parasites, they can survive as a species only if they have a mode of transmission to a new host, a mode of entry into the new host, the ability to survive for some time within the host, and a mode of escape from the host. These stages constitute a typical parasitic life cycle.

Although many protozoan and metazoan parasites have intricate life cycles, most fungi, bacteria, and viruses have relatively simple developmental stages. They are transferred, most often from host to host of the same species, by 1) direct contact, 2) droplet infection (inhalation of droplets from the upper respiratory tract), 3) ingestion (in food and drink contaminated directly or indirectly with infectious materials), and 4) indirect contact with contaminated objects. Some viruses and a few bacteria are transmitted by the bites of arthropods, in which the agent multiplies and may persist by transovarial transfer.

The importance of a suitable exit for the parasite

from a host is well illustrated in cases of aberrant parasitism. Tularemia, brucellosis, rabies, and trichinosis in man are all dead ends for the respective parasites, for there is no effective natural exit and means of transfer from man to man. Civilized man is an ineffective host for many insect-borne diseases because his cultural habits minimize contact with the vectors, and there are no other means for the respective agents to make an exit and be transferred to an uninfected individual.

Expression of Virulence Properties

The interaction of pathogens with the host varies from complete destruction of the microorganisms to complete overwhelming of the host (death). In between these extremes is the near stalemate that occurs in chronic or residual infections by pathogens. The pathogenic properties of the contaminating microorganisms are categorized by their involvement in 1) colonization of the host, 2) penetration of the host tissues, and 3) damage to host tissues. The host defense system may be directed against any of these groups of pathogenic properties and is divided into two categories: innate or nonacquired body defenses, and acquired (immunological) body defenses. Specific microbial pathogenic properties are described in this chapter.

Pathogenic Properties of Microbes

Colonization

The term *colonization* is synonymous with infection—the establishment and survival of a parasite on or within a host. Microbial colonization of man does not always lead to infectious disease, as evidenced by the existence of indigenous body floras. Colonization is, however, a prerequisite for subsequent damage to the body by most pathogens. Food poisoning with microbial toxins is an exception, for it does not require colonization but only ingestion of the harmful products produced in food by the growth of some clostridia and staphylococci. Nevertheless, colonization includes initial attachment to a body surface and subsequent multiplication within the body. Thus, attachment mechanisms and the ability to multiply within the body are considered to be important pathogenic properties of disease-producing microorganisms.

Attachment. Although some pathogens associate with the body by being mechanically trapped on a surface or by being accidentally injected or implanted into underlying tissues, most must attach to and multiply on skin or mucosal surfaces (or teeth, in the case of *Streptococcus mutans*) to become established. In doing so they must compete with the indigenous flora already present and with the body's natural defense mechanisms active at that site (e.g., the cleansing action of saliva, tears, respiratory secretions, and urine). Persistent colonization of mucous membranes, which continually undergo desquamation, presents additional problems. It involves initial attachment, multiplication, dislodgment of the progeny from desquamated epithelial cells, and reattachment to newly exposed epithelium.

Microbial attachment to body surfaces or tissues does have some degree of specificity, which helps explain why some organisms colonize or damage only certain tissues of the body. Tissue specificity has long been recognized for many viral diseases and is becoming quite obvious for many bacterial diseases as well. Specific structures or polymers on the bacterial surface are involved in the attachment mechanisms of many potential human pathogens, including *Streptococcus mutans, Streptococcus pyogenes, Neisseria gonorrhoeae, Vibrio cholerae, Salmonella typhimurium,* enteropathogenic *Escherichia coli, Klebsiella pneumoniae, Bacteroides asaccharolyticus, Fusobac-*

terium nucleatum, Corynebacterium parvum, Actinomyces viscosus, Actinomyces naeslundii, and *Mycoplasma.* For example, gonorrhoea is confined to the mucus-secreting epithelial surfaces of man and cannot be established on such surfaces of animals. Thus, the initial attachment is very specific and involves interaction between specific receptor sites on human epithelial surfaces and pili on the surface of the gonococci.

Multiplication. Multiplication is essential for colonization. It replenishes the attached cells that are removed by local host defense mechanisms. Multiplication begins soon after attachment and continues as long as suitable conditions exist, even after the pathogen has penetrated colonized mucous membranes. The successful colonizer must be able to derive all of its nutritional and physical requirements for growth from a specific host environment. Since the mere numbers of a pathogen within a host can determine whether damage to the host will occur (by overwhelming host defenses), the ability to multiply within the host is considered a determinant of virulence. It appears that most pathogens that attach to host surfaces can multiply there also. With human viruses the initial attachment or absorption to a host cell is an essential step for subsequent multiplication of the virus within that cell. Since a specific virus usually can attach to only certain types of host cells, subsequent multiplication at the initial site of attachment is a common event in viral infections. The relationship is less clear for bacteria, but some pathogens may have specific properties that favor their growth in vivo. For example, iron is required for growth by bacteria but may not be in a usable form within the host tissue fluids, since it is commonly bound to the protein transferrin. Some pathogenic bacteria such as *Mycobacterium tuberculosis* and some strains of *E. coli* have special iron scavenging systems that may overcome this problem. The tubercle bacillus produces a substance called mycobactin that releases iron from transferrin, and *E. coli* produces a catechol that can compete with transferrin for iron binding.

Penetration

Viruses and most bacterial pathogens that colonize mucous membranes must penetrate this surface and multiply in the underlying tissues before host damage occurs. Exceptions in the bacterial world are some enteric pathogens like the cholera organisms which colonize the intestinal mucosa, multiply on the surface, and produce toxic substances which then penetrate the tissue and cause damage. Little is known about specific mechanisms of microbial penetration. Viruses enter host cells by a process similar to phagocytosis or by direct penetration of the plasma membrane. Bacteria may produce enzymes (e.g., lecithinase, proteases) or other substances (e.g., endotoxin) that cause lysis or degeneration of the host cell, and the bacteria then proceed into the tissue space previously occupied by the host cells. Penetration of intestinal mucosa by *Shigella* is dependent on the presence and chemical composition of lipopolysaccharide (endotoxin). Some bacteria may produce enzymes like hyaluronidase that may destroy intracellular material and separate the host cells. Other bacteria such as *N. gonorrhoeae* actually may enter epithelial cells through a process similar to phagocytosis and then further invade the epithelium by repeated cycles of exocytosis and phagocytosis.

Resistance to Host Defenses

Successfully virulent pathogens must be able to at least partially withstand preexisting and subsequently mobilized body defense systems. This microbial capacity is especially important in the early stages of an infection when, in most cases, the protective reactions of the host are heavily weighted against the few invading organisms.

Resistance to Phagocytosis. Phagocytosis is one of the most important components of the innate body defense systems. Therefore, pathogens that resist phagocytosis are allowed to accumulate in the body at a less restricted rate. Many of the key factors related to the virulence and pathogenic mechanisms of bacteria involve surface components.

Early investigators observed capsules surrounding a variety of pathogenic bacteria in infectious exudates and inferred that these structures were important for virulence. In most instances the capsules consist of polysaccharides in the form of a hydrophilic gel, with a distinct chemical composition for each type of organism. However, peptide and glycoprotein capsules are present on some bacteria. *Streptococcus pneumoniae* is a representative example of a bacterium with a polysaccharide capsule.

In order for phagocytosis to proceed most efficiently, bacteria and other particulate matter must first be coated by opsonins. Fragments of complement components, many times generated by the alternate complement pathway, can act as opsonins for bacteria. The capsule of smooth virulent strains of *S. pneumoniae,* unlike that of rough strains, does not activate the alternate pathway, and therefore complement opsonins are not generated and these encapsulated strains are not phagocytosed. However, bacterial capsules are immunogenic (they will induce the formation of antibodies), and antibodies of the IgG and IgM classes specifically bound to the capsule also act as opsonins. Once antibodies are formed with their concomitant

opsonic activity, phagocytosis proceeds normally. Following penetration into tissue, it may take 5 or 6 days for antibody to appear, and during this period of time few, if any, of the invading organisms have been cleared from tissue. Under these circumstances, clinical illness is likely, and therefore encapsulated organisms are considered to possess increased virulence.

Resistance to phagocytosis may not totally depend on the presence of a capsule, for similar activity can be expressed by other surface components. For example, some *S. pyogenes* strains produce hyaluronic acid capsules that are less readily detectable than the capsules of the pneumococci. Virulence (resistance to phagocytosis) in these streptococci relates only in minor part to the somewhat labile capsule; it relates more to a cell wall antigen, the M protein, which is distributed over the surface of a streptococcal cell wall. M protein is involved in virulence since it is antiphagocytic and anti-M antibody is protective. The streptococci also have other surface antigens and components that are not related to virulence.

In most gram-negative bacteria, phagocytosis and the lytic action of serum are both neutralized by the cell wall endotoxins.

Although there can be no doubt of the importance of capsular and similarly active surface constituents for the pathogenicity of many bacteria, the presence of these surface constituents does not ensure pathogenicity (although it may still confer resistance to phagocytosis) and in some cases is not known to be contributory. Encapsulated but nonvirulent variants of pneumococci, *H. influenzae,* and *B. anthracis* have been discovered.

Resistance to Phagocytic Digestion. Once pathogenic bacteria invade a host, they may be divided into two types, depending on their resistance to phagocytic digestion. Bacteria in one group, the "intracellular pathogens," offer little resistance to engulfment by phagocytes, but once inside they often establish a complex relationship that allows both phagocyte and intracellular pathogen to exist in balance. Intracellular pathogens such as *M. tuberculosis* and *Brucella* are able to survive and multiply within the phagocytic cells, which facilitates their distribution within the body. *M. tuberculosis,* after it has been engulfed in a phagocytic vesicle, is able to inhibit the fusion of the phagocytic vesicle with lysosomes and thereby escape the microbicidal mechanisms of the phagocytic cell. Such pathogens are relatively inaccessible to chemotherapeutic agents and to antibodies.

Another group of invasive microorganisms, the "extracellular pathogens," are readily destroyed once they are phagocytized. For this group, which includes *S. pyogenes* and *S. pneumoniae,* the critical act of invasion is to escape or resist phagocytosis, which they do because they produce antiphagocytic capsules or because they have certain types of cell walls. Once phagocytized, however, the majority of such microorganisms are destroyed. As long as such microorganisms can remain outside of phagocytes they can cause disease. Their position outside of phagocytes allows them to stimulate the production of antibodies, which makes them susceptible to phagocytes and shortens the length of their infection.

Impairment of Neutrophil Functions. During an acute inflammatory reaction induced by an invading pathogen, leukocytes migrate toward the site of microbial proliferation as influenced by chemoattractants released at the infection site. At the site, the neutrophils (polymorphonuclear heterophilic leukocytes, PMNs) attempt to destroy the microorganisms. Although some bacteria interfere with phagocyte engulfment or digestion, others may have different effects on PMNs. Strains of several bacteria (e.g., *Staphylococcus, Streptococcus, Pseudomonas aeruginosa, Actinobacillus actinomycetemcomitans*) produce a leukocidin that specifically kills PMNs. The leukocidin from *Staphylococcus* is immunogenic and acts by increasing the permeability of PMNs through changes in the potassium pump. *Capnocytophaga,* a gram-negative anaerobic bacterium implicated in the pathogenesis of periodontal disease, produces changes in PMN morphology and impairs complement-induced PMN chemotaxis.

Several bacterial enzymes may damage many types of host cells, including PMNs. More specifically, neuraminidase produced by some strains (e.g., *Actinomyces, V. cholerae*) induces PMN cell membrane damage.

Exotoxins

Some bacteria produce special soluble proteins called *exotoxins,* which are among the most poisonous group of substances known to man. Exotoxins include a potent inhibitor of protein synthesis produced by *Corynebacterium diphtheriae;* the neurotoxins of *Clostridium tetani* and *Clostridium botulinum;* the enterotoxins of *Staphylococcus aureus, Vibrio cholerae,* enteropathogenic *Escherichia coli, Clostridium perfringens,* and *Shigella dysenteriae;* and the tissue necrosis toxins of *Staphylococcus aureus, Bordetella pertussis* and *Streptococcus pyogenes.*

Properties. Classic exotoxins have several distinctive characteristics, although they sometimes overlap with the characteristics of endotoxins or microbial lytic enzymes. They are usually labile, high molecular weight proteins that resemble enzymes, are strongly antigenic, and are excreted or readily separated from the bacterial cell that produced them. With the exception of botulinum toxin and the staphylococcus enterotoxin, most exotoxins are sensitive to proteolytic enzymes, particularly those of the gastrointestinal tract. They are also sensitive to heat and acids. These toxins may be divided into those that damage cytoplasmic membranes (phospholipases, hemolysins, and lysins) and those that act on some intracellular structure or process. The exotoxins with intracellular activity are composed of two distinct polypeptide chain components. One chain binds to an appropriate cell membrane receptor and the second chain mediates the biological activity of the exotoxin. Some of these exotoxins are synthesized in an inactive proenzyme form and must undergo proteolytic cleavage and reduction to release the biologically active fragment. It seems unlikely that mammalian cells would have evolved specific receptors for potentially fatal bacterial exotoxins. However, there is a striking structural resemblance between exotoxins and glycoprotein hormones.

Exotoxins are usually lethal, even in very small amounts, but they do have variable toxicity for different animals. Tetanus and botulinum toxins have more than 1 million guinea pig LD50/mg. On the other hand, diphtheria toxin contains about 3,500 guinea pig LD50/mg. Described in a different fashion, 218 g of botulinum type A toxin, if properly administered, would kill the entire world's population. The exposure of exotoxins to various chemicals eliminates their toxicity but preserves their antigenicity, producing toxoids, some of which are used to induce active immunity without dangers of toxicity.

Pharmacological Actions. At the subcellular level, diphtheria toxin, produced by *Corynebacterium diphtheriae* that carry the temperate bacteriophage β, interferes with protein synthesis by inhibiting cytoplasmic elongation factor 2 (EF-2). At the tissue level it acts on skeletal muscle, heart muscle, and the muscles of the diaphragm. Cells of *C. diphtheriae* are relatively nontoxic and remain in the localized pharyngeal lesion in typical diphtheria. However, the toxin itself is disseminated throughout the body via the blood. The net effect of the pharmacological action is to cause death from cardiac failure, or residual paralysis in individuals who recover.

The toxins of botulism and tetanus are both neurotoxins. Botulinum toxin affects impulse conduction through both presynapses and postsynapses of peripheral autonomic nerves by blocking the release of acetylcholine. The acid ester of choline is released from preganglionic and postganglionic endings of parasympathetic fibers and from preganglionic regions of sympathetic fibers. If acetylcholine is not released, impulses do not cross the affected synapses.

Tetanus toxin causes spastic paralysis by blocking the release of neurotransmitters from inhibitory synapses in spinal cord motor neurons. Tetanus toxin also may influence synaptic transmission at myoneural junctions, possibly by causing the accumulation of acetylcholine. Typical botulinal food poisoning results from ingesting the toxin previously produced in the food, although a recently described condition called infant botulism apparently involves ingestion of the spores with subsequent toxin production. In tetanus, the infecting *C. tetani* remain localized at the site of entry (e.g., puncture wound) but the toxin produced is disseminated to the central nervous system.

The shiga toxin of *Shigella dysenteriae* is cytotoxic, neurotoxic, and enterotoxic. Its primary biological activity appears to be inhibition of protein synthesis through inactivation of the 60S subunit of the eukaryotic ribosome. When introduced parenterally into animals, shiga toxin causes paralysis, diarrhea, and death. The *Staphylococcus aureus* enterotoxin of food poisoning apparently acts on neural receptors in the gut, causing a stimulation of the central nervous system with increased gut motility and powerful vomiting reactions.

Diarrhea-inducing enterotoxins (e.g., *Vibrio cholerae, Escherichia coli, Clostridium perfringens*) presumably function in a similar manner by increasing movement of water and ions from the intestinal tissues to the lumen of the bowels, causing diarrhea. Studies with the cholera toxin have shown that it binds to specific receptors on the mucosal cell membranes and stimulates adenyl cyclase activity, which reduces intracellular concentrations of cyclic adenosine monophosphate (cAMP). This alteration of tissue cAMP apparently causes excretion of water and ions from the tissue.

Besides producing enterotoxins and leukocidins, certain strains of staphylococci also produce exfoliative toxin, an exotoxin that causes exfoliation of skin in the scalded skin syndrome. Another tissue-necrotizing exotoxin from *B. pertussis* destroys upper respiratory tract epithelium in whooping cough. The erythrogenic toxin produced by strains of *Streptococcus pyogenes* causing scarlet fever produces necrosis of blood vessels.

The significance of exotoxin formation in bacterial physiology is uncertain. In some cases exotoxin production is a dispensable activity that is acquired by or expressed as a result of bacteriophage infection. For example, only those strains of *C. diphtheriae* that are lysogenic for β-phage that contains the *tox*⁺ gene produce the toxin. The erythrogenic toxin of *S. pyogenes* also is under the genetic control of a temperate bacteriophage. The same is probably true for botulinum toxin, since some toxigenic strains yield bacteriophages that infect and convert nontoxigenic strains to toxin producers.

Endotoxins

Properties. Endotoxins are lipopolysaccharides (LPS) complexed to proteins that occur in the outer membrane of the envelope of gram-negative bacteria. In contrast to exotoxins, endotoxins are heat stable, resistant to proteolytic enzymes, less toxic, have similar biological activities regardless of their source, are released from bacterial cells whose integrity has been disrupted, and cannot be converted to toxoids. The polysaccharide part of LPS is composed of a core, which is similar in all endotoxins, and the O-specific side chain, which varies in composition among endotoxins and determines the O-antigen specificity of the bacterial strain. The lipid A portion of LPS is generally accepted as responsible for the biological activity of endotoxin.

Biological Activities. Endotoxins have a number of biological actions. They elicit fever by causing the release of an endogenous pyrogen from PMNs. A more characteristic pharmacological activity of endotoxins is that they cause an increase in capillary permeability, together with hemorrhages. Another characteristic pharmacological reaction is to elicit inflammation when injected intradermally. Associated with the endotoxins' ability to elicit inflammation is their ability to cause the Shwartzman reaction. If endotoxin is injected into the skin of a rabbit, mild inflammation occurs at the site of the initial injection. If, after a day, the same or another endotoxin is administered intravenously, it provokes at the site of the original infection edema, hemorrhage, and necrosis. This is known as a localized Shwartzman reaction. If both injections are given intravenously, bilateral cortical necrosis of the kidneys will result, and death usually follows the second injection. Other reactions elicited by endotoxins are hyperglycemia, leukopenia followed by leukocytosis, and a wide variety of circulatory disturbances.

Other Toxic Substances

Bacterial Enzyme Toxins. Pathogenic bacteria sometimes produce enzymes capable of disorganizing host function by lysing host cells or the constituents of host tissue. Although it is often difficult to assess their exact significance, it is usually accepted that many of them contribute to the disease process.

Certain invasive strains, such as staphylococci, streptococci, and *C. perfringens,* produce hyaluronidase. This enzyme degrades hyaluronic acid, a mucopolysaccharide that is the cementing substance of connective tissues, thus allowing bacteria to penetrate such tissues and to be disseminated from the site of the initial infection. Enzymes in the plasma of normal individuals are antagonistic to hyaluronidase, which helps to establish an equilibrium between pathogen and host.

Pathogenic microorganisms sometimes produce enzymes (e.g., coagulase) that accelerate blood clotting, or they may produce kinases, which inhibit clotting or dissolve formed fibrin clots. Staphylococci are widely known for their ability to produce coagulase. It has been postulated that the ability of staphylococci to produce a fibrin clot assists them in establishing a localized circumscribed infection. It is sometimes suggested that staphylococci that produce coagulase are pathogenic and those that do not are not pathogenic, but the distinction is not always clear. A plasma factor with an action similar to prothrombin converts a staphylococcal product into active coagulase, which then induces fibrin clot formation. Animals that are resistant to staphylococcal infection, such as rats and mice, do not have the blood cofactor necessary for this type of clotting. Another factor involves inhibition of phagocytosis. Staphylococci that produce coagulase become coated with fibrin and are resistant to phagocytosis. The clotting plasma in the outer boundaries of a staphylococcal-induced infection physically restrains the phagocytes and prevents their contacting and engulfing the bacteria.

Bacteria such as streptococci produce enzymes or enzyme precursors known as kinases that indirectly inhibit fibrin clot formation by activating plasminogen of the blood plasma to form plasmin, which dissolves the clot. Staphylococci also are able to lyse fibrin clots by producing a staphylokinase, which is distinct from streptokinase. Several other bacteria lyse fibrin clots, probably by producing proteolytic enzymes rather than by producing kinases.

The role of the kinases in the nature of virulence seems rather straightforward with regard to staphylococci and streptococci. The pathogenic staphylococci, all of which produce a potent coagulase, are virulent and produce a localized, circumscribed lesion. They seldom invade the deeper tissue. Those staphylococci that seldom significantly disseminate from the localized infection do not produce significant amounts of staphylokinase, which would allow them to disseminate. On the other hand, streptococci are extremely invasive. They actively produce potent kinases, which may allow them to quickly break out of the local lesion and invade tissues.

Bacterial hemolysins are a group of substances that cause destruction of red blood cells. Hemolysins are antigenic and are often named after the bacteria producing them, e.g., streptolysin or staphylolysin.

In addition to the filterable or soluble bacterial hemolysins described above, bacteria also cause the hemolysis of erythrocytes about colonies on blood agar. Two types of reactions occur, green or α-type hemolysis, and clear or β-type hemolysis. The relationship has not been established between filterable hemolysins and blood-plate hemolysins, but it appears that different enzymes and different actions are involved. In most instances, a direct relationship has not been established between the ability of a microorganism to produce hemolysins and its ability to produce the symptoms of an infectious disease. A number of nonpathogenic bacteria also produce hemolysins.

Toxic Metabolites.   During bacterial growth and metabolism a variety of low molecular weight metabolites are released from the cells. If these substances accumulate in localized environments they may damage host cells or tissues. The best example is the tooth demineralization acids (e.g., lactic acid) produced by many types of cariogenic bacteria. Other examples are hydrogen sulfide and ammonia, which are cytotoxic and are products of protein metabolism, primarily by anaerobic bacteria.

Virulence of Viruses

The factors involved in the virulence of viruses are not so well defined as those of many bacteria. In general, virulence relates to the cellular changes viruses bring about as a result of their obligate intracellular parasitism. Host cell susceptibility to a given virus is primarily related to the presence or absence of receptors to which the virus particles can attach before entering the cell. Susceptibility may also be related to the inability of a virus to replicate within a cell as a result of nonspecific or specific host defense mechanisms such as interferon or antibody.

The cell responses to a viral infection include 1) no apparent damage, as in persistent infections, 2) cell transformation (hyperplasia with cell death or hyperplasia without cell death, as in transformation to cancer cells), 3) a cytopathic reaction with death of the infected cell, and 4) latent infections in which no viral replication occurs but the viral genome is present within the latently infected cell (see Chap. 34).

The mechanisms of the cytopathic changes caused by viruses relate to a number of possible reactions. Virulent DNA and RNA viruses respectively may inhibit host cell DNA or RNA synthesis. Viruses also act on lysosomes, causing either a reversible increase in permeability or an irreversible disruption. The latter results in the discharge of hydrolytic enzymes into the cell cytoplasm, resulting in the disruption and death of the host cell.

During an infection, enveloped viruses may incorporate a portion of their envelope into the cytoplasmic membrane of host cells, or more commonly, alter the host cell. The cell membrane of the altered host cell then has some of the antigenic characteristics of the infecting virus. As immunity to the virus develops during the course of an infection, the antigenically altered host cell reacts with the virus-induced effectors of the immune response, such as antibodies or lymphocytes, causing their inactivation or destruction. With some viruses, adjacent altered cells tend to fuse with each other and form giant cells.

Some viruses must replicate in host cells before they produce a cytopathic reaction. Other viruses in high concentration are toxic and rapidly produce cytopathic effects and death of cells without replicating. Vaccinia virus kills macrophages and mumps virus lyses erythrocytes without replicating in such cells. Syncytial cell formation by mumps virus relates to some action which it has on cytoplasmic membranes. Such actions relate to the viral capsid or envelope. Some viruses also may produce cytopathic effects when they replicate but produce an incomplete, noninfectious virion.

Another cytopathic effect occurring in host cells during virus infections is the development of inclusion bodies. Inclusion bodies consist of an accumulation of incompletely assembled units of viruses, virus-induced products, or of completely assembled virions. They may accumulate only in the nucleus of the host cell (e.g., adenovirus), only in the cytoplasm of host cells (e.g., rabies virus), or in both nucleus and cytoplasm (e.g., measles virus). In some instances, the inclusion bodies occurring in host cells contain neither unassembled subunits of virions nor completely assembled virions. Instead, the inclusion bodies seem to be a type of scar remaining at the site of a previous replication of virions that have left the area. An example of such an inclusion is the intranuclear eosinophilic inclusion body produced by herpes simplex virus.

Some viruses are oncogenic, causing tumors or leukemia, particularly in animals. In tissue cultures, such viruses are able to transform a normal cell to what resembles a malignant cell. The division of such malignant-type cells is no longer constrained by their contact with adjacent cells. If host cells are transformed by DNA viruses, they no longer continue to synthesize the infectious virus. However, they do retain some functional units of the infecting virus. Cells transformed by RNA viruses continue to produce complete virions. The exact mechanism of cell transformation by oncogenic viruses is not known; however, RNA tumor viruses, which have the ability to transform normal cells, possess an *src* gene that codes for a phosphoprotein that either has protein kinase activity or is very closely associated with a protein kinase. This kinase activity is unusual in that the amino acid tyrosine is phosphorylated rather than serine or threonine, which are phosphorylated by most other protein kinases. In addition, these viruses stimulate host cell DNA synthesis; they alter the cell surface, resulting in the incorporation of new antigens in the transformed cells; they cause chromosomal aberrations; and they remove the control of cell division that is due to a cell contacting adjacent cells (contact inhibition).

Virulence of Fungi

Only a few of the thousands of different fungi are pathogenic for man. The types of infectious diseases caused by fungi are classified according to the affected tissues: superficial infections (e.g., piedra), cutaneous infections (e.g., ringworm), subcutaneous infections (e.g., sporotrichosis), and systemic infections (e.g., histoplasmosis).

Fungal virulence determinants are not as well defined as those of bacteria (e.g., exotoxin and endotoxins). However, specific molds and yeasts do have known properties that could affect their pathogenicity. The yeast *Cryptococcus neoformans,* the cause of cryptococcosis, has a capsule that does impair phagocytic ingestion. Although the fungal world is a source of various pharmacologically active compounds including vitamins, antibiotics, adrenergic alkaloids, and hallucinogens, very little is known about potentially damaging products produced by the pathogenic yeasts and molds. Some may produce potentially damaging enzymes (e.g., *Sporothrix schenckii* produces neuraminidase), but in general they do not produce typical toxins during the infectious disease process. However, some fungi produce mycotoxins that may be fatal if ingested (e.g., the mushroom *Amanita phalloides*). Some strains of the mold *Aspergillus flavus* produce another mycotoxin, called aflatoxin, which is toxic and carcinogenic for animals. Outbreaks with high fatality rates in livestock after the ingestion of infected grain have been reported worldwide. The potential dangers for man also come from ingestion of foodstuffs contaminated with aflatoxins. However, the true risk to the human population is unknown. Sensitive techniques are used to monitor grains, peanuts, and other foods potentially contaminated with toxin-producing fungi.

One general property of fungi that may influence the course of mycoses is the relative inertness of the fungal cell wall polysaccharides (e.g., chitin, mannans, β-glucans). The cell walls are highly immunogenic, yet mammalian tissues lack the enzymes necessary to degrade the wall polysaccharides. Therefore, the cell wall is slowly removed from the tissues while continuing to stimulate the immune system. This, along with the production of other immunogenic products, contributes to the development of hypersensitivity, which is a regular occurrence in fungal disease.

ADDITIONAL READING

Joklik, W. K., Willett, H. P., and Amos, D. Bernard. (Eds.) 1984. *Zinsser Microbiology,* Ed. 18. Appleton-Century-Crofts, Norwalk, Conn.

Kaspar, D. L. 1986. Bacterial Capsule: Old Dogmas and New Tricks. J Infect Dis, **153,** 407.

Male, D., Champion, B., and Cooke, A. 1987. *Advanced Immunology.* J. B. Lippincott Co., Philadelphia.

Middlebrook, J. L., and Dorland, R. B. 1984. Bacterial Toxins: Cellular Mechanisms of Action. Microbiol Rev, **48,** 199.

Stites, D. P., Stobo, J. D., and Wells, J. V. (Eds.) 1987. *Basic and Clinical Immunology,* Ed. 6. Appleton and Lange, Norwalk, Conn.

Von Der Valk, P., and Herman, C. J. 1987. Biology of Disease Leukocyte Functions. Lab Invest, **57,** 127.

Part V

Bacterial Infections

16

Staphylococci and Staphylococcal Infections

George S. Schuster

Staphylococci are responsible for a significant proportion of the suppurative diseases encountered in medical and dental practice. Besides causing cutaneous infections, staphylococci may invade and produce severe infections in other parts of the body. There are three major species of staphylococci, *Staphylococcus aureus, Staphylococcus epidermidis,* and *Staphylococcus saprophyticus.* Of these, *S. aureus* is the most significant pathogen for man. *S. epidermidis,* a common inhabitant of the skin and mucous membranes, may produce abscesses, while *S. saprophyticus* is generally regarded as nonpathogenic.

Cell Structure and Colonial Morphology

Staphylococci are gram-positive, facultatively anaerobic, spherical bacteria that are widely distributed in the environment and on man and animals. They range from 0.5 to 1.5 μm in diameter. They seldom form chains but more often appear as irregular grapelike clusters of cells due to random divisions in multiple planes and failure to separate after division. They are nonmotile and do not form spores (Fig. 16.1). Colonial variants of the staphylococci may be mucoid, smooth, or rough. Many strains of *S. aureus* freshly isolated from staphylococcal disease produce golden yellow pigment, while the colonies of *S. epidermidis* are usually chalky or porcelain white; some staphylococcal colonies are lemon yellow in color. However, pigment production is a variable trait of staphylococci and is not reliable for differentiation.

The staphylococcal cell wall contains peptidoglycan and species-specific teichoic acids. In addition, *S. aureus* contains an antiphagocytic component known as protein A. Protein A has a strong affinity for the Fc portion of IgG molecules and can bind these molecules to the cell surface, leaving the specific antigen-binding portions exposed. This apparently has an

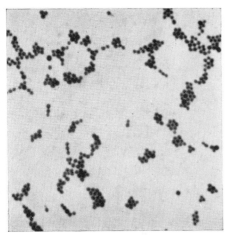

Figure 16.1: *Staphylococcus aureus.*

antiopsonic effect and interferes with phagocytosis. Some strains have an antiphagocytic polysaccharide capsule. Most strains also produce a surface "clumping factor" that converts fibrinogen to fibrin on the cell surface. This reaction is responsible for the clumping of *S. aureus* when the organisms are suspended in plasma.

Culture

Staphylococci grow well on most extract and infusion media and in sweat, urine, and tissue and plant extracts. Their metabolism is respiratory and fermentative and they utilize a wide variety of carbohydrates. Aerobically they can obtain energy and nitrogen from peptones, but anaerobically they seem to prefer glycolysis. Staphylococci grow on several differential media that restrict other microorganisms, often tolerating as much as 15% NaCl and 40% bile. Growth occurs over a wide range of temperature and pH, with optima of 30 to 37°C and pH 7.0 to 7.5, respectively.

Enzymatic Activity

Staphylococci produce a variety of enzymes and toxins, some of which contribute to the pathogenesis of staphylococcal infections (Table 16.1).

Proteolytic Activity. Staphylococci produce enzymes that are active on fibrin (clotted blood), inspissated serum, egg white, or gelatin. Collagenase is not produced by staphylococci.

Coagulase Activity. Pathogenic staphylococci produce an extracellular staphylocoagulase that acts on citrated or oxalated rabbit or human plasma. Nonpathogenic staphylococci are unable to coagulate plasma, but coagulase-negative staphylococci may be pathogenic. Staphylocoagulase clots fibrinogen in the presence of a coagulase-reacting factor (CRF), an apparent derivative of prothrombin. There are multiple antigenic types of coagulase, but there is no evidence that the antibodies are important in resistance to staphylococcal infections.

Staphylokinase. Most strains of staphylococci pathogenic for man can dissolve fibrin clots from man

Table 16.1: Extracellular Enzymes and Toxins

Product	Activity
Proteases	Degrade proteins
Coagulase	Enzyme that clots citrated plasma by converting prothrombin to thrombin, which converts fibrinogen to fibrin
Staphylokinase	Enzyme that degrades fibrin clots by converting plasminogen to a fibrinolytic enzyme; plasmin
Lipases	Lipid-splitting enzymes
Hyaluronidase	Enzyme that degrades hyaluronic acid
Lysozyme	Enzyme that breaks β1–4 links in murein of cell walls
β-Lactamase	Enzyme that breaks beta-lactam ring of penicillin
α-Toxin	Hemolysin
β-Toxin	Sphingomyelinase—hemolysin
δ-Toxin	Cytolytic
γ-Toxin	Hemolysin
Leukocidin	Damages macrophages and PMNs
Exfoliative toxin	Cleaves desmosomes in stratum granulosum of epidermis
Enterotoxin	Emetic
TSST-1 (toxic shock syndrome toxin)	Pyrogen; causes hypotension, rash

and a variety of animals. The lytic factor is produced as a kinase that activates serum or plasma protease. The active protease then lyses the fibrin of the clot. Staphylokinase has no relationship to staphylococcal virulence.

Lipases. Both pathogenic (99%) and nonpathogenic (30%) staphylococci produce lipases (phospholipases, lipoprotein–lipases, esterases). Lipases may assist *S. epidermidis* in being a consistent resident of the skin.

Hyaluronidase. Most pathogenic staphylococci produce hyaluronidase, which breaks down hyaluronic acid in connective tissue. It has a reputation as a "spreading factor" in bacterial infections, but its importance is limited to early stages of the infection because inflammation antagonizes the spreading action.

Phosphatase. Acid phosphatase is generally produced by pathogenic staphylococci. It could be used as a reasonably reliable indicator of staphylococcal virulence.

Lysozyme. Most coagulase-positive strains produce lysozyme, but the staphylococci are not sensitive to it.

Penicillinase. Staphylococci readily become resistant to penicillin by the production of penicillinase or beta-lactamase. Penicillinase inactivates penicillin by breaking its beta-lactam ring.

Toxins

The pathogenic staphylococci produce immunologically distinct toxins designated as alpha (α), beta (β), gamma (γ), and delta (δ). Commonly these toxins lyse erythrocytes, although they may be dermonecrotic, lethal, or leukocidic.

α-Toxin (Hemolysin). α-Toxin is a staphylococcal protein exotoxin that hemolyzes some animal erythrocytes, but not those of humans. It disrupts lysosomes and is cytotoxic for a variety of tissue culture cells, and it can damage human macrophages and platelets but not monocytes. It is also dermonecrotic, lethal, causes spasm of smooth muscle, aggregates blood platelets, injures renal cortex, and causes death by ventricular fibrillation. Current evidence suggests that α-toxin acts together with other virulence factors to play a role in development of staphylococcal disease.

β-Toxin (Sphingomyelinase). Staphylococci of animal origin produce a β-toxin that lyses goat, ox, and sheep erythrocytes but has only a slight effect on human erythrocytes. It acts on cell membrane sphingomyelin and on lysophosphatidyl choline, is lethal for rabbits and mice, and aggregates platelets.

β-Toxin produces hot–cold lysis of erythrocytes.

When allowed to act on blood agar at 37°C, it produces only a darkened zone and no hemolysis. If the culture is refrigerated overnight, lysis of the erythrocytes occurs.

γ-Toxin. Staphylococci produce a hemolysin termed γ-toxin. It is cytolytic for human and some animal erythrocytes but its precise mode of action is unknown. The presence of specific neutralizing antibodies in human staphylococcal bone disease suggests the possible contribution of this toxin to the disease state.

δ-Toxin. Staphylococci produce an antigenically distinct δ-toxin. It acts on phosphatidylserine but not sphingomyelin. δ-Lysin is slightly dermonecrotic and damages erythrocytes, macrophages, lymphocytes, neutrophils, and platelets.

Leukocidin. The nonhemolytic Panton–Valentine leukocidin produced by most pathogenic staphylococci attacks only macrophages and polymorphonuclear leukocytes. Its primary effect is to alter permeability to cations; other changes are secondary to this event. Although the leukocidin alone is not responsible for the pathogenicity of the staphylococci, it protects the organisms from host leukocytes.

Exfoliative Toxin (Epidermolytic Toxin). Strains of staphylococci belonging to phage group II are etiologic agents of a spectrum of dermatologic conditions that are termed staphylococcal scalded-skin syndrome. The causative strains of staphylococci produce an exotoxin, exfoliative toxin, that is responsible for the clinical manifestations of this condition. An intraepidermal cleavage plane at the stratum granulosum induces intraepidermal separation. This results in the severe exfoliation that is characteristic of these diseases.

Enterotoxin Action. Some coagulase-positive staphylococci produce heat-resistant, diffusible enterotoxins that are common causes of food poisoning and have been implicated in enterocolitis developing after antibiotic therapy. Such enterotoxins are produced in foods contaminated with toxigenic staphylococci. Food poisoning, which is an intoxication, occurs when the preformed toxins are ingested. The mechanism of action of the enterotoxins is unknown. The diarrhea has been attributed to inhibited water absorption and increased fluid flux into the lumen. The receptor for the emetic effect is the abdominal viscera, from which site the stimulus reaches the vomiting center via vagal and sympathetic nerves.

Toxic Shock Syndrome Toxin. Some strains of *S. aureus* have been shown to synthesize and release a protein that produces toxic shock syndrome. The exact role of the toxin in producing the clinical manifestations of rash, fever, and hypotension is not completely understood.

Antigenic Structure

Polysaccharides A and B.   Staphylococci contain two phosphorus-containing polysaccharide antigens designated A and B. The serologic determinants of both are teichoic acids, but of differing composition. Polysaccharide A, whose antigenic determinant is the *N*-acetyl glucosaminyl ribitol unit of teichoic acid, is found in the cell wall of *S. aureus,* while polysaccharide B, which is glycerol teichoic acid, is present in the cell wall of *S. epidermidis.*

Capsular Antigens.   Mucoid strains of staphylococci produce capsular antigens. One antigen is a polypeptide. Another capsular antigen, a polymer of glucuronic acid, is antiphagocytic.

Protein A.   *S. aureus* possesses a surface component called protein A that is linked to the peptidoglycan layer but also can be released extracellularly. Protein A has a strong affinity for the Fc portion of IgG molecules and can bind these molecules to the cell surface, leaving the Fab portions exposed and intact. For this reason protein A evidently has an antiopsonic effect and interferes with phagocytosis.

Bacteriophage Typing

Although some 30 type-specific agglutinogens have been identified, serological typing of staphylococci has not been useful in epidemiological studies.

A better method of typing coagulase-positive *S. aureus* is by determining the patterns of sensitivity exhibited by the various strains to bacteriophages. The phage patterns of the strains fall essentially into four large groups. Phage typing is particularly useful in epidemiological studies but it is not used for classifying staphylococci. The correlation of phage types with other properties of staphylococci has not been precise.

Genetic Variation

Genetic variation occurs readily in staphylococci. Loss of pigment is common and may occur independently of coagulase production. Staphylococci commonly undergo smooth–rough dissociation and loss of capsule. They mutate reversibly to form minute G colonies whose cells are relatively avirulent. Other variations include changes in susceptibility to bacteriophages, hemolytic abilities, toxin formation, and coagulase formation.

The development of resistance to drugs and antibiotics, both in vivo and in vitro, is a most important variation of staphylococci. Most antibiotic resistance appears to be plasmid mediated. Penicillin resistance is achieved by the production of penicillinase. Staphylococci may become resistant to "synthetic" penicillins that are not susceptible to penicillinase by means of lysogenic conversion. The facility with which the staphylococci become resistant to one or more antibiotics greatly complicates patient care in hospitals.

Staphylococcal Infections

Staphylococci cause a wide variety of diseases in man (boils, abscesses, furuncles, pyemia, meningitis, osteomyelitis, infection of wounds, and food poisoning). Such infections depend on the type, number, and route of introduction of the organisms, their toxic products, and previous exposure to staphylococci. In the human host, mediating factors are trauma, general health, nutritional status of the individual, toxemias, allergic reactions, and uncontrolled diabetes. Locally, mediating factors are changes in the capillary bed, the biochemical environment, and the inflammatory response.

Skin Infections.   Skin, the most common site of staphylococcal infection, is affected by furuncles, boils, carbuncles, wound complications, paronychia, and the generalized skin infection known as impetigo (Figs. 16.2 to 16.4). The furuncle is a circumscribed area of swelling that softens in the center and discharges pus. With a carbuncle the ulcerations are deep and involve wide areas of the skin, and the carbuncle is accompanied by fever and general malaise. Septicemias sometimes develop from severe carbuncles and may result in production of metastatic ab-

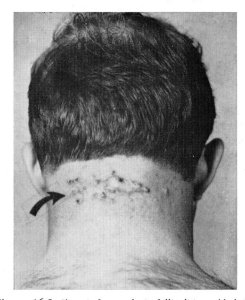

Figure 16.2: Chronic furunculosis, folliculitis, and keloidosis due to staphylococcal infection. (AFIP 53–12335.)

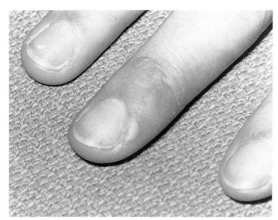

Figure 16.3: Staphylococcal infection of the finger.

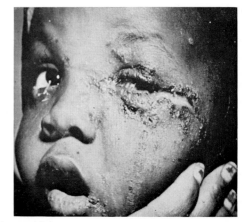

Figure 16.4: Impetigo of the face and lips due to staphylococci. (AFIP 13966–6.)

scesses throughout the body. Infections of the upper lip and nose are particularly dangerous, for staphylococci can easily invade the regional veins, causing cavernous sinus thrombosis, septicemia, and death.

In acne, staphylococci together with diphtheroid bacilli complicate and aggravate the changes that occur in the skin, and together they mediate the persistence and severity of the lesions.

It has recently been shown that *S. aureus* is a significant cause of angular cheilitis, an eroded and erythematous nonvesicular lesion radiating from the angle of the mouth. The staphylococcal disease often can be recognized by a yellow crust. *S. aureus* may be the sole infecting agent, or it may act in combination with streptococci or *Candida albicans*.

Coagulase-positive staphylococci of phage group II produce exfoliative toxin that has been associated with a dermatitis, characterized by intraepidermal separation, known as Ritter's disease in newborn infants and as toxic epidermal necrolysis in older individuals. In addition, these staphylococci may produce a scarlatiniform eruption. These diseases, together with bullous impetigo, have been termed staphylococcal scalded skin syndrome because of their resemblance to skin lesions produced by scalding. The syndrome usually is seen in infants and young children. The exfoliative disease generally presents with tenderness of the skin and abrupt onset of a diffuse erythema over most of the body. Mild edema of the face may be seen. Within 1 or 2 days the upper layers of the epidermis appear wrinkled or have peeled off, producing the Nikolski sign. There may be appearance of flaccid, fluid-filled bullae followed by separation of the epithelium, leaving a moist, red, glistening surface. The exfoliated areas then dry, yielding large flakes. The secondary desquamation lasts 3 to 5 days. Exfoliative lesions may be present on the face and mucous membranes of the oral cavity, lips, and

pharynx. In addition, there may be purulent lip lesions and fissures about the mouth. The clinical manifestations of the disease apparently are a result of toxin-induced cleavage of the desmosomes linking the cells in the stratum granulosum of the epidermis.

Staphylococci may produce a scarlatiniform rash with skin tenderness but without significant exfoliation. The rash resembles that produced by streptococci but there is no palatal exanthema or strawberry tongue. It resolves differently also. After 1 or 2 days of erythema, cracks appear in the creases of the skin, particularly around the eyes and mouth. After a few days, epidermal flakes desquamate, revealing healing skin beneath. In all cases the individuals are febrile, irritable, and anorectic during the exfoliative stage of disease.

Osteomyelitis. Staphylococci are commonly involved in osteomyelitis. They enter the bloodstream from a cutaneous lesion and are carried to one of the long bones where an abscess develops, causing tenderness and pain. Staphylococcal osteomyelitis is often chronic, with periods of regression and renewed activity continuing for years.

Respiratory Infections. Staphylococcal infections of the lower respiratory tract range from chronic bronchitis to acute bronchopneumonia. Staphylococcal infections of the lower respiratory tract occur more often in influenza epidemics, at which time they may reach epidemic proportions. Staphylococcal pneumonia is particularly serious because of the tendency of the organism to produce abscesses and parenchymal destruction. Staphylococcal pneumonia is also likely to occur in young children, debilitated individuals, and hospitalized individuals taking antibiotics.

Food Poisoning. Some strains of *S. aureus* produce an enterotoxin when they grow in foods held for some hours at a warm temperature. The foods appear normal in odor, taste, and appearance but, when eaten, cause vomiting, diarrhea, and prostration within 1 to 6 hours. The symptoms last for several hours. Recovery is usually complete within a day or two.

Enterocolitis. Broad-spectrum antibiotic therapy may upset the intestinal microbiota sufficiently for drug-resistant staphylococci to become the predominant intestinal bacteria, causing an enterocolitis. The manifestations include cramps, fever, diarrhea, dehydration, and electrolyte imbalance.

Toxic Shock Syndrome. This disease is produced by strains of *S. aureus* that produce a toxin called toxic shock syndrome toxin 1 (TSST-1). It is characterized by the rapid onset of fever, hypotension, and skin rash, with delayed epidermal desquamation of the palms and soles. Although men, children, and nonmenstruating women may develop the disease, the majority of cases have occurred during menstruation in women using tampons containing rayon fibers or polyester foam. Apparently these materials bind magnesium, which may enhance toxin production.

Hospital Infections. Staphylococcal infections in hospitals are of considerable concern because of their severity and incidence. Hospital patients and personnel are the principal reservoirs of the causative staphylococci. Of all microorganisms encountered in hospitals, staphylococci are the most likely to cause wound infections. Other staphylococcal hospital infections involve burns, bronchopneumonia, bacteremia (e.g., from a cellulitis arising from venipuncture or intravenous catheters), diarrhea, and enterocolitis. At best, aseptic precautions combined with sterilization and filtration of the air in the hospital environment can do no more than reduce the numbers of staphylococci to a noncritical level. Prophylactic treatment of the staff to reduce the staphylococci in the hospital environment is a doubtful control measure.

Staphylococcus epidermidis, a normal skin inhabitant, occasionally can cause endocarditis. It is a common cause of infection on or around prosthetic heart valves and hip replacements. *S. aureus* is the most common cause of infection of the latter site.

Staphylococcus saprophyticus is an opportunistic pathogen in compromised hosts. It may also be an agent in urinary tract infections in young women.

Pathogenesis

The pathogenesis of staphylococcal disease relates to resistance to phagocytosis, to the action of several staphylococcal enzymes, to the development of delayed hypersensitivity, and to the activities of the toxins. Man is constantly exposed to staphylococci from birth until death. Even so, the most virulent staphy-

lococci seldom cause serious infections in a human host unless resistance is drastically lowered by events such as severe burns, trauma, or surgery.

An important factor is the resistance of the virulent *S. aureus* to phagocytosis. The nature of the antiphagocytic action relates mostly to the in vivo formation of a capsule. Very few virulent staphylococci produce a detectable capsule in vitro, but anticapsular antibodies are present in most adults and particularly in those who have recently had a staphylococcal infection. Staphylococcal protein A may also be antiphagocytic.

Despite its role as an indicator of staphylococcal virulence, coagulase seems to have only a coincidental relationship to pathogenesis. A coagulase-negative mutant of a virulent coagulase-positive staphylococcus is just as virulent as the original staphylococcus. The mutant is able to elicit a lesion, surrounded by a fibrin barrier, that is identical to that produced by the coagulase-positive strain.

Staphylococcal lipase seems to relate to the production of boils and carbuncles. Lipase-positive staphylococci predominate in skin infections but seldom escape from the localized lesion.

α-Toxin is likely involved in the pathogenesis of staphylococcal infection through its hemolytic, dermonecrotic, leukocidal, and lethal actions. Leukocidins other than α-toxin also contribute to the pathogenesis of staphylococcal infections.

Delayed hypersensitivity is also a factor in the pathogenesis of staphylococcal infections. Repeated bouts of staphylococcal infections in experimental animals increase the severity of their skin lesions.

The enteritis caused by staphylococci is essentially a toxemia resulting from the ingestion of the enterotoxin released by staphylococci growing in contaminated food. Similarly, exfoliative skin disease is a result of the production and dissemination of a soluble toxin, and TSST-1 plays a role in toxic shock syndrome.

Immunity

Specific acquired immunity is an important addition to innate defenses in resistance to staphylococcal infections. Humoral antibodies are important, as indicated by the increased incidence of infection in patients with immunoglobulin deficiencies. Opsonization is likely a major factor in the antibody-mediated defense.

The barriers posed by fibrin, granulation tissue, and phagocytes are important in abscess formation and localization of infection, and broaching these barriers increases the chance of systemic infection. Delayed hypersensitivity contributes to tissue damage but also tends to help localize the disease, limiting spread throughout the body.

Laboratory Diagnosis

The laboratory diagnosis of staphylococcal infections involves their detection in purulent exudates and their culture on blood agar. Smears of purulent exudate are stained with gram stains. The detection of gram-positive cocci, not in chains, in such smears allows the presumptive diagnosis of a staphylococcal infection. Blood agar is most useful in cultural diagnosis. Selective media useful for the detection of staphylococci in heavily contaminated specimens are tellurite glycine agar, phenylethyl agar, or media containing 7.5% sodium chloride. Catalase production is useful to distinguish staphylococci from the catalase-negative streptococci. The virulence of an isolated colony can be established by demonstration of coagulase production. Mannitol fermentation is useful to distinguish *S. aureus* from *S. epidermidis,* which does not ferment that sugar. *S. saprophyticus* is resistant to novobiocin, making this test useful in its recognition. Enterotoxin in suspected food is demonstrated by immunological tests, although the usual diagnosis is on a clinical basis.

Treatment

Staphylococci are sensitive to penicillin, cephalosporins, macrolide antibiotics, novobiocin, chloramphenicol, and tetracyclines. Nevertheless, staphylococcal infections pose many problems in treatment. Because of the prevalence of antibiotic-resistant staphylococci, especially in hospital populations, and the ability of any of the pathogenic staphylococci to rapidly develop resistance to one or more antibiotics during treatment, it is essential that drug sensitivity of the infecting staphylococcus be established as soon as possible. Whatever the antibiotic used in treatment, the establishment of adequate drainage greatly facilitates treatment because antibiotics do not diffuse readily into areas of suppuration nor do they act effectively in such areas. In addition, organisms in purulent exudates may grow slowly or not at all. Several antibiotics such as penicillin are effective only against growing organisms, increasing the possibility of therapy failure.

Epidemiology and Control

Man is the principal reservoir of pathogenic staphylococci. Most infants become carriers soon after birth, and while the number of carriers fluctuates during the first few years of life, 50% to 60% of adults are continual or intermittent carriers. The anterior nares are the primary nidus for pathogenic staphylococci in the human body, but the skin is the residence of the other staphylococci. Many hospital personnel are nasal carriers of pathogenic and often antibiotic-resistant staphylococci. Such carriers widely disperse their staphylococci. The carrier state is usually established in the newborn within a few days of birth and becomes intermittent with age. The factors that determine the carrier state are not known. Immunological factors, both humoral and cell mediated, are likely contributors to immunity or lack thereof. The exclusion of nasal carriers from operating rooms, surgical wards, the burn ward, and infant wards and nurseries certainly lowers the rate of staphylococcal infection in hospitals. In addition, all surgical procedures and instrumentation should be performed with close attention to aseptic techniques, detection of carriers, control of airborne and fomite spread, and tracing of sources of infection.

Control of staphylococcal food poisoning depends mainly on proper food handling. Prompt refrigeration of food is essential to prevent growth of the organisms and toxin production. Food handlers who are carriers should not be in a situation where they can contaminate the food.

ADDITIONAL READING

Easmon, C. S. F., and Adlam, C. 1984. *Staphylococci and Staphylococcal Infections.* Academic Press, New York.

Hartman, A. A. 1978. Staphylococci of the Normal Human Skin Flora. Arch Dermatol Res, **261,** 295.

Kaplan, M. H., and Tenenbaum, M. J. 1982. *Staphylococcus aureus:* Cellular Biology and Clinical Application. Am J Med, **72,** 248.

Melish, M., and Glasgow, L. A. 1971. Staphylococcal Scalded-Skin Syndrome: The Expanded Clinical Syndrome. J Pediatr, **78,** 958.

Parisi, J. T. 1985. Coagulase-Negative Staphylococci and the Epidemiological Typing of *Staphylococcus epidermidis.* Microbiol Rev, **49,** 126.

Rogolsky, M. 1979. Nonenteric Toxins of *Staphylococcus aureus.* Microbiol Rev, **43,** 320.

Sheagren, J. N. 1984. *Staphylococcus aureus:* The Persistent Pathogen. N Engl J Med, **310,** 1368.

Verhoef, J., and Berbrugh, H. A. 1981. Host Determinants in Staphylococcal Disease. Annu Rev Med, **32,** 107.

Wise, R. I. 1973. Modern Management of Severe Staphylococcal Disease. Medicine (Baltimore), **52,** 295.

Wiseman, G. M. 1976. The Hemolysis of *Staphylococcus aureus.* Bacteriol Rev, **39,** 317.

17

Streptococci and Streptococcal Infections

George S. Schuster

Streptococcal Groups

Streptococci are spherical or ovoid, generally non-motile, nonsporulating, gram-positive bacteria that may occur singly, in pairs, in short chains, or in chains of eight to ten cocci when grown in appropriate media (Fig. 17.1). The cells average 1 μm and are less than 2 μm in diameter. Capsules are difficult to demonstrate in species other than *Streptococcus pneumoniae,* but occur in young cultures of many strains. Some capsules are polysaccharides, especially *S. pneumoniae,* while others, especially *S. pyogenes,* are hyaluronic acid.

Classification by Hemolytic Action. According to their hemolytic action on whole blood in an agar medium, streptococci can be divided into the following groups:

1. Alpha (α)-hemolytic streptococci, which cause an inner zone of green discoloration and an outer zone of complete hemolysis. Such streptococci are also called the viridans group after the Latin *viridis,*

meaning green. *Streptococcus salivarius* is the most common α-hemolytic streptococcus.

2. Beta (β)-hemolytic streptococci, which produce a clear zone of complete hemolysis about the colony (Fig. 17.2). The most common β-hemolytic streptococcus is *Streptococcus pyogenes.* However, some of the streptococci assigned to the β-hemolytic and immunologically related groups that are actually nonhemolytic include some members of Lancefield groups B, C, D, H, K, and O. All group N streptococci are nonhemolytic.

3. Nonhemolytic or, as they have been called, gamma (γ)-hemolytic streptococci produce no hemolysis on or in the medium. The most common nonhemolytic streptococcus is *Streptococcus faecalis.*

Immunological Classification. Streptococci that produce a group-specific carbohydrate (C substance) were divided after 1930 into 13 groups, designated by the letters A through O. Type antigens of the species, the diseases produced, and the primary habitats of these groups are shown in Table 17.1.

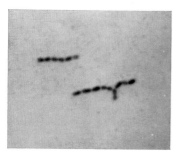

Figure 17.1: Cells of streptococci in a chain.

Anaerobic streptococci are generally nonhemolytic, but they are not grouped with the γ-hemolytic streptococci. They have been placed in a separate genus, *Peptostreptococcus*.

Morphology of Group A Streptococci

β-Hemolytic group A streptococci are gram-positive cocci that form long chains in vitro, especially in an unfavorable environment such as unsuitable media. In tissues they form diplococci or occur singly. The outermost layer of *S. pyogenes* is a capsule composed of hyaluronic acid, which is antiphagocytic. The organisms form short, fine fimbriae composed of M protein and lipoteichoic acid; the latter effects adherence to host cells by making the surface more hydrophobic, and binding to fibronectin on host cells.

The colonial forms of β-hemolytic streptococci are mucoid, matt, or glossy. Mucoid colonies are formed by streptococci that produce hyaluronic acid capsules. Matt colonies appear to be dried-out mucoid colonies. Small, glossy colonies are formed by streptococci that do not produce or retain a hyaluronic acid capsule. Group A streptococci also form L forms and protoplasts.

Streptococcal Metabolism

Facultatively anaerobic streptococci, when grown either aerobically or anaerobically, ferment carbohydrates, particularly glucose, forming lactic as well as formic and acetic acids and ethanol. They can be grown on complicated synthetic media. They grow well on beef infusion or other common media if it contains blood or serum. Potassium tellurite selectively permits the growth of nonhemolytic streptococci by inhibiting other bacteria; crystal violet (1:25,000) and sodium azide (1:1,000) inhibit most of the oral and respiratory microbial flora, permitting the growth of streptococci.

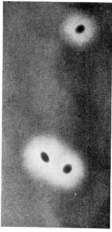

Figure 17.2: β-Hemolysis produced by appropriate streptococci growing in rabbit's blood agar.

Antigenic Structure of Streptococci

The antigenic components of group A streptococci and some of their characteristics are shown in Table 17.2. The principal streptococcal antigens are hyaluronic acid, group-specific C antigens, type-specific M antigen, T antigens, R antigens, P antigens, glycerol teichoic acids, murein, and antigens of the cytoplasmic membrane.

Hyaluronic Acid. Group A streptococci produce hyaluronic acid that is nonimmunogenic, probably because it is indistinguishable from the hyaluronate of ground substance. It is somewhat labile and readily diffuses away from the streptococcal cell. It is an important antiphagocytic factor.

Group-specific C Antigen. Hemolytic streptococci produce specific somatic antigenic polysaccharides, designated by the letter C, that are utilized to divide the β-hemolytic streptococci into 13 groups, designated A through O. C antigen is a component of the cell wall, making up about 10% of the dry weight of the organism. In the case of groups A and C, the antigen is composed of rhamnose and hexosamine. Its specificity depends mainly on the nature of the terminal sugar of the rhamnose side chain. It is not related to the development of streptococcal immunity. This antigen may be similar to heart valve glycoproteins, permitting cross-reactivity and contributing to the pathogenesis of rheumatic fever.

Type-specific M Antigens. Group A streptococci are divided into some 70 immunological types by cell wall protein antigens, designated M. Division is usually accomplished by precipitin tests, although other immunological reactions can be used. M protein is attached to fimbriae on the cell surface and is read-

Table 17.1: Immunological Groups of Streptococci and Their Usual Habitats

Group Antigen Designation	Type Antigen Designation	Chemical Nature Type Antigen	Location Type Antigen	Species Designation	Principal Type of Infection	Usual Habitat
A	M, R, T	Protein	Envelope	*S. pyogenes*	Acute pharyngitis, pneumonia, peritonitis, meningitis, peritonsillar abscesses, mastoiditis, otitis media, cervical adenitis, scarlet fever, rheumatic fever, acute nephritis, puerperal fever, erysipelas, acute hemorrhagic glomerulonephritis	Man
B	S (5 types)	Polysaccharide	Envelope	*S. agalactiae*	Mastitis	Cattle
C	(8 types)	Protein		*S. equisimilis*	Animal disease and human respiratory disease	Horses, man, lower animals
C	(1 type)	Protein		*S. equi*	Strangles	Horses
C	(8 types)	Protein		*S. zooepidemicus*		Animals
D	(1 type)	Protein		*S. equinus*		Horses
C	(3 types)	Protein		*S. dysgalactiae*		
D	(11 types)	Polysaccharide	Cell wall	*S. faecalis*	Human infection (urinary and wound) and food poisoning	Man, animals, dairy products
D	(19 types)			*S. faecium*		Mammalian feces
D				*S. durans*		
D				*S. avium*		
D	(many types)	Carbohydrate	Capsule	*S. bovis*		
D				*S. equinus*		
R, S, or T			Capsule	*S. suis*		
E	(1 type)	Carbohydrate		*Streptococcus* spp.	Pharyngeal abscess in swine	Milk, swine
F	I–V	Polysaccharide		*S. milleri (anginosus)*	Occasional human infection	Man
G	I–V	Carbohydrates		*Streptococcus* spp.	Human and Dog infection	Man, dog
H	(3 types)			*S. sanguis*	Occasional human infection	Man
K	(5 types)			*S. salivarius*	Occasional human infection	Man
L	I, II	Carbohydrates			Dog respiratory infection	Dog
M					Occasional dog infection	Dog
N	(many types)				None	Milk, cream
O					Occasional human respiratory tract infections; endocarditis	Man
Variable or none				*S. mutans*	Dental caries	Man, animals
None	(80 types)	Carbohydrates	Capsule	*S. pneumoniae*	Pneumonia	Man

Note. Only some of the more prominent species of oral streptococci are listed here. These are discussed in more detail in Chapter 49.

212

Table 17.2: Cellular Constituents of Group A Streptococci Involved in Antigenicity and Virulence*

Constituent	Serological Reactions	Chemical Composition	Certain Distinctive Properties
C	Group specific	Polysaccharide	Structural component of cell wall; composed of N-acetylglucosamine and rhamnose
M	Type specific	Protein	Alcohol soluble; resistant to heat at pH 2; destroyed by proteolytic enzymes; important factor in virulence; M antibodies confer protection
T	Usually common to several types; occasionally type specific	Protein	Resistant to proteolytic enzymes; destroyed by heating at pH 2; resists heating at slightly alkaline pH
R	Occurs in type 28 strains and in certain strains of groups A, B, C, and G	Protein	Resistant to proteolytic enzymes except pepsin; destroyed by heating at pH 2; resists heating at alkaline pH
Mucoid capsular substance	Nonantigenic	Hyaluronic acid	Occurs in groups A and C streptococci and animal tissues; composed of N-acetylglucosamine and glucuronic acid; depolymerized by hyaluronidase (probably two enzymes involved; some relation to virulence)

*Reproduced with permission from R. C. Lancefield: Cellular Constituents of Group A Streptococci Concerned in Antigenicity and Virulence. In *Streptococcal Infections,* chap. 1, p. 3, edited by M. McCarty. Columbia University Press, New York, 1954.

ily accessible to anti-M antibodies. Such antibodies are protective. M proteins are antiphagocytic, precipitate fibrinogen, and are toxic for platelets.

Other Streptococcal Antigens. A number of other streptococcal antigens exist, none of which are particularly related to virulence. Streptococcal T antigens are several immunologically distinct proteins that are resistant to proteolytic enzymes. T antigens are not related to virulence and their specific antibodies do not offer protection against streptococcal infection. R proteins, two of which are immunologically distinct, are present in streptococci as surface antigens. P, or nucleoprotein, antigen is present in both hemolytic and nonhemolytic streptococci, in which it is antigenically similar. Glycerolteichoic acid is a group-specific antigen for groups D and N. A glycosaminoglycan is present in streptococci that is somewhat similar antigenically to that of other bacteria. It causes reactions in humans similar to those produced by the endotoxin of gram-negative bacteria.

Extracellular Toxins and Enzymes

Immunoelectrophoretic analysis indicates that there are at least 20 extracellular antigens that are released when streptococci grow in human tissue. These substances include streptokinases, deoxyribonucleases (DNAses) or streptodornase, streptolysins S and O, erythrogenic toxin, proteinases, hyaluronidase, diphosphopyridine nucleotidase, amylase, and esterase.

All but streptolysin S, amylase, and esterase are immunogenic.

Streptokinases. Streptococci rapidly lyse fibrin clots of normal human blood by an agent that was found to be a kinase and was named streptokinase. It is an activator of plasminogen in serum, converting it to plasmin, a protease that digests fibrin. Streptokinase can be divided into two types, designated A and B. Streptokinases are produced by some streptococcal strains of groups A, C, G, and a few streptococci of groups B and F, as well as by some staphylococci and clostridia.

Deoxyribonucleases. Group A and some group C streptococci produce DNAses that are specifically active against highly viscous, extracellular DNA of purulent exudates. They do not penetrate into cells and have no action on the intracellular DNA of living cells.

Soluble Hemolysins. Group A streptococci and a few of group G and C streptococci of human origin produce distinct soluble hemolysins, O and S, which injure the cell membranes of erythrocytes and some tissue cells.

O hemolysin is an oxygen-labile, antigenic protein that is lethal for many laboratory animals and cardiotoxic for some. Its hemolytic activity can be neutralized by specific antibodies.

S hemolysin is bound to bacterial cells but can be extracted with serum. It is not antigenic and is not sensitive to oxygen, but it is inhibited by serum lipoproteins. It causes contraction of smooth muscle and is lethal for mice or rabbits. It is an important leuko-toxic factor. Once streptococci are phagocytized their leukotoxic factor acts on the leukocyte's cytoplasmic granules, releasing potent hydrolytic enzymes that cause irreversible damage, death, and disintegration of leukocytes. In turn, hydrolytic enzymes released from the disintegrated leukocytes damage host tissues.

Erythrogenic Toxins.   Group A and some strains of group C and G streptococci produce soluble erythrogenic toxins that cause the rash of scarlet fever and elicit headache, fever, and vomiting. Such toxigenic strains are lysogenic, and the toxin is probably produced under the direction of the temperate bacteriophage. The erythrogenic toxins can be used to determine susceptibility or resistance to scarlet fever by the Dick test, in which erythrogenic toxin is injected intracutaneously. If an erythematous area 10 to 30 mm in diameter develops within 6 to 24 hours, the individual is susceptible to the toxin. If antitoxin to the erythrogenic toxin is injected into the erythematous skin of a suspected case, local blanching indicates that the individual has scarlet fever. The blanching phenomenon is known as the Schultz–Charlton reaction.

Proteinase.   Some streptococci produce proteinases (or a proteinase) that hydrolyze gelatin, cooked meat, casein, M protein, streptokinase, hyaluronidase, and human γ-globulin. The proteinase that is active against M antigen reduces the immunogenicity of M antigen and interferes with streptokinase production or inactivates it. Immunization with proteinases affords no protection against streptococcal infection.

Hyaluronidase.   Some streptococci produce hyaluronidase, an enzyme that breaks down hyaluronic acid and has been thought to facilitate spread of streptococcal infections through tissues, or to interfere with localization of organisms in tissue. However, hyaluronidase is not essential to virulence, for some pathogenic group A streptococci do not produce it. The enzyme may remove the capsules of group A streptococci, increasing their susceptibility to phagocytosis.

DPNase.   Most streptococci that are nephritogenic produce diphosphopyridine nucleotidase (DPNase), also termed nicotinamide adenine dinucleotidase (NADase), which releases nicotinamide from NAD. NADase has no proven relation to the pathogenesis of streptococcal infections.

Genotypic Variations.   Streptococci undergo a smooth (mucoid) to rough (glossy) colonial variation, concurrent with the loss of capsules and virulence. Subcultured mucoid colonies lose capsules and emerge as glossy colonies. These will revert to a mucoid type by repeated animal passage. M protein, a virulence-related cell wall component, may be lost

from strains carried in the throat after an attack of streptococcal pharyngitis. Repeated animal passage will restore this component to the cell.

Hemolytic streptococci readily develop resistance to sulfonamides but not to penicillin, even after long clinical use. Streptococci that develop antibiotic resistance in vitro lose some of their virulence.

Streptococci vary in hemolysin production and in their capacity to form cell wall antigens other than M protein.

Streptococcal Diseases

Streptococci cause both suppurative diseases and nonsuppurative sequelae-type diseases. Suppurative diseases include pharyngitis (sometimes accompanied by scarlet fever), cervical adenitis, otitis media, mastoiditis, peritonsillar abscesses, meningitis, peritonitis, pneumonia, puerperal sepsis, cellulitis of skin and mucous membranes, impetigo contagiosa, and erysipelas. The principal nonsuppurative sequelae are acute glomerulonephritis, rheumatic fever, and erythema nodosum.

Pathogenesis and Pathology of Streptococcal Diseases.   The principal source of pyogenic streptococci is the human carrier. A streptococcal infection requires transmission of virulent antiphagocytic streptococci to a susceptible host. The antiphagocytic properties relate to the presence of M protein and a capsule. The nature of the lesion and the clinical manifestations also relate to the previous experience of the host with streptococci and streptococcal diseases.

The usual streptococcal infection in children from birth to about 12 years of age is an acute, purulent pharyngitis. This may be associated with various gradations of a syndrome composed of sore throat, fever, chills, headache, nausea, and vomiting. Infection may be followed by complications such as rheumatic fever, scarlet fever, infection of tissues or organs adjacent to the pharynx (cervical adenitis, otitis media, mastoiditis, peritonsillar abscesses), and more generalized infections such as meningitis, peritonitis, and pneumonia. Nonsuppurative sequelae such as acute glomerulonephritis, rheumatic fever, and erythema nodosum also may result.

Pharyngitis and Tonsillitis.   Group A β-hemolytic streptococci often cause pharyngitis and tonsillitis. Acute pharyngitis generally has a sudden onset with redness in the tonsillar area and on the mucous membranes of the pharynx and palate. Petechiae frequently appear on the soft palate, and in some patients elevated areas consisting of a normalcolored center surrounded by an erythematous border may be present on the palate. The mucous mem-

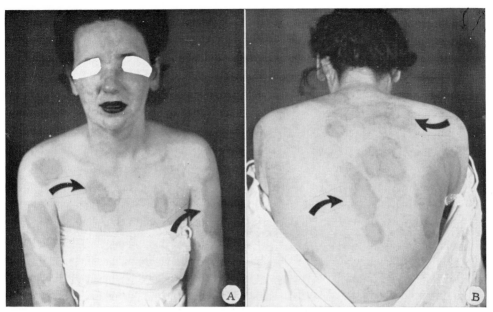

Figure 17.3: Erysipelas caused by streptococci. (AFIP 58–6180.)

branes and uvula often are edematous. The cervical lymph nodes may be enlarged and sore to the touch, and other regional lymph nodes may be involved. Group A streptococci are readily isolated from the mucosa in these patients.

Scarlet Fever. Scarlet fever, a highly contagious disease of childhood, has an incubation period of several days to a week. Onset is marked by a sore throat, fever, and vomiting, and in the early phase the cheeks become reddened. The throat becomes red and an exudate commonly develops. Within several days a rash appears, first on the trunk and then on the limbs and face. This facial rash spares the chin, nose, and lips. The oral mucosa often develops an enanthema that appears earlier and is more marked than the skin reactions. The mucosa is congested and red punctate mottling is present on the hard palate. The palate and uvula are frequently edematous and the uvula may become elongated, inducing coughing and regurgitation of fluids.

The tongue is also involved in scarlet fever. At first it has a milky white or gray appearance. The fungiform papillae become enlarged and swollen, projecting through the coat to appear as reddish protuberances, producing the so-called strawberry tongue. The tongue lesions subside after a time, followed by desquamation beginning at the tip and sides. The tongue eventually returns to normal size and appearance. Ulcerative glossitis also has been reported, as have other oral complications of scarlet fever.

Erysipelas. Erysipelas is an acute febrile disease that occurs most commonly in the elderly, although newborn infants are susceptible. It consists of an in-

flammatory reaction followed by invasion of the lymphatics by hemolytic streptococci, usually of group A. A minor lesion or abrasion often provides the initial entry site. However, this lesion often has healed by the end of the 3- to 7-day incubation period so that the initial portal is not evident. At the outset the skin around the initial site becomes red and swollen, but as the infection spreads outward the central point tends to clear. Organisms are found only toward the margins of the lesion and are readily isolated from excised tissue. Although erysipelas may develop on any part of the body surface, the face is the most common site. It may extend into the mucous membranes or, infrequently, originate in these tissues, particularly those of the pharynx or nose.

Facial erysipelas begins abruptly with a short period of malaise, headache, fever, and vomiting. After a few hours a local itching or burning sensation occurs at the affected area. Skin lesions appear around the nose or mouth as irregular, bright red, slightly raised areas. Lymphadenitis is a characteristic feature as the submaxillary lymph nodes enlarge. If untreated, the disease spreads at the periphery, extending over the face to produce a butterfly pattern (Fig. 17.3). The lips swell and become thick, the eyelids may become swollen, and the nose broadens, producing facial distortion. As the disease progresses a toxemia occurs, accompanied by fever and restlessness.

Erysipelas occasionally extends from the facial skin into the oral cavity, producing redness, pain, and swelling of the tongue. Infection originating in the upper respiratory tract results in throat pain, submaxillary lymphadenitis, and sometimes edema of the uvula and epiglottis. Although it may be fatal, erysipelas usually resolves after several days, leaving a dry desquamating skin.

Sequelae-type Diseases. *Glomerulonephritis.* Acute glomerulonephritis, caused by only a few strains of *S. pyogenes,* is preceded by an acute purulent infection of the pharynx or skin. It commonly follows type 12 infections, which are primarily pharyngeal, and type 49 infections, which occur primarily in the skin, although attacks may follow infection with other types. Strains of streptococci isolated from patients with poststreptococcal glomerulonephritis have been shown to secrete a nephritis strain–associated protein. It is not produced by strains isolated from individuals with other types of streptococcal disease. The manifestations are hematuria, edema, and hypertension and appear about a week after the onset of acute pyogenic infection.

The pathogenesis of the disease is not clear. Since antigen–antibody complexes have been found in the serum of patients with glomerulonephritis, many believe it is an immune complex disease. Others suggest that antibodies to streptococcal glycoprotein cross-react with related antigens of the glomerular basement membrane: these antigens may be found only in "nephritis-prone" individuals. Recent evidence indicates that antibodies against nephritis associated–proteins bind to glomeruli of patients with the disease but not those of nonstreptococcal glomerulonephritis patients, which suggests that the protein localizes in the glomeruli during the disease process. Morphologically the disease resembles immune complex disease. Acute disease usually resolves spontaneously, although some patients die within a year or progress to a chronic form of the disease.

Rheumatic Fever. Rheumatic fever is a serious sequela of infection with *S. pyogenes.* Its pathogenesis is not clear. It is acute in nature and terminates within a few weeks. Patients are prone to recurrent attacks and progressive heart valve damage whenever they subsequently develop *S. pyogenes* pharyngitis. When the disease occurs, infection is limited largely, if not exclusively, to the upper respiratory tract. The onset occurs 1 to 4 weeks or more after infection, and the signs and symptoms reflect widespread involvement of the heart and joints. Symptoms may include fever, malaise, leukocytosis, subacute nodular lesions, migrating polyarthritis, and sometimes abdominal pains and vomiting. Permanent cardiac damage, particularly of the mitral valve, often occurs, setting the stage for subsequent infection of damaged valves by other organisms, especially viridans streptococci, resulting in subacute bacterial endocarditis.

Rheumatic fever can follow infections with many types of *S. pyogenes* (except some strains found on the skin), and repeated attacks leading to progressive heart valve damage can occur over a period of years.

The initial infection usually subsides and organisms are cleared from the throat before the onset of rheumatic fever. Since organisms are usually not found locally or in the blood, development of the disease probably depends on postinfection events. It is seen only in humans but not in infants, follows upper respiratory tract infections but seldom skin infections, and is usually accompanied by a high antistreptolysin O titer and a persistent anti-group A polysaccharide titer. It develops in a small percentage of individuals within a population. There likely is a genetic component in susceptibility, and indeed it has been suggested that susceptible individuals may need to be infected by certain types of *S. pyogenes* for disease to occur. However, this is still speculative. One more widely held theory is that rheumatic fever represents an immune response to some streptococcal antigen(s). The long latent period, the abundance of lymphocytes and plasma cells in the lesions, and similarity between rheumatic fever and known immune disease make such a theory plausible. Another theory is that rheumatic fever is due to cross-reactivity between antibodies stimulated by streptococcal antigens with tissue antigens. Again, the exact pathogenesis and the role of the antibodies are not clear.

Erythema nodosum. Erythema nodosum is associated with diseases such as tuberculosis or coccidioidomycosis, and probably with streptococcal infections. It has been produced experimentally in rabbits in a form that may resemble the human disease. The toxic factor appears to be the peptidoglycan component of streptococcal cell walls.

Pathogenesis. The pathogenic mechanisms of streptococcal infections are not always known. Since streptococci are readily destroyed by phagocytes, their ability to resist phagocytosis due to surface components is likely an important determinant of pathogenesis. M protein production may play other roles in pathogenesis. Leukotoxin and adherence factors are also likely components of this complex set of reactions. The ability of streptococci to spread within tissues is an important factor to consider as well. This likely depends on one or more activities of the DNAse, hyaluronidase, leukotoxin, and tissue-toxic components, streptolysins O and S, NADase, M protein, and murein complex. The pathogenesis of sequelae diseases may well be a function of both toxic and immunologic reactions.

Immunity. Only anti-M antibodies protect significantly against streptococcal infections. Detectable anti-M antibodies develop after several weeks to months and may persist for years. There are at least 70 serological types in the group A streptococci, and it is likely that no single individual ever becomes immune to all streptococcal types. Since only a few streptococci cause acute glomerulonephritis, a single infection decreases the chances of a recurring infection.

Most group A streptococci can produce rheumatic fever, however, so that even multiple attacks do not greatly decrease the chances of subsequent rheumatic fever attacks. There are at least three immunologic groups of the erythrogenic toxin associated with scarlet fever. The presence of antibodies to one type will protect against infection with only that type. Recurrences of scarlet fever do occur with the other antigenic types.

Laboratory Diagnosis. The laboratory diagnosis of streptococcal infections requires culture and isolation, a description of cell and colonial morphology and action on blood. Diagnosis may also be reinforced by group A being more susceptible to bacitracin than are other groups. Serological reactions (complement fixation, agglutination) have been widely used in identification. Measurement of anti-M antibodies by bactericidal and mouse protection tests, the measurement of antistreptolysin antibodies, and the measurement of antibodies against other enzyme antigens are useful. β-Hemolytic streptococci of various Lancefield groups may be identified with specific antisera and the immunofluorescence test. Identification from wound infections is complicated because these are usually mixed infections. A variety of rapid (20 to 30 minute) tests are available for identification of group A streptococci from throat cultures. These should prove quite useful.

Treatment. Sulfonamides, penicillin, and broad-spectrum antibiotics have been used to treat streptococcal infections. Streptococci develop resistance to sulfonamides, and this class of drugs will not eliminate streptococci from the upper respiratory tract in acute pharyngitis. Penicillins are the drugs of choice; erythromycin also is useful for treatment. Many streptococci are resistant to tetracycline.

Epidemiology and Control. Transmission of respiratory infection occurs by aerosol or droplet spread and is favored by close contact and crowded living conditions. The overall carrier rate for S. *pyogenes* is about 5% to 10%, depending on the time of year. Carrier control and proper hygiene help prevent spread.

In the case of rheumatic fever patients, long-term prophylactic treatment with penicillin has been used to prevent repeated attacks. While prophylactic treatment of these patients to prevent endocarditis of dental origin is of great importance, preventive dentistry can help reduce the risk of disease of dental origin.

Streptococci of Other Groups

Much of the preceding discussion was devoted to S. *pyogenes;* however, streptococci of other groups are pathogenic as well.

The α-hemolytic streptococci, or viridans group, normally inhabit the oral cavity and upper respiratory tract of humans. S. *salivarius* is a common representative of this group. α-Hemolytic streptococci seem to belong to several different immunological groups, but only a few fit into groups A to O. Although relatively avirulent, they do cause disease in humans, chiefly subacute bacterial endocarditis. As inhabitants of the oral cavity, they cause repeated transient bacteremias that sometimes induce the endocarditis. The disease results from infection of an endocardial surface, such as the surface of the heart valves, which has already been damaged by congenital heart disease or rheumatic fever.

Streptococci of groups D and O are common causes of subacute bacterial endocarditis. These organisms are common members of the normal flora and reach the valves from the mouth and gut via the bloodstream. If untreated, this infection is usually fatal due to irreversible heart valve damage. Proper bacteriologic diagnosis and antibiotic susceptibility testing is crucial. Since the organisms may be resistant to antibiotics, successful therapy requires prolonged and rigorous treatment. Penicillin and streptomycin is the combination of choice for treating subacute bacterial endocarditis caused by enterococci. Enterococci of group D are a frequent cause of urinary tract infections.

Group B streptococci not infrequently cause serious infection in neonates, especially sepsis and meningitis. The rate is 1 to 3 cases per 100,000 births, with a mortality of 30% to 60%, depending on the time of onset. The source of infection is the vagina of the mother or nursery sources. The vaginal carrier rate is about 30%.

Streptococcus pneumoniae

Morphology. S. *pneumoniae* organisms are fairly large, ovoid, spherical, or lanceolate bacteria that are nonmotile, nonsporulating, aerobic and facultatively anaerobic, actively fermentative, and catalase negative (Fig. 17.4). Pneumococci are generally gram positive but become mostly gram negative and autolyze in older cultures. Pathogenic pneumococci are encapsulated with immunogenic, highly polymerized polysaccharides that serve as the basis for their subdivision into different types and for their pathogenicity. Heavily encapsulated types form mucoid colonies. Pneumococci cause α-hemolysis aerobically and β-hemolysis anaerobically.

Antigenic Structure. S. *pneumoniae* has distinctive polysaccharide capsular antigens and somatic antigens, R antigens, C substance, and M antigen, similar to other streptococci. Pneumococcal capsules are polysaccharide polymers that apparently are chemically distinct. They are used to divide the pneumo-

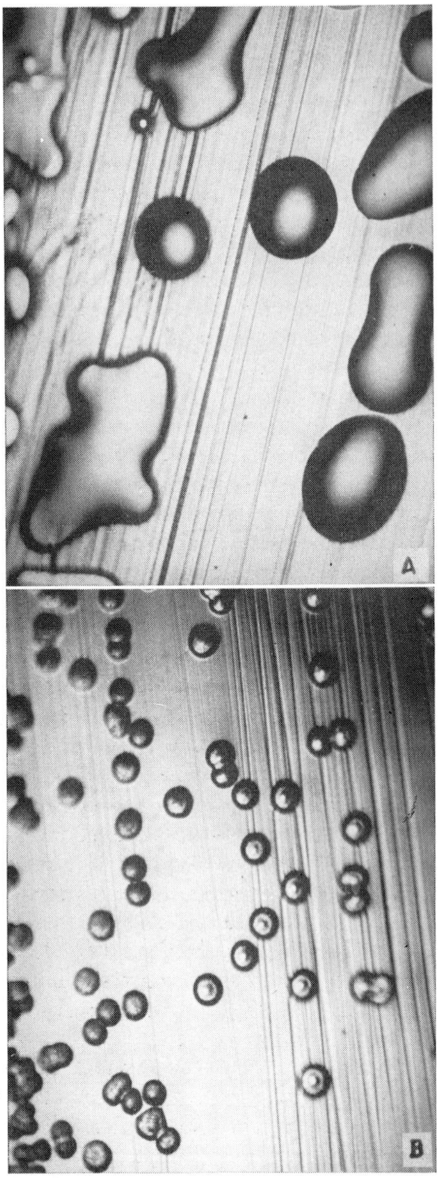

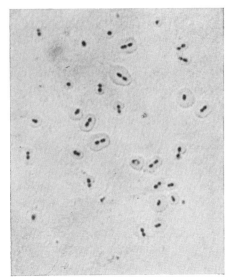

Figure 17.5: Quellung reaction of encapsulated type III pneumococci (×1100). (Reproduced with permission from R. Austrian: Morphologic Variation in Pneumococcus. *J Exp Med*, **98**, 21, 1953.)

Figure 17.4: Smooth and rough colonial forms of pneumococci. **(A)** Smooth, capsulated type III pneumococci in blood agar (×14). **(B)** Rough, noncapsulated pneumococci in blood agar (×12). (Reproduced with permission from R. Austrian: Morphologic Variation in Pneumococcus. *J Exp Med*, **98**, 21, 1953.)

cocci into 94 serological types. When the capsule is lost or not produced, pneumococci remain viable but become avirulent and easily phagocytized. Capsular polysaccharides are the basis for the quellung reaction (Fig. 17.5). When a given type of pneumococcus is exposed to its homologous type-specific antibody, the capsule appears to swell and becomes refractile. The test is a basis for the serological identification of pneumococcal types.

Pneumococci contain a somatic C substance (teichoic acid polymer) distinct from their capsular polysaccharide and antigenically distinct from the C substance of other streptococci.

Rough pneumococci have a protein antigen that is on or near the surface of the cell. They also possess type-specific somatic M antigens that are not antiphagocytic.

Genotypic Variations. If an encapsulated, virulent pneumococcus is cultured serially in the presence of its specific antipolysaccharide, it retains its viability but loses its capsule and becomes noncapsulated, nonvirulent, and nonspecific as to type. It also changes its colonial form from smooth to rough. If a rough colonial strain is grown in the presence of its homologous anti-R serum, a smooth type of pneumococcus is soon derived whose type specificity is identical with that from which the rough strain was originally derived. The mechanism involved seems to be a selective process.

Pneumococcal Transformation. In culture, smooth virulent pneumococci mutate at a low but definite rate, lose their capsule, and become rough and avirulent. By transfer of DNA, a virulent pneumococcus can be transformed into another smooth type by way of the rough form. This can take place either in vivo or in vitro.

Toxins. No significant soluble toxin has been described for *S. pneumoniae* that could be related to its invasiveness or virulence. Two toxins are produced in vitro. Pneumolysin is an oxygen-labile intracellular toxin possessing β-hemolytic and general cytotoxic activity. Another internal toxin that is released on autolysis produces purpura when inoculated into experimental animals. Leukocidin and hyaluronidase are produced in small quantities.

Pneumococcal Infection

The predominant pneumococcal infection is pneumonia. Pneumococci also cause primary infection in sinusitis, otitis media, osteomyelitis, arthritis, peritonitis, meningitis, and possibly gingivitis. Pneumococcal septicemia, empyema, endocarditis, pericarditis, meningitis, and arthritis occur as secondary complications of pneumococcal pneumonia.

Pneumococcal Pneumonia. Pneumococcal pneumonia is characterized by its sudden onset and, even early in the disease, by both local manifestations (acute inflammation of the lungs, pleurisy) and systemic manifestations (general constitutional symptoms, chills, high fever, and frequently a bacteremia). Untreated patients with uncomplicated pneumococcal pneumonia are acutely ill for 7 to 10 days. Then circulating antibodies increase and there is a crisis, after which the temperature and symptoms abate, usually quite rapidly. Once infection is established, neutrophils function as the major phagocytic defense. Neutrophils readily kill ingested pneumococci. The critical immune forces involve primarily opsonin-dependent phagocytosis. Optimum killing requires both alternate and classical complement pathways. Therefore, availability of adequate amounts of specific antibody is critical in the determining outcome of infection. The outcome essentially depends on the balance of specific antibody versus organisms producing capsular polysaccharide. Free opsonins are usually found in the blood at or near the time of crisis. Specific immunity lasts for decades, and second attacks by the same serologic type are rare. The symptoms of pneumococcal pneumonia patients treated with antibiotics abate within several days, but all signs of pneumonia usually do not disappear for three or four weeks.

Pneumococcal Bacteremia. Pneumococcal bacteremia has been associated with the appearance of gingival lesions in infants. Affected children develop fever, leukocytosis, and lesions in the posterior maxillary tuberosity area, the buccal surface of the alveolar ridge, and the posterior area of the hard palate. The lesions initially appear as a "boggy" fluid-filled erythematous area that later becomes ulcerative and necrotic; then the swelling subsides and the lesions resolve. The relationship between the pneumococcal bacteremia and gingival lesions is not clear, but the lesions are characteristic enough that pneumococcal bacteremia should be suspected in infants with unexplained fever and leukocytosis in association with a gingival lesion similar to that described.

Pathogenesis. The pneumococci are strict parasites that are found in the human nasopharynx. They are disseminated in droplets of nasopharyngeal secretions. Infection depends considerably on whether an individual is a carrier of a particular pathogenic pneumococcus at a given time and on some concurrent factor that sufficiently lowers resistance. Most epidemics of pneumococcal pneumonia co-occur with other epidemics (e.g., common cold or influenza) or occur in relatively closed communities such as hospitals, asylums, prisons, and military installations when resistance is low and carrier and contact rates are high.

Factors Affecting Mortality. Mortality in pneumonia is influenced by age, the existence of concomitant disease, the type of causal pneumococcus, the extent of lung involvement, and the presence of bacteremia. Concomitant diseases of special importance are circulatory disturbances, chronic chest diseases, diabetes mellitus, cirrhosis of the liver, and leukemia.

Complications. Complications of pneumococcal pneumonia are concerned either directly with the disease in the chest or with an extension of the infection to other organs or areas of the body. Complications of the disease in the chest are a prolonged febrile course despite treatment (in alcoholics and debilitated individuals), pleural effusion, empyema, superinfection, delayed resolution, and relapse.

Pneumococcal meningitis sometimes occurs in individuals with pneumonia who develop a bacteremia. Pneumococcal endocarditis can be expected to occur in as many as one third of all patients with pneumococcal meningitis. It is more common in elderly individuals than in younger persons.

In addition to meningitis and endocarditis, other complications of pneumococcal pneumonia caused by bacteremia are metastatic localization in the peritoneal or synovial cavities and direct extension of the original infection to cause sinusitis, otitis media, pericarditis, or empyema.

Laboratory Diagnosis. Laboratory diagnosis is important in the treatment of pneumococcal infection. Sputum is stained by the gram method to determine if lanceolate diplococci are present, then cultured on blood agar for isolation and more positive identification. If antisera are available, a capsular swelling test is a rapid and reasonably reliable test for early diagnosis. A blood culture should be done before antibiotic therapy is instituted. Serous and spinal fluids should be examined for diplococci and cultured on adequate media. Diagnosis may also be made by injecting sputum or saliva intraperitoneally into mice. If pathogenic pneumococci are present, the mice will usually die within 48 hours.

Treatment. Pneumococci are most sensitive to penicillin and erythromycin, moderately susceptible to carbomycin, chlortetracycline, oxytetracycline, and tetracycline, less susceptible to chloramphenicol, bacitracin, and streptomycin, and relatively insusceptible to neomycin and polymyxin B. In treatment, penicillin, the tetracyclines, and erythromycin are the antibiotics of choice. Antibiotic therapy has reduced mortality in pneumococcal pneumonia from about 30% to about 5% or less. Early treatment is important to stop the growth and spread of organisms.

ADDITIONAL READING

Baddour, L. M., and Bisno, A. L. 1986. Infective Endocarditis Complicating Mitral Valve Prolapse: Epidemiologic, Clinical, and Microbiologic Aspects. Rev Infect Dis, **8,** 117.

Beachey, E. H., Simpson, W. A., Ofek, I., et al. 1983. Attachment of *Streptococcus pyogenes* to Mammalian Cells. Rev Infect Dis, **5,** S670.

Broughton, R. A., and Baker, C. J. 1983. Role of Adherence in the Pathogenesis of Neonatal Group B Streptococcal Infection. Infect Immun, **39,** 837.

Facklam, R. R. 1977. Physiological Differentiation of Viridans Streptococci. J Clin Microbiol, **5,** 184.

Fischetti, V. A., Jones, K. F., Hollingshead, S. K., and Scott, J. R. 1988. Structure, Function, and Genetics of Streptococcal M Protein. Rev Infect Dis, **10,** S356.

Fleming, H. A. 1987. General Principles of the Treatment of Infective Endocarditis. J Antimicrob Chemother, **20,** Suppl A, 143.

Fox, E. N. 1974. M Proteins of Group A Streptococci. Bacteriol Rev, **38,** 57.

Freedman, L. R. 1987. The Pathogenesis of Infective Endocarditis. J Antimicrob Chemother, **20,** 1.

Kaplan, M. H. 1979. Rheumatic Fever, Rheumatic Heart Disease and the Streptococcal Antigens Cross-Reactive with Heart Tissue. Rev Infect Dis, **1,** 988.

McCarty, M. 1971. The Streptococcal Cell Wall. Harvey Lect, **65,** 73.

Patterson, M. J., and Hafeez, A. E. B. 1976. Group B Streptococci in Human Disease. Bacteriol Rev, **40,** 774.

Peters, G., and Smith, A. L. 1977. Group A Streptococcal Infections of the Skin and Pharynx. N Engl J Med, **297,** 311.

Reed, W. P., Selenger, D. S., Albright, E. L., et al. 1980. Streptococcal Adherence to Pharyngeal Cells of Children with Acute Rheumatic Fever. J Infect Dis, **142,** 803.

Tylewska, S. K., Fischetti, V. A., and Gibbons, R. J. 1988. Binding Selectivity of *Streptococcus pyogenes* and M-Protein to Epithelial Cells Differs from that of Lipoteichoic Acid. Curr Microbiol, **16,** 209.

Unny, S. K., and Middlebrooks, B. L. 1983. Streptococcal Rheumatic Carditis. Bacteriol Rev, **47,** 97.

Wannamaker, L. W. 1983. Streptococcal Toxins. Rev Infect Dis, **5,** S723.

Washington, J. A. 1987. The Microbiological Diagnosis of Infective Endocarditis. J Antimicrob Chemother, **20,** Suppl A, 29.

18

Neisseria

George S. Schuster

The genus *Neisseria,* with one exception, consists of small gram-negative cocci, usually occurring in pairs with adjacent sides flattened. They may have capsules and fimbriae but have no flagella and hence are nonmotile, although some piliated species may show a "twitching motility." Their optimum temperature for growth is 35 to 37°C. For the most part they are oxidase positive and catalase positive, the former feature being quite useful for identification. *Neisseria* species other than *N. meningitidis* and *N. gonorrhoeae* grow on relatively simple nutrient media; *N. meningitidis* and *N. gonorrhoeae,* which respectively cause meningitis and gonorrhea, require more complex media. In addition to *Neisseria* the family Neisseriaceae includes *Branhamella catarrhalis,* a species found in the nasal cavity of man that may participate in respiratory infections or otitis media of infants.

Neisseria: **Gonorrhea and Meningitis**

Neisseria gonorrhoeae

General Characteristics. *N. gonorrhoeae* organisms (commonly gonococci) are gram-negative,

nonmotile, aerobic, nonsporulating cocci that occur singly in culture but in body exudates and phagocytes are diplococci with adjacent sides flattened. Individual cells range from 0.6 to 1.0 μm in diameter. They may possess a capsule of unknown composition. Gonococci may have pili, and these have been related to their virulence.

The colonies of gonococci, which usually develop after 48 hours of incubation, are at first small and transparent but after incubating for several days become grayish white and have a lobate margin.

Cultivation and Metabolism. Gonococci grow best on enriched media containing heated blood or on defined media. Typical media for other bacteria contain fatty acids and trace elements that are inhibitory to growth. Carbon dioxide is an absolute requirement for growth, and a CO_2 concentration as high as 4% to 8% may be necessary during initial isolation. Cultures are difficult to maintain even under the most favorable conditions.

The formation of indophenol oxidase by gonococci is useful for their detection in primary, mixed cultures. Agar plates on which the organisms have grown are treated with a 1% solution of tetramethyl- or dimethyl-*p*-phenylenediamine by flooding or spraying; alternately, single colonies can be tested with a drop of the reagent. Colonies that produce indophenol oxidase become pink, then black. However, many other bacterial species from the genital tract also produce indophenol oxidase.

Glucose is the only carbohydrate ordinarily fermented by gonococci, with the production of acid but no gas.

Antigenic Composition. There are multiple serotypes of gonococci, based on differences in the principal outer membrane proteins. By immunofluorescence involving the intact cell surface, the gonococci have been classified into eight types and subtypes. The pili that have been isolated consist primarily of a single kind of protein subunit. Several serologically distinct types have been found. Also, it appears that there are several serologically heterogeneous determinants of the gonococcal lipopolysaccharide. Tests for these are important in epidemiological studies of gonorrhea. Gonococcal lipopolysaccharide also has endotoxic activity.

Clinical Course of Gonorrhea. Gonococci have a predilection for the mucous membranes of the genital tract. Very shortly after contact with the mucosal surface they attach by pili to the surface cells, thus establishing the infection. Within a few days they penetrate between cells of the mucous membrane to subepithelial connective tissue, where they cause an inflammatory reaction of varying severity consisting of a dense infiltration of polymorphonuclear leukocytes (PMNs). This produces the characteristic mucopurulent discharge. The incubation period is usually 3 to 5 days but may range from 1 to 30 days. In men the onset is typically sudden with a purulent discharge from the urethra (Fig. 18.1) and painful urination; the patient may be febrile. Approximately 10% of cases are asymptomatic, although the individual may transmit the disease.

In women, infection is not as evident since a high proportion are asymptomatic. Also, cases in women are not as easily diagnosed. Signs of the disease include burning and frequency of urination, vaginal discharge, and fever. Infection of the fallopian tubes may produce pelvic inflammatory disease that causes blocking of the tubes, resulting in sterility and fluid accumulation. Gonococcal infection of the birth canal is transmitted to the eyes of newborn infants, producing ophthalmia neonatorum, which frequently results in blindness if untreated.

Gonococcal infection of the oral cavity occurs in adults as a primary infection from oral–genital sex or as a secondary infection transmitted by the hands carrying the gonococci from infected genitalia to the oral cavity or from gonococcemia (Fig. 18.2). In the oral cavity, the incubation period varies from 1 or 2 days to a week or more. Several types of lesions may subse-

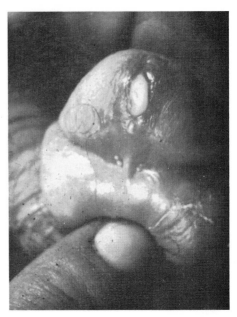

Figure 18.1: Acute gonorrhea. (AFIP 218663.)

quently develop. They range from sharply localized whitish or yellowish white patches to a more generalized lesion covering a large area of the oral mucosa with a grayish adherent membrane that eventually sloughs off, leaving bright areas with numerous bleeding points. The gingivae are usually inflamed and swollen. Pain in the area is a prominent symptom. Areas of the oral cavity most often affected are the gingiva, tongue, and soft palate. Patients with oral gonococcal infection are ill, sometimes seriously so, usually with a temperature above 100°F.

Local lesions and symptoms of oral gonococcal infection may simulate those of Vincent's infection,

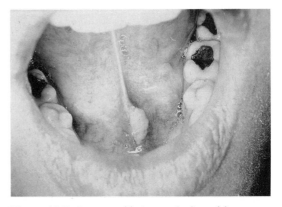

Figure 18.2: Gonococcal lesion on the lingual frenum resulting from gonococcemia. (Reproduced with permission from H. W. Merchant and G. S. Schuster: Oral Gonococcal Infection, *J Am Dent Assoc,* **95,** 808, 1977.)

and pharyngeal streptococcal infection or pharyngeal diphtheria may have a similar superficial appearance. Without a concurrent genital infection, the differential diagnosis may be quite difficult to make and may finally depend on isolation of gonococci from the area.

Gonococci invade tissues and the circulatory system during gonorrheal infections, establishing metastatic infections involving the heart (endocarditis); joints (arthritis); skin (dermatitis), especially on the elbows and dorsal surfaces of the wrists; salivary glands (parotitis); central nervous system (meningitis); and reproductive glands (sterility). Other complications include conjunctivitis and lesions on the oral mucous membranes.

Pathogenesis. Fimbriae are important in the attachment of gonococci to host cells and they are also important in pathogenesis of these organisms, although nonpathogenic species may also possess such structures. Once attached, the gonococci elaborate cytotoxic substances that can damage mucosal cells. Antibodies to these structures are opsonic and also prevent attachment of gonococci to epithelial cells. They may play an antiphagocytic role. Freshly isolated gonococci appear to be encapsulated. This structure also is antiphagocytic. Pathogenic species of *Neisseria* produce an extracellular protein that cleaves the heavy chain of IgA, interfering with its role as an antibody. This enzyme may play a role in pathogenesis.

Diagnosis. The diagnosis of gonorrhea requires the isolation of gram-negative, oxidase-positive diplococci from pus or other exudate and their identification as gonococci by sugar fermentation tests (Fig. 18.3). Microscopic observations of PMNs and intracellular gram-negative diplococci in exudates are valuable but may be misleading in women, owing to the presence of similar-appearing saprophytes in cervical materials. Culture on Thayer-Martin medium or chocolate agar is useful for growing and recognizing

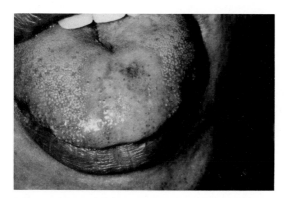

Figure 18.3: Lesion of the tongue in a 25-year-old man. The localized white patch resembled a lesion caused by *Neisseria gonorrhoeae* but by fermentation reactions the causative organism was identified as *Neisseria sicca*.

Neisseria from clinical specimens, for subculture, and for performing an oxidase test. Distinction between species of *Neisseria* is usually based on sugar fermentation: *N. gonorrhoeae* produces acid from glucose but not maltose, sucrose, or lactose. Immunofluorescent staining of exudates and other serological tests are valuable adjuncts to the cultural demonstration of gonococci. The most significant clinical manifestation for diagnosis is a purulent urethral discharge.

Treatment. Uncomplicated gonococcal infections are best treated by intramuscular aqueous procaine penicillin G together with probenecid by mouth. Alternatively, ampicillin by mouth together with probenecid may be used, but this regimen seems to have a slightly lower cure rate than penicillin. For patients who are allergic to penicillin, tetracycline by mouth or spectinomycin intramuscularly are alternative therapies.

Penicillinase-producing gonococci have been recognized in the United States. Patients infected with these strains do not respond to penicillin therapy. If such organisms are isolated, alternate therapies must be used.

Neisseria meningitidis

General Characteristics. Meningococci are aerobic, gram-negative, nonmotile, nonsporulating cocci or diplococci, ordinarily 0.8 μm or less in diameter. Fresh isolates of most serogroups are encapsulated. Like the other neisseriae, meningococci are very susceptible to adverse environmental conditions such as drying or unfavorable pH. Isolates should be put in culture without delay. *N. meningitidis* is difficult to grow, primarily because of complex nutritional requirements and toxic components in ordinary media. The addition of starch or albumin to media reduces toxicity. Organisms from normally sterile sites can be grown on chocolate agar, but if other organisms are present the selective Thayer-Martin medium should be used. Like gonococci, meningococci are oxidase positive.

Antigenic Composition. Virulent meningococci have been divided into groups on the basis of their capsular antigens. Some groups have distinctive protein antigens in the outer membrane that may contribute to induction of host immunity. The somatic antigens are closely related to other *Neisseria* species. These include nucleoprotein, a somatic carbohydrate, and an endotoxin. Meningococci and gonococci also share at least six other heat-stable somatic antigens.

Genetic Variations. Meningococci undergo genetic variation, producing strains that are highly resistant to sulfonamides, and to a lesser degree to penicillin. Penicillin-resistant strains revert to penicillin-sensitive strains when cultured in a penicillin-free medium. When grown in the presence of streptomycin, streptomycin-dependent strains develop whose virulence in experimental animals is enhanced by the presence of streptomycin. Meningococci go quickly from a virulent, smooth form to an avirulent, rough-colony form with loss of the surface antigens.

Meningococcal Infection

Pathogenicity.   The pathogenicity of the meningococcus relates to antiphagocytic and endotoxic mechanisms. The antiphagocytic activity of *N. meningitidis* relates to capsular polysaccharides that inhibit phagocytosis. Meningococci are extracellular parasites that are phagocytized and destroyed in the presence of specific antibody. If they are to produce disease they must be able to resist phagocytosis.

The other virulence factor is the meningococcal endotoxin, which can cause vascular damage. Successive injections of endotoxin elicit the local Shwartzman phenomenon, while single injections produce venous thrombi in bone marrow and lungs and degenerative changes in heart, liver, and spleen. This lipopolysaccharide suppresses leukotriene B_4 synthesis in human PMNs. This loss deprives the leukocyte of a strong chemotactic and chemokinetic factor.

Epidemiology.   The primary habitat of the meningococcus is the nasopharynx of symptomless human carriers. Some 1% to 2% of the population are chronic carriers; an additional 5% to 20% are intermittent carriers. Preceding and during epidemics, carrier rates rise 70% to 90%. Less than 0.1% of an exposed population develops overt disease, indicating that a high carrier rate is not the only determinant.

Meningococcal disease occurs mostly in the young and in the aged. The rate in men is double that in women. In children, infection is related to a high carrier rate but not to the seasons or to a social class. Meningococcal infection is not one of the effective "immunizing infections of childhood."

The Clinical Types of Meningococcal Disease.   The nasopharynx is the point of entry for the meningococci and this precedes hematogenous spread. A local infection occurs in capillaries of the skin and other organs, from which the bacteria are carried to the central nervous system.

Dissemination via the bloodstream results in lesions in various areas such as the skin, meninges, joints, and lungs. Clinical manifestations depend on the site of localization. These include a mild febrile illness accompanied by pharyngitis. Systemic disease is characterized by fever and prostration. An erythematous macular rash may be observed, followed by a petechial eruption that leads to ecchymosis. This is characteristic of fulminant meningococcal disease.

Meningococcemia may be accompanied by meningitis, pericarditis, or arthritis. There may be a suppurative infection of the membranes surrounding the brain and spinal cord. Surviving patients may have permanent sequelae, especially of the nervous system. Pharyngeal lesions due to meningococci but resembling those produced in gonococcal infection have been described. Thus, infections produced by neisseriae must be diagnosed with special care because of possible social and legal implications.

Diagnosis.   The laboratory diagnosis of meningococcal infections consists of the demonstration of meningococci in stained smears from the fluid of the petechial lesions of the skin or in cultures of blood, spinal fluid, and nasopharyngeal secretions on Thayer-Martin medium, chocolate agar, or other appropriate media.

Immunity.   Man is inherently resistant to meningococcal disease. Newborns rarely contract the disease but become susceptible to it as they lose their maternal antibodies. It is likely that they then develop resistance from repeated exposure to subinfective doses of meningococci, or to a nonencapsulated strain, or to an encapsulated strain of low virulence. Recovery from meningococcal disease or the development of a carrier state is accompanied by the appearance of antibodies against both the capsular group-specific polysaccharide and the endotoxin.

Prevention.   The introduction of sulfonamides in 1939 provided a successful prophylactic measure for both civilian and military populations. In time, however, sufficient numbers of the virulent meningococci became resistant to the sulfonamides that this class of drugs was rendered useless. No other chemotherapeutic agent has emerged for widespread prophylaxis, but rifampin is the current drug of choice. Group A and group C capsular polysaccharide vaccines are available and provide good immunity against these serogroups. This is via complement-mediated bactericidal antibodies.

Treatment.   Penicillin is the drug of choice for active disease. In the event of penicillin sensitivity, chloramphenicol is an effective alternative. In systemic infections, supportive therapy is important to the patient's care.

Branhamella catarrhalis

Branhamella catarrhalis is a gram-negative coccus that resembles *Neisseria*. Its normal habitat is the mucous membranes of mammals. Although it is a component of the human flora, it is not totally harmless. Rather, it is a significant cause of systemic infection such as endocarditis, pneumonia, and meningitis, as well as a variety of infections in immunocompromised patients. It has been implicated in acute sinusitis and otitis media in children, and it may cause clinical syndromes indistinguishable from those caused by gonococci.

ADDITIONAL READING

Britigan, B. E., Cohen, M. S., and Sparling, P. F. 1985. Gonococcal Infection: A Model of Molecular Pathogenesis. N Engl J Med, **312,** 1683.

Doern, G. V., and Gantz, N. M. 1982. Isolation of *Branhamella (Neisseria) catarrhalis* from Men with Urethritis. Sex Transm Dis, **9,** 202.

Doern, G. V., Miller, M. J., and Winn, R. E. 1981. *Branhamella (Neisseria) catarrhalis* Systemic Disease in Humans. Arch Intern Med, **141,** 1690.

Duerden, B. I. 1988. Meningococcal Infection. J Med Microbiol, **26,** 161.

Eisenstein, B. I., Sox, T., Biswas, G., Blackman, E., and Sparling, P. F. 1977. Conjugal Transfer of the Gonococcal Penicillinase Plasmid. Science, **195,** 998.

Fiumara, N. J. 1972. The Diagnosis and Treatment of Gonorrhea. Med Clin North Am, **56,** 1105.

Handsfield, H. H., Lipman, T. O., Harnisch, J. P., Tronca, E., and Holmes, K. K. 1974. Asymptomatic Gonorrhea in Men: Diagnosis, Natural Course and Prevalence. N Engl J Med, **290,** 117.

Handsfield, H. H., Sandstrom, E. G., Knapp, J. S., et al. 1982. Epidemiology of Penicillinase-Producing *Neisseria gonorrhoeae* Infections. N Engl J Med, **306,** 950.

Herbert, D. A., and Ruskin, J. 1981. Are the "Nonpathogenic" Neisseriae Pathogenic? Am J Clin Pathol, **75,** 739.

Nankervis, G. A. 1974. Bacterial Meningitis. Med Clin North Am, **58,** 581.

Noble, R. C., and Cooper, R. M. 1979. Meningococcal Colonization Misdiagnosed as Gonococcal Pharyngeal Infection. Br J Vener Dis, **55,** 336.

Swanson, J. 1983. Gonococcal Adherence: Selected Topics. Rev Infect Dis, **5,** 5678.

Yow, M. D., Baker, C. J., Barrett, F. F., and Ortigoza, C. O. 1973. Initial Antibiotic Management of Bacterial Meningitis (Selection in Relationship to Age). Medicine, **52,** 305.

19

Corynebacterium and Diphtheria

George S. Schuster

Although the genus *Corynebacterium* contains many species parasitic to man and animals, the only major pathogen of humans is *C. diphtheriae*, the cause of diphtheria. *C. diphtheriae* is maintained in man, its only natural host, by a small population of chronic carriers who harbor the organism in the nose or nasopharynx. Nonpathogenic corynebacteria, termed diphtheroids, are found on the mucous membranes of the oral cavity, upper respiratory tract, urogenital tract, and eyes. Many diphtheroids have not been adequately characterized or categorized. Two of the defined ones, *C. hofmanni* and *C. xerosis*, are found in the respiratory tract and on the conjunctiva, respectively.

Corynebacterium Diphtheriae

General Characteristics. *C. diphtheriae* are gram-positive, nonmotile, nonsporulating, nonencapsulated, somewhat pleomorphic bacteria. They occur as straight, slightly curved, crooked, or seemingly branched rods. The cells are 2 to 6 μm long and 0.5 to 1 μm in diameter. Under less than optimal growth conditions the organisms may be club-shaped and appear in pallisades or clumps, with angular aggregates resembling Chinese characters. The cells contain bands or beads that stain with methylene or toluidine blue. These are called metachromatic granules or Babès–Ernst granules and are composed of highly polymerized polyphosphates.

C. diphtheriae can be divided into three distinct morphological and cultural types: gravis (rough), mitis (smooth), and intermedius (rough or smooth). There is no relationship between morphological type and virulence.

Growth and Nutrition. The diphtheria bacillus, an aerobe and facultative anaerobe, will grow on a simple medium, but a medium enriched with animal protein is more suitable. Media commonly used are Loeffler's serum medium, or selective media such as blood or chocolate agar containing potassium tellurite. In the latter case, the tellurite is reduced to tellurium and the colonies appear gray to black. *C. diphtheriae* grows over a wide temperature (15 to 40°C) and pH (7.2 to 8.0) range.

Antigenic Composition. *C. diphtheriae* contains thermolabile, alkali-soluble surface protein (K) antigens that are responsible for agglutination reactions. Less specific thermostable carbohydrate (O) antigens have been found in the interior of the bacterial cell. Various combinations of O and K antigens constitute the antigenic structure of the serotypes of *C. diphtheriae*. Lipid antigens are also present but are less specific than the agglutinogens.

Diphtheria Toxin. Pathogenic diphtheria bacilli produce a lethal exotoxin. Toxigenicity is characteristic only of diphtheria bacilli lysogenized by β-prophage or a closely related phage that carries the *tox$^+$* gene for formation of diphtheria toxin. Loss of prophage by a toxigenic strain converts it to a nontoxigenic strain, which in turn can be made toxigenic by reinfection. While the *tox$^+$* gene controls the synthesis of toxin, expression also relates to the physiology and metabolism of the diphtheria bacillus: toxin is synthesized in high amounts when exogenous Fe^{2+} is depleted.

In man and rabbits, diphtheria toxin is lethal in doses of less than 100 μg/kg. When exposed to formalin, the toxin is converted to a toxoid that has no toxicity but is antigenically indistinguishable from the toxin. Vaccines prepared from toxoid elicit protective antibodies against all diphtheria toxins. Diphtheria toxin is a heat-labile protein consisting of a single polypeptide chain with a molecular weight (MW) slightly greater than 61,000 daltons. It may be nicked into a two-fragment complex yielding activated toxin which consists of two polypeptides, A (MW = 21,150) and B (MW = 40,000), linked by two disulfide bridges. Whole toxin liberated by *C. diphtheriae* is converted into the activated complex by enzymes, after which the B fragment binds to receptors on the cell surface. The complex is then cleaved and the A fragment gets into the cytoplasm where it catalyzes a reaction resulting in inactivation of elongation factor 2 (EF-2). Inactivation of EF-2 stops assembly of the polypeptide chain. Apparently only a few hundred molecules of toxin can kill a cell. This may take only a few hours.

Diphtheritic Infections

Man is the sole host and main reservoir of *C. diphtheriae*. Infections are commonly acquired from a patient, a carrier, or a person with subclinical infection via respiratory droplets or direct contact. Contami-nated fomites, dust, or milk are other sources. Infections are most frequent in young children. Following a 2- to 7- day incubation period, pharyngeal infection is usually characterized by headache and a sore throat of slight to moderate intensity. Unlike streptococcal infection, erythema and pain are absent, although prostration out of proportion to the findings is usually present. The course of disease depends on the host's resistance, microbial virulence, and whether respiratory tract obstruction occurs.

Apparently organisms reach and colonize the mucosal surface of the throat before lesions appear. The initial amount of toxin kills underlying epithelial cells and induces a local inflammatory exudate in which organisms grow further. The initial small, yellowish white lesions coalesce and darken; they may spread and include wide areas over the tonsils, posterior pharynx and nares, uvula, soft palate, larynx, and trachea. The tough, grayish white pseudomembrane that forms consists of necrotic cells embedded in a fibrinous exudate. Membranes may loosen and separate, obstructing the respiratory tract.

The cervical lymph nodes become swollen and tender and massive edema of the neck may develop, producing the so-called bull neck. The organisms tend to be largely restricted to mucosal layers and only occasionally spread to lymph nodes and blood. The reason for this failure to invade deep tissues is unknown.

There are two principal causes of death, the systemic effects of toxin and local obstruction of the airway. The most serious effects of the systemic toxemia are cardiac damage and respiratory depression. Cardiac failure results from fatty degeneration of the myocardium or peripheral circulatory collapse. Myocarditis usually manifests after the second week, and death may occur up to several months later. Paralysis of the soft palate due to cranial nerve damage often appears after the third week and leads to regurgitation of fluid through the nose during swallowing. Later complications include paralysis of oculomotor, facial, pharyngeal, diaphragmatic, and intercostal muscles. Respiratory paralysis may result in death in some instances.

Obstruction of the airway is due to excessive edema or a detached pseudomembrane. The latter can occur with great suddenness and requires emergency intubation or tracheotomy.

Patients who recover from diphtheria usually show no permanent effects. Organisms may not be eliminated immediately after recovery but persist for a month or two, producing a convalescent carrier state.

Complications involving the oral cavity directly are rare. Cases have been described in which the entire mucous membrane of the oral cavity was covered with a thick, firmly attached, yellowish membrane. A case has been reported in which a lesion covered with a whitish membrane developed on the lower lip of a child. The site of erupting deciduous teeth and the corners of the mouth also have been the sites for diphtheritic involvement.

Localized diphtheritic infections may occur on lips, nares, and, less often, conjunctiva. Membrane formation is rare and the systemic symptoms are usually mild, but occasionally they are severe. The middle and external ears may be affected by a chronic otitis media of diphtherial origin.

Diphtheria bacilli are also involved in ulcerative, indolent, chronic cutaneous infections in warm or tropical climates (Figs. 19.1 and 19.2). This infection, often called desert sore or tropical ulcer, according to the circumstances of its occurrence, arises at the site of a minor injury. It develops into a persistent ulcer, often lasting for months.

Immunological Aspects. Immunity to infection by diphtheria bacilli is primarily antitoxic, mainly antibodies of the IgG and IgA classes. However, total immunity to toxigenic strains also involves antibac-

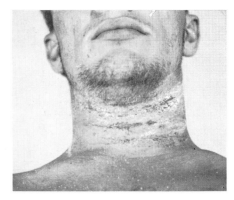

Figure 19.1: Cutaneous diphtheria of the neck. (AFIP A44723–1.)

terial immunity. The nature of this immunity is unknown, but it may be related to blocking of microbial adherence. The human infant is naturally immune to diphtheria only by passive transfer of antitoxin from an immune mother. Where immunization is not practiced, immunity in older children and in adults is de-

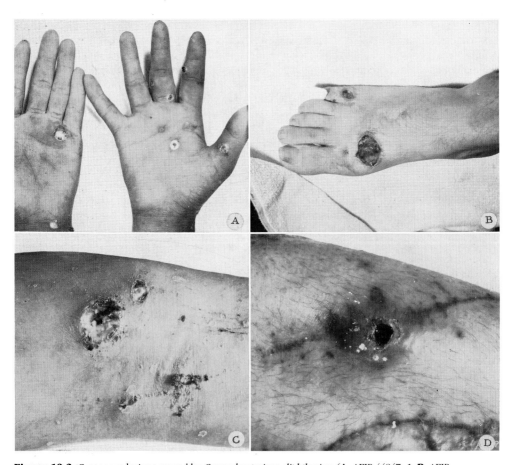

Figure 19.2: Cutaneous lesions caused by *Corynebacterium diphtheriae*. (**A**, AFIP 44847–1; **B**, AFIP L–4360–1; **C**, AFIP 44847–2; **D**, AFIP A–45659–1.)

pendent on natural contact with diphtheria toxin. Recovery from an untreated initial infection with a highly virulent strain is possible only if the individual can survive until antibodies develop. Immunity develops with less danger when the diphtheritic infection is caused by a moderately virulent strain. The degree of immunity achieved by natural immunization is variable and transient and diminishes with time unless boosted by repeated antigenic stimuli.

Mass artificial immunization is effective in substantially reducing the prevalence of diphtheria. In an artificially immunized population, however, most mothers are not sufficiently immune to provide significant passive protection to their offspring. Thus, artificial immunization is effective in controlling diphtheria only when about 70% of a population is effectively immunized.

The Schick Test. The degree of immunity to diphtheria can be measured by the Schick test. In the Schick test diphtheria toxin and a control are injected intracutaneously into the flexor surface of the arms. A positive reaction, negative reaction, pseudoreaction, or combined reaction occurs at the test sites. In a positive reaction, erythema, superficial necrosis, and a brownish pigmentation develop at the test site in 24 hours and last for more than a week. There is no reaction at the control site. In a negative reaction, there is a brief transient response at either the test or control site. In a pseudoreaction, an erythema develops at both control and test sites within 18 hours, increases for not more than 48 hours, and disappears within 3 or 4 days. This reaction indicates immunity plus an allergy. In the combined reaction, the control and test sites both go through the successive stages of an allergic reaction but the reaction at the control site subsides within 3 or 4 days whereas the reaction at the test site persists, indicating an absence of immunity.

Immunization. Active immunization to diphtheria is accomplished by administering various preparations of toxoid. These consist essentially of a purified toxoid administered as fluid or an alum-precipitated compound. The toxoid is given in three successive doses for the immunization of children. It is less suitable for immunization of adults because of a systemic reaction to the bacillary proteins, which is not likely to occur in children. Severe local and systemic reactions may result from the use of toxoids, even when a preliminary skin test indicates no sensitivity to them. A combined tetanus, pertussis, and diphtheria toxoid (DPT) is available for primary immunization in young children, and a highly purified toxoid preparation is now available for administration to older children and adults.

Passive immunity to diphtheria can be established by the injection of antitoxin. The immunity is of short duration but has the somewhat restricted usefulness of protecting highly susceptible individuals exposed directly to the disease.

Laboratory Diagnosis. Prompt treatment in the form of antitoxin administration is critical to recovery. Delays of hours or even minutes may be critical. Thus, diagnosis is usually made on a clinical basis, with laboratory diagnosis serving for confirmation. There are no rapid, reliable, routine laboratory methods available.

Specimens are obtained from the primary lesion. Initial growth and isolation is accomplished on Loeffler's medium, tellurite medium, and blood agar. Growth on blood agar and no growth on tellurite agar indicates no diphtheria bacilli. Growth of typical diphtheria bacilli on tellurite agar indicates their presence. Diagnosis should be made also by injecting the suspected bacteria subcutaneously or intracutaneously into protected and unprotected guinea pigs or rabbits. If the bacteria are toxigenic, a local lesion with superficial necrosis develops in unprotected animals, which then die in 1 to 4 days. The gel diffusion test is also used to determine toxigenicity. In this test a paper impregnated with diphtheria antitoxin is incorporated in agar containing serum. Suspected bacilli are streaked on the agar surface. If diphtheria bacilli are present a line of antigen–antibody precipitate forms.

Treatment. Immediate therapy for diphtheria is imperative. It should be instituted as soon as tests for serum sensitivity are completed. Toxin is quickly bound by tissues and is soon unavailable for antibody neutralization. Antitoxin given on the first day is usually effective, but its effectiveness decreases thereafter and by day 4 it is of little or no value. Suspected diphtheria should be treated immediately with 100 to 500 units of antitoxic serum/lb, depending on the severity of the symptoms. Bacteriological diagnosis should be completed as quickly as possible for confirmation of the clinical diagnosis. Penicillin, cephalosporin, erythromycin, or the tetracyclines are useful adjuncts in the treatment of diphtheria since they tend to discourage continued toxin formation.

Control. The control of diphtheria requires the active immunization of children. Immunization should be done universally by the time the child is 3 months old, at 1 year of age, and again at school age. Such a regimen provides adequate protection until adolescence. Further immunization or boosting of immunity in adults is complicated by their reaction to some component of diphtheria vaccine and is dependent on their immunity status as determined by Schick testing. Although untoward reactions to the vaccine are seldom fatal, they are prevalent enough to preclude mass immunization of adults. Thus, it is important to detect and control carriers and institute emergency prophylactic measures in the case of outbreaks of disease: this includes quarantine, booster immunization, and administration of antibiotics to contacts.

ADDITIONAL READING

Brubaker, R. R. 1985. Mechanisms of Bacterial Virulence. Annu Rev Microbiol, **39**, 21.

Collier, R. J. 1975. Diphtheria Toxin: Mode of Action and Structure. Bacteriol Rev, **39**, 54.

Gill, D. M., Pappenheimer, A. M., Jr., and Uchida, T. 1973. Diphtheria Toxin, Protein Synthesis, and the Cell. Fed Proc, **32**, 1508.

Groman, N. B. 1984. Conversion of Corynephage and Its Role in the Natural History of Diphtheria. J Hygiene (Cambridge), **93**, 405.

Hatano, M. 1956. Effect of Iron Concentration in the Medium on Phage and Toxin Production in a Lysogenic, Virulent *Corynebacterium diphtheriae*. J Bacteriol, **71**, 121.

Maximescu, P., Oprisan, A., Pop, A., and Potorac, E. 1974. Further Studies on *Corynebacterium* Species Capable of Producing Diphtheria Toxin (*C. diphtheriae, C. ulcerans, C. ovis*). J Gen Microbiol, **82**, 49.

Maximescu, P., Pop, A., Oprisan, A., and Potorac, E. 1974. Diphtheria *Tox*[+] Gene Expressed in Corynebacterium Species Other than *C. diphtheriae*. J Hygiene Epidemiol Microbiol Immunol, **18**, 324.

Pappenheimer, A. M., Jr. 1977. Diphtheria Toxin. Annu Rev Biochem, **44**, 69.

Shubil, A. M. 1985. Effect of Antibodies on Adherence of Microorganisms to Epithelial Cell Surfaces. Rev Infect Dis, **7**, 51.

20

Enterobacteriaceae and the Enteric Gram-Negative Microbial Flora

George S. Schuster

Enterobacteriaceae

The family Enterobacteriaceae contains several groups of saprophytic and pathogenic bacteria that inhabit the intestinal tract of man and animals. Other members of the family are plant parasites or soil inhabitants and decomposers of organic material. There are several groups that have similar habitats—i.e., they inhabit the intestinal tract or the soil—but are not Enterobacteriaceae. These include *Bacteroides* species, *Clostridium* species, *Pseudomonas* species, *Vibrio* species, and *Wolinella*. *Bacteroides* and *Clostridium* are discussed in Chapters 21 and 22, respectively, while the remainder will be discussed in this chapter as part of the enteric gram-negative flora. The typical enteric bacilli are gram-negative rods that may vary considerably in size and shape. They are glycolytic, producing acid or acid and gas. Nearly all species reduce nitrate to nitrite. These common characteristics cannot be used to differentiate individual members from each other.

Even when all the differential characteristics available are applied, individual species cannot be clearly differentiated and the groups blend into one another, with many intergrading types. Table 20.1 follows closely but not completely the classification of *Bergey's Manual of Determinative Bacteriology,* 9th edition in listing some of the most important enteric bacteria. Based upon nucleic acid hybridization studies several changes have been proposed in the taxonomy of the Enterobacteriaceae, mostly in *Klebsiella* and *Proteus,* and in *Pseudomonas* species of the family Pseudomonadaceae. These are being incorporated into the current literature and may provide a basis for later reclassification. Indeed, the entire taxonomy of the Enterobacteriaceae is in a state of flux since DNA relatedness studies have shown unexpected homologies that will result in considerable changes in groupings and nomenclature.

The Morphology of the Enterobacteriaceae. The Enterobacteriaceae are small, gram-negative, non-spore-forming rods. They may be motile by peritri-

Table 20.1: Enteric Bacteria

1. Coliform bacilli: *Escherichia coli, Enterobacter aerogenes, Klebsiella pneumoniae, Klebsiella pneumoniae* subsp. *ozaenae, Klebsiella pneumoniae* subsp. *rhinoscleromatis, Serratia marcescens, Edwardsiella tarda, Citrobacter freundii*
2. *Proteus–Providencia* group: *Proteus vulgaris, Proteus mirabilis, Morganella morganii, Proteus rettgeri*, genus *Providencia*
3. *Salmonella:*
   a. Causing human diseases: *Salmonella typhi, Salmonella paratyphi* A, *Salmonella schottmulleri, Salmonella hirschfeldii*
   b. Causing diseases in animals, birds, and humans: *Salmonella typhimurium, Salmonella cholerasuis, Salmonella enteritidis, Salmonella gallinarum, Salmonella arizonae, Salmonella salamae, Salmonella boutenae*
      Note: Attempts have been made to reduce the salmonellae to three species: *Salmonella choleraesuis, Salmonella typhi,* and *Salmonella enteritidis,* with about 1800 serotypes
   c. Causing diseases in animals and birds only: *Salmonella anatum, Salmonella gallinarum, Salmonella pullorum*
4. *Shigella: Shigella dysenteriae, Shigella boydii, Shigella flexneri, Shigella sonnei*
5. *Vibrio: Vibrio cholerae*
6. *Aeromonas* group: *Aeromonas hydrophila, Aeromonas punctata, Aeromonas salmonicida*
7. *Pseudomonas aeruginosa,* and at least 30 other recognized species
8. *Flavobacterium:* Seven species widely distributed in the environment

chous flagella, or nonmotile. Enteric bacteria may possess a well-defined capsule, a loose capsule or slime layer, or no capsule. Many species have pili (fimbriae) for attachment to surfaces or transfer of genetic information.

Physiological and Cultural Characteristics. Enterobacteriaceae are facultative organisms that have diverse biochemical properties. Under anaerobic conditions they ferment carbohydrates, but aerobically they utilize the tricarboxylic acid (TCA) cycle. The different organisms vary in the carbohydrates they ferment, although all ferment glucose. The pathway used in metabolism and the end products produced, such as gas formation, are useful in speciation. Gram-negative enteric bacilli are resistant to some bacteriostatic dyes and surface-active compounds such as bile salts. Use of selective media containing such compounds facilitates the isolation of the enteric bacilli from fecal specimens. A variety of biochemical characteristics have been applied to differentiate the coliform–dysentery–typhoid groups. Especially useful are characteristics collectively known as the IMViC reactions: *i*ndole production, *m*ethyl red acid determination, acetylmethylcarbinol production (*V*oges–Proskauer reaction), and the utilization of *c*itrate. Antigenic analysis also has been used to differentiate coliform–dysentery–typhoid groups.

Antigenic Structure of the Enterobacteriaceae. The antigenic characteristics of enterobacteria are important in their classification and epidemiology. Enterobacteria contain three types of antigens: H, O, and K. Those that are motile contain the protein H antigen in their flagella. The variations in flagella antigen are likely due to differing amino acid sequences.

The polysaccharide O antigen is a somatic antigen present in the cell wall. Within some genera the O antigens are structurally diverse and can be used for serological subgrouping.

The K or capsular antigens are acidic polysaccharides. They may exist as a true capsule or as an overlying layer that blocks O antigen from reacting with homologous antibodies. Vi antigen is a type of K antigen found in only certain species, such as *Salmonella typhi*. It plays a role in the pathogenesis of typhoid fever.

In addition to differential antigens, all enterobacteria possess a common antigen (EAC) that appears to be present on the outer surface of the bacteria and may play a role in host–bacteria interactions. It can be detected by hemagglutination or hemolysis of antigen-covered erythrocytes.

Colicins. Enteric bacilli produce colicins that are able to attach themselves to specific receptors on other susceptible enteric bacilli. They then kill the susceptible bacteria by a variety of means such as blocking phosphorylation, inhibiting protein synthesis, or degrading nucleic acids. They are selective in their activity, attacking only susceptible strains. This helps to stabilize the enteric microbiota.

Coliform Bacilli

Escherichia coli. *E. coli* universally inhabits human and animal intestinal tracts. These organisms are gram-negative, nonsporulating, occasionally encapsulated, variably motile bacilli. *E. coli* is aerobic or facultatively anaerobic and is easily grown on common laboratory media.

E. coli is not very pathogenic for either man or animals, ordinarily serving a useful purpose in the intestinal tract. It is a major source of vitamin K and in some persons a secondary source of B vitamins. It is an opportunist, however, and produces disease when the resistance of the intestinal tract or adjacent areas is lowered sufficiently for it to invade the tissues.

E. coli diarrheal disease is contracted orally by ingesting contaminated food and water. Enterotoxigenic *E. coli* diarrhea occurs in all age groups but mortality is highest in infants, especially undernourished infants. Adults may experience traveler's diarrhea, also caused by enterotoxigenic strains. The pathogenesis is a two-step process: intestinal colonization followed by toxin elaboration. Colonization is achieved by fimbriae. The diarrhea results from hypersecretion of water and electrolytes caused by a heat-stable enterotoxin, a heat-labile enterotoxin, or both. The latter is a protein that acts in a manner similar to *Vibrio cholerae* toxin and shares some antigenic determinants with it.

Diarrheal disease of infants and young children caused by *E. coli* and resembling shigella may also occur. It appears as a bloody diarrhea containing mucus; epithelial destruction is evident. The infection centers in the large intestine and the invasive organisms do not produce either heat-stable or heat-labile enterotoxins.

Diarrheal disease of infants and young children may occur in an epidemic form. This infection resembles *Salmonella* infection in that the bacteria exhibit limited invasion (as far as the lamina propria of the intestinal villi, but not causing massive tissue destruction). It may be that they attach and cause a localized degeneration of epithelial cells. There may be a cytotoxin involved, possibly due to acquisition of an *ent* plasmid, but most strains of the type involved do not produce enterotoxins as determined by the standard assays.

E. coli is often the cause of urinary tract infections. It gains entrance to the urinary tract via the urethra, bladder, and ureters. It commonly causes cystitis (infection of the bladder), but its suppurative infections of the kidney are persistent and difficult to control. *E. coli* often relates to infections of the gallbladder, peritonitis, appendicitis, and other infections along the intestinal tract, including wounds. *E. coli* is frequently encountered in gram-negative bacteremias and septicemias.

E. coli diarrheal disease is transmitted from person to person with no known animal vectors. Transmission is clearly related to poor hygiene and poor general sanitation. Besides cases of traveler's diarrhea and common-source diarrhea, *E. coli* diarrheal disease often occurs as a nosocomial infection in infants.

Control is best achieved by preventing transmission and by proper sanitation. Because death is usually due to dehydration, rehydration in severe cases is an important aspect of treatment. In severe or chronic cases and in the very young, antibiotics may be appropriate. While *E. coli* is generally sensitive to most antibiotics used to treat gram-negative infections, single or multiple resistance to such agents is often present or soon develops in treatment. As a lifesaving measure, more toxic agents are used such as gentamicin, kanamycin, streptomycin, polymyxin, or colistin. Maintenance of fluid balance is critical in management of diarrhea.

Enterobacter. The genus *Enterobacter* has been well characterized only relatively recently. Previously it was not distinguished, especially in clinical isolates. *Enterobacter* organisms are short, frequently encapsulated, gram-negative rods that are usually motile.

The two main species are *Enterobacter aerogenes* and *Enterobacter cloacae*. They can cause similar infections, often of the urinary tract. *E. aerogenes* is often found as a secondary pathogen superinfecting a primary infection. *E. aerogenes* may be found in wound infections, blood, and sputum, as a primary agent or a commensal.

Klebsiella pneumoniae. *K. pneumoniae,* at one time called Friedländer's bacillus, is a gram-negative, nonsporulating, nonmotile, facultatively anaerobic rod. *Klebsiella* species are classified serologically into at least 80 antigenic types.

K. pneumoniae is present in less than 5% of all normal human respiratory tracts. It is also present in the feces of about 5% of normal individuals. It is the cause of less than 3% of all cases of pneumonia and is associated with a few inflammatory suppurative infections. Pneumonia caused by *K. pneumoniae* is highly fatal if untreated and may be attended by such profound changes in the lung as necrosis, abscess formation, and cavitation. The residual lung damage may be so great as to require surgical intervention.

K. pneumoniae is susceptible to most antibiotics that act on gram-negative bacteria except ampicillin and carbenicillin. Cephalosporin is usually effective. Nalidixic acid and nitrofurantoin are effective in treating infections of the urinary tract.

Serratia. The genus *Serratia,* of which *Serratia marcescens* is best known, is composed of gram-negative motile rods that form a red pigment, prodigiosin. They have long been considered to be nonpathogenic but it now seems more likely that they are opportunistic pathogens. They are susceptible to aminoglycoside antibiotics, chloramphenicol, and trimethoprim–sulfamethoxazole.

Members of the *Enterobacter, Klebsiella,* and *Serratia* genera are frequently causes of bacteremia in hospitals. They are also involved frequently in infections associated with respiratory tract manipulations such as tracheotomy, and following the use of contaminated inhalation equipment. *Klebsiella* and *Serratia* are commonly involved in infections following intravenous and urinary tract catheterization and infections complicating burns.

Edwardsiella. A relatively new genus, *Edwardsiella,* was created in 1965 to include a group of motile, gram-negative, lactose-negative bacilli that resemble but are considered distinct from salmonellae. They are found in humans and other mammals and reptiles. They cause acute gastroenteritis and serious septic infections. *Edwardsiella tarda* is the type species.

Citrobacter. The genus *Citrobacter* contains three species, *C. amalonaticus, C. diversus,* and *C. freundii.* At one time these bacteria were called paracolon bacilli. The citrobacteria resemble but are distinct from salmonellae. Although these bacilli are found in normal feces and are not considered true enteric pathogens, they also are associated with human diarrhea, urinary tract infections, and assorted septic infections. They are sensitive to chloramphenicol and the aminoglycoside antibiotics.

Proteus–Providencia Group. The Proteus–Providencia group of the Enterobacteriaceae consists of gram-negative, lactose-negative, motile bacilli that deaminate phenylalanine. *Proteus* species produce abundant urease and grow at an alkaline pH, the latter property helping distinguish them from other enteric bacilli.

The genus *Proteus* contains two clinically important species, *Proteus vulgaris* and *Proteus mirabilis.* Also of importance is *Morganella* (formerly *Proteus*) *morganii* and *Providencia rettgeri.* The most important pathogens of the *Proteus–Providencia* group are *Proteus vulgaris* and *Morganella morganii. Proteus vulgaris* and *Proteus mirabilis* have the peculiar characteristic of "swarming" or intermittent spreading while growing on a moist agar surface. Swarming complicates isolation of other bacterial species mixed with *Proteus* species.

The *Proteus* species are antigenically heterogeneous and have been subdivided on the basis of O, H, and K antigens, but thus far this is not a useful epidemiological tool. Certain strains, designated by the letter X, contain three O antigenic components by which they are divided into OX2, OX19, and OXK groups. These react with antibodies of individuals with rickettsial infections. The cross-reaction (Weil–Felix test) is used in the diagnosis of such rickettsial infections as typhus.

Proteus strains are widely distributed and are involved in the decay of protein. They are rarely found in large numbers in the intestinal tract except when there is some disturbance, as in diarrhea. Collectively, coliform bacilli and *Proteus* are responsible for 40% of all nosocomial infections. *Proteus* is a frequent cause of urinary tract, surgical wound, and lower respiratory tract infections. It may also be a significant cause of bacteremia, most often in elderly patients. *Proteus* species are sensitive to aminoglycosides and trimethoprim–sulfamethoxazole. Only *P. mirabilis* is sensitive to ampicillin and cephalothin.

The genus *Providencia* contains enteric bacteria that occur in the feces of normal individuals as well as those with diarrhea.

Pseudomonas

Organisms of the genus *Pseudomonas* appear as straight or slightly curved rods, 0.5 to 1.0 by 1.5 to 5.0 μm. They are gram negative and usually motile by one or several polar flagella. They are aerobic, having a strictly respiratory type of metabolism with oxygen as the terminal electron acceptor.

The genus *Pseudomonas* contains more than 140 species, most of which are saprophytic. Of the more than 25 species associated with humans, most known to cause human disease are associated with opportunistic infections. *P. aeruginosa* and *P. maltophilia* account for approximately 80% of those recovered from clinical specimens. *P. aeruginosa* receives the most attention. It is a ubiquitous, free-living organism that can be found in most moist environments and is a major threat to hospitalized patients. It seldom causes disease in healthy individuals.

Biochemical and Cultural Characteristics. *P. aeruginosa* is an extremely adaptable organism that can utilize over 80 different organic compounds for growth, and ammonia can serve as a nitrogen source. It can grow at 42°C, although 35°C is optimal. Clinical isolates often are β-hemolytic.

P. aeruginosa is more resistant to chemical disinfection than other vegetative bacteria. In the presence of adequate moisture it can survive in a variety of places such as respiratory equipment, humidifiers, floors, baths, and water faucets. Most of the commonly used antimicrobials are ineffective against *P. aeruginosa.* It has been isolated from quaternary ammonium compounds and hexachlorophene soaps. Phenolics and glutaraldehyde are usually effective disinfectants.

Pathogenesis and Pathology. The mechanisms by which *P. aeruginosa* produce disease are not understood. There are a number of enzymes and toxins that cause pathologic effects in animals but whose role in human disease is not clear. Two proteases may be responsible for the hemorrhagic skin lesions in some infections, and in eye infections may cause destruction of corneal tissue. There are two hemolysins, one of which is a phospholipase that also may contribute to invasiveness of the lung. There are at least three exotoxins, one of which inhibits protein synthesis. Their role in disease is unclear. In addition a pigment termed pyocyanin is produced. It may contribute to overall disease through its effect on oxygen uptake of cells, including leukocytes.

P. aeruginosa infections occur in individuals with altered host defenses. These include burn patients, patients with malignant or metabolic disease, or those who have undergone surgical manipulations. Localized lesions occur at the site of burns or wounds. Infection of corneal tissues can result in loss of the eye. The organisms can spread and by septicemia initiate focal lesions in other tissues. With septicemia, mortality may reach 80%. Empyema is common. Since the major body defense against *Pseudomonas* infection is a functioning phagocytic system, mortality is high in patients with leukemia, especially when they become severely leukopenic.

Diagnosis and Treatment. Diagnosis is made by isolating the organisms. *P. aeruginosa* will grow on almost any laboratory medium. Most antimicrobials are ineffective against *P. aeruginosa,* so prevention of infection is the major means of control. Many strains are susceptible to aminoglycosides but resistant forms develop, especially during prolonged treatment. Some strains are sensitive to carbenicillin. Gentamicin and carbenicillin appear to act synergistically and may be useful in combination for serious infection. Ciprofloxacin has proved to be quite useful to treat *Pseudomonas* pneumonia.

Eikenella

The genus *Eikenella* currently contains one species, *E. corrodens*. The *Eikenella* are straight rods, 0.3 to 0.4 by 1.5 to 4.0 μm. They are gram-negative, non-sporeforming, facultative anaerobes. They lack flagella and are nonmotile in the typical sense, although a "twitching motility" may occur on agar surfaces. The organisms are oxidase positive and negative for catalase, urease, and indole. No acid is formed from glucose or other carbohydrates. The colonies appear to corrode the surface of agar, although noncorroding strains may occur. They are nonhemolytic, although a slight greening of blood media may occur around the colonies.

E. corrodens is a normal inhabitant of the human intestine and oral cavity. It is sometimes pathogenic, and when isolated from lesions it often is in mixed culture with other facultative bacteria or with anaerobes. It may become the predominant or sole survivor of antibiotic-treated mixed infections. Infection of the sinuses, oral cavity, and upper and lower respiratory tract is not uncommon. Serious infections reported include Ludwig's angina and brain abscesses,

as well as liver abscesses, peritonitis, and wound infections. Meningitis, endocarditis, and osteomyelitis also have been described. In general, *E. corrodens* is regarded as an opportunistic pathogen.

Most strains of *E. corrodens* are usually sensitive to penicillin G, ampicillin, and some cephalosporins, but resistant to others. They often are sensitive to tetracyclines and rifampicin but are constantly resistant to lincomycin and clindamycin.

Salmonella

Taxonomy of *Salmonella*. The genus *Salmonella* comprises a biochemically and serologically diverse group of organisms that infect humans and many animal species. Most are motile, produce H_2S from thiosulfate and gas from glucose fermentation; they rarely ferment lactose. The genus *Salmonella* has been classified by a variety of ways due to the large number of serotypes. One of the more useful is the scheme of Kauffman and White. By use of H, O, and Vi antigens about 1,800 serotypes of salmonellae have been identified. These have been grouped into five so-called subgenera designated I to V. These are further divided into serotypes or serovars, some of which have specific names while others are designated only by their antigenic formula. An alternative scheme classifies them into three species, *S. typhi, S. choleraesuis,* and *S. enteritidis,* with various antigenic types as serotypes.

Poultry products are the largest source of nontyphoid salmonellosis. Improperly cooked or stored meat may permit growth of the organisms, resulting in infection. Dried eggs may also act as a source, either directly or as a contaminant when used in other food products. Household pets including turtles may harbor *Salmonella* and act as a source of infection.

The clinically distinct diseases resulting from *Salmonella* infections depend on the species involved, the number of microorganisms ingested, and the resistance of the susceptible individual. These diseases are gastroenteritis, typhoid and other enteric fevers, and septicemia. The latter condition usually arises from a localized focus of infection in some organ.

Salmonella gastroenteritis is usually caused by *S. enteritidis,* serotype *typhimurium,* although any species can cause it. It has an incubation period of about 24 hours and is characterized by the sudden onset of abdominal pain, nausea, vomiting, diarrhea, and fever. It usually lasts 2 to 5 days and is self-limiting.

Typhoid fever is exclusively a human disease caused by *S. typhi.* Milder enteric fevers are caused by *S. paratyphi, S. schottmulleri,* and *S. hirschfeldii.* Typhoid fever has an incubation period of less than 14 days, during which the bacteria multiply intracellularly in lymphoid tissue. Onset is insidious with headache, malaise, anorexia, and a febrile period in which body temperature increases stepwise to an average of 104°F (40°C). The disease continues for about 3 weeks, with the temperature returning to normal after a period of gradual remission during the third week.

The incubation period of the milder enteric fevers is usually less than 10 days and the duration is similar to or less than that of typhoid fever. The symptoms are similar to those of typhoid fever but less severe.

Salmonellae may localize in joints, heart, lungs, or other organs and produce local abscesses. From such foci, salmonellae enter the bloodstream, causing a septicemia with a high, rheumatic-type fever.

Immunity to *Salmonella*. A lasting immunity develops during an attack of typhoid fever. Immunity to salmonellosis relates to anti-O and anti-Vi antibodies. Anti-H antibodies have no apparent protection. However, a high antibody titer may be present during relapses or fatal, terminal stages of the disease due to the bacilli multiplying intracellularly.

Pathogenicity of *Salmonella*. In man, *Salmonella* species are transmitted from sick humans, infected animals, or healthy carriers to susceptible individuals. Temporary and permanent carriers are common. Salmonellae leave the infected or carrier individual in feces or urine which contaminates milk, food, or water and gain entrance into the body through the intestinal tract. The organisms pass through the epithelium into the subepithelial tissues. After penetration, the organisms are ingested by macrophages, where they multiply and may be carried to other sites. The ability of the organisms to survive intracellularly may be due to surface O antigens or the Vi antigen, since organisms containing the latter antigen are more virulent than those lacking it.

The exact role of endotoxin in *Salmonella* infections is not clear but it may be responsible for fever and possibly shock during bacteremia. It also may cause localization of leukocytes in the tissue due to activation and resulting chemotactic properties of complement. Several species of *Salmonella* contain enterotoxin, although its role in salmonellosis is not understood.

Major epidemics of typhoid fever are caused by contaminated drinking water or food. Wherever adequate sanitary measures have been applied, typhoid fever has nearly disappeared. Small outbreaks are sometimes traced to typhoid carriers among institutional or restaurant food handlers. Vaccines prepared from *S. typhi* cells have long been used prophylactically. The vaccines have proved somewhat successful in children but none has proved entirely effective in preventing disease.

Laboratory Diagnosis of *Salmonella*. The laboratory diagnosis of *Salmonella* infection consists principally in the isolation and identification of the causative microorganisms or the demonstration of a rise in specific agglutinins within 1 or 2 weeks after the onset of the disease. Stool specimens are the best source of organisms during acute gastroenteritis. Blood cultures are best for detection of enteric fevers and septicemia. In typhoid bone marrow cultures may be positive, even after blood becomes negative. Urine also may be positive.

Treatment of *Salmonella* Infections. The treatment of typhoid fever and other *Salmonella* infections centers on generalized supportive care of the patient and antibiotics. Ampicillin or chloramphenicol are the drugs of choice, although resistance to these has occurred. In such cases trimethoprim–sulfamethoxazole has proved effective. Ampicillin, possibly with cholecystectomy, may be used in chronic carriers.

Prevention and Control of *Salmonella* Infections. Considerable success has been achieved in *Salmonella* control by modern methods of livestock slaughter, better control and supervision of meat, eggs, and other animal products consumed by man, proper sewage disposal, and a carefully controlled water supply. The detection and control of human *Salmonella* carriers have greatly helped to control typhoid fever and other human salmonelloses. Active immunization is not as effective as are sanitary procedures and the elimination of carriers.

The Shigellae

Shigellae are primarily human pathogens that cause infections of the intestinal tract characterized primarily by diarrhea. Although fermentation reactions are useful for separation and differentiation, final identification of the various species is dependent on their antigenic structure. The recognized species are *Shigella dysenteriae*, *Shigella boydii*, *Shigella flexneri*, and *Shigella sonnei*. *S. flexneri* and *S. dysenteriae* are the most common causes of dysentery.

Bacteriological Characteristics of the Shigellae. The morphology of the shigellae closely resembles that of the other enteric bacteria. Shigellae are facultatively anaerobic, having both respiratory and a fermentative type of metabolism. They are gram-negative, nonmotile, nonsporulating rods. The shigellae are not very resistant to either physical or chemical agents and do not survive for long in the environment. They are particularly sensitive to acids; hence, if they are to be isolated from feces they must be cultured promptly or they will die from the acid produced by other fecal bacteria.

Pathogenicity of *Shigella*. The causal organisms are usually transmitted to the digestive tract of the susceptible individual in contaminated food or water. They penetrate the epithelial cells of the terminal ileum and colon, multiply, and cause cell death and sloughing of the lining. The incubation period may be as short as 24 hours. The onset of the disease is characterized by abdominal pain and cramps caused by an acute inflammatory reaction of the mucous membranes of the large bowel and occasionally the terminal ileum. Ulceration may occur, with hemorrhage and the production of mucin. Septicemia does not occur and the infection is self-limited. During the severe diarrhea, dehydration and disturbance of the electrolyte balance are frequent concomitants. Shigellae produce a heat-labile enterotoxin that can cause fluid accumulation in ileal loops of rabbits. The role of the toxin in disease is not clear since invasive but nontoxigenic strains of *S. dysenteriae* can cause disease. It may be responsible for the watery diarrhea that occurs in *Shigella*-induced dysentery.

Immunity to *Shigella*. Abundant humoral antibodies are formed during a dysentery infection. However, recovery from the disease does not correlate with the appearance of specific antibodies. Individuals living in regions where the dysentery bacilli are indigenous become resistant if not immune to recurrent attacks of bacillary dysentery. Local tissue immunity may be the most important protective factor. Although *Shigella* vaccines have been prepared that induce a high antibody titer, they are not effective.

Laboratory Diagnosis of *Shigella*. The laboratory diagnosis of dysentery consists principally of the isolation and identification of the causal microorganisms. Diagnosis of dysentery retrospectively by the demonstration of specific agglutinin formation is not very practical. The demonstration of a rise in antibody titer during the course of the disease is the only significant demonstration of specific antibody formation. Serological typing and biochemical studies are necessary for complete diagnosis and identification.

Treatment of *Shigella*. Although many do not seek treatment and the disease may be self-limiting, antimicrobial therapy decreases severity and mortality of the disease. Especially in the debilitated and in young children and the elderly, antibiotic therapy is indicated. While ampicillin is the drug of choice, most shigellae are sensitive to tetracyclines, streptomycin, sulfonamides, kanamycin, chloramphenicol, nalidixic acid, and colistin. However, trimethoprim–sulfamethoxazole also is effective. *Shigella* is notorious for its ability to quickly develop drug resistance.

Prevention and Control of *Shigella*. The control of bacillary dysentery requires careful disposition of excreta. Careful consideration must also be given to the detection of subclinical or symptomless cases that may become carriers. No convalescent patient should be released while still discharging dysentery bacilli. Food and water must be protected and flies must be controlled.

The Vibrios

The genus *Vibrio* is composed of 22 recognized species and a number of biotypes that are variously parasitic, pathogenic, and widely distributed as saprophytes in water and soil. *Vibrio cholerae* causes cholera, a waterborne gastrointestinal disease in areas of inadequate sanitation, which normally affects only human beings. *Vibrio* strains not capable of producing true cholera have been isolated in tropical areas. Nontoxigenic strains of *V. cholerae* may be isolated from the environment. Other *Vibrio* species that are not pathogenic for man produce disease in birds, animals, or fish.

Vibrio cholerae. *V. cholerae* is a gram-negative, nonsporulating, slightly curved rod that is markedly pleomorphic under adverse conditions. The cells are actively motile by a single polar flagellum. It is considered a facultative anaerobe. A biotype of *V. cholerae* was first isolated at the El Tor quarantine station on the Sinai Peninsula. It is antigenically similar but differs from *V. cholerae* by being hemolytic and less virulent. El Tor vibrios produce a more mild diarrheal disease. Other similar types were isolated and for a time these bacteria were considered to be distinct species.

Pathogenesis of Cholera. Cholera is primarily acquired by the ingestion of the *V. cholerae* in contaminated water or food. The incubation period ranges from 1 to 5 days but is commonly no longer than 3 days. At the end of the incubation period cholera begins suddenly with the development of abdominal cramps, nausea, vomiting, and diarrhea. In the more severe form there is a voluminous liquid feces (rice water stools) discharged that is composed of mucus, epithelial cells, and 10^6 or more vibrios per milliliter, but it contains practically no protein. Patients with cholera may discharge as much as 10 to 15 L of fluid per day, resulting in an extracellular fluid deficit, metabolic acidosis, and hypokalemia of sufficient severity to quickly produce shock and death. In either mild or severe cholera, the vibrios do not invade or disrupt the intestinal mucosa. They are able to maintain themselves in large numbers on the surface of the intestinal mucosa where they produce the cholera enterotoxin, which at submicrogram levels is able to stimulate a net flow of fluids and electrolytes from cells into the lumen of the gut, producing symptoms characteristic of the disease.

Laboratory Diagnosis of *Vibrio*. Laboratory procedures essential to the exact diagnosis of cholera are the detection and identification of the organisms. Essential to diagnosis is the cultivation of *V. cholerae* from stools, but not from vomitus, in which they are inconstant. Many types of media have been used for cultivation, but the usual enteric media are suboptimal for growth and isolation. Specialized media are available for growth of *V. cholerae*. Once isolated the organisms can be identified by staining with fluorescein-labeled specific antisera and by biochemical and agglutination tests.

Treatment of *Vibrio*. The current treatment of cholera consists of the restoration of lost liquids and electrolytes, usually resulting in dramatic recovery. This is accomplished by the intravenous administration of isotonic sodium chloride containing appropriate amounts of sodium bicarbonate or sodium acetate and potassium chloride. The administration of tetracycline will also assist in preventing intestinal fluid loss by decreasing the number of organisms. Although antibiotics are useful in the treatment of cholera, they are not a complete substitute for fluid and ion restoration.

Prevention and Control of Cholera. The prevention and control of cholera are problems of public and private hygiene, mostly concerned with removing factors that favor the spread of the disease. Certainly, decontamination of drinking water is an important measure, as is the improvement of environmental sanitation. Safeguarding food and drinks by control of manufacturing processes or conditions under which they are sold, particularly during epidemics, is important in checking the spread of the disease. The early detection and isolation of cholera victims, particularly those without severe signs, are important life-saving and control measures. Various methods have been used to treat convalescent and contact carriers. Many of those concerned with prevention and control of cholera believe that the parenteral administration of killed vaccines is useful.

Campylobacter

Campylobacter organisms are slender, spirally curved rods, 0.2 to 0.5 by 0.5 to 5 μm, although as cultures age coccoid forms appear. They are motile with a corkscrew-like motion by means of a single polar flagellum at one or both ends. They are microaerophilic, with a respiratory type of metabolism. Carbohydrates are neither fermented nor oxidized. *Campylobacter* is found in the reproductive organs, intestinal tract, and oral cavity of man and animals. There are five species, *C. fetus, C. jejuni, C. coli, C. sputorum,* and *C. concisus. C. fetus* and *C. sputorum* have named subspecies. *C. jejuni* and *C. coli* cause diarrheal disease; *C. fetus* subsp. *fetus* causes systemic illness, mostly in debilitated individuals; *C. sputorum* subsp. *sputorum* is found in the gingival crevice of humans; and *C. concisus* is found in the gingival crevice of humans with gingivitis and periodontitis.

Pathogenesis and Pathology. *C. jejuni* is probably the most frequent pathogen of this group.

The attack rate varies with the ingested dose. In enteritis the incubation period ranges from 1 to 7 days, with most cases falling in the range of 2 to 4 days. In the intestine there is an acute exudative and hemorrhagic inflammation, and the lesions may appear identical to those in ulcerative colitis. The mechanisms of pathogenesis are not known, although bacteremia and tissue invasion are likely factors. Many isolates produce a cytotoxin and enterotoxin but their clinical significance is unknown.

C. jejuni infections often appear as acute gastroenteritis with fever, diarrhea (perhaps bloody), and abdominal pain, which may be quite severe. Nausea and vomiting are less common. The illness may last from 1 day to several weeks, although it frequently is self-limited within 7 days.

Diagnosis. *Campylobacter* enteritis is not easily distinguished clinically from illness due to other enteric pathogens. Presence of gram-negative organisms and the appearance of darting motile strains in a fresh fecal specimen may permit a presumptive diagnosis to be made. Definite diagnosis is made by isolation from a fecal culture.

Epidemiology and Control. *Campylobacter* enteritis is usually acquired from contaminated food or water, or from products from animals that carry the organisms in their intestinal tract. In some countries, usually underdeveloped, up to 40% of healthy children may be carrying and excreting the organism. This is an age-related phenomenon with the highest excretion rates in very young children. The reasons for the difference in developed and developing countries is not known. In developed countries where infection is usually associated with illness the highest rate occurs during summer months and in persons 10 to 29 years old. Infection may be acquired by drinking untreated water, eating undercooked foods such as chicken, beef, or turkey, or eating raw clams. Direct contact with infected domestic animals and wild birds also has been implicated in transmission. Person-to-person transmission appears to be uncommon.

Control involves avoiding contaminated food or drink, proper cooking of food, and good personal hygiene. Individuals with severe or prolonged symptoms may be treated with antimicrobials; erythromycin and tetracycline appear to be the agents of choice.

Orofacial Infections

Gram-negative enteric bacteria may inhabit the oropharynx and, as a result, produce infections of this region. These are a particular problem in elderly and chronically ill patients and those in whom antibiotic therapy has depressed the gram-positive bacterial population. In the chronically ill patient, such infections become more common as the level of illness increases and the level of self-care decreases. The organisms found include *Escherichia coli, Enterobacter* species, *Pseudomonas aeruginosa, Proteus* species, *Klebsiella* species, and other members of the Enterobacteriaceae. These have been isolated from soft tissue infections and osteomyelitis, most often as a component of a mixed infection. The pattern of infections suggests that many are secondary infections or exacerbations of subacute infections. Many patients have received antibiotics for several days or weeks in association with some oral surgical procedure or infection. Acute infections with the enteric bacteria appear usually as a low-grade fever and an obvious swelling filled with thick, possibly foul-smelling purulent material. Treatment usually entails drainage and adjunctive antibiotic therapy. However, since these organisms are resistant to many antibiotics, the antibiotic must be selected with particular care.

ADDITIONAL READING

Carpenter, C. C. J. 1971. Cholera: Diagnosis and Treatment. Bull NY Acad Med, **47,** 1192.

Carpenter, C. C. J. 1972. Cholera and Other Enterotoxin-related Diarrheal Diseases. J Infect Dis, **126, 551.**

Clementi, K. J. 1975. Treatment of *Salmonella* Carriers with Trimethoprim-Sulfamethoxazole. Can Med Assoc J, **112,** 28S.

Collins, C. M. 1973. Importation of Cholera into New Zealand, 1972. NZ Med J, **78,** 105.

Costerton, J. W., Ingram, J. M., and Cheng, K. J. 1974. Structure and Function of the Cell Envelope of Gram-Negative Bacteria. Bacteriol Rev, **38,** 87.

Donta, S. T. 1975. Changing Concepts of Infectious Diarrheas. Geriatrics, **30,** 123.

Dupont, H. L. 1978. Enteropathogenic Organisms. Med Clin North Am, **62,** 945.

Dupont, H. L., Formal, S. B., Hornick, R. B., Snyder, M. J., Libonati, J. P., et al. 1971. Pathogenesis of *E. coli* Diarrhea. N Engl J Med, **285,** 1.

Dupont, H. L., Hornick, R. B., Snyder, M. J., Libonati, J. P., Formal, S. B., and Gangarosa, E. J. 1972. Immunity in Shigellosis: Parts I and II. J Infect Dis, **125,** 12.

Etkin, S., and Gorbach, S. L. 1971. Studies on Enterotoxin from *Escherichia coli* Associated with Acute Diarrhea in Man. J Lab Clin Med, **78,** 81.

Finegold, D. C. 1970. Hospital-Acquired Infections. N Engl J Med, **283,** 1384.

Formal, S. B., Semski, P., Jr., Giannella, R. A., and Austin, S. 1972. Mechanisms of *Shigella* Pathogenesis. Am J Clin Nutr, **25,** 1427.

Gangarosa, E. J. 1971. The Epidemiology of Cholera: Past and Present. Bull NY Acad Med, **47,** 1140.

Gangarosa, E. J., Beisel, W. R., Chanys, B., Sprinz, H., and Prapont, P. 1960. The Nature of the Gastrointestinal Lesion in Asiatic Cholera and Its Relation to Pathogenesis: A Biopsy Study. Am J Trop Med Hyg, **9,** 125.

Gangarosa, E. J., and Faich, G. A. 1971. Cholera: The Risk to American Travelers. Ann Intern Med, **74,** 412.

Garroway, R. Y., and Ordway, C. B. 1980. *Serratia marcescens* Osteomyelitis: Report of Two Cases. J Trauma, **20,** 1007.

Goodwin, C. S. 1986. *Campylobacter pyloridis,* Gastritis and Peptic Ulceration. J Clin Pathol, **39,** 353.

Gorbach, S. L. 1971. Intestinal Microflora. Gastroenterology, **60,** 1110.

Gyles, C. L. 1972. Plasmids in Intestinal Bacteria. Am J Clin Nutr, **25,** 1455.

Holmgren, J., and Lonnroth, I. 1976. Cholera Toxin and the Adenylate Cyclase-Activating Signal. J Infect Dis, **133,** S64.

Hornick, R. B., Greisman, S. E., Woodward, T. E., Dupont, H. L., Dawkins, A. T., and Snyder, M. J. 1970. Typhoid Fever: Pathogenesis and Immunologic Control. N Engl J Med, **283,** 686.

Keusch, G. T., and Grady, G. F. 1972. The Pathogenesis of *Shigella diarrhea:* I. Enterotoxin Production by *Shigella dysenteriae.* J Clin Invest, **51,** 1212.

Kurosky, A., Markel, D. E., Touchstone, B., and Peterson, J. W. 1976. Chemical Characterization of the Structure of Cholera Toxin and Its Natural Toxoid. J Infect Dis, **133** (Suppl), S14.

Laforce, F. M., Hopkins, J., Trow, R., and Wang, W. L. L. 1976. Human Oral Defenses against Gram-Negative Rods. Am Rev Respir Dis, **114,** 929.

Lifshitz, F. 1977. The Enteric Flora in Childhood Disease-Diarrhea. Am J Clin Nutr, **30,** 1811.

Marshall, B. J. 1986. *Campylobacter pyloridis* and Gastritis. J Infect Dis, **152,** 650.

Mathewson, J. J., Johnson, P. C., Dupont, H. I., et al. 1985. A Newly Recognized Cause of Traveler's Diarrhea: Enteroadherent *Escherichia coli.* J Infect Dis, **151,** 471.

Mills, J., and Drew, D. 1976. *Serretia marcescens* Endocarditis: A Regional Illness Associated with Intravenous Drug Abuse. Ann Intern Med, **84,** 29.

Morris, J. G., Jr., and Black, R. E. 1985. Cholera and Other Vibrioces in the United States. N Engl J Med, **312,** 343.

Pierce, N. F., Greenough, W. B., and Carpenter, C. C. J. 1971. *Vibrio cholerae* Enterotoxin and Its Mode of Action. Bacteriol Rev, **35,** 1.

Polin, K., and Shulman, S. T. 1982. *Eikenella corrodens* Osteomyelitis. Pediatrics, **70,** 462.

Pollack, M. 1984. The Virulence of *Pseudomonas aeruginosa.* Rev Infect Dis, **6,** S617.

Rose, H. D., Heckman, M. G., and Unger, J. D. 1973. *Pseudomonas aeruginosa* Pneumonia in Adults. Am Rev Respir Dis, **107,** 416.

Rosenbaum, B. J. 1972. Modern Concepts in the Treatment of Cholera. Milit Med, **137,** 26.

Sack, D. A., Wells, J. G., Merson, M. H., Sack, R. B., and Morris, G. K. 1975. Diarrhoea Associated with Heat-Stable Enterotoxin-producing Strains of *Escherichia coli.* Lancet, **2,** 239.

Steffen, R., van des Linde, F., Gyr, K., and Schar, M. 1983. Epidemiology of Diarrhea in Travelers. JAMA, **249,** 476.

Stein, K., Nersasian, R. R., O'Keefe, P., et al. 1978. *Eikenella* Osteomyelitis of the Mandible Associated with Anemia of Chronic Disease. J Oral Surg, **36,** 285.

Walker, R. I. 1986. Pathophysiology of *Campylobacter* Enteritis. Microbiol Rev, **50,** 81.

Washington, J. A., II. 1976. Laboratory Approaches to the Identification of Enterobacteriaceae. Hum Pathol, **7,** 151.

21

Anaerobic Bacteria

George S. Schuster

Bacteroides and *Fusobacterium*

Bacteroides and *Fusobacterium* are gram-negative bacilli that are important members of the normal body flora. They are involved in a variety of infectious processes at various sites. There are numerous species, especially in the gastrointestinal tract and the oral cavity. *Bacteroides fragilis* is one of the most commonly encountered enteric pathogens. Many of the oral species are associated with disease processes in the orofacial region, although their role is not always clear. *Fusobacterium nucleatum* is the most commonly encountered species in this genus. *F. necrophorum*, although less frequently encountered, may produce serious disease. In addition, other species in both of these genera can produce disease, although less frequently.

General Characteristics of *Bacteroides*

Organisms of the genus *Bacteroides* are gram-negative, obligately anaerobic, non-spore-forming rods. They are nonmotile or motile by peritrichous flagella. The cells have rounded ends and, depending on the species, are about 0.5 to 0.8 µm in diameter and 1.6 to 8.0 µm long. Terminal or central swellings, vacuoles, or filaments are common in many species, and some are encapsulated. Cells may be more pleomorphic when grown under less than ideal conditions. *Bacteroides* organisms require relatively complex media. Carbon dioxide is required or utilized and is incorporated into succinic acid. Hemin is required or stimulatory for growth of many species, especially the saccharoclastic ones. Some species produce a brown to black pigment, which is a heme derivative that colors the colony. Similarly, vitamin K is required or highly stimulatory for growth of some species, and both of these supplements are routinely added to culture media.

The cellular composition of *Bacteroides* is much like that of other gram-negative rods. Of particular interest is the endotoxin, which is different from that of the typical gram-negative species such as *E. coli. Bacteroides* endotoxins contain no heptose or

Table 21.1: *Bacteroides* Species Detected in the Human Mouth*

Nonpigmented Species	Pigmented Species
B. oralis	B. gingivalis
B. buccae	B. intermedius
B. oris	B. melaninogenicus
B. zoogleoformans	B. endodontalis
B. forsythus	B. loescheii
B. gracilis	B. denticola
B. ureolyticus	
B. capillosus	
B. pneumosintes	
B. fragilis	

*B. pneumosintes and *B. fragilis* are not commonly found.

2-ketodeoxyoctonate. The lipid A component is absent or different from that of the typical endotoxin as well. The endotoxins show little chemotoxic activity: what is shown is complement dependent, using the alternate pathway.

The guanine plus cytosine (G + C) content of the DNA is quite variable, ranging from 28 to 61 mol%. The DNA of black-pigmented *Bacteroides* strains isolated from the human oral cavity shows 47 to 49 mol% G + C, whereas that of nonoral strains has between 52 and 53 mol% G + C.

The ninth edition of *Bergey's Manual* lists 39 species of the genus *Bacteroides*. There is some confusion in the nomenclature of these organisms because of new isolates, and several investigators have given different names to what may be the same species. The nonoral species most frequently encountered as pathogens are *B. fragilis*, followed by *B. thetaiotaomicron*. Those currently believed to make up part of the oral microflora can be broadly divided into black (or brown)-pigmented and nonpigmented types. Table 21.1 lists names of *Bacteroides* species found in the mouth. Because of the rapidly changing classification and nomenclature, the literature regarding the locale and role of these species in disease, especially of the oral cavity, is confusing. As molecular probes for identification become more common, the classification of these organisms will become clearer. It is already known that the DNAs of oral and nonoral strains have no significant homology.

Bacteriophages active against *Bacteroides* species, especially *B. fragilis*, are not uncommon. Plasmids have been found in about one-half the strains tested. For some of these plasmids the significance is unknown; however, some do code for antibiotic resistance to a wide variety of antimicrobials.

General Characteristics of Fusobacteria

Members of the genus *Fusobacterium* are obligately anaerobic, gram-negative, non-spore-forming rods. The cells may be spindle-shaped or have parallel sides and rounded ends. All described species are nonmotile. The size range is about 0.4 to 0.7 by 3 to 10 μm. There may be central swellings and intracellular granules. Cells of *F. necrophorum* are elongated or filamentous and curved.

The lipopolysaccharide of *F. necrophorum* is in a multilayered external coat. The 2-ketodeoxyoctonate and sugar content of the endotoxin varies from strain to strain. Biological activity also varies, with many strains showing strong activity.

The ninth edition of *Bergey's Manual* lists 10 species in the genus. *Fusobacterium nucleatum* is the most commonly encountered species, but *F. necrophorum* is not infrequent and can produce serious disease.

Pathogenesis

Bacteroides and *Fusobacterium* are present as indigenous flora on mucosal surfaces. When they penetrate this barrier under appropriate conditions, they will establish an infection. Thus, most infections are of endogenous origin. Many infections are mixed and include streptococci, staphylococci, or other indigenous organisms. A variety of conditions such as surgery, malignancy, use of cytotoxic drugs, or vascular damage may predispose to infection by these anaerobes; anything that lowers the oxidation–reduction potential favors their growth. Antimicrobial agents to which anaerobes are resistant (e.g., aminoglycosides) may facilitate the infection. Once anaerobes establish an infection in tissue and begin to multiply they maintain the reduced oxygen tension by excreting end products of fermentation. In a mixed infection, facultative organisms may potentiate the process by scavenging oxygen and providing nutrients that facilitate growth of the anaerobe.

Bacteroides and *Fusobacterium* produce enzymes that contribute to pathogenesis. *B. melaninogenicus* and *B. gingivalis* produce collagenase, which may result in a more acute process. Several strains of *Bacteroides* produce high levels of neuraminidase, and *B. fragilis* and *B. melaninogenicus* strains can produce hyaluronidase. Other enzymes that may contribute to pathogenesis include DNAse, phosphatase, heparinase, phospholipase A, and a variety of proteases.

F. necrophorum produces a leukocidin and a hemolysin and will agglutinate erythrocytes. An animal strain produces a phospholipase A and lysophospholipase.

Other virulence factors include an ability to inhibit phagocytosis. The capsule of some *Bacteroides* species also may be a virulence factor. The mechanism for capsular virulence is not clear, but it appears to interfere with phagocytosis and opsonophagocytic killing and possibly to facilitate adherence of the organism to tissues.

Immunity

Polymorphonuclear leukocytes have oxygen-dependent and oxygen-independent microbicidal systems. They are capable of killing some *Bacteroides* species under aerobic or anaerobic conditions.

Immunoglobulin and complement components can participate in chemotoxis and killing of anaerobes such as *Bacteroides*. Antibody to capsular polysaccharide of some species is induced by infection, and such immunization may confer protection against abscess development. T-cells also may be involved in immunity to *Bacteroides*. Fusobacteria may persist in the liver for extended periods. Here its proliferation in Kupffer cells impairs macrophage functions.

Clinical Infections

Since *Bacteroides* and *Fusobacterium* organisms are inhabitants of mucosal surfaces, infections usually are of endogenous origin. They tend to be slowly developing and may become chronic, with brief acute episodes, and they often produce viscous, foul-smelling purulent material. The infections usually appear as abscesses with extensive necrosis. These features are not unique to infections with *Bacteroides* or *Fusobacterium* but are typical of infection by gram-negative anaerobic rods.

Infections are seen in areas where there is low oxygen tension due to impaired blood supply, and some tissue necrosis may already be present. Thus, they may follow an initial acute infection caused by aerobes or facultative organisms and may occur at a variety of sites.

Intraabdominal Infections. These usually result from perforation of the gut, such as wounds, appendicitis, or surgery, and the organisms enter the peritoneum. The first manifestation is peritonitis, followed by abscess formation. The usual isolates are *Bacteroides* species, mainly *B. fragilis*, and fusobacteria, although clostridia and anaerobic gram-positive cocci may be present.

Pleuropulmonary Infections. These usually result in lung abscesses, necrotizing pneumonia, and empyema. They often follow tissue damage by other organisms and are due to aspiration of organisms found in the oral cavity. Such infections may also follow progressive dental infections or other extrapulmonary disease, bronchogenic carcinoma, or pulmonary embolus. The infecting agents frequently are mixed and include oral *Bacteroides* species and gram-positive cocci.

Upper Respiratory Tract Infection. Such infections take the form of peritonsillar abscesses, otitis media, mastoiditis, and sinusitis. The latter can spread to the central nervous system and result in brain abscesses.

Soft Tissue Infection. Anaerobic infections of the skin and more superficial tissues usually result from trauma, surgery, or ischemia due to vascular disease. Bite wounds are especially serious and usually contain *Bacteroides* and *Fusobacterium* species as predominant members of the flora.

Oral Infection. Black-pigmented *Bacteroides* species have been associated with periodontal disease and endodontic infections; they will be discussed in the appropriate chapters. They can be isolated from orofacial abscesses that develop following endodontic or periodontic lesions, pericoronitis, or complications of tooth extraction. Following periodontal abscesses, *B. gingivalis, B. intermedius,* and *B. melaninogenicus* are usual isolates. Pericoronitis and abscesses as a complication of extraction are associated with *B. intermedius* and *B. gingivalis*, although *B. endodontalis* has occasionally been found. Such infections can be serious since they involve tissue spaces and can spread along fascial planes.

Fusobacteria were first observed in ulcerative gingivitis and have been associated with other organisms in infections of the tissue spaces. They also have been associated with acute necrotizing gingivitis.

Diagnosis

The clinical features of *Bacteroides* and *Fusobacterium* infections are similar to those of other anaerobic infections. These features are distinctive enough to suggest such a problem, as they include foul smell, tissue necrosis, and association with trauma, malignancy, surgery or circulatory problems.

The definitive diagnosis requires demonstration or isolation of the responsible organism. Samples should be isolated under anaerobic conditions. This involves aspiration or tissue specimens; swabs, smears, etc. are often unusable. Samples should be transported to the laboratory immediately under anaerobic conditions. Because of the relatively slow growth of some strains, a direct smear and gram stain is very useful. The organisms are grown in appropriate media in the laboratory and identified using a variety of identification schemes. Gas–liquid chromatography is a particularly sensitive and useful method for specific identification. Direct gas–liquid chromatography of clinical samples may provide clues to the presence of certain organisms, e.g., large amounts of butyric acid in the absence of isobutyric or isovaleric acid suggest *fusobacterium* species. Immunofluorescence is also useful for detecting *Bacteroides* and fusobacteria in clinical specimens. Tests for antibody development are not practical.

Epidemiology

Bacteroides and fusobacterial infections are of endogenous origin and follow trauma or other disease. Thus, it is important for the clinician to know whether these organisms are present at the sites, so as to anticipate possible infection. In addition, the pathogenicity of the various species must be considered, as well as various ecological determinants such as oxygen tension, ability to adhere, and the presence of synergistic species that would enhance growth.

Bacteroides and *Fusobacterium* species are present in many oral cavities by 12 months of age and become more common and numerous with time. *Bacteroides* are almost invariably found in quantity in the feces of adults, while *Fusobacterium* is found in 18% of adults. Species of both have been found in vaginal flora and on the external genitalia. Although *Bacteroides* has occasionally been recovered from the environment, the source of infection with both of these organisms is the indigenous flora.

Control

Infections by *Bacteroides* and *Fusobacterium* are best controlled by prevention, i.e., by avoiding conditions that reduce tissue redox potential and by preventing the introduction of organisms into susceptible sites. Prophylactic antibiotic therapy is effective in some situations. Anaerobic infection following dental procedures may be managed by prophylaxis with penicillin. Before bowel surgery, neomycin plus erythromycin or neomycin plus tetracycline is useful.

Appropriate therapy of established infections can control them and prevent their spread. The effectiveness of antibiotics varies. Aminoglycosides such as gentamicin are generally ineffective. The activity of erythromycin is variable. Most penicillins and cephalosporins are less active than penicillin G, but there is increasing resistance to this agent. Ampicillin, carbenicillin, and penicillin V are about equally as effective as penicillin G. Cefotoxin is active against *B. fragilis*, and cefmandole is active against most species except *B. fragilis*. Generally the oral species are susceptible to penicillin, chloramphenicol, clindamycin, erythromycin, and metronidazole. The *B. fragilis* group is most susceptible to chloramphenicol, clindamycin, and metronidazole.

In addition to antimicrobials, draining of abscesses and the removal of obstructions and necrotic tissue are useful adjuncts. Hyperbaric oxygen is not useful.

Resistance to penicillin is usually due to beta-lactamase, which may be transferable. Indeed, plasmid-mediated resistance to several antibiotics has been demonstrated with several species of *Bacteroides*.

Anaerobic Cocci

The anaerobic cocci are part of the normal microbial flora of healthy individuals; however, they can cause infections of traumatized tissues or in the compromised host. They are opportunistic pathogens that cause a variety of infections, often as part of a mixed infection. They can, however, be significant pathogens in and of themselves, since about 15% of isolates are found in pure culture. The organisms are part of the oral, cutaneous, intestinal, and genitourinary tract flora.

Included in this group are both gram-positive and gram-negative organisms. They are physiologically diverse as well: their common links are anaerobiosis, morphology, and role as opportunists. In this group we include members of the genera *Peptostreptococcus, Peptococcus, Veillonella,* and some species of *Streptococcus*. The organisms may be saccharolytic, proteolytic, or both. Some are more aerotolerant than others, e.g., *Streptococcus intermedius*.

General Properties

There are five species of obligately anaerobic streptococci: *Peptostreptococcus anaerobius; Peptostreptococcus productus, Peptostreptococcus lanceolatus, Peptostreptococcus micros,* and *Peptostreptococcus parvulus*. Anaerobic streptococci have been isolated from Ludwig's angina, pleurisy, sinusitis, pelvic cellulitis, pulmonary abscesses, pleural empyema, cerebrospinal meningitis, from the uterus and bloodstream in puerperal infections, and from wound infections. They seem to prefer necrotic or gangrenous lesions. Most of the recognized species are part of the normal flora of the mouth, intestine, and perhaps more consistently of the female genital tract. They cannot be demonstrated regularly in the upper respiratory tract and intestinal tract.

Anaerobic streptococci include small chain-forming cocci that vary widely in function and activity, except for their anaerobic nature. Colonial forms range from coal black to translucent and grayish white colonies. Some anaerobic streptococci disintegrate fresh fibrin, blood, and fresh organs, causing green or black discoloration and fetid odors. It has been impossible to classify the anaerobic streptococci by serological methods, but some antigenic relationship exists between anaerobic streptococci and groups A, B, and C hemolytic streptococci.

Organisms of the genus *Peptococcus* are gram-positive cocci that occur in pairs or chains. They do not require fermentable carbohydrate. There are several clinically significant isolates, including *P. asaccharolyticus, P. magnus, P. prevotii,* and *P. saccharolyticus. Veillonella parvula* is a small gram-negative coccus that appears in pairs, clumps, or short chains. It is a member of the normal oral flora but is also found in the gastrointestinal and genitourinary tracts. Veillonellae are isolated from clinical specimens (0.5% to 2% of anaerobic isolates), but little is known of their role in production of infection.

Pathogenesis and Pathology

In general, like the anaerobic bacilli, the anaerobic cocci do not produce a distinct disease entity. Rather, their manifestations are nondistinct, appearing as mild skin abscesses, deep tissue abscesses, necrotizing pneumonia, septic abortion, or even brain abscesses.

Skin and soft tissue infections may resemble clostridial infection (gas gangrene). They take the form of myonecrosis, necrotizing fascitis, a chronic burrowing ulcerative lesion, or cellulitis. They are characterized by purulent exudate, varying degrees of tissue necrosis involving the skin, fascia, or muscles, and perhaps systemic toxicity. Not infrequently they are found in infections of the tissue spaces of the head and neck as well as in osteomyelitis of the mandible and sinusitis. Often such infections also involve *Staphylococcus aureus* and/or *Streptococcus pyogenes,* as well as *Fusobacterium* and *Bacteroides.* Such mixtures of organisms produce myonecrosis and necrotizing cellulitis.

The peptococci are isolated more frequently from soft tissue infections. Such infections of the head and neck region may be of endodontic origin, from periodontal lesions such as pericoronitis, or following surgery.

Pleuropulmonary infections include lung abscesses, necrotizing pneumonia, aspiration pneumonia, and empyema. Aspiration of the oral flora is often the inciting incident for these infections. Important clinical features include a putrid odor of discharge or sputum and the presence of tissue necrosis. Underlying conditions include dental infections, bronchogenic carcinoma, pulmonary embolus with infarction, and bronchiectasis. Anaerobic cocci account for about 40% of the isolates; *Fusobacterium* and *Bacteroides* species are often isolated concomitantly. Anaerobic pulmonary infections frequently develop slowly and may be chronic.

Anaerobic cocci are significant pathogens in puerperal fever and septic abortion, as well as in pyomet-

ria, tuboovarian abscesses, and postoperative wound infections following gynecologic surgery. *Peptococcus prevotii, Peptostreptococcus anaerobius,* and *Streptococcus intermedius* are the cocci most frequently isolated. These organisms are part of the normal flora of the affected area or surrounding tissues.

Anaerobes, including anaerobic cocci, *Bacteroides,* and *Fusobacterium,* are the predominant groups isolated from brain abscesses. The cocci have been isolated in pure culture. Chronic otitis media or mastoiditis frequently are the source of organisms, the infection resulting from direct extension into the brain.

Peptococcus magnus, the most frequently isolated anaerobic coccus (as high as 12% of isolates) is often associated with chronic bone and joint infections and ankle ulcers, and it is not infrequently isolated in infections of prosthetic joints.

Diagnosis

Establishing a definite role for anaerobic cocci in infection is sometimes difficult because these organisms are a significant part of the normal flora and can contaminate samples taken from a lesion or site. This is less of a problem where it is the sole isolate, especially from a deep lesion. Once isolated, the organisms can be identified by methods like those used for other anaerobes, including metabolic products, especially organic acids.

Epidemiology and Control

Since anaerobic cocci are part of the normal flora, they often cause or contribute to an infection after trauma or surgery, where there is disruption of the normal barriers, and in compromised patients, including cancer patients. Persons with diabetes, circulatory disturbances, or who have undergone radiation or immunosuppressive drug therapy also are candidates for such infections.

Treatment consists of drainage and tissue debridement accompanied by antibiotic therapy. Penicillin is the drug of choice, although clindamycin is also useful. Some strains may be less susceptible to these drugs than others. Another problem is that in mixed infections other organisms may be present that produce beta-lactamase, thus protecting the cocci from the action of penicillin.

ADDITIONAL READING

Bartlett, J. G. 1983. Recent Developments in the Management of Anaerobic Infections. Rev Infect Dis, **5,** 235.

Bartlett, J. G., and Gorbach, S. L. 1976. Anaerobic Infections of the Head and Neck. Otolaryngol Clin North Am, **9,** 655.

Brook, I. 1985. Enhancement of Growth of Aerobic and Facultative Bacteria in Mixed Infections with *Bacteroides* Species. Infect Immun, **50,** 929.

Brook, I. 1986. Isolation of Capsulate Anaerobic Bacteria from Orofacial Abscesses. J Med Microbiol, **22,** 171.

Brook, I. 1987. Comparison of Two Transport Systems for Recovery of Aerobic and Anaerobic Bacteria from Abscesses. J Clin Microbiol, **25,** 2020.

Brook, I., and Walker, R. I. 1984. Pathogenicity of Anaerobic Gram-Positive Cocci. Infect Immun, **45,** 320.

Brook, I., and Walker, R. I. 1984. Significance of Encapsulated *Bacteroides melaninogenicus* and *Bacteroides fragilis* Groups in Mixed Infections. Infect Immun, **44,** 12.

Finegold, S. M. 1980. Anaerobic Infections. Surg Clin North Am, **60,** 49.

Finegold, S. M. 1982. Pathogenic Anaerobes. Arch Intern Med, **142,** 1988.

Finegold, S. M., and Wexler, H. M. 1988. Therapeutic Implications of Bacteriologic Findings in Mixed Aerobic-Anaerobic Infections. Antimicrob Agents Chemother, **32,** 611.

Goldstein, E. J. C., Citron, D. M., and Finegold, S. M. 1984. Role of Anerobic Bacteria in Bite-Wound Infections. Rev Infect Dis, **6,** S177.

Gorbach, S. L., and Bartlett, J. G. 1974. Anaerobic Infections. N Engl J Med, **290,** 1177.

Hnatko, S. I. 1983. Epidemiology of Anaerobic Infections. Surgery, **93,** 125.

Kannangara, D. W., Thadepalli, H., and McQuister, J. L. 1980. Oral Surg, **50,** 103.

Lewis, R. P., Sutter , V. L., and Finegold, S. M. 1978. Bone Infections Involving Anaerobic Bacteria. Medicine, **57,** 279.

Sigeti, J. S., Guiney, D. G., Jr., and Davis, C. E. 1983. Mechanism of Action of Metronidazole or *Bacteroides fragilis.* J Infect Dis, **148,** 1083.

Talley, F. P., and Gorbach, S. L. 1979. Clinical Aspects of Anaerobic Infection. J Infect, **1,** 25.

22

Clostridium

George S. Schuster

Clostridia

The genus *Clostridium,* composed of gram-positive, obligately anaerobic, sporulating rods, is divided into more than 60 species. Some are frankly pathogenic, but many of the saprophytic species inhabit the soil, where they decompose organic matter and fix nitrogen. A few species are important in industrial fermentations. Pathogenic species inhabit soils and the intestinal tracts of man and domesticated animals. They cause tetanus, gas gangrene, enterocolitis, and botulism. Tetanus and botulism are each caused by single species, *Clostridium tetani* and *Clostridium botulinum,* respectively. Enterocolitis may be caused by several different species, and at least five or six species are primarily involved in gas gangrene.

The clostridia associated with human or animal disease are identified by 1) cultural characteristics, 2) biochemical activities, 3) spore formation and the morphology of the spore, 4) the production of specific toxins and their identification by neutraliza-tion with homologous antitoxins, and 5) the requirements for special media and conditions.

The pathogenicity of the clostridia for the most part depends on their production of powerful exotoxins, either outside the body in foodstuffs or in local infections in the tissues. Disease production by the gas gangrene group is partly attributable to the production in vivo of lytic enzymes, which assist in the spread of infection and the dissemination of the breakdown products of tissue.

Clostridium tetani

Morphology of C. tetani. *C. tetani* is a gram-positive, obligately anaerobic, sporulating rod with a spherical, terminal spore. The organisms are about 3 to 5 μm long and 0.3 to 0.7 μm in diameter. They are flagellated and therefore motile. The terminal spores give the cells the appearance of drumsticks. The bacteria and their spores are normal inhabitants of the soil and the intestinal tract of man and animals. The spores of *C. tetani* are very resistant to physical and chemical agents.

Growth and Metabolism of *C. tetani*. The tetanus bacillus grows optimally at 37°C if the oxidation–reduction potential is reduced sufficiently. Carbohydrates are not fermented by the tetanus bacillus but the complex nutritional requirements can be met by blood agar or cooked meat medium. Swarming occurs on blood agar, with growth spreading over the surface of the agar, making colony isolation difficult.

Antigenic Structure of *C. tetani*. *C. tetani* has been divided into at least 10 serotypes, based on their flagellar (H) antigen. Other antigens include a somatic (O) antigen and a spore antigen. Tetanus toxins are antigenically identical, regardless of the serotype from which they are derived.

Tetanus. Tetanus, commonly called lockjaw, is essentially a tonic spasm of striated muscle caused by the neurotoxin of *C. tetani*.

The chief reservoir of tetanus cells or spores is the soil, from which they find their way into wounds, burns, and other injuries. If conditions are suitable, as in traumatized tissue or puncture wounds with a sufficiently low oxidation–reduction potential, the spores germinate in 2 to 50 days and the bacilli multiply locally, producing a toxin that usually is disseminated to nearby peripheral nerves and eventually to the central nervous system (CNS). The toxin probably travels within the nerve trunk in the tissue spaces between individual nerve fibers, as well as via the bloodstream; it is not clear how it enters the CNS. Tetanus occasionally occurs in a localized form, adjacent to the site of inoculation, but more frequently it is generalized in nature.

The earliest manifestation of tetanus is muscle stiffness, usually in the muscles near the infected wound, followed by spasm of the masseter muscles, trismus or lockjaw, the classic symptoms of tetanus. As the disease progresses, tetanic spasms cause clenching of the jaws, flexing of the arms, extension of the legs, and arching of the back. These spasms are brief but may be frequent. Occasionally the spasms are severe enough to produce bone fracture, including fractures of the vertebral bones. The patient assumes a rigid position with an arched back and the weight borne on the head and heels (opisthotonus). Respiratory complications such as aspiration pneumonia are common. The disease may persist over several weeks, and death may occur during one of the spasms due to contractions of the muscles of respiration. Injuries close to the head have a poor prognosis. In nonfatal cases the symptoms progress to a point, then gradually regress. Patients who recover usually have no permanent sequelae.

Tetanus toxin is released mostly after cessation of cellular growth. The toxin, a single protein chain with a molecular weight of about 150,000 daltons, is among the most poisonous produced by bacteria. When crystallized it contains more than 50 to 75 million lethal doses for mice per milligram of protein. It is readily converted by formaldehyde into a stable toxoid, which is useful for active immunization. Upon release the toxin molecule is nicked, leaving 50,000- and 100,000-dalton moieties. Tetanus toxin acts at the synaptosome. It binds to the gangliosides in the synaptic membranes. This is dependent upon the number and position of sialic acid residues. Toxin produces excitation of the CNS by blocking synaptic inhibition in the spinal cord, presumably at inhibitory terminals. Such elimination of inhibitory responses of the nerve fibers permits the uncontrolled spread of impulses initiated in the CNS, resulting in an exaggerated reflex response of the skeletal muscles. The pattern of response is determined by the strongest muscles at a given joint. A second toxin, tetanolysin, causes lysis of erythrocytes and kills neutrophils. It does not contribute significantly to the pathogenesis of tetanus.

Laboratory Diagnosis of *C. tetani*. The initial diagnosis and the treatment of tetanus depend on the presence of certain clinical symptoms. Time is of the essence, and treatment should not wait on the few days required to isolate and identify *C. tetani*. Nevertheless, the causative bacteria should be cultured and isolated. Identification of *C. tetani* relates to morphological, serological, and cultural characteristics, especially sporulation and the type of terminal spore produced, hemolysis of blood, swarming, staining with fluorescent antibodies, toxin production, and toxin neutralization in a mouse protection test.

Treatment of *C. tetani* Infection. Initial treatment consists of immediate excision of the lesion to expose it to air, followed by the administration of antitoxin to neutralize as much as possible of the toxin before it becomes fixed to the tissues. Large doses of penicillin, or a suitable alternate, should be administered. These antibiotics not only act on the clostria but also restrict growth of contaminating aerobes, which help maintain anaerobic conditions that favor clostridial growth. Supportive care to maintain respiratory functions and control spasms is also important.

Prevention and Control of Tetanus. Some time after World War I, toxoid came into use for active immunization against tetanus. The usual practice is to immunize during the first year of life with a multiple vaccine containing tetanus toxoid, diphtheria toxoid, and pertussis vaccine in a course of three injections about a month apart. A booster dose is given a year later and when the child enters elementary school. Booster vaccinations are given at 10-year intervals to those who are regularly exposed to a risk of infection. Previously immunized individuals who are wounded should receive an immediate booster dose of toxoid. Wounded individuals not previously immunized should be given human tetanus immune globulin as well as toxoid injections for future protection.

Histotoxic Clostridial Infections

Gas Gangrene. Gas gangrene is essentially a rapidly spreading edematous myonecrosis accompanied by profound toxemia and prostration, that results from the infection of severe wounds and the invasion of muscle by species of *Clostridium,* especially *C. perfringens, C. novyi, C. bifermentans, C. histolyticum,* and *C. septicum. C. perfringens* type A, the most frequent cause of gas gangrene in man, produces a variety of extracellular toxins with necrotizing and hemolytic activity. Alpha toxin, which is lecithinase C, is the major toxin; others include proteinase, hyaluronidase, and collagenase.

The cells of the principal species of *Clostridium* involved in gas gangrene are all relatively large, gram-positive rods that form oval, subterminal spores greater in diameter than the vegetative cell.

Wound Infection and the Pathogenesis of Gas Gangrene. The development of gas gangrene is intimately related to the general problem of wound infection. The organisms most commonly found in wounds are the *Clostridium* species, nonsporulating bacteria of fecal origin (enterococci and enterobacteriaceae), and pyogenic cocci (staphylococci and streptococci). Factors that influence the course of a wound infection are the nature of the contaminating bacteria; the location, nature, and severity of the wound; the presence of extraneous material in the wound; the condition of the patient, including immune response; and perhaps most important of all, the promptness and adequacy of treatment. Infected wounds that do not develop into gas gangrene, but appear as abscesses or cellulitis, exhibit approximately three phases. In the primary stage, which lasts about a week, clostridia and streptococci predominate. In the secondary stage, which lasts from 2 to 3 weeks, there is a gradual transition from the primary anaerobic infection to one dominated by pyogenic cocci, accompanied by enterococci and enterobacteriaceae. Finally, the latter gradually disappear, leaving a simple pyogenic infection by staphylococci and streptococci.

Cytotoxic clostridial infections usually result from the introduction of the causal clostridia or their spores by contamination of wounds with soil. The intensity of the infection can vary from simple wound contamination of short duration without frank disease,

to anaerobic cellulitis, to the most serious condition of all, clostridial myonecrosis or gas gangrene, which can develop within several hours. In simple wound contamination the clostridia may be present without obvious pathology. Anaerobic cellulitis occurs when the clostridia infect tissue damaged by direct trauma or ischemia. Organisms spread through subcutaneous tissue and along fascial plans but do not invade healthy tissue. There is extensive clostridial growth, and gas is a prominent feature. Extreme toxemia, such as occurs in clostridial myonecrosis, is not present.

In myonecrosis, during the first few hours after the initiation of the infection, there is at first connective tissue destruction adjacent to healthy muscle. Characteristic of the onset of the infection is a rapidly spreading edema that first involves subcutaneous connective tissue and then the connective tissue of muscles. Accompanying the edema, gas may develop and distend the tissue (Fig. 22.1). The resulting pressure tends to spread the infection. As the disease progresses, more and more tissue is involved and muscle tissue adjacent to the wound is discolored. The infection is rapidly destructive and more foul-smelling if the proteolytic species are present. Gas gangrene results in a severe toxemia and prostration caused by the absorption of the products of tissue injury and dissolution. Although the patient usually remains mentally alert, coma and delirium sometimes precede death. Characteristically there is a reduced blood pressure and death results from circulatory failure.

Streptococcal myositis may appear similar to gas gangrene except that it is caused by anaerobic streptococci, there is only focal muscle involvement, the discharge from the wound is purulent, and toxemia is inconstant.

C. perfringens is also a cause of food poisoning. A self-limited gastroenteritis is induced some 12 hours after the ingestion of foods, particularly meat, that are contaminated with *C. perfringens.* A more serious enteric infection, enteritis necroticans, has been described. It is an acute inflammatory infection of the small intestines that causes a high mortality.

Laboratory Diagnosis of Cytotoxic Clostridial Infections. The demonstration of typical gram-positive bacilli in exudate from infected wounds is indicative of cytotoxic clostridial infections. It is also useful to culture specimens, both aerobically and anaerobically. Growth of typical gram-positive bacilli anaerobically but not aerobically indicates a clostridial infection. Positive identification of clostridia requires the determination of their biochemical characteristics.

Treatment of Cytotoxic Clostridial Infections. The treatment of clostridial wound infections requires surgical debridement and, in the case of gas gangrene, the complete removal of infected muscle. Polyvalent antitoxin is useful, as is hyperbaric oxygen

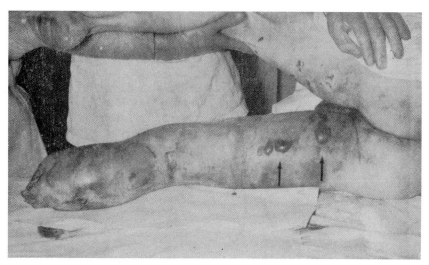

Figure 22.1: Gas gangrene. Note gas bubbles that have formed beneath the skin. (AFIP.)

in the treatment of clostridial myonecrosis. Penicillin prevents spread of the infection and prevents a bacteremia.

Antibiotic-Associated Colitis

Certain antibiotics, including clindamycin, ampicillin, and neomycin, have been associated with the development of diarrhea and pseudomembranous enterocolitis. This appears to be due to enterotoxin-producing strains of *Clostridium difficile. C. difficile* is usually present in low numbers in the normal intestinal flora of some individuals and may be resistant to various antibiotics. Administration of these drugs selects for the resistant strains that overgrow in the gastrointestinal tract. Production of the enterotoxins results in symptoms, but the toxins' modes of action are not known. Cessation of the use of the antibiotic will result in resolution in most cases. Vancomycin has been successfully used to treat *C. difficile* enterocolitis, although there have been reports of deaths after the vancomycin was stopped.

Botulism

Bacteriological Characteristics of *Clostridium botulinum.* *C. botulinum,* widely distributed in soils, is a gram-positive, spore-forming, motile, anaerobic rod, 3 to 8 μm long by 0.5 to 1.3 μm wide. The organisms under strictly anaerobic conditions produce a characteristic and very potent lethal exotoxin.

Botulinum Toxin. Botulism normally is an intoxication resulting from the consumption of food in which *C. botulinum* has grown and produced exotoxin. There are eight serologically distinct types of the organism, based on the type of toxin produced. The toxins are designated A, B, C α, C β, D, E, F, and G, of which A, B, E, and F are the types apparently involved in human illness. Production of C and D toxins depends on lysogeny by certain bacteriophages. Some strains of *C. botulinum* produce both A and F toxins. Botulinum toxin is the most potent toxin known. One microgram of purified toxin is lethal for man and contains about 20,000 minimum lethal doses for a mouse. The toxins are relatively heat-labile, being inactivated at 100°C for 10 minutes. They are resistant to the gastric acids and intestinal proteolytic enzymes. The powerful neurotoxin is released as the organisms die and undergo autolysis. Following its ingestion, the toxin is absorbed largely from the small intestine, appearing in the lymphatics, then the bloodstream. The toxin acts at the myoneural junction to produce paralysis of the cholinergic nerve fibers at the point of release of acetylcholine. It suppresses release of acetylcholine. Death occurs following paralysis of respiratory organs.

Clinical Manifestations. Typically symptoms of botulism begin 12 to 36 hours after ingestion of contaminated food. The onset of the disease is relatively gradual. The following symptoms are characteristic of the disease in man:

1. Either an arrest of secretion or the hypersecretion of salivary glands and the glands in the buccopharyngeal mucosa.
2. More or less complete inability to hold the eyelids open, dilation of pupils, paralysis in accommodation, diplopia, and internal strabismus.

3. Dysphagia, aphonia, constipation, and retention of urine.
4. General weakness of all voluntary muscles.
5. An absence of fever and sensory and mental disturbances.
6. Depression of respiration and circulation.

Death is caused by asphyxia resulting from respiratory paralysis or heart failure.

Until recently it was assumed that botulism could be caused only by ingestion of preformed toxin. However, botulism in infants may occur following elaboration of toxin from organisms in the gastrointestinal tract. In many instances, the cases have followed ingestion of honey contaminated with botulinum spores, suggesting this food as a possible source of the illness in these children. Death is caused by a paralyzed tongue or pharyngeal muscles that occlude the airway or by paralysis of the diaphragm and intercostal muscles.

Laboratory Diagnosis of *C. botulinum*. Diagnosis of botulism is mainly done by clinical determinations. The demonstration of *C. botulinum* as a cause of food poisoning depends on detecting the toxin or the bacilli either in the contents of the intestinal tract of the victim or in the food eaten by the victim.

Prevention and Control of *C. botulinum*. On the whole, the prevention of botulism is simple. All preserved foods that are obviously spoiled should be avoided, but *C. botulinum* often toxifies food without obvious signs of spoilage. Thus, suspect food should never be put in the mouth, since that may allow toxin absorption. Since growth of *C. botulinum* does not occur at pH values below 4.5, highly acidic foods do not cause botulism. Exposure to 100°C for 15 minutes or its equivalent can be relied on for detoxification. The botulinal toxins can be converted into effective toxoids by formaldehyde but no clear-cut indications have been defined for their general use. Polyvalent type A, B, and E antitoxin should be administered intravenously or intramuscularly as a prophylactic to all who have consumed a known toxified food but have not yet exhibited symptoms of botulism. The therapeutic value of the antitoxins has not been convincingly demonstrated.

ADDITIONAL READING

Allen, S. D., Dunn, G. D., Page, D. L., et al. 1977. Bacteriological Studies of a Patient with Antibiotic-Associated Pseudomembranous Colitis. Gastroenterology, **73,** 158.

Bartlett, J. G., Chang, T., Taylor, N. S., and Onderdonk, A. B. 1979. Colitis Induced by *Clostridium difficile*. Rev Infect Dis, **1,** 370.

Bartlett, J. G., Tedesco, F. J., Shull, S., Lowe, B., and Chang, T. 1980. Symptomatic Relapse after Oral Vancomycin Therapy of Antibiotic Associated Pseudomembranous Colitis. Gastroenterology, **78,** 431.

Bartlett, J. G., Willey, S. H., Chang, T., and Lowe, B. 1979. Cephalosporin-Associated Pseudomembranous Colitis Due to *Clostridium difficile*. JAMA, **242,** 2683.

Blake, P. A., Feldman, R. A., Buchanan, T. M., Brooks, G. F., and Bennett, J. V. 1976. Serologic Therapy of Tetanus in the United States, 1965–1971. JAMA, **235,** 42.

Boroff, D. A., and Gupta, D. 1971. Botulinum Toxin. In *Microbial Toxins,* Vol. IIA, p. 1, edited by S. Kadis, T. C. Montie, and S. J. Ahl. Academic Press, New York.

Finegold, S. M. 1980. Anaerobic Infections. Surg Clin North Am, **60,** 49.

George, W. L., Rolfe, R. D., Sutter, V. L., and Finegold, S. M. 1979. Diarrhea and Colitis Associated with Antimicrobial Therapy in Man and Animals. Am J Clin Nutr, **32,** 251.

Gorbach, S. L., and Thadepalli, H. 1975. Isolation of *Clostridium* in Human Infections: Evaluation of 114 Cases. J Infect Dis, **131,** S81.

Gunn, R. A. 1979. Epidemiologic Characteristics of Infant Botulism in the United States. Rev Infect Dis, **1,** 642.

Hobbs, B. C. 1974. *Clostridium welchii* and *Bacillus cereus* Infection and Intoxication. Postgrad Med J, **50,** 597.

Ito, K. A., Chen, J. K., Lerke, P. A., Seeger, M. L., and Unverferth, J. A. 1976. Effect of Acid and Salt Concentration in Fresh-Pack Pickles on the Growth of *Clostridium botulinum* Spores. Appl Environ Microbiol, **32,** 121.

Kellett, C. E. 1939. The Early History of Gas Gangrene. Ann Med Hist, **1,** 452.

Kwan, P. L., and Lee, J. S. 1974. Compound Inhibitory to *Clostridium botulinum* Type E Produced by a *Moraxella* Species. Appl Microbiol, **27,** 329.

Lenner, S. 1943. Experience with Gas Gangrene in Field Hospitals on the Western Front. War Med, **3,** 660.

Lerner, P. I. 1974. Antimicrobial Considerations in Anaerobic Infections. Med Clin North Am, **58,** 533.

Maclennan, J. D. 1962. The Histotoxic Clostridial Infections of Man. Bacteriol Rev, **26,** 177.

Marrie, T. J., Faulkner, R. S., Bodley, B. W. D., et al. 1978. Pseudomembranous Colitis: Isolation of Two Species of Cytotoxic Clostridia and Successful Treatment with Vancomycin. CMA J, **119,** 1058.

McClung, L. S. 1956. The Anaerobic Bacteria with Special Reference to the Genus *Clostridium*. Ann Rev Microbiol, **10,** 173.

Merson, M. H., and Dowell, V. R., Jr. 1973. Epidemiologic, Clinical, and Laboratory Aspects of Wound Botulism. N Engl J Med, **289,** 1005.

Nakamura, M., and Schulze, J. A. 1970. *Clostridium perfringens* Food Poisoning. Annu Rev Microbiol, **24,** 359.

Niilo, L. 1975. Measurement of Biological Activities of Purified and Crude Enterotoxin of *Clostridium perfringens*. Infect Immun, **12,** 440.

Peterson, D. R., Eklund, M. W., and Chinn, N. M. 1979. The Sudden Infant Death Syndrome and Infant Botulism. Rev Infect Dis, **1,** 630.

Polin, R. A., and Brown, L. W. 1979. Infant Botulism. Pediatr Clin North Am, **26,** 345.

Price, A. B., Larson, H. C., and Crow, J. 1979. Morphology of Experimental Antibiotic-Associated Pseudomembranous Colitis in the Hamster: A Model for Human Pseudomembranous Colitis and Antibiotic-Associated Diarrhea. Gut, **20,** 467.

Prince, A. S., and Neu, H. C. 1979. Antibiotic-Associated Pseudomembranous Colitis in Children. Pediatr Clin North Am, **26,** 261.

Sakaguchi, G., Ohishi, I., Kozaki, S., Sakaguchi, S., and Kitamura, M. 1974. Molecular Structures and Biological Activities of *Clostridium botulinum* Toxins. Jpn J Med Sci Biol, **27,** 95.

Sellin, L. C. 1981. The Action of Botulinum Toxin at the Neuromuscular Junction. Med Biol, **59,** 11.

Silva, J., Jr., and Fekety, R. 1981. Clostridia and Antimicrobial Enterocolitis Annu Rev Med, **32,** 327.

Smith, L. D. S. 1979. Virulence Factors of *Clostridium perfringens*. Rev Infect Dis, **1,** 254.

Smith, M. J. A., and Myall, R. W. T. 1976. Tetanus: Review of the Literature and Report of a Case. Oral Surg, **41,** 451.

Van Beek, A., Zook, E., Yaw, P., Gardner, R., Smith, R., and Glover, J. L. 1974. Nonclostridial Gas-forming Infections: A Collective Review and Report of Seven Cases. Arch Surg, **108,** 552.

Van Heyningen, W. E., and Mellanby, J. 1971. Tetanus Toxin. In *Microbial Toxins,* Vol. IIA, p. 69, edited by S. Kadis, T. C. Montie, and S. J. Ajl. Academic Press, New York.

23

Mycobacteria

George S. Schuster

Most human mycobacterial disease is caused by *Mycobacterium tuberculosis* or by *M. leprae*. Nevertheless, a significant number of infections are caused by the "atypical" mycobacteria: *M. tuberculosis* causes tuberculosis in humans, *M. bovis* is the bovine tubercle bacillus, *M. paratuberculosis* (Johne's bacillus) causes an enteric infection in cattle, and *M. leprae* causes leprosy in humans. The collective term "atypical mycobacteria" encompasses all mycobacteria except those of the tuberculosis complex and *M. leprae*. Atypical mycobacteria produce a variety of clinical conditions, including lesions of the skin and mucosa, especially in compromised patients.

More than 50 species of mycobacteria have been recognized. Some grow rapidly, others grow slowly. The species commonly pathogenic for humans are slow-growers and outnumber the nonpathogenic species. Among the rapidly growing species only two, *M. fortuitum* and *M. chelonae*, are significant human pathogens.

M. tuberculosis is the most frequently encountered mycobacterium in clinical practice. It is far more con-

tagious than the atypical mycobacteria, and it is more susceptible to chemotherapeutics than most atypical mycobacteria.

Mycobacterium tuberculosis

Morphological Characteristics. *M. tuberculosis* usually appears as a slender, curved rod that is nonmotile, nonsporulating, forms no demonstrable capsule, but contains characteristic glycogen and polymetaphosphate granules and large mesosomes. Up to 60% of the cell walls of tubercle bacilli may be lipid, compared with 20% of the cell walls of gram-negative organisms and 1% to 4% of the cell walls in gram-positive organisms. They are somewhat hydrophobic and relatively impermeable to basic dyes. However, at the boiling point of water, appropriate dyes penetrate the cell wall and stain the interior. Tubercle bacilli retain such dyes even when exposed to acidified solvents (Ziehl-Neelsen or acid-fast method of staining, Chap. 3), and for this reason they are called acid-fast microorganisms. Under certain conditions these organisms can be made to stain with the gram stain, in which case they appear gram positive.

Cultivation and Nutrition. The human tubercle bacillus can be cultured on three general types of media. The first type is an enriched solid medium that is used for initial isolation of tubercle bacilli from an infection. Biotin and catalase may be incorporated to stimulate revival of damaged bacilli in clinical specimens. This may facilitate initial isolation. A second type of medium contains a nonionic detergent or wetting agent and provides dispersed growth of tubercle bacilli that have been adapted to artificial cultivation. A third type of medium for tubercle bacilli is chemically defined. Growth is slow, but maximal growth is eventually achieved with this medium. Because growth is rather slow, initial identification may be done by microscopy.

Chemical Composition. The pathogenicity of tubercle bacilli has been studied with regard to proteins, polysaccharides, and lipids. Proteins make up half the dry weight of the cell. When administered to nontuberculous animals in very large amounts, they cause fever, hemorrhage, and a slight anemia. In very small amounts they are extremely toxic for tuberculous humans or animals. Such protein is an essential component of the hypersensitivity reaction that occurs in tuberculosis. When linked to a waxy factor of the tubercle bacillus and injected into animals, proteins cause a typical tuberculin hypersensitivity.

The polysaccharide fraction of the tubercle bacillus constitutes only a small portion of its substance. Tuberculocarbohydrates are not primarily toxic for the healthy human or animal body, do not cause the formation of tubercles, and do not produce the tuberculin type of hypersensitivity. Anaphylactic hypersensitivity to the carbohydrates may develop when they are linked to proteins.

The cells of tubercle bacilli and other mycobacteria contain from 20% to 40% lipid that is composed of neutral fats, phospholipids, and waxes; as much as 60% of the cell wall is composed of lipids. The lipids include an interesting group of large saturated fatty acids known as mycolic acids. These are covalently linked to carbohydrates to form mycosides. Virulence of the tubercle bacillus is especially associated with one of these mycosides, 6,6'-dimycolyltrehalose. This mycoside has the ability to inhibit polymorphonuclear leukocyte (PMN) migration in vitro, elicit granuloma formation, and damage mitochondrial membranes; it is toxic to cells. It also activates the alternate complement pathway and is lethal to mice. Wax D, another mycoside of high molecular weight, has the capacity to enhance the immunogenicity of many antigens. It is commonly used in a water-in-oil emulsion known as Freund's complete adjuvant. When wax D is mixed with the proteins of the tubercle bacillus or even saprophytic mycobacteria, it readily induces a delayed-type hypersensitivity reaction. Another lipid fraction, which is quite firmly bound in the cell wall, is related to acid fastness. In addition, there is a group of sulfolipids, trehalose 2'-sulfates esterified to fatty acids, that seem to enhance the toxicity of 6,6'-dimycolyltrehalose and prevent the fusion of phagosomes and lysosomes.

Tuberculosis

Tuberculosis is an infection with tubercle bacilli that principally affects the lungs but may involve the lymph nodes (scrofula), meninges (meningeal tuberculosis), kidneys (renal tuberculosis), bone or spine (Pott's disease), skin (lupus; Fig. 23.1), and oral cavity. It may take the form of a general infection (miliary tuberculosis) involving one or more of the organs, or it may appear to be nothing more than a mild bronchitis. In the individual with little resistance, tuberculosis is sometimes a fulminating disease, with much destruction of the affected organs.

Clinical Appearance and Pathogenesis: Primary Infection. When tubercle bacilli enter the tissues of a nonimmune individual, usually by inhalation, they reach the alveolar spaces and establish a localized primary infection, usually in the lower lobes and anterior segments of the lungs. The first reaction is negligible. Once in the alveolar space, the bacilli are ingested by pulmonary alveolar macrophages and the majority are soon destroyed. It is not clear how macrophages kill tubercle bacilli, and whether they actually do so is questionable. It has been suggested that macrophages kill tubercle bacilli

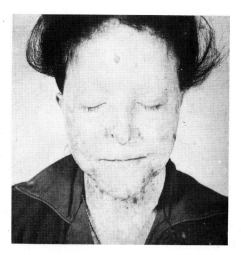

Figure 23.1: Recurrent lupus vulgaris. (AFIP 58–15052–15.)

by producing hydrogen peroxide. At the same time lysosomes would be important in this process, so the ability of the organisms to inhibit phagosome–lysosome fusion must be considered. The outcome of the interaction between organism and cell (and whether disease results) may depend on the balance between such activities. Some organisms may survive and multiply intracellularly and eventually kill the phagocyte. The released organisms chemotactically attract macrophages from the bloodstream, forming a small tubercle. Such blood-borne macrophages readily ingest the organisms but cannot kill them until they become activated. Alveolar macrophages determine whether the lesion becomes established but do not have any significant effect on the subsequent course. The activation of blood-borne macrophages accumulating in the newly formed tubercle occurs as a result of stimulation by lymphocytes that were also attracted to the developing tubercle. The lymphokines of importance in the process are chemotactic, migration inhibitory, and mitogenic factors that cause lymphocyte and macrophage infiltration, macrophage activation, and macrophage and lymphocyte division. Cellular hypersensitivity is manifested by a local accumulation of lymphoctyes and macrophages caused at least in part by T-cell and perhaps B-cell chemotactic lymphokines.

The patient at this initial stage is asymptomatic or has only mild symptoms of fatigue and irritability. After 2 to 8 weeks, seroconversion occurs and the patient has a positive reaction to the tuberculin skin test. This corresponds to activation of the macrophage response, which helps limit the primary infection. When delayed hypersensitivity develops and granulomatous inflammation occurs, the characteristic lesions known as tubercles are formed. Not all macrophages in a tuberculous granuloma have the same function. Some may present antigen and stimulate lymphocytes. Some may secrete proteases, while some may produce factors to stimulate production of monocytes and granulocytes in the bone marrow.

Tubercle bacilli in pulmonary lesions may drain into the hilar lymph nodes and establish new lesions there. The pulmonary focus and the lesions in the hilar nodes together are called the primary complex. Caseation necrosis, wherein the necrotic centers of lesions become semisolid and may remain so, occurs in these lesions. The efferent lymph from these infected nodes may drain organisms into the bloodstream, causing secondary foci in the lungs. In addition, the organisms can enter the circulation when small vessels are eroded by the caseation process. Secondary foci may develop in other organs such as the liver, spleen, and kidneys. Where these develop depends on whether the organisms enter the pulmonary or systemic circulation and whether they multiply at these secondary sites. Secondary foci will progress if the accumulating blood-borne macrophages cannot limit growth of the organisms and will arrest if the accumulating macrophages are able to stop microbial growth. Primary tubercles, particularly in young people, may heal by fibrosis and calcification, producing characteristic radiographic findings. These are called the Ghon complex.

Due to cell-mediated hypersensitivity, macrophages and lymphocytes rapidly accumulate and may become activated wherever tubercle bacilli or their antigens exist in the tissues. The reaction causes accelerated tubercle formation that facilitates destruction of inhaled organisms that were not destroyed by alveolar macrophages. Thus it can stop the progression of exogenous reinfection and also can stop progression of lesions arising by hematogenous spread. In most cases the infection is contained, and because of lymphocyte memory the patients retain tuberculin reactivity and resistance to primary reinfection for life. Thus, when a relatively small number of organisms is present in a tissue site and cell-mediated hypersensitivity controls them, this is beneficial to the patient.

When large numbers of organisms and antigens are present in the tissue, the immunological response can be detrimental. The hypersensitivity reaction itself causes cell death and tissue destruction. Thus, the reaction that is responsible for cell-mediated immunity of tuberculosis is, with large quantities of antigen, responsible for much of the tissue damage present in the disease, specifically caseation, liquefaction, and tuberculous pneumonia. The detrimental reaction is produced by the cells and tissues of the host itself, i.e., lymphocytes and cytotoxic lymphokines, macrophage and granulocyte products (e.g., lytic enzymes and oxygen-derived free radicals), and the blood coagulation process. The toxicity of the bacterial components depends on the degree of hypersensitivity of the host.

In approximately 10% of primary infections, immunity is inadequate to contain the infection and regional parenchymal multiplication is followed by progressive tissue destruction and liquefaction, followed by discharge of lesions, producing cavitation. This may result in extension of the disease via the bronchi.

Reactivation of Disease. Much adult tuberculosis is due to reactivation of dormant foci remaining after primary infection. These foci frequently are in the lung and persist owing to a favorable environment, especially good oxygenation. Reactivation may or may not be associated with identifiable factors such as malnutrition, diabetes, silicosis, or corticosteroid therapy. Once reactivation has occurred the lesion undergoes liquefaction and cavitation and the organisms proliferate. They may enter the bronchi and spread to other parts of the lung and be transmitted to other individuals by aerosol. Extrapulmonary lesions usually develop as a result of reactivation of dormant lesions seeded during primary infection. Indeed, almost 15% of tuberculosis cases involve extrapulmonary sites. Almost any organ may be the site of lesions but especially the lymph nodes, pleura, bones and joints, genitourinary system, and peritoneum. The oral cavity is not infrequently involved. If a lesion ruptures into a pulmonary vein, miliary or disseminated tuberculosis may result.

Tuberculous lesions heal when the growth of the organisms in them is inhibited by host defenses with or without chemotherapeutic assistance. The fibrosis that walls off the lesions and closes the cavity is part of the healing process.

There are several types of lesions in tuberculosis, including the encapsulated nodule, which may be caseous, liquified, or calcified (Fig. 23.2). Liquefaction is the most harmful response and, like caseation, is linked to delayed hypersensitivity. It is due to hydrolysis of tissue, including caseous tissue, by lytic enzymes of macrophages and possibly granulocytes. These cells accumulate around the caseous focus because

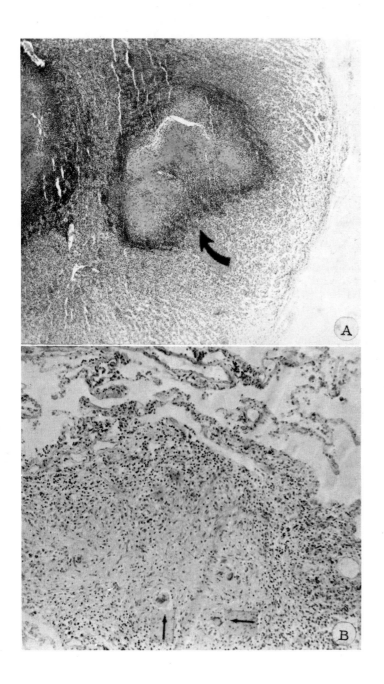

Figure 23.2: Generalized tuberculosis. (**A**) Tubercles, with central caseation about which there is extensive cellular infiltration with erythrocytes and mononuclear cells. Alveoli filled with hemorrhagic exudate. (**B**) Higher magnification of tubercle showing fibrosis and numerous giant cells. (AFIP 162451.)

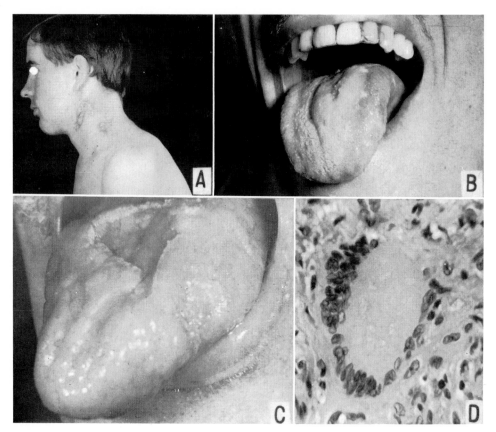

Figure 23.3: Tuberculosis about the oral cavity. (**A**) Tuberculosis of lymph nodes, and scrofula; (**B**) and (**C**) tuberculosis of the tongue; (**D**) tubercle. (**A,** AFIP 13926; **B,** AFIP AMH8680; **C,** AFIP 218869; **D,** AMH8680.)

the host is hypersensitive to antigens that may be within the caseous material. During liquefaction the organisms multiply extracellularly and may reach large numbers. When the lesion ruptures into the bronchial tree, organisms spread to other parts of the lung and to the environment. The large antigen load overwhelms the existing immunity. At this time the hypersensitivity to microbial antigens becomes more detrimental overall, because when liquefaction and rupture into the bronchial tree occur, cavity formation and aerosolization result, and spread of infection is more likely. When fibrous encapsulation occurs the lesions tend to arrest and stop progressing.

Proliferative types of lesions contain tuberculous granulation tissue. They will heal when a good host defense is present.

Exudative types of lesions occur when contents of a cavity enter the bronchi. Large amounts of antigenic material enter the bronchial tree and cause exudation of plasma components and leukocytes into the pulmonary alveoli.

The tuberculous cavity is a cavity in which large numbers of organisms are growing. It is often a site

for the development of antibiotic resistance. Several types of lesions are recognized; commonly, two or more of these lesion types coexist in the same patient.

Oral Tuberculosis

Tuberculous lesions, usually circumscribed and walled-off, may occur in any oral tissue or organ. Oral tuberculosis lesions have been reported in the tongue, mandible, maxilla, lip, alveolar process, alveolar sockets, gingiva, cheeks, pharynx, tonsils, salivary glands, and nasal cavity (Fig. 23.3). The types of lesions encountered have been described as ulcers, gummata, fissures, lupus, hypertrophic gingivitis, tuberculoma, "mouse-eaten" furrowed ulcerations, and granulomas.

Tubercular infection of oral tissues may arise, under appropriate conditions, from either an exogenous (from disseminated tubercle bacilli in the oral cavity) or endogenous (via the circulatory system) source of microorganisms. Usually, oral infection is dependent on a generalized pulmonary involvement, influenced by a concurrent lowering of resistance to infection and a possible increase in virulence of the involved microorganisms. Oral tuberculosis has been reported to occur in 3.5% of patients with systemic lesions, and rarely in those without systemic infection. Primary infection of the oral tissues does occur without systemic infection, but it is rare. The amount of lymphoid tissue in the area influences the site of tuberculous infection, for the incidence is much less in the anterior than in the posterior part of the oral cavity, coinciding with the distribution of lymphoid tissue in these areas. Much protection is afforded against tubercular infection by the flushing and antibacterial action of saliva, and undoubtedly by the antagonistic action of other oral microorganisms. Trauma or constant low-grade infection predisposes to oral tuberculous infection at a site if other conditions are favorable.

Tuberculous infection is found in periapical areas or in tooth sockets after extraction in patients with long-standing pulmonary infection. The frequency of this type of infection is about 8% in such populations. In tuberculous patients, after extraction, healing is delayed and the socket is filled with a mass of granulation tissue that is sometimes called "tuberculous granulations." This tissue is characterized by numerous small pink or dark-red elevations that bleed easily if disturbed. If the granulation tissue is removed by curettage, a healthy blood clot forms, usually followed by normal healing.

Tuberculosis of the oral mucous membranes often follows advanced pulmonary infection, where it has been found to occur in approximately 20% of consecutive autopsies of tuberculous patients. The incidence overall of clinically discernible oral lesions in patients with pulmonary tuberculosis has been reported as up to 1.5%. The more common pathological lesions of oral mucosa are ulcerative, miliary, and infiltrative, and the less common are the granuloma, tuberculous fissure, and cold abscess. The ulcerative type is most common. The mucous membranes of the soft and hard palate are most often affected. The surface of the tongue is occasionally affected, with the lesions occurring near the base, where they are not likely to be discovered on the usual clinical examination. Lesions are found less often on the buccal mucosa. The oral tuberculous lesion of soft tissue is initiated in lymphoid tissue, where it produces chronic inflammation, loss of stratified squamous epithelium, and ulceration. Hyperplasia, degeneration, and leukocyte infiltration of the deeper tissues occur, together with granulation and tubercle formation.

Tuberculous lesions also occur, though rarely, in the maxilla and mandible, where they usually cause an osteomyelitis. Swelling is characteristic of the disease, and there may or may not be pain. When fully developed, the swelling ruptures s[...] nuses are established through [...] are discharged. The mandible [...] more often than the maxilla, b[...] data to indicate how often in[...] occurs. Infection of the mand[...] garded as primary if the mucous membrane is attacked first with subsequent involvement of the underlying bone.

Several cases of tuberculosis of the salivary glands have been reported in the literature, affecting mostly people in the second and third decades of life. The parotid gland is affected most often and the sublingual gland is seldom affected. In more than three fourths of the cases there was no family or personal history of tuberculosis. There appear to be two types of salivary tubercular lesions. One is chronic and encapsulated and requires many years to develop, the other is acutely inflammatory and requires only a few days or weeks to develop. Clinically, the lesions first appear as small swellings or tumors that are usually freely movable.

Resistance

It is apparent from what is generally known about tuberculosis that humans are susceptible to infection but resistant to disease. Tuberculosis is less infectious than the common communicable diseases of childhood. Frequent and perhaps prolonged contact may be needed during routine exposure. Of all persons newly infected, about 5% will develop clinical disease within a year. For the remainder, the chance of clinical disease occurring depends on a variety of factors. Race, sex, and age are factors. Case rates in males tend to increase with age, whereas case rates in females are likely to be highest during childbearing ages; in this age group rates in females may be higher than in males. Generally there has been a shift toward increasing disease with age. Socioeconomic status also appears to be related to tuberculosis rates. A high proportion of persons who are poorly educated, poorly paid, or poorly housed have high rates. Persons who are exposed to large amounts of dust, especially mineral dust, also have higher rates.

Genetic factors play a role in tuberculosis, as in other diseases, although the role in human disease is not clear. Blacks with HLA antigen Bw15 have a higher incidence of tuberculosis and more advanced disease than blacks with other genotypes. Whether blacks on the whole are more susceptible than whites has not been determined. Different genetic types may exhibit differences in the type or extent of immune responses, which may influence disease. In addition, different tissues or organs may respond differently to the presence of organisms.

...ion appears to influence resistance, but is of-...ifficult to separate from socioeconomic factors. It ...s been suggested that resistance may be related to protein consumption but not to vitamin or total caloric intake.

Active Immunization. Most current attempts at active immunization of man use a vaccine composed of living, attenuated tubercle bacilli. An attenuated bovine strain developed by Calmette and Guérin (BCG) is used almost universally, but a live vaccine is also made of strains of the vole bacillus (*Mycobacterium microti*). The efficacy of such vaccines has ranged from 0% to 80% in several studies; the reasons for such variation are not clear. Even with a vaccine, the necessity of vaccination remains questionable, especially in Western populations. Furthermore, BCG has been associated with a variety of adverse reactions. Such reactions, coupled with tuberculin conversion, make the tuberculin skin test virtually useless for screening, thus the recommendation that vaccination against tuberculosis be used only under limited circumstances seem prudent.

Tuberculin and Tuberculin Reaction. An experimental animal or a human sensitized to tubercle bacilli through infection or by vaccination reacts characteristically to several soluble components of the cells, termed tuberculins. The active constituents are the proteins of the bacilli. There are several types of tuberculin, the most important of which are:

1. Original or old tuberculin (OT), which is prepared by evaporating a 6-week broth culture to approximately 1/10th its original volume, after which any remaining intact cells are removed by filtration.

2. Purified protein derivative (PPD), which is a protein fraction precipitated by trichloroacetic acid or ammonium sulfate from the autoclaved supernatants of cultures of tubercle bacilli grown in synthetic media.

A method of testing for tuberculin sensitivity (the Mantoux test) entails injecting PPD intracutaneously on the flexor surface of the forearm. The test is positive if within 24 to 48 hours an indurated area of inflammation, 10 mm or more in diameter, develops at the site.

In active but nonterminal tuberculosis the size of the tuberculin reaction is of no prognostic significance because of the variety of factors that impinge on its appearance. However—and especially in the United States—the size of the reaction is predictive of the probability of infection. Thus, in individuals not showing disease, the risk of subsequent tuberculosis is directly related to the size of the reaction. In one study the risk of subsequent tuberculosis was approximately ten times greater among persons with large tuberculin reactions.

A less sensitive method of tuberculin testing is the patch test, in which a small piece of filter paper, impregnated with tuberculin, is taped to the skin. The test is positive if an inflammatory, often vesiculated, reaction develops after several days.

A single positive tuberculin reaction indicates present or previous infection with tubercle bacilli but tells nothing of the current activity of the process. A positive test within several months of previously negative tests indicates that the individual is undergoing or recovering from an initial infection. A negative test is particularly useful in excluding tuberculosis during diagnosis and in epidemiological studies.

Bacteriological Diagnosis. Tubercle bacilli may be found in the sputum or urine, in the intestinal tract (from swallowed sputum), or in infected tissue. They may be detected in sputum, intestinal contents, or urine by examining a direct smear for acid-fast bacilli. The tubercle bacilli may be cultured on appropriate media, with visible growth occurring after incubation for 2 to 5 weeks, or they may be inoculated into the groin or thigh muscle of a guinea pig.

Epidemiology. For the most part, the incidence of tuberculosis has gradually decreased in the United States in the last 100 years. At the beginning of the decline, the incidence of tuberculosis and the mortality were highest in children, but active disease and mortality were lowest in old age. Since that time, the risk of exposure has decreased in children and the mortality has shifted from a peak in childhood to its current peak in elderly individuals. This group had a high rate of exposure to tuberculosis in childhood and most acquired a primary infection that established a dormant focus of viable tubercle bacilli. The relatively high incidence of infection in the present elderly group is caused principally by reactivation of the dormant tuberculous foci.

Although the overall incidence of tuberculosis in the United States has decreased, recently the rate of decrease has slowed and indeed, the incidence of tuberculosis appears to be increasing in some areas, especially Texas, New York, California, and Florida. This apparently is linked to the incidence of acquired immunodeficiency syndrome (AIDS) in a population that is more susceptible to tuberculosis.

Treatment. After 1940, several chemicals came into use that radically changed the treatment of tuberculosis. Streptomycin and *p*-aminosalicylic acid (PAS), either singly or in combination, were put into common use in the United States. PAS requires relatively large oral doses to be effective in the treatment of tuberculosis and produces gastrointestinal side effects. Thus, it is not generally used as a primary drug. Streptomycin, which is rapidly active against tubercle bacilli, was considered most effective against tuberculosis in the exudative phase. However, the organisms may become resistant to it, for the treatment of tuberculosis is necessarily prolonged. Consequently, there is also serious danger of permanent damage to the eighth cranial nerve. Isonicotinic acid hydrazide (isoniazid, or INH) then came into use as the single most effective drug for the treatment of tuberculosis. It is relatively inexpensive, has low toxicity, and is effective when given orally, even in small doses. Rifampin has also come into use as a very effective drug for treating tuberculosis, particularly when used in combination with isoniazid. Rifampin is absorbed well when given orally and is relatively nontoxic. Similarly, ethambutol hydrochloride is effective when used in combination with isoniazid. Other chemotherapeutic agents can be used in the treatment of tuberculosis, although they are usually used when the primary drugs cannot be used because of allergy or the development of microbial resistance. These drugs include pyrazinamide, ethionamide, cycloserine, viomycin, capreomycin, and kanamycin.

Isoniazid can be used successfully for prophylactic chemotherapy of tuberculosis. It has brought about a 50% decrease in active cases of tuberculosis when applied to persons who had recently become tuberculin positive. Its use has been particularly effective in household contacts.

Mycobacterium leprae

The cells of *M. leprae* are acid-fast, gram-positive, nonsporulating, nonmotile rods. They stain more easily and are less acid-fast than *M. tuberculosis. M. leprae* is an obligate parasite of man, in whom it grows profusely in tissues and organs, causing leprosy. *M. leprae* has not been cultured in vitro and is not readily transmitted to laboratory animals or higher primates. By serial passage in certain strains of mice, transmissible mutants arise that eventually establish a progressive infection. *M. leprae* also infects the foot pad of mice, but even after serial passage remains confined to the foot pad. Recent evidence indicates that the armadillo is susceptible to infection with the leprosy bacillus.

Leprosy

Course and Appearance. At present, leprosy is prevalent in Central and South America, Southeast Asia, China, Africa, India, and Central Africa. It is estimated that there are as many as 5,000,000 lepers in the world today.

Transmission of leprosy usually requires long and close contact between a person with the disease and a susceptible person, children being the most susceptible. The incubation period ranges between 2 and 3 years but may be as long as 30 years.

Pathogenesis and Pathology. Leprosy has been divided into five clinical types: tuberculoid, borderline tuberculoid, borderline, borderline lepromatous, and lepromatous. The following discussion considers only the tuberculoid and lepromatous types.

Tuberculoid leprosy appears as granulomas in the dermis, consisting of epithelioid cells, giant cells, and an extensive lymphocytic infiltrate. Organisms invade nerves and selectively colonize Schwann cells. Cutaneous nerve fibers are obliterated, accounting for the anesthesia seen, and larger nerves become swollen and eventually destroyed by the granulomas. This is related to a cell-mediated immune response.

In lepromatous leprosy the epithelioid and giant cells are not evident and lymphocytes are rare. There are many histiocytes filled with bacterial lipid and there are large numbers of organisms in the macrophages. Organisms invade the vascular system and there is a continuous bacteremia. There is also neurological damage and the Schwann cells are involved, but to a lesser extent than in tuberculoid leprosy.

The earliest form of leprosy is usually an asymptomatic macule, several centimeters in diameter, on the trunk or extremities. For the most part these lesions heal, but in some patients they progress. To a great extent the prognosis depends on the immunological status. In tuberculoid leprosy there are few skin lesions but these may be quite large. In borderline leprosy the lesions are more numerous and nerve involvement is more severe. In the lepromatous form the lesions are multiple and distributed bilaterally. Lesions then coalesce and there is a folding of the skin, especially on the face, and a general distortion of the tissues. Deformities of the hands and feet often occur (Figs. 23.4, 23.5, and 23.6).

In oral disease, the initial lesions are swellings on the lips that then become flat nodules. Later the tongue may be affected by lesions ranging from mild

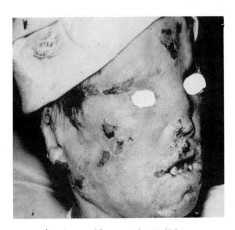

Figure 23.4: Advanced leprosy. (AFIP 43.)

glossitis to nodules along the anterior one-half or perhaps the whole tongue. In the late stages lesions may appear on the soft and hard palates and uvula. Palatal perforation may result. As damage progresses, anesthesia and paralysis occur. Loss of facial expression and inability to close the eyes follow. As leprosy progresses there is an increased incidence of trauma due to the paralysis and anesthesia, and an increase in secondary infections as a result.

Diagnosis.   The diagnosis of leprosy is by clinical examination and by the microscopic demonstration of leprosy bacilli in tissue from suspected lesions or in scrapings from the nasal mucosa. Leprosy may be confused with syphilis, yaws, tuberculosis of the skin, ringworm, and neuritis.

Lepromin, analogous to tuberculin, is used in a skin test for leprosy. It is more useful in determining prognosis or phase of the disease than in actual diagnosis because of possible false positive reactions.

Control of Leprosy.   The control of leprosy by segregation is still in current use, even though the disease is not very communicable. The modern forms

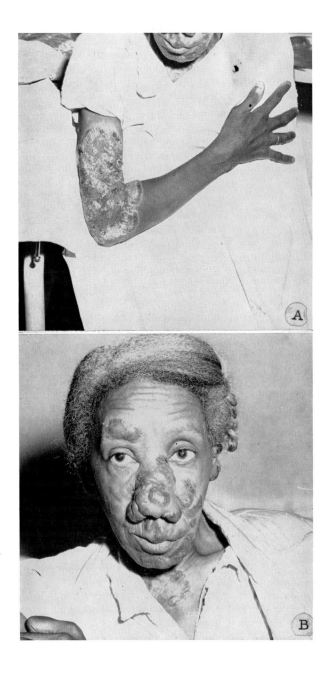

Figure 23.5: Advanced lepromatous leprosy. (**A,** AFIP 54–18444; **B,** AFIP 54–18443.)

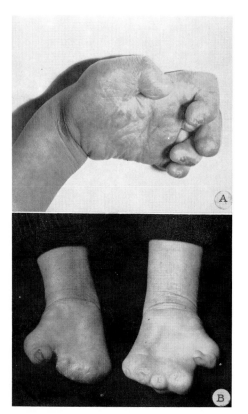

Figure 23.6: Lepromatous leprosy showing "claw" hand (**A**) and extensive destruction of the fingers (**B**). (AFIP 45–14075.)

of segregation are institutional or in the home. It might seem that compulsory segregation would eliminate leprosy in one generation, but it does not. The detection of early leprosy is difficult, and it is during this stage that the disease is most easily transmitted to children. Since compulsory segregation is akin to corporal punishment, lepers often attempt to escape detection and will resist segregation as long as possible, thereby defeating the attempt at prevention.

Since 1921 a modified form of compulsory segregation has been practiced in the United States, with lepers being confined to the National Leprosarium at Carville, Louisiana. The National Leprosarium receives and cares for lepers who are referred to it by local or state health authorities or who go there voluntarily to receive treatment. Home segregation of lepers is difficult and not very satisfactory.

Treatment. Diaminodiphenylsulfone or related sulfone compounds are the drugs of choice in the treatment of leprosy. They produce a gradual improvement over several years, although resistance may occur after prolonged treatment. There is some indication that rifampin may be useful in the treatment of leprosy.

Atypical Mycobacteria

A variety of mycobacterial species that are not common human pathogens are capable of causing human disease under certain circumstances. The most frequently encountered of these opportunistic mycobacterial species are *M. avium, M. intracellulare, M. scrofulaceum, M. kansasii, M. xenopi, M. marinarum, M. chelonae,* and *M. fortuitum.*

The *M. avium* complex, as presently described, comprises strains of two species, *M. avium* and *M. intracellulare.* The taxonomic relationship between the two species is not clear. Morphologically they are typical mycobacteria, but *M. avium* is occasionally filamentous with true branching. These organisms are ubiquitous in nature, based on immunological surveys. Occasionally these organisms produce serious pulmonary disease that is slowly progressive but difficult to treat. Of more concern recently is the observation that progressive infection of all organs may be seen with apparently unrestrained growth of these organisms in tissues of patients with AIDS.

M. scrofulaceum, like the *M. avium* complex, is widely distributed in nature. It may be associated with pulmonary disease but is more commonly seen in localized lesions of cervical adenitis in children. *M. kansasii* is most frequently associated with pulmonary disease but may affect other organs. *M. marinarum* usually is associated with localized, self-limiting skin lesions that develop at sites of cuts or abrasions acquired in infested swimming pools. *M. fortuitum* and *M. chelonae* are opportunistic pathogens that may be associated with pulmonary disease, meningitis, or, most frequently, with severe abscess at the sites of trauma or surgical procedures, including prosthetic implants.

There have been reports of infections by these atypical mycobacteria in transplant patients. They were mostly noted in renal transplant patients and usually manifested as lesions of the skin and mucosa.

ADDITIONAL READING

Addington, W. W. 1979. The Treatment of Pulmonary Tuberculosis. Arch Intern Med, **139,** 1391.

Banner, A. S. 1979. Tuberculosis: Clinical Aspects and Diagnosis. Arch Intern Med, **139,** 1387.

Blumberg, B. S., Melartin, L., Guinto, R., and Lechat, M. 1970. Lepromatous Leprosy. J Chronic Dis, **23,** 507.

Collins, C. H., Grange, J. M., and Yates, M. D. 1986. Unusual Opportunist Mycobacteria. Med Lab Sci, **43,** 262.

Comstock, G. W. 1982. Epidemiology of Tuberculosis. Am Rev Respir Dis, **125,** 8.

Dannenberg, A. M. Jr. 1982. Pathogenesis of Pulmonary Tuberculosis. Am Rev Respir Dis, **125,** 25.

Dannenberg, A. M., Jr., Ando, M., and Shima, K. 1972. Macrophage Accumulation, Division, Maturation, and Digestive and Microbicidal Capacities in Tuberculous Lesions: III. The Turnover of Macrophages and Its Relation to

Their Activation and Antimicrobial Immunity in Primary BCG Lesions and Those of Reinfection. J Immunol, **109**, 1109.

Jolly, H. W., Jr. 1975. Atypical Mycobacterial Infections of the Skin: Treatment. Dermatol Dig, **14**, 16.

Lowrie, D. B. 1983. How Macrophages Kill Tubercle Bacilli. J Med Microbiol, **16**, 1.

Miller, R. L., Krutchkoff, D. J., and Grammara, B. S. 1978. Human Lingual Tuberculosis. Arch Pathol Lab Med, **102**, 360.

Read, J. K., Heggie, C. M., Meyers, W. M., and Connor, D. H. 1974. Cytotoxic Activity of *Mycobacterium ulcerans*. Infect Immun, **9**, 114.

Reich, C. V. 1987. Leprosy: Cause, Transmission, and a New Theory of Pathogenesis. Rev Infect Dis, **9**, 590.

Shapiro, C. D. K., Harding, G. E., and Smith, D. W. 1974. Relationship of Delayed-type Hypersensitivity and Acquired Cellular Resistance in Experimental Air-borne Tuberculosis. J Infect Dis, **130**, 8.

Wayne, L. G. 1982. Microbiology of Tubercle Bacilli. Am Rev Respir Dis, **125**, 31.

Wayne, L. G. 1985. The "Atypical" Mycobacteria: Recognition and Disease Association. CRC Crit Rev Microbiol, **12**, 185.

West, B. C., Todd, J. R., Lary, C. H., *et al.* 1988. Leprosy in Six Isolated Residents of Northern Louisiana. Arch Intern Med, **148**, 1987.

Wolstenholme, G. E. W., and O'Connor, M. (Eds.) 1963. *Pathogenesis of Leprosy.* Little, Brown & Co., Boston.

24

Actinomycetes and Actinomycosis

George S. Schuster

A number of pathogenic microorganisms resemble both bacteria and fungi. Some of these microorganisms are included in the order Actinomycetales, which contains the genera *Actinomyces, Arachnia, Bifidobacterium, Bacterionema,* and *Rothia.* They resemble in many ways both the pathogenic fungi and the corynebacteria and diphtheroids. The *Nocardia,* members of a different family in this order, more closely resemble the mycobacteria (some are acid-fast) and have less resemblance to fungi, while the *Streptomyces* species more closely resemble the fungi than do the others.

Actinomycosis is a disease of human beings and some species of animals that is caused by species of *Actinomyces,* although there have been reports of cases due to *Arachnia* and *Bifidobacterium.* It is generally recognized that *Actinomyces bovis,* the type species, is the cause of actinomycosis or lumpy jaw in cattle. The human oral species are generally considered to be *Actinomyces israelii,* the principal cause of human actinomycosis; *Actinomyces naeslundii,* an essentially nonpathogenic species, although human in-

fections have been reported; *Actinomyces viscosus,* which has been implicated in periodontal disease and may play a role in some cases of human actinomycosis; and *Actinomyces odontolyticus,* an isolate from deep dentinal caries. Other species include *A. meyeri, A. pyogenes, A. denticolens, A. howellii,* and *A. hordeovulneris.* The last three are animal pathogens, as is *A. pyogenes,* although it can cause disease in humans.

In some characteristics the *Actinomyces* strains resemble both bacteria and fungi, and they have often been considered to be transitional between the two groups of microorganisms. Most of the more fundamental characteristics of the actinomycetes indicate that they are, in fact, bacteria. They are anaerobic or facultative, in contrast to the pathogenic fungi, which are uniformly aerobic. Because their cell membranes contain no sterols, they are not sensitive to the polyene antibiotics, which can act on pathogenic fungi. They are sensitive to antibacterial chemotherapeutic agents, which have no effect on pathogenic fungi. The cell walls of the actinomycetes are similar to those of bacteria in that they contain muramic acid and do not

263

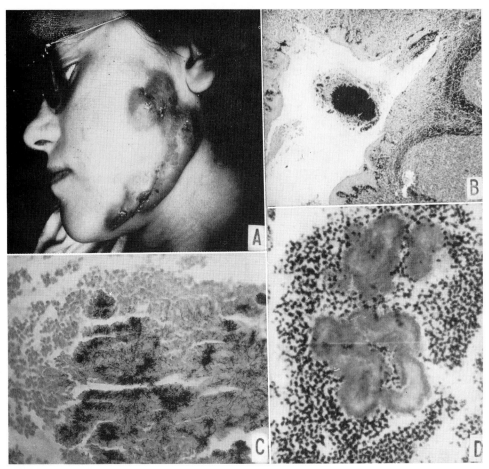

Figure 24.1: (**A**) Facial actinomycosis. (**B**) "Sulfur" granule in tissue (×35). (**C**) *Actinomyces* in the skin (×160). (**D**) "Sulfur" granule in tissue (×340). (**A,** AFIP 88; **B,** AFIP 137912; **C,** courtesy of Max Poser, Bausch and Lomb Optical Company; **D,** AFIP 89.)

contain the chitin or glucans that are typical of the cell walls of fungi. They are prokaryotic, for they lack a nuclear membrane. The actinomycetes form mycelia in tissue or in culture and can form branching filaments. However, the diameter of these filaments is similar to that of the cells of bacilli and is not as wide as those of fungi. Thus, the actinomycetes are more correctly considered to be bacteria rather than fungi.

Clinical Course and Manifestations

Human actinomycosis may involve almost any area of the body. Primary lesions occur most frequently in the oral cavity, face, or neck (Figs. 24.1 and 24.2). The abdominal cavity and the lungs are other frequent sites of infection. Clinically, five types of actinomycosis have been distinguished, according to the area of ini-

tial infection: cervicofacial, abdominal, cutaneous, thoracic, and genital.

The initial lesion of the more prevalent cervicofacial infection is usually found in the oral cavity. The onset of the disease is insidious, and, if it does not follow some surgical procedure or injury, is first noticed as a persistent swelling, usually in the parotid or mandibular regions. The swelling is not painful, although it may be if secondarily infected. If the disease develops soon after surgery, the wound heals slowly, and swelling persists or even increases. With such symptoms the diagnosis of actinomycosis is difficult, for the symptoms are those of cellulitis or residual osteitis with a different or more common etiology. A dark red or purplish skin overlying a very hard, board-like swelling is characteristic of actinomycosis. As the infection progresses, points of fluctuation develop extraorally, abscesses form, and multiple sinuses appear. Bone involvement is rare in the early stages of the disease, but later a true osteomyelitis may develop, with considerable bone destruction. When this occurs the infection may burrow upward toward the spine or cranial region, often causing death.

Primary thoracic actinomycosis is not uncommon and may be caused either by *A. israelii* or by aerobic *Nocardia* species. The pulmonary infection occurs with low-grade fever, coughing, and expectoration of bloody sputum. As the disease progresses, draining sinuses, extending to the external chest wall or to the heart, are established by direct invasion. The patient gradually loses weight, becomes anemic, and has a severe pulmonary infection.

Cutaneous infections are usually the result of traumatic implantation of organisms. They are first seen as small subcutaneous swellings that slowly enlarge and soften. The lesions rupture to the surface

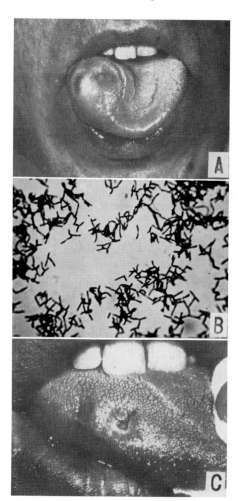

Figure 24.2: Actinomycosis. (**A**) Lesion involving the tongue. (**B**) Causal actinomycetes. (**C**) Lesion after treatment. (Reproduced with permission from L. Dorph-Petersen and J. J. Pindborg: Actinomycosis of the Tongue. *Oral Surg, Oral Med, Oral Pathol*, **7,** 1178, 1954.)

and sinus tracts form. They also can burrow deeper into the tissues, invading and destroying bone.

Abdominal actinomycosis may be caused by the invasion of the intestinal mucosa by actinomycetes from the oral cavity, or by the extension of a pulmonary infection. It initially appears as a palpable abdominal mass that simulates appendicitis. Infection may spread to the liver, spleen, or spinal column.

Recently, genital actinomycosis has been described in women using intrauterine devices. The diagnosis is based on histology of the infected tissues and isolation of the organisms from tissues and devices.

Actinomycosis is a persistent disease that may show signs of regression, only to recur with renewed vigor. The actinomycetes elicit an immunological reaction that is not very consistent. Opsonins, agglutinins, precipitins, and complement-fixing antibodies occur, but they are not useful in diagnosis, and their role in resistance is unknown.

Pathogenesis of Actinomycosis

Since *A. israelii* normally inhabits tonsils, carious teeth, and calculus deposits, any open wound in the mouth such as those caused by extraction of teeth, accidents, or pulp exposure provides a pathway for the introduction of the organisms into susceptible tissue. However, the simple introduction of potentially pathogenic actinomycetes into oral tissues does not necessarily lead to infection. Several factors seem to be involved in actinomycosis. A single inoculation of actinomycetes into susceptible animals seldom causes infection, whereas repeated inoculation frequently does, indicating that some form of tissue sensitization may play a role in the process of infection. Trauma associated with surgery, injury, or less often such chronic irritation as calculus beneath the gingival margin predisposes to infection.

During an infection, the pathogenic actinomyces form characteristic but not necessarily specific granules that are commonly visible by ordinary observation. These granules, often called sulfur granules because of their resemblance to precipitated sulfur, are present in the tissues of the lesion but are most easily found in the exudate and pus of the lesion. Sulfur granules may vary considerably in size and composition, but their central portion consists of delicate intertwining filaments. The peripheral filaments are surrounded by gelatinous sheaths, giving them a clublike appearance. Granules are found, however, without any peripheral clubs. The tiny branching filaments in granules stain positive with gram stain or may appear as gram-positive beads. When stained with hematoxylin–eosin, the central portion is basophilic, while the periphery is eosinophilic.

Laboratory Diagnosis of Actinomycosis

A laboratory method for diagnosing actinomycosis consists of detecting sulfur granules in pus or exudate from a suspected lesion by ordinary visual observation. Pus for observation of the granules can be collected directly into a sterile test tube or obtained indirectly from deeper lesions by aspiration with needle and syringe and then placed in a tube. Rotation of the tube will distribute the pus thinly over its surface so that the larger granules can be more easily observed directly. Or the pus can be crushed between a cover glass and slide and stained with gram stain for observation of granules too small to see by direct vision.

Cultivation is also useful for diagnosis. Specimens of exudate or tissue should be cultured in enriched media and incubated both aerobically and anaerobically at 37°C. Thioglycollate broth is especially useful for distinguishing *A. israelii* from other species by the hard colonies it produces versus the more easily disrupted colonies of the others. Except for *A. viscosus,* the catalase test can be used to distinguish the catalase-negative *Actinomyces* from *Corynebacterium* and *Propionibacterium.*

Treatment of Actinomycosis

Treatment of actinomycosis is complicated by the large tissue areas involved and the hard swelling, but exploration and drainage of sinus tracts and excision of damaged tissue greatly facilitates chemotherapy. Combined treatment consisting of surgical intervention and chemotherapy has effected an 80% to 90% cure rate. Antibiotic therapy should be intensive and prolonged, perhaps weeks to months. Treatments with penicillin, erythromycin, tetracycline, cephalosporin, clindamycin, and lincomycin have been reported as successful.

ADDITIONAL READING

Bach, M. C., Monaco, A. P., and Finland, M. 1973. Pulmonary Nocardiosis. JAMA, **224,** 1378.

Brock, D. W., Georg, L. K., Brown, J. M., and Hicklin, M. D. 1978. Actinomycosis Caused by *Arachnia propionica:* Report of 11 Cases. Am J Clin Pathol, **59,** 66.

Bujak, J. S., Ottesen, E. A., Dinarello, C. A., and Bremer, V. J. 1973. Nocardiosis in a Child with Chronic Granulomatous Disease. J Pediatr, **83,** 98.

Coleman, R. M., Georg, L. K., and Rozzell, A. R. 1967. *Actinomyces naeslundii* as an Agent of Human Actinomycosis. Appl Microbiol, **18,** 420.

Cran, J. A., and Haunam, A. G. 1963. Cervico-facial Actinomycosis. Aust Dent J, **8,** 106.

Eastridge, C. E., Prather, J. R., Hughes, F. A., Jr., Young, J. M., and McCaughan, J. J., Jr. 1972. Actinomycosis: A 24-Year Experience. South Med J, **65,** 839.

Ellen, R. P., and Balcerzak-Raczkowski, I. B. 1975. Differential Medium for Detecting Dental Plaque Bacteria Resembling *Actinomyces viscosus* and *Actinomyces naeslundii.* J Clin Microbiol, **2,** 305.

Eng, R. H. K., Corrado, M. L., Cleri, D., Cherubin, C., and Goldstein, E. J. C. 1981. Infection Caused by *Actinomyces viscosus.* Am J Clin Pathol, **75,** 113.

Engel, D., Van Epps, D., and Clagett, J. 1976. *In Vitro* and *In Vivo* Studies on Possible Pathogenic Mechanisms of *Actinomyces viscosus.* Infect Immun, **14,** 548.

Fillery, E. D., Bowden, G. H., and Hardie, J. M. 1978. A Comparison of Strains Designated *Actinomyces viscosus* and *Actinomyces naeslundii.* Caries Res, **12,** 299.

Gutshik, E. 1976. Case Report: Endocarditis Caused by *Actinomyces viscosus.* Scand J Infect Dis, **8,** 271.

Hamner, J. E. 1965. Anterior Maxillary Actinomycosis: Report of Case. J Oral Surg, **23,** 60.

Hertz, J. 1957. Actinomycosis: Oral, Facial, and Maxillary Manifestations. J Int Coll Surg, **28,** Part I, 539.

Kuranutsu, H. K., and Paul, L. 1980. Role of Bacterial Interactions in the Colonization of Oral Surfaces by *Actinomyces viscosus.* Infect Immun, **29,** 83.

Laca, E. 1964. Primary Actinomycosis of the Parotid Gland. Thorax, **13,** 234.

Langenegger, J. J. 1965. Actinomyces and Their Effects on Oral Tissues. J Dent Assoc South Afr, **20,** 1.

Larsen, J., Bottone, E. J., Dirkman, S., and Saphir, R. 1978. Cervicofacial *Actinomyces viscosus* Infection. J Pediatr, **93,** 797.

Leafstedt, S. W., and Gleeson, R. M. 1977. Cervicofacial Actinomycosis. Am J Surg, **130,** 496.

Peabody, J. W., Jr., and Seabury, J. H. 1957. Actinomycosis and Nocardiosis. J Chronic Dis, **5,** 374.

Reiner, S. L., Harrelson, J. M., Miller, S. E., et al. 1987. Primary Actinomycosis of an Extremity: A Case Report and Review. Rev Infect Dis, **9,** 581.

Saunders, J. M., and Miller, C. H. 1980. Attachment of *Actinomyces naeslundii* to Human Buccal Epithelial Cells. Infect Immun, **29,** 98.

Slack, J. M., Landfried, S., and Gerencser, M. A. 1971. Identification of *Actinomyces* and Related Bacteria in Dental Calculus by Fluorescent Antibody Technique. J Dent Res, **50,** 78.

Sprague, W. G., and Shafer, W. G. 1963. Presence of Actinomyces in Dentigerous Cyst: Report of Two Cases. J Oral Surg, **21,** 243.

Thadepalli, H., and Rao, B. 1979. *Actinomyces viscosus* Infection of the Chest in Humans. Am Rev Respir Dis, **120,**203.

Vasarinsh, P. 1968. Primary Cutaneous Nocardiosis. Arch Dermatol, **98,** 489.

25

Spirochetes and Spirochetal Diseases

George S. Schuster

The spirochetes are classified in the order Spiro-chetales. The ninth edition of *Bergey's Manual of Determinative Bacteriology* lists two families in this order, the Spirochetaceae and the Leptospiraceae. In the first family the only members that are pathogens for humans are in the genus *Treponema* and the genus *Borrelia*. The genus *Treponema* contains several species of significance, including *T. pallidum, T. pertenue,* and *T. cunniculi.* Several species occur as part of the oral and intestinal flora. For the most part these appear to be nonpathogenic, although some of the oral strains have been associated with periodontal disease. These are discussed elsewhere. The genus *Leptospira* has two species, *L. interrogans* and *L. biflexa,* with numerous serological variants. *Leptospira* organisms are readily differentiated by being obligate anaerobes that are tightly coiled and have hooked ends.

Treponema pallidum and Related Spirochetes

Morphology of *T. pallidum*. The causative agents of venereal and endemic syphilis (*T. pal-lidum*), yaws (*T. pertenue*), pinta (*T. carateum*), rabbit syphilis (*T. cuniculi*), and some of the oral spirochetes (*T. microdentium* and *T. mucosum*) cannot be wholly differentiated morphologically. They do differ in the diseases or lack of diseases they produce. *T. pallidum,* as well as the other related spirochetes, is a thin, spiral microorganism (Fig. 25.1). Since the cells are 0.1 to 0.4 μm in diameter and 5 to 15 μm long, their visualization with an ordinary light microscope is difficult. Staining is not particularly helpful for observing the spirochetes unless the dye or some component such as silver is deposited to increase their volume and breadth. Spirochetes can be seen by dark-field or phase-contrast microscopy. Electron microscopy has revealed much of the internal morphology of spirochetes.

T. pallidum is similar structurally to other spirochetes (Fig. 25.2). It consists of a multilayered cytoplasmic membrane, six thin fibrils that are located between the cytoplasmic membrane and the cell wall, a muramic acid–containing cell wall, and a thin outer envelope. Pathogenic strains also appear to have a dense capsule-like layer not present in nonpathogens. *Treponema* species also contain intracytoplasmic

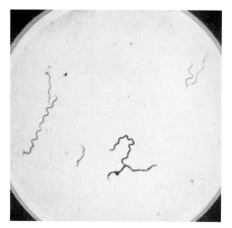

Figure 25.1: *Treponema pallidum* (× 1,000). (Courtesy of Max Poser, Bausch and Lomb Optical Company.)

tubules located on the inner surface of the cytoplasmic membrane that contribute to the cell's morphology.

The cells of *T. pallidum* are flexible and elastic and have distinctive movement and motility, undergoing a sustained movement that involves rapid rotation about a longitudinal axis and bending and flexing about the length. Their flexibility allows them to move among intercellular spaces.

Metabolism and Cultivation of *T. pallidum*.
Most attempts to culture fully pathogenic *T. pallidum* have been unsuccessful. Tissue cultures have been a problem because they are inherently aerobic, whereas *T. pallidum* is considered anaerobic. Recent evidence suggests that *T. pallidum* is microaerophilic and requires low (1% to 4%) oxygen concentrations. There have been unconfirmed reports of successful cultivation in tissue culture under reduced oxygen. The problem with in vitro growth is that the human and some other mammalian bodies may offer a nutritional factor that is not supplied in vitro.

Serial infection of the testicles of living rabbits has been the most successful method of propagating and maintaining virulent strains of *T. pallidum*. The Syrian hamster is also useful, but the infection is not so characteristic as it is with the rabbits.

Cultural procedures and animal inoculation have resulted in the isolation of several treponemal strains, some of which have maintained their pathogenicity in susceptible animals for considerable time. Cultured strains are antigenically heterogeneous, whereas the pathogenic Nichols and Noguchi strains resemble *T. pallidum*. Cultured strains are considered not to be identical with *T. pallidum*.

The fully virulent *T. pallidum* can be kept viable for about a week in an anaerobic maintenance medium

but it does not reproduce. The organisms apparently do metabolize in it, for penicillin, even at very low concentrations, will kill them after being exposed to it for 5 hours or so.

The cultured strains of spirochetes that resemble *T. pallidum* metabolize glucose and require exogenous fatty acids, co-enzymes, bicarbonate, a variety of amino acids, and purines and pyrimidines.

T. pallidum is sensitive to temperature, for its survival time decreases as the temperature increases between 20°C and 40°C. The sensitivity of *T. pallidum* to increased temperature was used as the basis for fever therapy of syphilis. In blood or blood products at refrigerator temperature, the spirochetes do not survive for more than 48 hours. Contaminated whole blood used in transfusions is not a source of infections after it has been maintained for 4 days at refrigerator temperature.

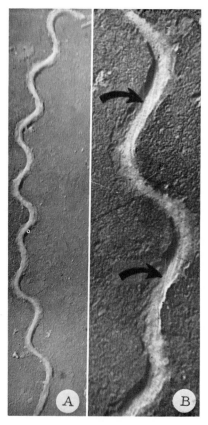

Figure 25.2: (**A**) *Treponema pallidum* from exudate of primary chancre. (**B**) The same spirochete at higher magnification showing an axial band (*arrows*) around which the main body of the spirochete is wound. (Reproduced with permission from R. H. A. Swain: Electron Microscopic Studies of the Morphology of Pathogenic Spirochetes. *J Pathol Bacteriol,* **69,** 117, 1955.)

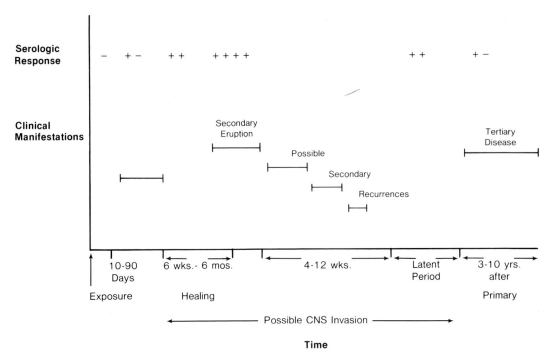

Figure 25.3: Time course of clinical events in syphilis and serological response at the various stages of disease.

Syphilis

Venereal Syphilis. Syphilis, caused by *T. pallidum*, is a venereal disease with a long clinical course and protean manifestations. It occurs naturally only in humans and is usually transmitted by sexual contacts between adults or congenitally from mother to fetus. In the Middle East and the Balkan states, endemic syphilis occurs that is propagated by nonvenereal contact between children or children and adults.

In the primary and secondary stages of syphilis, *T. pallidum* grows and survives well in the oral cavity and the genitalia. Genital transmission of *T. pallidum* accounts for 90% to 95% of syphilitic infections. The overwhelming proportion of primary extragenital infections occur about the mouth as a result of transmission of the organisms from the oral cavity when kissing or by oral-genital contact. Oral lesions may also result from localization of spirochetes in the tissues following dissemination by the blood or lymphatics. Syphilis is seldom but occasionally transmitted indirectly by fomites. There are many organisms in the primary lesions that can be readily transmitted. All secondary lesions of the skin and mucous membranes are highly infectious. In the later stages of syphilis, an individual may disseminate few or no spirochetes. The treponemes may be transmitted through the placental barrier of an infected pregnant woman to a fetus. However, *T. pallidum* does not always infect the fetus.

The number of organisms necessary to initiate infection is quite small. After inoculation the organisms move between cells, undergo rapid multiplication, and are widely disseminated via the perivascular lymphatics and the systemic circulation. This takes place before development of the primary lesion. The time course of syphilis is shown in Figure 25.3. In man the incubation time required to produce an initial lesion averages about 3 weeks. The shortest incubation periods have resulted from accidental inoculation of individuals with contaminated instruments. At the end of the primary incubation period a chancre develops, although a generalized systemic, syphilitic infection may occur without its appearance. The chancre is usually single and painless (Fig. 25.4). It appears first as an erythematous macule, then as a papule that enlarges, becomes infiltrated, and eventually erodes. The base of the chancre is reddish brown. When fully developed it has a narrow, copper-colored, beveled border and is well demarcated from the surrounding skin or mucous membrane. It is indurated and hence is called a hard chancre. The floor of the chancre produces a serosanguineous discharge and is covered by an adherent fibrinous membrane.

In the oral region, the most frequent sites for the development of a chancre are the lips and tongue; the

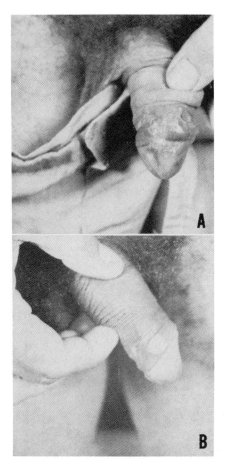

Figure 25.4: Chancre of the penis. (**A,** AFIP 59–12783; **B,** AFIP 59–12654.)

gingiva is seldom involved (Fig. 25.5). When chancres occur on tonsils, they are often mistaken for diphtheria. Extraorally, initial infection and chancre formation may occur in or about the eyes of dentists or health personnel. The chancre, if not secondarily infected, usually heals within 2 weeks but may persist for as long as 6 weeks after initial onset. As the lesion subsides healing occurs with or without scarring.

Two to 10 weeks after the primary disease appears the patient may experience secondary disease. There is a systemic or generalized infection and the integument teems with spirochetes. Prominent findings include fever, sore throat, generalized lymphadenopathy, headache, rash, and malaise. Involvement of palms and soles of the feet is common (Fig. 25.6); cutaneous eruptions manifest as macules and papules (Fig. 25.7). On mucous membranes such as those of the oral cavity the lesions are papules or mucous patches (Figs. 25.8 and 25.9). The latter is due to a local vasculitis. The lesions appear as white or small gray, slightly raised areas. They sometimes appear as split papules at the commissures. Condylomata lata occur around moist areas such as the anus and vagina. The mucosal and cutaneous eruptions persist or recur for 2 to 3 years. Recurrent outbreaks of secondary lesions become less extensive and further apart as the infection becomes latent. Other signs of this stage of disease are often secondary to a generalized immune response. Nephrotic syndrome with immune complex nephritis results from deposition of antigen–antibody complexes in the glomerular basement membrane. Arthritis and arthralgia may have a similar etiology.

After the last episode of secondary disease the patient enters the latent stage. The first 2 years of this phase of disease are considered early latent stage, the subsequent time late latent stage. Persons in the late latent stage are seroreactive but have no signs or symptoms of active disease. Approximately 60% of untreated patients in the late stage have an asymptomatic course, while 40% develop symptoms. Progression from late latent to late symptomatic syphilis is often preventable if appropriate therapy is instituted at this stage. During secondary disease, as immunity develops the number of spirochetes decreases.

From 3 to 10 years after disappearance of last evidence of secondary disease the symptomatic patient may develop tertiary disease. The slow but persistent reactions occurring during this period may be hyperergic, chronic, proliferative, inflammatory, and destructive; they involve viscera and the skeletal, cardiovascular, and central nervous systems. A very characteristic lesion of late syphilis is the gumma, probably arising from an immunological reaction. This lesion is quite destructive and may affect any tissue or organ of the body (Fig. 25.10). Very few spirochetes are present in a gumma, certainly insufficient to produce the extensive damage found unless an allergic reaction of the tissues to spirochetes is involved.

The principal lesions of late syphilis are gummas and nodular or nodulo-ulcerative syphilids of the skin. These lesions are similar histologically but differ in gross appearance. The lungs, bronchi, and trachea are seldom affected in late syphilis. Gummas occur frequently in the oral cavity and in the larynx and vocal cords, however, resulting in a painless but persistent hoarseness. During this period a glossitis may be present. Next to the skin, the skeleton is most commonly involved in late syphilis. The changes in bone are usually a destructive osteitis or hypertrophic periosteitis, to which no bone is immune. The joints may be involved, commonly with hydroarthrosis.

Central Nervous System Syphilis. The central nervous system may be invaded by *T. pallidum* at any time from 10 days or more before the chancre appears until 4 or 5 years after latency develops, but not thereafter, apparently due to the development of

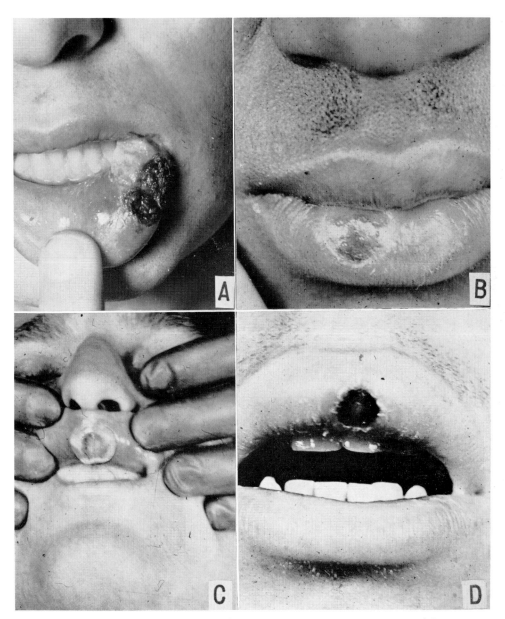

Figure 25.5: Primary syphilitic chancres of the lip. (**A**, AFIP B251B; **B**, AFIP 358; **C**, AFIP LS360.)

an immunity. About 30% of those initially involved develop asymptomatic neurosyphilis, but only about half develop late symptomatic neurosyphilis if untreated.

Asymptomatic neurosyphilis is characterized by any of the following changes in the cerebrospinal fluid: an increase in the number of lymphocytes; an increase in the protein content, principally globulin, which can be detected by the colloidal gold reaction; and the appearance of a positive complement-fixation test.

The reactions occurring in symptomatic neuro-syphilis are acute or subacute meningitis, meningovascular syphilis, tabes dorsalis, general paresis, and optic atrophy. Acute meningitis is rare, develops more often in early than in late syphilis, and resembles bacterial meningitis. Subacute meningitis may extend for weeks or months. Meningovascular syphilis is usually chronic and mild with prominent vascular changes consisting of narrowing, occlusion, or rupture of blood vessels. Tabes dorsalis, sometimes called locomotor ataxia, results from degeneration of the posterior roots and columns of the spinal cord and malfunction of certain cranial nerves. General

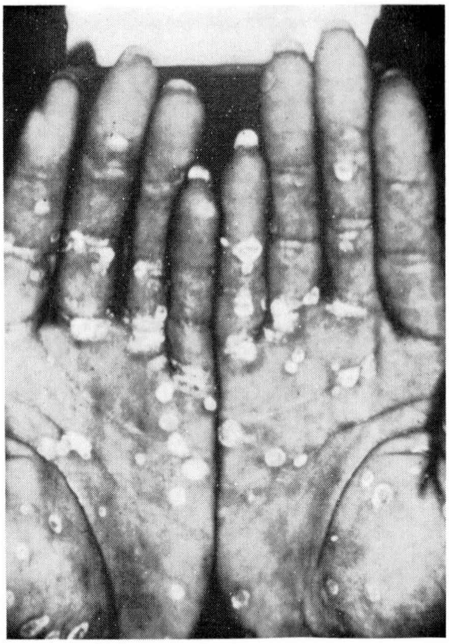

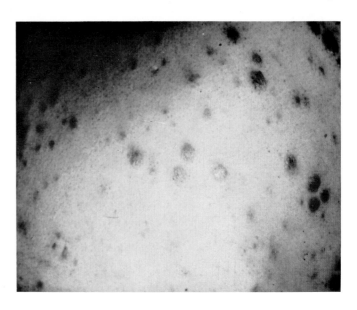

Figure 25.6: Palmar cutaneous manifestations of secondary syphilis. (AFIP 56–7603–9.)

paresis is produced by a chronic meningoencephalitis, resulting in progressive atrophy of the brain and loss of motor and mental function. If untreated the disease is usually fatal within 3 to 4 years. Late neurosyphilis may present as a variety of other neurologic diseases.

Cardiovascular Syphilis. Approximately 10 to 40 years after primary syphilis, untreated patients may develop signs of cardiovascular involvement. The structures most commonly involved are the great ves-

sels of the heart, in which arteritis may develop. The inflammatory reaction also may cause stenosis, angina, myocardial insufficiency, and death.

Congenital Syphilis. Another form of syphilis arises from prenatal infection. Infection may be transmitted from a syphilitic mother to the fetus through the placental circulation at any time before birth. Syphilitic infection interferes with normal fetal growth and development. A syphilitic newborn may exhibit a variety of manifestations of varying degrees of severity. These include hepatosplenomegaly, jaundice, hemolytic anemia, skin lesions, and damage to the long bones. The infant may have no lesions or may be dead at birth.

Congenital syphilis may manifest in the oral cavity as delayed dentition and abnormal development of two groups of teeth, the upper central incisors and the first permanent molars. These abnormal teeth have been termed Hutchinsonian teeth and mulberry molars, respectively. Hutchinsonian incisors are widely separated, with crowns that converge toward the incisal edge, giving rise to the term "pegged teeth" (Figs. 25.11 and 25.12). The incisal edges of Hutchinsonian teeth are usually notched, often singly. The mulberry molar does not develop correctly, resulting in defective cusps that are not properly oriented and are covered by defective enamel. Dental defects occur in about 38% of all children with prenatal syphilis.

Immunological Aspects of Syphilis

Immune Response. During the initial infection with *T. pallidum,* humoral antibodies are detectable by the time the chancre appears. IgG and IgM antibodies persist for a long time in untreated pa-

Figure 25.7: Cutaneous eruptions of the secondary syphilis. (AFIP 58–13966–45.)

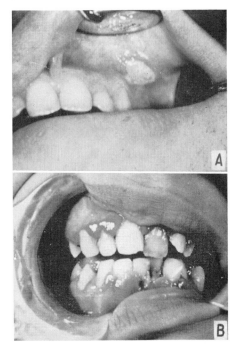

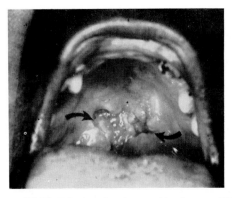

Figure 25.10: Palatal perforation resulting from syphilitic gumma. (AFIP 218663.)

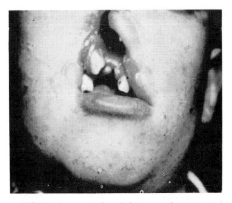

Figure 25.8: Secondary syphilitic manifestations. (**A**) Mucous patch adjacent to the mucobuccal fold. (**B**) Mucous patch in the upper right maxillary gingiva. (**A**, AFIP 363; **B**, AFIP.)

Figure 25.11: Congenital syphilitic manifestations in an adult. (AFIP 356.)

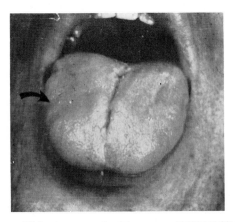

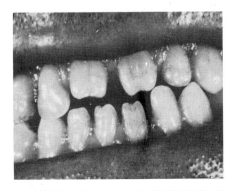

Figure 25.9: Mucous patch of the tongue. (AFIP 218663.)

Figure 25.12: Hutchinsonian teeth. (AFIP 218547–4.)

tients. It is not clear how the organism persists in the face of such a strong response. It may be that the outer layers of the virulent treponemes are so dense that they protect the organism against the effects of antibody attachment. In treated patients IgM levels decline but IgG persists for many years. Syphilis proceeds through its clinical stages despite the presence of humoral antibodies.

In early syphilis, cell-mediated immunity is in-hibited. Lymphocytes demonstrate a reduced response specifically to treponemal antigens. However, individuals with late secondary and tertiary syphilis do exhibit cell-mediated immunity to treponemal antigens. These antigens can inhibit migration of leukocytes from syphilitic individuals.

Thus, neither humoral nor cell-mediated immunity is sufficient to provide protection against syphilis. However, persons with untreated syphilis have a relative resistance to syphilis, and chancre development following a second infection is unusual.

Serological Reactions: Wassermann Antigen. Complement is fixed by syphilitic sera. This is due to Wassermann antibody, which is stimulated to appear during the disease. The original complement-fixation tests used as antigen an alcoholic extract of the livers of stillborn syphilitic infants. Subsequently it was found that the alcoholic extracts of a wide variety of tissues were equally effective as antigen. The specific principal is a phospholipid, termed cardiolipin (diphosphatidyl glycerol), which is fully reactive only when supplemented with lecithin and cholesterol. Mostly a highly purified preparation is used, termed VDRL antigen, after the Venereal Disease Research Laboratory.

Two theories have been proposed to explain the occurrence of the Wassermann antibody in man in response to Wassermann antigen. One explanation holds that it is a true antibody to a lipoidal component of *T. pallidum.* A different explanation is that treponemes and other bacteria cause the disintegration of human tissue during an infection, releasing cardiolipin as a hapten. According to this theory, the appearance of the Wassermann antibody is an autoimmune response. The antigen may bind to a protein carrier, perhaps of microbial origin, becoming a complete antigen capable of eliciting an antibody response.

Over the years two common types of serological tests have been devised using cardiolipin-lecithin antigen, the Wassermann and Kolmer complement-fixation tests and the flocculation test, of which there are numerous modifications. Both complement-fixation and flocculation tests are known as serological tests for syphilis (STS). It has become evident that the Wassermann antibody occurs in high titer during a more or less definite period in individuals with a variety of infectious and noninfectious diseases. Thus, these tests may lead to a high proportion of false positive and some false negative results in late untreated syphilis. In some individuals with no treponemal infection, the Wassermann antibody titer may remain high for months or years. However, the tests are inexpensive and demonstrate changing antibody titers in the individual.

Immobilization Phenomenon of *T. pallidum.* Syphilitic serum contains an antibody specific for an antigenic component of *T. pallidum,* which immobilizes it in the presence of complement. The *T. pallidum* immobilization (TPI) test was devised for the detection of syphilitic infections. This test is particularly useful in detecting biologically false positive cases as determined by STS but otherwise is not used very much clinically. The TPI test is specific for syphilis and yaws but does not differentiate between them or other treponemal infections.

Immunofluorescence Tests.   Fluorescent antibody tests are being utilized to a greater extent now in the diagnosis of syphilis and are available in several forms. Fluorescent treponemal antibody (FTA) tests use lyophilized organisms of the Nichols strain of *T. pallidum* as an antigen. This is fixed to a slide, followed by test serum. After any reaction has occurred, fluorescein-labeled antihuman immunoglobulin is applied and the presence of reacting antibody in the patient's serum is determined by fluorescent microscopy. A currently used variation of this test is the FTA–ABS (fluorescent treponemal antibody absorption) test. In this test the patient's serum is absorbed with another species of *Treponema* to remove shared antibodies, i.e., antibodies to nonspecific group antigens. The absorbed serum is reacted with nonviable Nichols strains of *T. pallidum,* followed by labeled antihuman globulin, and if serum contains specific antibody, which is usually against *T. pallidum,* it reacts in this indirect immunofluorescence test as in the FTA test. Another variation is the IgM–FTA–ABS test, which is specific for IgM antibodies and is useful for differentiating between passively transferred antibodies and actively formed antibodies in possible cases of congenital syphilis.

Hemagglutination Tests.   A hemagglutination method for serodiagnosis of syphilis is available and is particularly useful for screening. This test, the TPHA test, involves sensitizing tanned erythrocytes with treponemal antigens. When these react with specific antispirochetal antibodies, the erythrocytes are agglutinated. This test may be performed by microtitration.

Thus, there are a variety of immune reactions associated with syphilis. Both humoral and cell-mediated immune reactions have protective functions, and some may participate in the pathogenesis of the disease. However, the immune responses are also very useful in diagnosis of these infections.

Laboratory Diagnosis of *T. pallidum.* The inability to culture *T. pallidum* on laboratory media hampers the laboratory diagnosis of syphilis. An early method of laboratory diagnosis was the dark-field examination of an exudate from a suspected lesion for spirochetes, and this test still may be useful if the individual has not turned seroreactive. It is not useful for oral lesions, owing to the presence of indigenous treponemes that are morphologically indistinguishable from *T. pallidum.* Positive identification has been made of *T. pallidum* in smears of exudate from a suspected lesion on slides by the fluorescent antibody technique (FTA test). This technique differentiates *T. pallidum* from other spirochetes, especially nonpathogenic contaminants.

The wide variety of serological tests described above are useful for the laboratory diagnosis of syphilis. The World Health Organization recommends screening sera with the VDRL test, the rapid plasma reagenic (RPR) test, or the automated reaginic test (ART), and confirming positive sera with the FTA–ABS test. The hemagglutination tests are also useful for confirmation.

Treatment of *T. pallidum* Infection. Penicillin is the drug of choice in the treatment of syphilis. Slowly absorbed or repository types of penicillin are most widely used. Intramuscular injection of penicillin G- benzathine, 2.4 million units per week for 2 weeks, is quite effective. Patients allergic to penicillin may be given 500 mg of tetracycline four times a day for 12 days. About the only drawback to the use of penicillin is the Jarisch–Herxheimer reaction, which is caused by the release of spirochetal endotoxin following lysis of the spirochetes. This toxic reaction is usually seen following treatment of primary or secondary syphilis and is uncommon in late syphilis. It usually manifests as headache, fever, and malaise. It resolves in a day, although reactions in late syphilis may result in cardiovascular or nervous system damage.

Epidemiology and Control. The incidence of syphilis declined from 1941 to 1956, at which time it began to increase. There was a modest decrease in cases from 1982 to 1985, but the number then began to increase again. Overall the trend has been up. The major increase has been in men and has been not only in actual number of cases but also in cases per 100,000 population. The increase has been in primary, secondary, and congenital syphilis.

A syphilitic person is highly contagious during the primary and secondary stages. The disease is acquired principally by sexual contact, but dental and medical personnel may acquire it accidentally during their treatment of syphilitic patients. Occasionally, the disease may be acquired by nonsexual contact in barber shops and beauty parlors. Another factor complicating the control of syphilis is that many syphilitics, particularly women, are unaware that they have the disease. If such an individual is sexually promiscuous, he or she may transmit the disease to many contacts. Control relates to early identification and treatment of all syphilitic persons and their contacts. Several prophylactic procedures, including the use of a condom, cleansing of the genitalia with soap and water, application of calomel ointment, and vaccines, have not controlled syphilis. Although penicillin is quite successful in treating syphilis, it is not a prophylactic.

Treponema pertenue and Yaws

Treponema pertenue. The causative agent of yaws is morphologically indistinguishable from *T. pal-*

lidum. T. pertenue has not been satisfactorily cultivated in artificial media. In rabbits, it does not reproduce as rapidly as *T. pallidum,* and few cells can be obtained for study. Our knowledge of this organism is limited. No significant immunological difference has been demonstrated between *T. pertenue* and *T. pallidum.*

Yaws. Yaws is an endemic disease of worldwide distribution in hot and wet climates; it seldom occurs in the temperate zone. It is found in the tropics of Central and South America, the West Indies, Africa, India, Southeast Asia, Indonesia, Northern Australia, and the islands of the South Pacific. Worldwide, an estimated 50 million people have yaws.

There are several modes of yaws infection. Usually it is acquired by contact, the organisms entering the body through abrasions in the integument. The incubation period of yaws is about 2 weeks to a month. The initial lesion, known colloquially as the "mother yaw," appears as single or multiple papules or granulomas that ulcerate, crust over, and heal with scarring over the next 1 to 2 months, while evidence of a generalized infection develops.

Usually after 1 to 3 months, secondary flat-topped granulomas as large as 3 cm in diameter diffusely involve the skin. The secondary lesions, which may persist for years, teem with spirochetes and are known as "daughter yaw" or papillomatous frambeside, which gives to yaws the synonym frambesia. These lesions may heal without scarring, but recurrences may continue for several years. The palms of the hand and the plantar surfaces of the feet may be affected with painful and incapacitating frambesides, known as "crab yaws" from the crablike gait of such individuals. Bones and joints may be involved with arthritis and hydroarthrosis, respectively. As the disease progresses, the lesions in the skin, bone, and joints tend to become very destructive. Yaws persists throughout the lifetime in about 25% of cases, without per se causing death.

The symptoms of yaws are quite diagnostic. Laboratory diagnosis is similar to that for syphilis. Penicillin is the choice treatment for either control or eradication.

Endemic Syphilis or Bejel

The causal spirochete of endemic syphilis or bejel is morphologically identical with *T. pallidum* and *T. pertenue.* The disease it produces in humans differs slightly from venereal syphilis and yaws.

Endemic syphilis occurs throughout the Middle East and in the Balkan states. It is acquired primarily in childhood but occasionally is transmitted congenitally.

The initial lesion of endemic syphilis seldom occurs on the genital organs but is often oral or cutaneous. The course of the disease is somewhat similar to that of venereal syphilis, except that the stages are likely to be more prolonged and late lesions have a predilection for bone and mucous membranes. The best treatment is penicillin, administered as in venereal syphilis.

Treponema carateum and Pinta

Treponema carateum. *T. carateum,* the cause of pinta, is morphologically and serologically similar to *T. pallidum* and *T. pertenue.* It has not been cultured but has been successfully transferred to chimpanzees and experimentally from person to person to establish its causal relationship to pinta.

Pinta. Pinta, which has been described by many synonyms such as mal del pinto, carate, and azul, was for years thought to be a cutaneous mycosis. In 1938 a spirochete was discovered in active lesions and subsequently shown to be the causal organism. Pinta is prevalent in tropical and subtropical areas of the Western hemisphere, where there are an estimated 1,400,000 cases, but it also occurs in Africa, the Middle East, India, and the Philippines. Pinta is not venereal but is transferred from person to person by contact. It affects all age groups and if not treated it may persist for a lifetime.

Pinta progresses through three distinct stages. The incubation period is from 7 to 20 days and the primary stage extends to a year or more. The primary lesion is a papule that slowly develops into an erythematosquamous patch that spreads slowly around the affected area. Adjoining patches develop and coalesce with the original one. The secondary stage begins 6 to 12 months or more after onset with skin rashes and papules for which the name "pintid" has been proposed. Primary and secondary stages are not sharply delineated, for secondary lesions may occur simultaneously with the primary lesions. After several years or more, the tertiary stage begins, usually to continue for life if untreated. The lesions of this stage are characterized by achromic or pigmented spots, erythema, follicular keratosis, and keratoderma.

The treatment of pinta is similar to that for syphilis and yaws. The drug of choice is penicillin.

The Leptospirae and Leptospirosis

Morphology. *Leptospira* species range from pathogenic types causing human fevers and infections of a wide variety of animals (collectively termed leptospiroses) to harmless parasites. They are distinguishable from other spirochetes by their very fine spirals and by their tapered and curved or hooked ends.

Growth and Cultivation of *Leptospira*. The leptospirae are the least difficult of the pathogenic spirochetes to cultivate, growing aerobically on a simple medium. They grow best in liquid or on semisolid media; they do not grow satisfactorily on most solid media. Cultivation on simple media decreases virulence, which can be maintained or even revived by the addition of emulsions of fresh tissue such as liver. The leptospirae utilize long chain unsaturated fatty acids as a source of carbon and energy and can use inorganic ammonium salts as a nitrogen source.

Species and Classification of *Leptospira*. The genus *Leptospira,* first established by Noguchi in 1917, was divided into saprophytic and parasitic species. The saprophytic types are classified as *L. biflexa,* while according to the ninth edition of *Bergey's Manual of Determinative Bacteriology,* those parasitic in man and animals are classified as *L. interrogans.* The leptospirae are divided into several serological groups, which in turn are separated into serotypes. The etiological agents of the various leptospiroses are considered to be the various serogroups of *L. interrogans.* For example, Weil's disease is due to the serogroup *icterohaemorrhagiae.*

Antigenic Structure. *Leptospira* includes a large number of serologically distinct groups. These serogroups are differentiated and characterized by agglutination reactions. The serogroups are not recognized taxons but have been given names that imply that they are different species. The serogroups serve primarily for diagnostic purposes and no formal classification has been established. Nineteen serogroups have been proposed for *L. interrogans:* each serogroup is made up of one or more serotypes, and there are more than 175 serotypes. The immunological forms appear to be quite stable and are widely distributed geographically and among various hosts.

Epidemiology of *Leptospira*. The leptospirae are widely distributed in rodents and wildlife mammals, which are their natural hosts, but their geographic distribution is variable. They can survive for several weeks in surface waters under optimal conditions.

Human leptospiral infections are usually acquired directly or indirectly from infected rodents or other mammals. The spirochetes persist in the renal tubules of small rodents and larger wild mammals and are shed in urine. The organisms gain entrance through the mucosa of the eyes, nose, mouth, throat, or abraded skin. Infection is related to occupation (agricultural workers, slaughterhouse workers, sewer workers, and miners). Leptospiral infection that occurs when swimming is common. It may also occur in soldiers who must live in close contact with their environment.

Clinical Types of Human Leptospirosis. Human leptospiroses range from extremely severe to moderate and relatively mild infections. The classic severe form of leptospirosis is spirochetal fever, spirochetal jaundice, or more commonly Weil's disease. A more moderate form of leptospirosis is canicola fever. In addition, a large number of diseases are produced in particular geographical locations; they are given such local names as canefield fever, seven-day fever, autumnal fever, Fort Bragg fever, mud fever, and ricefield fever. They correspond to either Weil's disease or canicola fever.

Weil's Disease. Weil's disease, the most virulent leptospirosis, is caused by several *Leptospira* serotypes, especially of the serogroup *icterohaemorrhagiae*. The organisms gain entrance into the body through the skin or mucous membranes. The incubation period is usually 7 to 13 days. Onset, marked by fever and rigor, is usually sudden and dramatic. The disease occurs in three stages. The first stage, in which a leptospiremia occurs, lasts about a week. It is characterized by a high temperature (104°F; 40°C), malaise, debility, headache, muscular pain, and sore throat, and sometimes pneumonia near the end of the first stage.

The second stage of Weil's disease, which occupies a few days, is the most critical period of the infection and is characterized by the initiation of the immunological response. Death is most frequent during the second stage, though it may occur earlier. Acute renal failure is not unusual and is the cause of death in most cases. Jaundice is pronounced, the temperature is lower, and a rash occurs in 10% of patients.

In the third stage, beginning in the third week, fever may persist or recur but signs and symptoms abate, jaundice decreases, kidney function increases, the antibody titer increases, cardiac action improves, and convalescence begins. This stage lasts from 6 to 12 weeks or as long as 6 months. Mortality ranges from 5% to 30%, perhaps averaging about 10%.

Canicola Fever. Canicola fever is a milder type of leptospirosis than Weil's disease. It is transmitted by direct contact, by contact with excreta, or by bathing in contaminated water. The course of the disease and the symptoms are similar to those of Weil's disease but less severe.

Laboratory Diagnosis. The bacteriological diagnosis of the leptospiral fevers consists of the demonstration of the causal organisms and the detection of specific antibodies for the involved serotype. The organisms can be demonstrated by culture of body fluids or tissues in suitable fluid or semisolid media. *Leptospira* may be isolated from contaminated specimens by intraperitoneal inoculation of hamsters and guinea pigs. Direct demonstration by microscopic techniques may be a useful adjunct. Antibodies can be detected by agglutination tests. The number of antigens used in the test depends in part on the number of serotypes in a given geographic area. The microscopic agglutination test is the most useful strain-specific serologic test. Negative immunological tests throughout the course of an illness indicate the absence of leptospirosis. The presence of leptospiral antibodies indicates a leptospiral infection or residual antibodies from past leptospiral infection.

Treatment. Leptospiral infections may be treated with penicillin, tetracycline, the macrolide antibiotics, and streptomycin. Recovery is enhanced if treatment is started during the first 2 days after onset. If delayed past the fourth or fifth day, the course of the illness may not be altered.

Borrelia

The *Borrelia* are rather large spirochetes, having a diameter of about 0.2 to 0.5 µm and length of 4 to 18 µm, and fewer coils than the leptospirae. In addition, they have 7 to 20 periplasmic flagella originating at the ends and overlapping at the center of the cell. Because of their greater diameter, they are more readily stained and visualized with aniline dyes than are other spirochetes. *Borrelia* organisms are unusual in that they contain cholesterol; the only other bacteria in which this occurs are the mycoplasma. The *Borrelia* are relatively slow-growing microaerophilic organisms requiring complex media.

Pathogenesis and Pathology. Borreliae cause generalized infection after entering the host. *B. recurrentis* and the related spirochetes causing relapsing fever are widely distributed in rodents, foxes, and dogs: rodents are likely the primary reservoir. Man becomes infected through the vectors, lice or ticks. Onset of the disease is sudden, with fever, headache, and muscle pain that persists for 4 to 10 days, followed by a 5- to 6-day afebrile period. In louse-borne disease there usually is a single relapse. The mortality rate of untreated cases may be as high as 40%, and myocarditis is probably the most common cause of death. Tick-borne relapsing fever is similar but less severe than louse-borne disease. The fatality rate is from 0 to 8% but there usually are several relapses of decreasing intensity. Relapses are due to the ability of the organisms to undergo antigenic variations. Thus, as antibodies to the predominant type appear, the organisms disappear from peripheral blood and are replaced by a different type.

Lyme disease is caused by the spirochete *B. burgdorferi,* of which there appears to be only one antigenic type, and it does not undergo antigenic variations. It is transmitted to humans by hard ticks, the deer tick *Ixodes dammini* or *I. pacificus*. Lyme disease typically begins in summer with a unique skin lesion called erythema chronicum migrans (ECM), a migrating annular lesion, which may be accompanied by headache, stiff neck, fever, arthralgia and myalgia, malaise, fatigue, or lymphadenopathy. Weeks or months later some patients may develop meningoencephalitis, peripheral or cranial neuropathy, myocarditis or atrioventricular node block, or migrating musculoskeletal pain. Such reactions may occur for years. Actual arthritis may develop later and become chronic, with erosion of bone and cartilage. The mechanisms by which *Borrelia* produces disease are not known since the cells produce no known toxins.

Diagnosis. Diagnosis of relapsing fevers is usually based on demonstration of spirochetes in the patient's blood by dark-field examination or other means. Lyme disease is suspected on the basis of clinical manifestation, especially the characteristic red skin lesion of EMC, although lesions are not found in all cases. It can be diagnosed serologically by immunofluorescence.

Epidemiology. *Borrelia* are transmitted by the body louse or ticks. Transovarial transmission does not occur in lice, thus they serve as vectors while humans are the reservoirs. In tick-borne disease all tissues are involved; thus there is transovarial transmission of the microbes. Only a short feeding time is necessary to transmit infection via their secretions. People may not be aware of having been bitten.

Control. Avoidance of the vectors is the best way to prevent these infections. In endemic areas, proper precautions to prevent tick bites and good personal hygiene are important. Tetracycline is the drug of choice for relapsing fever and Lyme disease. The latter is susceptible to penicillin and these drugs, if given early in the illness, will shorten the course of disease and can prevent some of the major late complications of Lyme disease such as cardiac abnormalities. Indeed, late complications of Lyme disease respond to tetracycline, suggesting that spirochetes persist in infected persons.

ADDITIONAL READING

Ackerman, A. B., Goldfaden, G., and Cosmides, J. C. 1972. Acquired Syphilis in Early Childhood. Arch Dermatol, **106,** 92.

Benack, J. L., Bosler, E. M., Honrahen, J. P., et al. 1983. Spirochetes Isolated from the Blood of Two Patients with Lyme Disease. N Engl J Med, **308,** 740.

Cave, V. G., and Nikitas, M. A. 1976. Venereal Disease: Clinical and Laboratory Diagnosis. Mt Sinai J Med, **43,** 795.

Chapel, T. A. 1980. The Signs and Symptoms of Secondary Syphilis. Sex Transm Dis, **7,** 161.

Fitzgerald, T. J. 1981. Pathogenesis and Immunology of *Treponema pallidum.* Annu Rev Microbiol, **35,** 29.

Fiumara, N. J. 1976. Venereal Diseases of the Oral Cavity. J Oral Med, **24,** 1.

Fiumara, N. J., and Berg, M. 1974. Primary Syphilis in the Oral Cavity. Br J Vener Dis, **50,** 463.

Garner, M. F. 1972. The Serological Diagnosis of Treponemal Infection. NZ Med J, **75,** 353.

Habicht, G. S., Beck, G., and Benach, J. L. 1987. Lyme Disease. Sci Am, **257,** 78.

Harwood, C. S., and Canale–Parola, E. 1984. Ecology of Spirochetes. Annu Rev Microbiol, **38,** 161.

Holt, S. C. 1978. Anatomy and Chemistry of Spirochetes. Microbiol Rev, **42,** 114.

Masacola, L., Pelosi, R., Blount, J. H., et al. 1985. Congenital Syphilis Revisited. Am J Dis Child, **139,** 575.

Reif, J. S., and Marshak, R. R. 1973. Leptospirosis: A Contemporary Zoonosis. Ann Intern Med, **79,** 893.

Schell, R. F., and Musher, D. M. 1983. Pathogenesis and Immunology of Treponemal Infection. In *Immunology Series,* edited by N. B. Rose. Marcel Dekker, New York.

Sell, S., and Norris, S. J. 1983. The Biology, Pathology, and Immunology of Syphilis. Int Rev Exp Pathol, **24,** 203.

Steere, A. C., Grodzicki, R. L., Kornblatt, A. M., et al. 1983. The Spirochetal Etiology of Lyme Disease. N Engl J Med, **308,** 733.

Taber, L. H., and Feigin, R. D. 1979. Spirochetal Infections. Pediatr Clin North Am, **26,** 377.

Titche, L. L. 1972. Tertiary Syphilis of the Mouth. Arch Otolaryngol, **96,** 460.

26

The Aerobic Spore-Forming Bacilli

George S. Schuster

Bacillus anthracis

B. anthracis is the only member of the aerobic genus *Bacillus* that is considered a significant pathogen. However, *Bacillus cereus, Bacillus subtilis,* and *Bacillus sphaericus* have been reported to cause meningitis, endocarditis, and osteomyelitis. *B. anthracis* is a large aerobic, gram-positive, encapsulated spore-forming rod (Fig. 26.1). It is nonhemolytic, which differentiates it from most other members of the genus *Bacillus.* Sporulation occurs readily under almost all conditions except in the living host, where encapsulation is most prominent. Spores are very resistant, contaminating soils, the chief source of animal infection, for many years. They withstand boiling water for 10 minutes and dry heat (140°C) for 3 hours.

Anthrax bacilli possess capsular and somatic antigens and antigens that make up a complex exotoxin. The capsule is unusual in that it is a high molecular weight polypeptide consisting of D-glutamic acid. The somatic antigen is a polysaccharide component of the cell wall. The immunogenic toxin has been divided into three distinct, antigenically active components: protective antigen, lethal factor, and edema factor.

B. anthracis exhibits genetic variation with regard to spore formation, virulence, sensitivity to chemotherapeutic agents, nutritional requirements, bacteriophages, and lysozyme. Virulence essentially relates to two factors, capsule formation and exotoxin production, and only strains that produce both are fully virulent. The capsule interferes with phagocytosis and is important in pathogenesis, especially in the early stages of infection. Anticapsular antibodies, however, are not protective. The signs and symptoms of anthrax are due to the toxin's cumulative effects on the central nervous system. Toxemia can result in respiratory failure, anoxia, and death.

Anthrax

In animals, the spores of *B. anthracis* enter the body through some break in the oral or intestinal mucosa or by inhalation. The incubation period is only a day

279

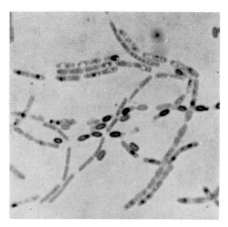

Figure 26.1: Anthrax bacilli undergoing sporulation (× 1850). (Courtesy of Max Poser, Bausch and Lomb Optical Company.)

or two, followed by an acute, fulminating disease that may terminate fatally within a few hours and usually in less than 1 day. In man, the organisms enter the body through breaks or wounds of the skin and the oral and intestinal mucosa or by inhalation. In the skin, a vesicle called a malignant pustule develops 2 to 5 days after infection (Fig. 26.2). It begins as a papule that becomes filled with bluish black fluid. This ruptures, revealing a black eschar surrounded by an inflammatory ring. The infection may remain localized or disseminate. In the pulmonary infection, the primary manifestation is an acute pneumonia that leads to respiratory distress and cyanosis. Pulmonary anthrax is almost always fatal. The rapid (24-hour) toxin-caused death usually sets in before therapy can be instituted. Inhaled spores are transported to lymph nodes by alveolar macrophages where they germinate, resulting in septicemia. In the intestinal tract *B. anthracis* causes an acute enteritis.

Anthrax infection of the oral cavity has been caused by unsterilized toothbrushes made from bristles contaminated with anthrax spores. In a typical case, the hard palate was initially infected, causing considerable swelling and eventually discharging a straw-colored fluid. The patient was quite ill with a temperature that ranged from 100 to 102°F (38 to 39°C). The bone of the area became involved, and as the infection progressed, most of the palatal and alveolar bone was destroyed. As the lesion developed, more and more of the area was involved with extensive edema. The teeth were overly erupted and apparently without bony support. Pustules with bright red bases appeared on the mucosa surface; many developed into vesicles that broke and scabbed, with eventual resolution. Treatment with antianthrax serum halted the symptoms, and the patient gradually recovered. Animals and humans that survive an attack of anthrax are usu-

ally resistant to reinfection. Vaccines have proved useful for controlling outbreaks.

Pathogenesis. The spores of *B. anthracis* are engulfed by macrophages but not destroyed. The spores germinate, escape, and multiply extracellularly. In systemic disease the organisms usually remain in the lymphatics and blood vessels. Toxin is a major component of the pathogenesis of anthrax, being toxic for the CNS, leukocytes, and other cells, although it is not clear what cell types may be attacked to account for the edema, hemorrhage, and necrosis of the local lesion or the hemoconcentration, anoxia, and renal and respiratory failure of systemic shock. Anthrax toxin consists of three components, which are proteins or lipoproteins. Factor I is designated edema factor, factor II is designated protective antigen since it induces protective antibodies in guinea pigs, and factor III, termed lethal factor, is essential for the lethal effect. In addition to cell toxicity caused by the toxin, including toxicity for phagocytes, the capsule contributes to virulence by being antiphagocytic.

Laboratory Diagnosis of Anthrax. The laboratory procedures useful for the diagnosis of anthrax are demonstration of characteristically large bacilli in gram-stained tissue specimens, culturing, and inoculation of samples into guinea pigs or mice.

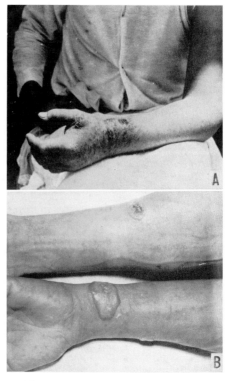

Figure 26.2: The cutaneous lesions of anthrax. (**A,** AFIP 218885–7; **B,** AFIP D45409–10.)

Treatment of Anthrax.   The anthrax bacillus is sensitive to penicillin, tetracycline, erythromycin, and chloramphenicol. Penicillin is the drug of choice and tetracycline is the best alternate. Cutaneous anthrax responds favorably to chemotherapy. Pulmonary anthrax is quite resistant to chemotherapy, and the mortality from this infection is very high.

Prevention and Control of Anthrax.   Anthrax is epidemic in Asia, Africa, and the Middle East, where it causes heavy loss. Cases have occurred in Texas, Louisiana, South Dakota, Nebraska, and California. Worldwide, the human cases are estimated to range up to 100,000 annually. The few cases of anthrax that occur in the United States are acquired by contact with infected livestock or with imported hair, wool, or hides. The most successful control of animal anthrax relates to the use of attenuated vaccines. A vaccine made of antigens that stimulate protective antibodies is also useful for workers who may come into contact with infected animal products and for veterinarians.

Other *Bacillus* Species

Other members of the genus *Bacillus* may be pathogens, often in compromised patients. *B. cereus* causes two types of food poisoning. One type occurs about 4 hours after eating and is characterized by severe nausea and vomiting; it resembles staphylococcal food poisoning. The other type occurs 16 to 18 hours after ingestion of the contaminated food and resembles clostridial food poisoning. It is characterized by abdominal cramps and diarrhea. The food is usually contaminated by spores that survive cooking, germinate, multiply, and produce enterotoxins. *B. cereus* also produces opportunistic infections in patients with implanted prosthetic devices and in immunocompromised patients.

B. subtilis is found in air, soil, dust, and organic material. Like *B. cereus,* it can cause opportunistic infection in immunocompromised patients and produces septicemia in drug users exposed to contaminated narcotics.

ADDITIONAL READING

Brachman, P. S. 1970. Anthrax. Ann NY Acad Sci, **174,** 577.

Brachman, P. S. 1980. Inhalation Anthrax. Ann NY Acad Sci, **353,** 83.

Centers for Disease Control. 1969. Anthrax in New Jersey. MMWR, **18,** 212.

Centers for Disease Control. 1969. Cutaneous Anthrax in North Carolina. MMWR, **18,** 40.

Christie, A. B. 1973. The Clinical Aspects of Anthrax. Postgrad Med J, **49,** 565.

Lincoln, R. E., and Fish, D. C. 1970. Anthrax Toxins. In *Microbial Toxins,* Vol. VIII, p. 369, edited by S. J. Ajl, et al. Academic Press, New York.

McKendrick, D. R. 1980. Anthrax and Its Transmission to Humans. Cent Afr J Med, **26,** 126.

Plotkin, S. A., Brachman, M., Utell, M., Bumford, F. H., and Atchison, M. M. 1960. An Epidemic of Inhalation Anthrax: The First in the Twentieth Century. I. Clinical Features. Am J Med, **29,** 992.

Ronaghy, H. A., Azadeh, B., Kohout, E., and Dutz, W. 1972. Penicillin Therapy of Human Anthrax. Curr Ther Res, **14,** 721.

Sirisanthana, T., et al. 1984. Outbreak of Oral-Oropharyngeal Anthrax: An Unusual Manifestation of Human Infection with *Bacillus anthracis.* Am J Trop Med Hyg, **33,** 144.

Tuazon, C. U., Murray, H. W., Levy, C., Solny, M. N., Curtin, J. A., and Sheagren, J. N. 1979. Serious Infections from *Bacillus* sp. JAMA, **241,** 1137.

Turnbull, P. C. B. 1981. *Bacillus cereus* Toxins. Pharmacol Ther, **13,** 453.

27

Haemophilus and *Bordetella*

George S. Schuster

Haemophilus Species

The genus *Haemophilus* is a group of facultatively anaerobic, gram-negative coccoid bacilli that cannot synthesize essential components of their enzyme systems, which are furnished by blood. These include the X (heat-stable) factor (hemin), which supplies porphyrins, and the V (heat-labile) factor, or NAD. Of the 16 recognized species, *Haemophilus influenzae, Haemophilus aegyptius* (Koch–Weeks bacillus), *Haemophilus parasuis,* and *Haemophilus haemolyticus* require both X and V factors. *Haemophilus ducreyi* requires only X factor, whereas *Haemophilus parainfluenzae* and *Haemophilus parahaemolyticus* require only V factor. *H. influenzae* is associated with acute respiratory infections and causes purulent meningitis. *H. ducreyi* produces soft chancre or chancroid. *H. aegyptius* causes a highly contagious conjunctivitis termed pinkeye.

Haemophilus influenzae

Morphology and Metabolism. Fully virulent *H. influenzae* organisms are small encapsulated coccobacilli, but it is not unusual to see cocci, bacilli, and long filaments in a single culture. Primary isolation of *H. influenzae* is best accomplished on chocolate blood agar in which both the X and V factors have been released from the red blood cells. On chocolate agar, fully virulent, encapsulated strains form relatively small, mucoid, transparent colonies that exhibit a characteristic iridescence when viewed by oblique light during the first 6 to 8 hours of incubation.

Antigenic Structure. The encapsulated strains have been divided into six immunological types designated a, b, c, d, e, and f, based on capsular swelling and agglutination and precipitation reactions. Antigenically, *H. influenzae* resembles the pneumococcus, for all of the type-specific capsules are carbohydrates. Nonspecific somatic, protein antigens are also present in *H. influenzae*. The virulence of *H. influenzae* is at least partially related to the polysaccharide capsule, which interferes with phagocytosis.

Genetic Variations. *H. influenzae* undergoes smooth to rough variations at a relatively rapid rate. The species undergo transformations mediated by DNA with regard to drug resistance and to formation of specific capsular antigens.

Diseases Caused by *H. influenzae*. *H. influenzae* and its close relatives *H. haemolyticus, H. parainfluenzae,* and *H. parahaemolyticus* are indigenous to the human pharynx. *H. haemolyticus* and *H. parainfluenzae* are essentially nonpathogenic, except for rare cases of subacute endocarditis. *H. parahaemolyticus* is frequently associated with acute pharyngitis and occasionally with subacute endocarditis. *H. influenzae* is associated with pharyngitis, sinusitis, and otitis media; less frequently it is involved in primary pneumonia, empyema, endocarditis, pyroarthrosis, and obstructive laryngotracheal infection with bacteremia in young children. A less frequent but very serious disease mediated by *H. influenzae* is primary pyogenic meningitis in children less than 3 years old. Another disease is a secondary complication of infections of the respiratory tract, notably in pandemic influenza.

It has been reported that children between the ages of 6 months and 2 years may develop a buccal cellulitis as a result of infection by *H. influenzae* type b. This begins as a swelling of the cheek with central erythema that rapidly progresses to a lesion without a distinct border but having a reddish discoloration surrounded by a purplish area. Occasionally the entire lesion is purple-red in color. There may be regions of erythematous buccal mucosa accompanying the buccal lesion. These must be differentiated from trauma, erysipelas, and streptococcal cellulitis, usually by blood cultures. Another condition usually seen in children is epiglottitis, a cellulitis of the loose tissues of the epiglottis. It begins with a sore throat and rapidly progresses to shortness of breath, airway obstruction, and respiratory arrest.

Diagnosis. Prompt bacteriological diagnosis of infections with *H. influenzae* is essential to therapy. *H. influenzae* may be identified rapidly in spinal fluid, exudate from the middle ear or joints, empyema fluid, nasopharyngeal mucus, or sputum; identification techniques include staining, capsular swelling, and a precipitin test for type-specific polysaccharide. Cultures should be made of such specimens and the blood, and the diagnosis verified by demonstration of capsular swelling by type-specific antiserum.

Treatment. Before 1938, nearly all patients with *H. influenzae* meningitis died. Ampicillin is useful in treating infections with *H. influenzae* but an increasing proportion of isolates produce beta-lactamase. Chloramphenicol was the drug of choice for penicillin-resistant strains in meningitis, but third-generation cephalosporins are also quite effective.

Immunity. Immunity develops with increasing age from inapparent exposure to *H. influenzae* during the normal course of life. During the first 3 years, when there is relatively little immunological resistance, the individual is most susceptible. A polysaccharide vaccine given in conjunction with another vaccine that can provide an adjuvant effect may prove useful in this young population. Resistance to *H. influenzae* parallels development of other immunological protection, suggesting its importance.

Haemophilus aegyptius

A bacterial species was observed by Koch in 1883 and isolated by Weeks in 1887 from a human conjunctivitis known as pinkeye. It was named the Koch–Weeks bacillus and was indistinguishable from nonencapsulated *H. influenzae*. However, it is immunologically distinct and also differs in rather subtle cultural characteristics. It is now recognized as *H. aegyptius*.

Haemophilus ducreyi

H. ducreyi, commonly called Ducrey's bacillus, is a small gram-negative rod with the common characteristics of the genus *Haemophilus. H. ducreyi* is the cause of about 10% of all venereal infections, producing soft chancre or chancroid on the genitalia and lymphatic swellings (buboes), and abscesses in the groin (Figs. 27.1 and 27.2). This disease is often con-

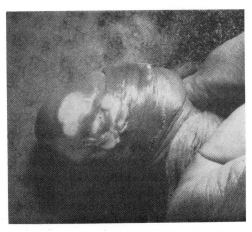

Figure 27.1: The soft chancre or chancroid caused by *Haemophilus ducreyi.* (AFIP.)

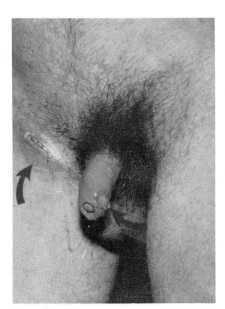

Figure 27.2: New, acute chancroid, showing the involvement of adjacent lymph node. (AFIP.)

fused clinically with syphilis. Hypersensitivity to the bacillus is used as the basis for a diagnostic cutaneous test. Immunity to chancroid does not develop, and untreated infections may persist for years. Two thirds of isolates of *H. ducreyi* produce beta-lactamase. However, most isolates seem susceptible to erythromycin and this drug produces excellent clinical results.

Bordetella

The genus *Bordetella* is made up of three species of strictly aerobic gram-negative coccobacilli (*Bordetella pertussis, Bordetella bronchiseptica,* and *Bordetella parapertussis*).

Morphology and Metabolism. *B. pertussis,* the cause of whooping cough, is a short, ovoid, gram-negative, nonmotile, and nonsporing bacillus that does not require either X or V factors. Cell morphology is also more constant than that of *H. influenzae.* Encapsulated and noncapsulated types occur, the former having smooth colonial characteristics. Complex media (e.g., Bordet–Gengou agar media) are required for the growth of virulent *B. pertussis.* It has little or no action on most carbohydrates and develops a marked alkalinity in broth.

Antigenic Structure and Variation. Freshly isolated *B. pertussis* organisms are antigenically homogeneous. When initially isolated, the encapsulated coccobacillus is termed a phase 1 type. It is fully virulent, has pili-type appendages, and requires enriched media. Subsequent culturing brings about variations,

analogous to smooth to rough variation, that result in a stepwise change through phase 2 and 3 types to phase 4 cells, which are pleomorphic and will grow on unenriched media. Phase 4 cells are not virulent and have no filaments or capsules. Several types of toxin have been identified, including a heat-labile toxin, a lipopolysaccharide endotoxin, a histamine-sensitizing factor, a lymphocytosis promoting factor, hemagglutinins, and possibly an islet activating protein. These are intimately involved in infection, disease, and immunity.

Whooping Cough. *B. pertussis* is transmitted in droplets from one human respiratory tract to another; no intermediate vectors or fomites of importance have been demonstrated. Human infection has three clinical phases, each lasting about 2 weeks: the catarrhal, the paroxysmal or spasmodic, and the convalescent. From 7 to 14 days after exposure, the catarrhal stage begins with coryza, sneezing, and mild but progressive cough. The bacilli multiply on the epithelium of the trachea and bronchi and their toxic components cause irritation and coughing. The pertussis toxin apparently impairs the normal action of the cilia of the epithelial cells in the trachea and bronchi. The paroxysmal stage is characterized by violent repetitive coughing, which forcefully empties the lungs and is followed by sudden forceful croaking or whooping inspiration. The infection may spread even to the alveoli and often results in interstitial pneumonia or secondary infection. Thick, ropy, mucinous bronchial secretions may obstruct the lower airways and produce atelectasis. Allergy to protein fractions of *B. pertussis* may contribute to the clinical manifestations of whooping cough.

Immunity. The immunity that develops from an attack of whooping cough prevents a second attack except in rare instances. During convalescence, antibodies to *B. pertussis* appear in the serum, persist for several months, and gradually decrease or even disappear. The relationship of humoral antibodies to immunity to whooping cough is uncertain. Clinical immunity may be partially cellular. There is no satisfactory way to measure individual immunity to whooping cough. Nevertheless, immunization with killed phase 1 *B. pertussis* is an effective protective measure.

Laboratory Diagnosis. The bacteriological diagnosis of whooping cough entails the obtaining of a culture of the causal organisms on a Bordet–Gengou agar plate containing penicillin to inhibit grampositive bacteria. Identification is made by microscopic examination of gram-stained smears and by agglutination with specific antiserum. Since agglutinins for *B. pertussis* do not appear in the serum of a patient until the third week of infection or later, it has no practical diagnostic value. A rapid diagnosis is possible by immunofluorescence using nasopharyngeal smears.

Treatment. *B. pertussis* is sensitive in vitro to erythromycin, with chloramphenicol and tetracyclines as alternative agents. If administered early enough, erythromycin may shorten the paroxysmal manifestations. Supportive treatment is very important.

Prevention and Control. Whooping cough affects 90% of the nonimmunized population, usually in childhood. The disease is controlled by active immunization of infants (age 2 months) in a primary course of three injections at monthly intervals and with booster shots given at 1 year of age and again 5 years later. The immunizing agent consists of killed, smooth (phase 1) organisms or extracts of these organisms. These preparations are combined with diphtheria and tetanus toxoids to form a vaccine. The use of such vaccines has greatly reduced morbidity due to whooping cough caused by *B. pertussis*. It does not protect against whooping cough caused by *B. parapertussis*.

ADDITIONAL READING

Aftandelians, R., and Connor, J. D. 1973. Bactericidal Antibody in Serum During Infection with *Bordetella pertussis*. J Infect Dis, **128**, 55.

Aftandelians, R. V., and Connor, J. D. 1974. *Bordetella pertussis* Serotypes in a Whooping Cough Outbreak. Am J Epidemiol, **99**, 343.

Bennett, N. 1973. Whooping Cough in Melbourne. Med J Aust, **2**, 481.

Borska, K., and Simkovicova, M. 1972. Studies on the Circulation of *Bordetella pertussis* and *Bordetella parapertussis* in Populations of Children. J Hyg Epidemiol Microbiol Immunol, **16**, 159.

Davies, J. L., Laughton, C. R., and May, J. R. 1974. An Improved Test for *Haemophilus influenzae* Precipitins in the Serum of Patients with Chronic Respiratory Disease. J Clin Pathol, **27**, 265.

Farooki, Z. O., Henry, J. G., and Green, E. W. 1974. *Haemophilus influenzae* Pericarditis Associated with Meningitis: A Treatable Fatal Disease. Clin Pediatr, **13**, 609.

Holt, L. B. 1972. The Pathology and Immunology of *Bordetella pertussis* Infection. J Med Microbiol, **5**, 407.

International Symposium on Pertussis. 1978. National Institutes of Health, Bethesda, Md.

Khan, W., Ross, S., Rodriquez, W., Controni, G., and Saz, A. K. 1974. *Haemophilus influenzae* Type B Resistant to Ampicillin. JAMA, **229**, 298.

Kulenkampff, M., Schwartman, J. S., and Wilson, J. 1974. Neurological Complications of Pertussis Inoculation. Arch Dis Child, **49**, 46.

Norden, C. W., and Michaels, R. 1973. Immunologic Response in Patients with Epiglottitis Caused by *Haemophilus influenzae* Type B. J Infect Dis, **128**, 777.

Morse, S. I., and Morse, J. H. 1976. Isolation and Properties of Leukocytosis and Leukocytosis Promoting Factor of *Bordetella pertussis*. J Exp Med, **143**, 1483.

Parton, R., and Wardlaw, A. C. 1974. Cell-Envelope Proteins of *Bordetella pertussis*. J Med Microbiol, **8**, 47.

Pittman, M. 1970. *Bordetella pertussis*: Bacterial and Host Factors in the Pathogenesis and Prevention of Whooping Cough. In *Infectious Agents and Host Reactions*, edited by S. Mudd. W. B. Saunders, Philadelphia.

Rapkin, R. H., and Bautista, G. 1972. *Haemophilus influenzae* Cellulitis. Am J Dis Child, **124**, 540.

Roap, R. M., et al. 1987. Virulence Factors of *Bordetella bronchiseptica* Associated with the Production of Infectious Atrophic Rhinitis in Experimentally Infected Neonatal Swine. Infect Immun, **55**, 217.

Ross, R., Munoz, J., and Cameron, C. 1969. Histamine Sensitizing Factor, Mouse Protective Antigens and Other Antigens of Some Members of the Genus *Bordetella*. J Bacteriol, **99**, 57.

Sims, W. 1972. Pathogenicity of Human Oral Strains of Haemophili: Enzymes, Anaerobiosis and Effects on Mice and Rabbits. Arch Oral Biol, **17**, 745.

Smith, A. L. 1983. *Haemophilus influenzae* Pneumonia. Semin Infect Dis, **5**, 56. Thieme-Stratton, New York.

Turk, D. C., and May, J. R. 1967. *Haemophilus influenzae:* Its Clinical Importance. English Universities Press, London.

28

Brucella and Brucellosis

George S. Schuster

Brucella

The genus *Brucella* comprises six recognized species, of which *Brucella melitensis, Brucella abortus,* and *Brucella suis* are the most common. The other species described are *Brucella neotomae,* found in desert wood rats; *Brucella ovis,* which causes epididymitis and abortion in sheep; and *Brucella canis,* which causes epididymitis and abortion in dogs.

Morphology and Metabolism. All *Brucella* organisms are gram-negative, non-acid-fast, nonsporulating, usually nonmotile, sometimes encapsulated cells that occur singly, in pairs, or in short chains. Although the cells are typically short rods, cocci or coccobacilli may predominate. Brucellae form smooth (S), intermediate (I), rough (R), mucoid (M), and G type colonies. The virulent and strongly antigenic *Brucella* is the S type, which undergoes spontaneous smooth to rough variation. Loss of virulence and changed antigenicity correlate with changes in co-

lonial morphology in the R type. The transition from S to R type may be sudden and complete, but a transient or intermediate (I) type may arise. The colonies of the mucoid (M) type mutate to the R type either in liquid or on solid media. G type colonies appear infrequently among S type colonies during initial isolation of brucellae from infected uteri. *Brucella* is difficult to grow on initial isolation, and *B. abortus* requires 5% to 10% CO_2 for initial isolation. Several components of media inhibit the growth of *Brucella*.

Antigenic Composition. S strains have distinctive antigenic compositions that progressively lose specificity during the usually gradual transformation from S to R phases in culture. S forms of the three *Brucella* species contain two characteristic heat-stable antigens, termed A and M. These antigens are toxic polysaccharide–lipid–protein complexes. A and M antigens of the three species are closely related but not identical. Furthermore, their amounts and distribution on the cell surfaces allow antigenic variations to occur among species.

Animal Brucellosis

Animal brucellosis is primarily an infection of goats, sheep, swine, and cattle. It causes great economic loss in livestock because of decreased milk supply, failure to produce offspring because of loss of fertility or abortion, and an overall decrease in market value. Although it is a secondary disease of man and is seldom if ever transmitted from person to person, it can pose a threat to human health.

Human Brucellosis

Human brucellosis (undulant fever) is usually acquired through contact with infected animals or materials. The route of infection with *Brucella* is through the alimentary tract (ingestion), conjunctiva and skin (contact), and lungs (inhalation). Organisms entering a host can gain access to lymphatics. Often there is local lymphadenopathy, and bacteremia may subsequently develop following bacterial multiplication and dissemination from the primary involved nodes. The organisms then localize, particularly in the reticuloendothelial system. Brucellae have been observed inside phagocytes, where they are protected from antibodies and antibiotics. There is a granulomatous response in infected tissues that may in some cases lead to abscess formation. After an extremely variable incubation period, ranging from 3 to 60 days, the disease begins either insidiously or abruptly. Symptoms of the disease are weakness, an evening rise in temperature, chills, sweats, anorexia, headaches, loss of weight, backache, splenomegaly, abdominal tenderness, rheumatism, arthritis, and anemia. The nonspecific symptoms may be accompanied by nervousness and mental depression. Many of the symptoms of human brucellosis result from the reaction of host defenses, since hypersensitivity develops quickly. In humans, brucellosis may assume many forms, ranging from an acute or undulant form to a recurrent type of disease that may persist for years. The human disease is generally divided into two types, acute or undulant and chronic. The acute type relates to the occurrence of focal lesions in the vascular or central nervous system. The chronic granulomatous type occurs when the organisms exist intracytoplasmically. Patients recovering from brucellosis may develop complications related to chronic granulomatous lesions in bones, joints, bursae, meninges, endocardium, lungs, liver, spleen, epididymis, testes, and kidneys. In many instances these lesions cannot be differentiated histologically from those of tuberculosis. A chronic localized pulmonary brucellosis occurs in humans. The symptoms are fever, productive coughing, chest pains, choking sensations, hoarseness, and chills, together with many of the other usual symptoms of generalized brucellosis. Joints are often involved as a complication of brucellosis, with the most common manifestation being polyarthritis. Spondylitis is an infrequent complication of brucellosis, resembling tuberculosis of the spine.

Brucella sometimes causes ocular lesions. The central nervous system is involved not infrequently, with *Brucella* invading cerebrospinal fluid or cerebral tissue. Other complications of brucellosis are granulomatous panarteritis, miliary peritonitis, urinary infections, salpingitis, epididymitis, and orchitis.

Immunity. While serum antibodies, as measured by agglutination, precipitin, opsonin, or bactericidal tests, occur early in the disease, they do not prevent reinfection by brucellosis.

Hypersensitivity. Hypersensitivity plays a significant role in human brucellosis. In nonsensitized individuals most organisms are phagocytized, but some survive to pass to the regional lymph nodes. Some take up an intracellular existence within liver, spleen, lymph nodes, and bone marrow. Subsequently the organisms are killed, releasing endotoxin, which elicits the characteristic clinical symptoms of the disease. Hypersensitivity also seems to be an important factor mediating chronic brucellosis, for affected individuals are quite sensitive dermally and systemically to *Brucella* antigens.

Laboratory Diagnosis of Brucellosis. The laboratory diagnosis of human brucellosis depends on isolation and identification of the causal organisms and the performance of agglutination tests. Diagnosis by culture is difficult because the organisms are present in the blood, urine, and feces only intermittently and in small numbers. Usually blood or other tissue is cultured for as long as a month in tryptose or trypticase soy broth. It is useful to inoculate the cultures into guinea pigs. The injection of suspected material into the yolk sacs of embryonated eggs is sometimes superior to either of the above procedures.

Perhaps the most commonly used laboratory diagnostic procedure is the agglutination test. A titer of 1:160 in individuals with appropriate symptoms is usually considered significant. A fluctuating or rising titer is particularly suggestive of infection. Antigenic cross-reactions may occur between *Brucella* and *Francisella tularensis* or *Vibrio cholerae*.

The *Brucella* skin test is mostly for detection of hypersensitivity. Antigen is injected intradermally into the forearm and observed in 24 to 48 hours. In a hypersensitive individual, usually not in the early stages of the disease, an edematous area develops, usually not larger than 2.5 cm in diameter.

Treatment and Control. The antibiotics that

have been used in the treatment of brucellosis are the tetracyclines and streptomycin. Several regimens have been devised to overcome the high relapse rate and to treat brucellosis more effectively. One entails the administration of a tetracycline and streptomycin. Such combinations of antibiotics have resulted in a significantly lower relapse rate.

Prevention of human brucellosis is mainly dependent on control of the animal sources of infection. Available vaccines are suitable mainly for animals. Control of dairy product processing as well as animal surveillance and immunization have greatly reduced the dangers of brucellosis in the United States.

ADDITIONAL READING

Alton, G. G., Maw, J., Rogerson, B. A., and McPherson, G. G. 1974. The Serological Diagnosis of Bovine Brucellosis: An Evaluation of the Complement Fixation Serum Agglutination and Rose Bengal Tests. Aust Vet J, **51,** 57.

Bertrand, J. L., and Gueyffier, C. 1974. *Brucella endocarditis.* A General Review with Reference to 46 Observations from Medical Literature and One Personal Observation. Lyon Med, **231,** 123.

Brucellosis: A Symposium. 1950. American Association of the Advancement of Science, Washington, DC.

Buchanan, T. M., Baher, L. C., and Feldman, R. A. 1974. Brucellosis in the United States, 1960–72: An Abattoir-Associated Disease. Part I. Clinical Features and Therapy. Medicine, **53,** 403.

Busch, L. A., and Parker, R. L. 1972. Brucellosis in the United States. J Infect Dis, **125,** 289.

Coghlan, J. D., and Longmore, H. J. A. 1973. The Significance of Brucella Antibodies in Patients in a Rural Area. Practitioner, **211,** 645.

Elberg, S. S. 1973. Immunity to Brucella Infection. Medicine, **52,** 339.

Farrell, I. D., Robertson, L., and Hinchliffe, P. M. 1975. Serum Antibody Response in Acute Brucellosis. J Hyg (Cambridge), **74,** 23.

Foley, B. V., Clay, M. M., and O'Sullivan, D. J. 1970. A Study of a Brucellosis Epidemic. Ir J Med Sci, **3,** 457.

Kulshreshtha, R. C., Atal, P. R., and Wahi, P. N. 1973. A Study on Serological Tests for the Diagnosis of Human and Bovine Brucellosis. Indian J Med Res, **61,** 1471.

Mann, P. G., and Richens, E. R. 1973. Aspects of Human Brucellosis. Postgrad Med J, **49,** 523.

McCullough, N. B. 1970. Microbial and Host Factors in the Pathogenesis of Brucellosis. In *Infectious Agents and Host Reactions,* edited by S. Mudd. W. B. Saunders, Philadelphia.

Robertson, L., Farrell, I. D., and Hinchliffe, P. M. 1973. The Sensitivity of *Brucella abortus* to Chemotherapeutic Agents. J Med Microbiol, **6,** 549.

Young, E. J. 1983. Human Brucellosis. Rev Infect Dis, **5,** 821.

Young, E. J., and Suvannoparrat, U. 1975. Brucellosis Outbreak Attributed to Ingestion of Unpasteurized Goat Cheese. Arch Intern Med, **135,** 240.

29

Yersinia, Francisella, and *Pasteurella*

George S. Schuster

The organisms described in this chapter are all gram-negative, facultative or aerobic rods. They cause zoonoses, infections that are naturally transmitted between lower vertebrates and man. Included are *Yersinia,* which causes plague and other infections; *Francisella,* which causes tularemia; and *Pasteurella.*

Yersinia pestis

Morphology and Cultivation. *Y. pestis* is a gram-negative, nonmotile rod or coccobacillus, usually 1 to 2 μm long and 0.5 to 0.8 μm in diameter, that shows bipolar staining. Under less than optimal growth conditions, plague bacilli are pleomorphic. Virulent strains produce a large capsule that is more like a slime layer.

The plague bacillus is facultative, growing either aerobically or anaerobically at an optimum temperature of 28°C. A large inoculum is required to initiate growth in ordinary nutrient media, so complex media have been devised for obtaining growth from small inocula and for primary isolation. Repeated subculturing of the plague bacillus anaerobically reduces its virulence.

Virulence. *Y. pestis* is highly virulent. When freshly isolated from human or rodent infections, only a few plague bacilli are fatal in a guinea pig. Virulence can be maintained by repeated passage in susceptible animals, by storing cultures at 4°C, or by drying from the frozen state. Virulence is diminished by rapid, repeated subculturing, by culturing in the presence of ethanol, by passage through immune animals, and by bacteriophage action.

Plague bacilli contain a toxin that resembles an exotoxin in that it can be easily converted into a toxiod. It also produces a lipopolysaccharide endotoxin that behaves pharmacologically similar to those of enteric bacilli but has a greater LD^{50} for animals.

Antigenic Structure. Virulent plague bacilli possess at least ten different antigens. Immunological methods have defined an envelope or capsular (F1) antigen, a somatic antigen, and the toxin. Virulent strains produce more of the envelope antigens than

289

do avirulent strains. The envelope antigen, composed of a heat-labile protein, is antiphagocytic, highly soluble in water, difficult to demonstrate as a definite capsule, and thermolabile. It seems to be an essential immunizing antigen. The somatic antigen is of unproved immunological significance.

Bacteriophages. Numerous bacteriophages specific for the plague bacillus have been isolated. Attempts to use bacteriophage in the treatment of experimental plague have not been successful, in part because the phage may lyse the infecting plague bacilli enough to release lethal amounts of the toxin.

Plague

Plague in the United States. Plague has existed in Hawaii since 1899 and has occurred in several cities in the continental United States since 1900. Wild rodent or sylvatic plague is now prevalent in the western United States. The three groups of rodents constituting the primary reservoirs are ground squirrels, wood rats, prairie dogs, and occasionally sagebrush voles and meadow mice. Human plague has been contracted throughout the western states from wild rodents directly or through their fleas.

Human Plague. Plague is transmitted to man from infected rats or other rodents by the bite of infected fleas. Except in pneumonic plague, direct transfer of *Y. pestis* from person to person rarely if ever occurs. Following the flea bite type of infection, the organisms enter the lymphatics and reach the lymph nodes, usually in the groin, where they cause them to become enlarged and tender, forming buboes (literally a swelling in the groin). An initial bacteremia may distribute the bacilli to the spleen, liver, and bone marrow. If the action of the reticuloendothelial system is sufficient to remove the circulating bacilli, the initial bacteremia or septicemia develops.

Bubonic plague has an average incubation period of 3 or 4 days. It is characterized by sudden onset, high fever, unusually rapid pulse, disturbed sensorium, and prostration. Mortality averages 60% to 90% within 3 to 5 days. As plague bacilli die they release toxin, which causes widespread hemorrhagic and degenerative changes.

A less common but very dangerous type of human plague is the primary pneumonic variety. Originating in the pneumonia secondary to bubonic plague, this highly contagious disease is transmitted from person to person by droplets of infected sputum. The plague bacilli multiply uninhibited in the lungs, release large quantities of toxin, and cause death within 2 days.

Immunity. In humans, recovery from an attack of plague produces solid immunity and reinfection is rare. Acquired immunity is essentially anti-infectious and to a lesser extent antitoxic.

Several types of vaccines consisting of formalin- or heat-killed virulent bacilli or living avirulent bacilli have been used to immunize against plague infection. The degree of vaccine efficacy under field conditions is not certain.

Antisera for passive immunization are commonly obtained from rabbits and horses. A variety of antigens have been used: killed plague cultures, filtrates of broth cultures, live virulent bacilli, live avirulent bacilli, toxoids, envelope antigens, and F1 antigen.

Laboratory Diagnosis. Culture of organisms for the laboratory diagnosis of plague is dangerous and maximal care must be exercised. The diagnostic methods used must produce rapid results. Bacteriological diagnosis consists of the identification of *Y. pestis* in gram-stained smears of sputum or tissue exudate from a bubo. *Y. pestis* can be isolated by culturing on blood agar. Plague bacilli can be rapidly identified by fluorescent antibody staining or lysis with appropriate bacteriophage. Animal inoculation, particularly into guinea pigs, is sometimes used if the specimen is grossly contaminated with other bacteria.

Treatment. The early use of streptomycin, chloramphenicol, or tetracyclines reduces the mortality from plague to below 5%. A few strains of *Y. pestis* become resistant to streptomycin; this resistance may be overcome by the concurrent administration of either chloramphenicol or tetracycline.

Control and Prevention. The best method for the control of plague is the eradication of commensal rats, other rodents, and fleas. The rodent–flea–rodent cycle can be broken at least temporarily by insecticides and rodenticides.

Yersinia pseudotuberculosis and *Yersinia enterocolitica*

Y. pseudotuberculosis and *Y. enterocolitica* are both relatively large pleomorphic, gram-negative, sometimes motile rods that exhibit bipolar staining. They are distinguished from each other by differences in biochemical characteristics, susceptibility to bacteriophages, the pathogenicity of *Y. pseudotuberculosis* for guinea pigs, by antigenic differences, and by differences in susceptibility to antibiotics.

The most common manifestation of *Y. enterocolitica* is an acute gastroenteritis or enterocolitis, especially in children. It may also cause terminal ileitis or mesenteric lymphadenitis. The organisms are usually transmitted in food or water, but person-to-person transmission may occur as well.

Y. pseudotuberculosis infection usually manifests as terminal ileitis or mesenteric lymphadenitis. Humans probably acquire the infection by ingestion of food contaminated with animal excreta.

Francisella and Tularemia

Francisella tularensis. *F. tularensis* is a gram-negative, pleomorphic microorganism that is primarily rod-shaped, although coccoid forms predominate in young cultures and rods in older cultures. It is an obligate aerobe. *F. tularensis* stains satisfactorily with crystal violet and carbol fuchsin but not with methylene blue.

F. tularensis is cytotropic and accordingly difficult to cultivate. There are divergent views on its reproduction. Budding forms are seen, but electron microscopy shows constrictions suggesting binary fission. It will grow on initial isolation on cysteine–glucose–blood agar or in enriched broth media. After initial isolation, simpler media can be used for growth. *F. tularensis* can also be cultured in chick embryo tissue, in embryonated eggs, where it grows mostly in the yolk sac, and in albino mice.

Both smooth and rough colonial variants of *F. tularensis* occur. Most nonsmooth strains are avirulent and most smooth strains are virulent.

Antigens. Several kinds of antigens have been extracted from *F. tularensis,* but only a single antigenic type has been identified. The cell wall antigens demonstrated include soluble specific polysaccharide antigen that gives a wheal type of reaction in the skin of convalescent human patients, a protein antigen that elicits agglutinins, and an endotoxin whose role in pathogenesis is similar to that of *Salmonella typhi.*

Tularemia. Tularemia occurs most frequently in the United States and Russia, although it has been reported from European countries, Canada, Mexico, Venezuela, and Japan. It has occurred in virtually every state of the United States. Tularemia occurs seasonally, in the summer in the western United States and in the winter months in the eastern United States.

In the United States, tularemia is primarily an infection of wild mammals, but the principal sources of human infection are the cottontail rabbit and, in the western states, the jack rabbit. Tularemia is usually transmitted from animal to animal (and occasionally to humans) by bloodsucking insects. *F. tularensis* survives in the environment, in water and soil, and in animal products, which serve as alternative media for its transmission to humans. It is unusually hazardous to work with in the laboratory, and a pneumonic form may result from inhalation of infected droplets.

The clinical manifestations of tularemia generally resemble those of bubonic plague. Tularemia may simulate several other diseases such as influenza or pneumonia. In man the clinical forms of disease are ulceroglandular, typhoidal, oculoglandular, glandular, pulmonary, and ingestive. The mortality varies with the type of disease.

The incubation period of tularemia is usually 2 to 5 days but may extend to 10 days. Prodromal symptoms are rare and the onset is sudden. The disease has a febrile, influenza-like nature, with headaches, fever, chills, profuse sweats, body pain, nausea, vomiting, and prostration. Fever of 102 to 104°F (39 to 40°C) is constantly present during the first 2 to 4 weeks of infection, although it may persist for months with an initial rise, a remission, and a secondary rise. A significant percentage of victims develop a rash that is macular, papular, or blotchy.

In the ulceroglandular type of tularemia, a primary lesion in the form of a small red papule usually but not always develops at the site of infection, which is commonly on the upper extremities, face, or conjunctiva. This papule enlarges and ulcerates, forming an indolent ulcer with raised edges and a ragged floor (Fig. 29.1). From the site of the initial infection, *F. tularensis* invades along superficial and deep lymphatics, producing dermal lymphangitic nodules, regional lymphadenitis, and buboes.

Oculoglandular disease is similar to ulceroglandular except that the conjunctiva is the primary site. Infection manifests with a granulomatous conjunctivitis that may suppurate. The preauricular, parotid, submaxillary, and cervical lymph nodes often become involved. The two forms that do not manifest with a primary ulcer—glandular and typhoidal disease—must be differentiated from other diseases.

In most cases with a favorable prognosis, the antibody titer begins to rise about 1 week after the onset of the disease, coinciding with the disappearance of the initial bacteremia and the beginning of the abatement of lesions and symptoms. In unfavorable cases, a septicemia develops from foci of necrosis or is continually present, producing miliary foci of necrosis in many organs and glands.

Eighty percent of primary lesions of tularemia, when acquired by contact, occur on the fingers, but initial lesions may occur at any site about the body, including the oral cavity and face. Primary infection of the oral cavity usually results from eating flesh infected with *F. tularensis,* or it may be carried by contaminated hands to the face or oral cavity. The initial oral lesion of tularemia closely resembles the chancre of syphilis, which often leads to delayed diagnosis of the disease. In addition to primary lesions of the oral cavity, secondary lesions associated with tularemic infection may occur. Such secondary infection of the

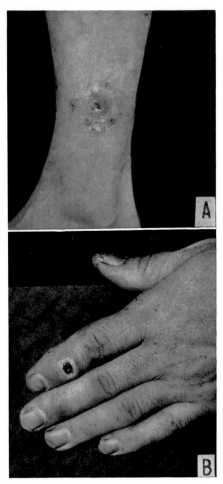

Figure 29.1: Tularemia. (**A**) Leg lesion; (**B**) lesion on the index finger. (**A,** AFIP 218885–1; **B,** AFIP 85387–2.)

oral cavity usually produces small grayish white areas on the tongue, gingiva, and buccal mucosa that eventually become ulcerated. These ulcers are superficially coated with thin layers of fibrin and only a few contaminating microorganisms. If tularemic infection is continued, the oral lesions may simulate Vincent's infection, or Vincent's infection may be superimposed on the tularemic infection. If the pharyngotonsillar region is involved, the lesions may resemble those of diphtheria. The continuation of oral lesions is dependent on the systemic disease, for the ulcers regress on the abatement of the systemic disease, following adequate treatment. Facial lesions heal with scarring but oral lesions heal without residual tissue changes.

Diagnosis. The diagnosis of tularemia is based on a history indicative of exposure to the infection, clinical findings, culture of *F. tularensis,* particularly from blood, and serological tests. A definitive diagnosis of tularemia requires identification of organisms from exudates or on special culture media, such

as cystine–glucose–blood agar, by specific fluorescent antibodies or by an agglutination test. Allergic tests have also been used. During the first week of tularemia, intracutaneous injection of homologous antiserum produces a wheal-and-erythema response. After antibodies appear, a similar response is elicited by the polysaccharide. A delayed-type hypersensitivity reaction also is demonstrable by intracutaneous injection of protein antigen. An attack of tularemia results in immunity sufficient to either prevent or greatly mitigate a second infection.

Treatment and Control. Streptomycin effectively cures tularemia. The tetracyclines and chloramphenicol also are effective, but since they are bacteriostatic, relapse may result if treatment is halted prematurely. Immunization with attenuated vaccines provides some resistance in man, especially against respiratory infections. Successful control requires elimination of insect vectors as well as precautions against contamination of skin with infected blood or meat.

Pasteurella multocida and Pasteurellosis

Bacteriology of *Pasteurella multocida.* *P. multocida,* the species name implying the killing of many kinds of animals, is a common cause of fowl cholera in birds and mammalian hemorrhagic septicemia, syndromes generically called pasteurellosis. The organisms are short, ellipsoidal, gram-negative, nonmotile, nonsporulating rods that exhibit bipolar staining and possess polysaccharide capsules. Their chemical composition varies among serogroups.

Pasteurellosis. *P. multocida* normally parasitizes the upper respiratory tract and less often the intestinal tract of mammals and fowl. It is considered a true commensal in cats, dogs, and some rodents. The ordinarily innocuous strains produce disease when they acquire virulence from repeated animal passage or because of lowered host resistance, usually due to debilitation. Low resistance and high virulence result in fowl cholera, or acute hemorrhagic septicemia in a variety of animals. Evidently an endotoxin causes many of the symptoms seen in pasteurellosis. It is now recognized that *P. multocida* can infect humans, although the number of proved human infections is quite small. The most common known source of human infection is the bite of an animal, usually a cat, dog, or rabbit. The clinical manifestations of the human infection are quite variable, ranging from localized swelling and abscess formation to bronchiectasis, pneumonia, meningitis, and septicemia. Diagnosis of human pasteurellosis rests on clinical findings, cultivation, and identification of the causative organism; infection of animals; agglutination with specific antisera; and penicillin sensitivity tests. Most strains of *P. multocida* are sensitive to ampicillin and tetracycline. However, infections can usually be controlled with penicillin.

ADDITIONAL READING

Bennett, L. G., and Tornabene, T. G. 1974. Characterization of the Antigenic Subunits of the Envelope Protein of *Yersinia pestis.* J Bacteriol, **117,** 48.

Bradford, W. D., Noce, P. S., and Gutman, L. T. 1974. Pathogenic Features of Enteric Infection with *Yersinia enterocolitica.* Arch Pathol, **98,** 17.

Butler, T. 1975. Plague and Tularemia. Pediatr Clin North Am, **26,** 355.

Chen, T. H., and Meyer, K. F. 1974. Susceptibility and Antibody Response of *Rattus* Species to Experimental Plague. J Infect Dis, **129** (Suppl), S62.

Cooper, A., Martin, R., and Tibbles, J. A. R. 1973. Pasteurella Meningitis. Neurology, **23,** 1097.

Cueva, R. A., Davidson, T. M., and Dickinson, D. 1986. Pasteurella Infections of the Head and Neck. Arch Otolaryngol Head Neck Surg, **112,** 207.

Foshay, L. 1950. Tularemia. Annu Rev Microbiol, **4,** 313.

Francis, D. P., Holmes, M. A., and Brandon, G. 1975. *Pasteurella multocida:* Infection after Domestic Animal Bites and Scratches. JAMA, **233,** 42.

Hannuksela, M., and Ahvonen, P. 1975. Skin Manifestation in Human Yersiniosis. Ann Clin Res, **7,** 368.

Hawes, S. C. 1973. Bubonic Plague. NZ Med J, **77,** 389.

Jacobs, R. F., and Narain, J. P. 1983. Tularemia in Children. Pediatr Infect Dis, **2,** 487.

Johnson, R. H., and Rumans, L. W. 1977. Unusual Infections Caused by *Pasteurella multocida.* JAMA, **237,** 146.

Klock, L. E., Olsen, P. F., and Fukushima, T. 1973. Tularemia Epidemic Associated with the Deerfly. JAMA, **226,** 149.

Kohl, S. 1979. *Yersinia enterocolitica* Infections in Children. Pediatr Clin North Am, **26,** 433.

Marshall, J. D., Jr., Bartelloni, P. J., Cavanaugh, D. C., Kadull, P. J., and Meyer, K. F. 1974. Plague Immunization: II. Relation of Adverse Clinical Reactions to Multiple Immunizations with Killed Vaccine. J Infect Dis, **129** (Suppl), S19.

Massey, E. D., and Mangiafico, J. A. 1974. Microagglutination Test for Detecting and Measuring Serum Agglutinins of *Francisella tularensis.* Appl Microbiol, **27,** 25.

Meyer, K. F., Cavanaugh, D. C., Bartelloni, P. J., and Marshall, J. D. 1974. Plague Immunization: I. Past and Present Trends. J Infect Dis, **129** (Suppl), S13.

Meyer, K. F., Smith, G., Foster, L. E., Marshall, J. D., Jr., and Cavanaugh, D. C. 1974. Plague Immunization: IV. Clinical Reactions and Serologic Response to Inoculations of Haffkine and Freeze-Dried Plague Vaccine. J Infect Dis, **129** (Suppl), S30.

Ohara, S., Sato, T., and Homma, M. 1974. Serological Studies on *Francisella tularensis, Francisella novicida, Yersinia philomiragia,* and *Brucella abortus.* Int J Syst Bacteriol, **24,** 191.

30

Legionella and Legionnaire's Disease

George S. Schuster

Legionella

Legionella organisms are gram-negative rods 0.3 to 0.9 μm in diameter and 2 to 20 μm long. They are non-spore-forming, nonencapsulated, and motile by one or more straight or curved polar or lateral flagella. The organisms are aerobic. L-Cysteine and iron salts are required for growth. Carbohydrates are neither fermented nor oxidized. Branched chain fatty acids predominate in the cell wall. The organisms are usually isolated from surface water, mud, and polluted lakes and streams.

There is one genus in the family Legionellaceae, *Legionella*. Six species are recognized in the ninth edition of *Bergey's Manual of Determinative Bacteriology,* although later work recognizes 24 species, 9 of which have been implicated in human disease.

Legionellae are fastidious and do not grow on commonly employed media such as nutrient or standard blood agar, but the latter medium, supplemented with cysteine and iron has been used to cultivate *L. pneumophila.* Several complex and semisynthetic broth media are now available. Growth occurs between 25 and 43°C, with an optimum at 36°C. The optimum pH is 6.8 to 7.0.

Motile strains of all *Legionella* species possess cross-reacting H antigens. O antigens are largely unique for each species, and more than one such antigen group is present in *L. pneumophila* and *L. longbeachae.*

Legionnaire's Disease

Clinical Manifestations and Pathogenesis. Legionnaire's disease is primarily associated with *L. pneumophila,* although illness has been associated with *L. micdadei.* It is usually considered a severe pneumonic illness, but in addition to the lungs the central nervous system, gastrointestinal tract, liver, and kidneys may be involved. The disease is usually airborne or waterborne. There is no clear documentation of person-to-person spread. Early clinical manifestations are headache, malaise, and myalgia, often accompanied by a sharp temperature rise within 24 hours, followed by chills or rigor. A nonproductive cough is common, frequently with mucoid bronchial secretions. Diarrhea, abdominal pain, or both are fairly common symptoms that may precede the pneumonia. The pneumonia is frequently confluent and may resemble lobar pneumonia. The pathology is that of an acute, purulent, fibrinous lobar pneumonia with large amounts of fibrin and many neutrophils and macrophages in the alveoli. Death is usually preceded by shock or respiratory failure.

The neurological manifestations include delirium, disorientation, confusion, and hallucinations. Cerebrovascular disease may compound these responses. The cerebrospinal fluid appears normal and it seems unlikely that the central nervous system is invaded, suggesting action of a toxin.

Gastrointestinal complaints include nausea, vomiting, and diarrhea. These are usually short-lived and self-limited. Liver function tests may show elevated SGOT or bilirubin. Proteinuria, azotemia, and serum creatinine elevations also may occur but usually return to normal quickly. Mild hematuria also occurs.

Pontiac fever is a less severe illness that is characterized by a short (6 to 48 hours) incubation period, fever, headache, myalgia, and dry cough but no evidence of pneumonia. It appears to be a self-limited disease, not associated with documented mortality.

The mechanisms of pathogenesis are not clear. Several species of *Legionella* produce hemolysis in vitro. Lecithinase also is produced, but there is no proof that these show in vivo toxicity. There is no evidence to show typical endotoxin; however, cytolytic exotoxin, phospholipase c, and small peptides capable of destroying monocytes have been reported.

L. pneumophila is able to survive phagosomal engulfment and multiply therein, ultimately destroying the macrophage and releasing numerous daughter cells. Similarly, it can multiply within human peripheral blood monocytes.

There is little evidence to suggest that the manifestations of Legionnaire's disease are linked to an immunopathological mechanism, but data on this aspect are limited. Humans produce antibody, and some of this is protective. The organism is subject to the bactericidal effect of complement, and specific antibody may be opsonizing. There is an intense cellular interaction of the organisms with neutrophils and macrophages in the lungs. Delayed hypersensitivity to the organisms can be induced in guinea pigs. It is not known if the cellular immunity responses are protective or have another role.

Diagnosis. Although the organisms can be cultured, diagnosis is usually done immunologically. Immunofluorescence is the current method of choice.

Serological diagnosis may be done using paired sera. Specimens are collected 3 weeks apart. Those showing a fourfold rise in titer, to at least 128, combined with a suggestive clinical history and physical findings are indicative of legionellosis. Similarly, a titer of 256 or greater on a single serum sample is usually indicative of legionellosis if the patient's history and physical findings are also suggestive. The development of new media has increased the feasibility of diagnosis by culturing blood, sputum, or tracheal aspirates.

Epidemiology and Control. Legionnaire's disease came to the attention of the medical community in 1976 when almost 200 individuals attending an American Legion convention in Philadelphia developed an illness ranging from cough and fever to severe pneumonia. Twenty-nine of these individuals died. After the cause was identified, review of stored specimens showed that prior outbreaks had occurred in other places. Several thousand cases have been reported subsequent to the 1976 outbreak. Surveillance studies suggest that between 1% and 4% of previously undiagnosed cases of pneumonia may have been caused by *L. pneumophila*. Of the many subsequent outbreaks, some were associated with central air conditioning systems, some with aerosolized water in various other forms, and one with an excavation. Sporadic cases have been reported in all states and in 50 countries. Cases have been reported year-round, although most occur in warmer months. The organism exists in nature; it has been found in water in cooling towers, streams, lakes, and mud. These organisms or antigenically related ones have been found in soil insects and earthworms. This suggests that legionellae are widely distributed in nature and that man is an accidental host.

The most effective control measures appear to be preventive, i.e., regular maintenance of air conditioning systems, addition of biocides to cooling towers, and extra chlorination of water supplies in buildings. Vaccines are feasible but not available.

Species other than *L. pneumophila* have been associated with human disease. In addition to the named species, several have been isolated but are currently unnamed. They behave much like *L. pneumophila* and have similar growth requirements. Their distribution, habitats, and disease potential also appear similar. The full disease spectrum of the legionellae is not known.

Treatment. Supportive treatment consists of oxygen supplementation and possibly renal dialysis if necessary. Erythromycin is the drug of choice although this may be supplemented by other antibiotics. The organism is susceptible to rifampin, which may be of use if erythromycin fails. *L. pneumophila* produces beta-lactamase, which is more active on cephalosporins than penicillins, so these are not recommended for treatment.

ADDITIONAL READING

Broome, C. V. 1983. Pneumonia Due to *Legionella* Species. In *Seminars in Infectious Disease,* edited by L. Weinstein and B. N. Fields. Thieme-Stratton, New York.

Gregory, D. W., Schaffner, W., Alford, R. H., et al. 1979. Sporadic Cases of Legionnaire's Disease: The Expanding Clinical Spectrum. Ann Intern Med, **90,** 518.

McDade, J. E., Shepard, C. C., Fraser, D. W., et al. 1977. Legionnaire's Disease: Isolation of a Bacterium and Demonstration of Its Role in Other Respiratory Diseases. N Engl J Med, **297,** 1197.

Ward, P. A. 1979. Immunology and Immunopathology of Legionnaire's Disease. Ann Intern Med, **90,** 506.

31

Miscellaneous Pathogenic Bacteria

George S. Schuster

The Mycoplasmas

In 1898 Nocard and Roux found the etiological agent of a type of bovine pleuropneumonia to be a small, highly pleomorphic, very fragile microorganism cultivable in a cell-free medium. Twenty-five years later a similar microorganism was found to cause agalactia, an inflammatory disease of the udder in sheep and goats. Similar microorganisms have been isolated from animals, the genitourinary tracts of humans, and from nearly all healthy human mouths and throats. Similar saprophytic organisms have been isolated from sewage, manure, humus, and soil. Based on their resemblance to the etiological agent of bovine pleuropneumonia, these microorganisms were called pleuropneumonia-like organisms, or, more commonly, PPLO.

The mycoplasmas belong to the family Mycoplasmataceae, which has two genera, *Mycoplasma* and *Ureaplasma*. Several species in these genera are present as part of the normal flora of man. *M. pneu-*

moniae, M. hominis, and *U. urealyticum* are human pathogens, the latter two mainly as opportunists.

Physical and Chemical Characteristics. Mycoplasmas range in size from 200 to 300 nm in diameter. They are bounded by a trilaminar membrane but lack a rigid wall, causing them to appear as cocci, cocci with tubules, filaments and pear-shaped cells (Figs. 31.1 and 31.2). The cells are rich in lipids, mostly sterols derived from the environment. These lipids provide the major rigidity to the cell, enabling it to withstand osmotic pressure differences. The general biosynthetic capacities of the mycoplasmas are limited. The genome consists of a single, circular, double-stranded DNA molecule of approximate molecular weight of 5×10^8 daltons.

Physiology and Metabolism. Most *Mycoplasma* species are facultative anaerobes, although they grow better under aerobic conditions. The organisms can be divided into two broad groups, fermentative and nonfermentative. In the former, adenosine triphosphate (ATP) is derived from gly-

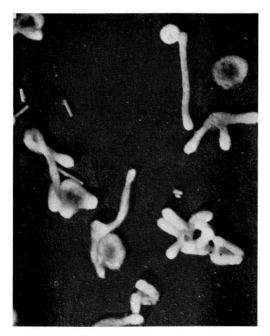

Figure 31.1: Various cellular forms of the mycoplasma of goat pleuropneumonia seen in a 24-hour serum broth culture (× 10,080). (Reproduced with permission from E. Klieneberger–Nobel and F. W. Cuckrow: A Study of the Organisms of Pleuropneumonia Group by Electron Microscopy. *J Gen Microbiol,* **12,** 95, 1955.)

colysis, while in the latter group other pathways provide ATP.

The mycoplasmas can be cultured in or on infusion or digest media. Essential growth factors for mycoplasmas are present in ascitic fluid and animal sera. Except for *M. laidlawii,* the mycoplasmas require fatty acids and cholesterol. Saprophytic species of the mycoplasmas grow in media containing no sera or similar growth factor. On solid media mycoplasmas form colonies that are 20 to 600 μm in diameter and have the appearance of a fried egg with a dense, embedded central core.

Penicillin, crystal violet, and potassium tellurite may facilitate the isolation of mycoplasmas from mixed cultures.

Mycoplasmal Disease in Man. The principal human disease definitely related to *Mycoplasma* is an atypical pneumonia caused by *M. pneumoniae. M. pneumoniae* is immunologically distinct from other human mycoplasmas. After an incubation period of 2 to 3 weeks, there is a gradual onset of fever, headache, and a nonproductive cough. In the early stages physical findings may be minimal. As the disease progresses, loud rales become prominent. Untreated disease may last up to 3 weeks. There is a late elevation in the white blood cell count, and cold agglutinins appear at 2 to 3 weeks. The initial diagnosis is made on

clinical grounds. Laboratory diagnosis is made by direct culturing of sputum or pharyngeal swabbings, and the bacteria are identified by hemadsorption, β-hemolysis of guinea pig erythrocytes, staining with homologous fluorescein-labeled antibody, or inhibition of growth by specific antibody. Tetrazolium also inhibits the organism's growth. The best treatment for primary atypical pneumonia is uncertain, although tetracyclines do affect the course of the disease. Erythromycin is also used for treatment.

Mycoplasma-induced mild respiratory infections characterized by sore throat and pharyngitis particularly occur in the 1- to 5-year-old age group. *M. pneumoniae* also produces allergic reactions such as a bullous eruption of mucous membranes (Stevens–Johnson syndrome).

The pathogenesis of mycoplasma disease is poorly understood. There are no toxins in *M. pneumoniae* infection. However, the organisms may attach to respiratory epithelial cells, which interferes with the cells' ciliary action. The cells die and desquamate, resulting in inflammation. Local accumulation of H_2O_2 may cause cell damage as well.

Listeria monocytogenes

Listeria monocytogenes is a widely distributed saprophyte that infects many species of mammals, birds, crustaceans, and ticks. In man it is usually an opportunistic pathogen, causing meningitis, febrile pharyngitis, as well as other disease forms.

Physical and Chemical Characteristics. *Listeria monocytogenes* is a pleomorphic, non-spore-forming, gram-positive rod that ranges in size from 0.2

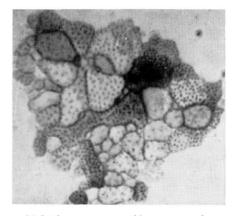

Figure 31.2: Pleuropneumonia-like organisms from a lung of a bronchiectatic rat, showing intracellular granules. (Reproduced with permission from E. Kleineberger–Nobel: Methods for the Study of the Cytology of Bacterial and Pleuropneumonia-like Organisms. *Q J Microsc Sci,* **91,** 340, 1950.)

to 0.4 μm in diameter by 0.5 to 2.0 μm long. It possesses peritrichous flagella. A chloroform-soluble lipid can be extracted that produces a marked monocytosis when injected into mice and that likely causes the monocytosis seen in human infections. *Listeria* produces an oxygen-labile hemolysin that has cardiotoxic activity and a toxic protein that is lethal for mouse macrophages. This hemolysin contributes to the pathogenesis of human infection. The organisms are facultatively anaerobic and grow on blood agar over a wide range of temperatures.

Infections in Man. Listeriosis is mainly seen in immunocompromised individuals. It most commonly appears as a leptomeningitis. Healthy individuals may develop the disease on sufficient exposure. A marked monocytosis is characteristic of listeriosis in man as well as animals. Infections in newborns range from meningitis to a disseminated disease that manifests with respiratory distress, vomiting, diarrhea, hepatosplenomegaly, and disseminated abscesses in a variety of organs.

Diagnosis and Treatment. Diagnosis depends on isolation and identification of *L. monocytogenes.* No serological tests are available. In untreated individuals the mortality is as high as 70%. Sulfonamides, penicillins, tetracyclines, and erythromycin are useful to treat listeriosis, but ampicillin is the drug of choice. Prevention requires pasteurization of milk and elimination of diseased animals.

Streptobacillus moniliformis

It is now generally agreed that a group of gram-negative bacilli isolated from humans who develop a fever after animal bites, and to which a multitude of names have been applied, belong to a single species, *Streptobacillus moniliformis.*

Bacteriological Characteristics of *Streptobacillus.* *S. moniliformis* is a CO_2-requiring, facultatively anaerobic, gram-negative, pleomorphic, nonencapsulated, nonmotile, sometimes pathogenic microorganism. It occurs in vivo and under optimal culture conditions as a bacillus. Under less satisfactory culture conditions it occurs as long chains of relatively large, irregular vegetative bacilli interspersed with cocci and coccoid swellings. It also occurs as the small filterable L type first described by Klieneberger–Nobel in 1935, specifically as L_1.

The L_1 colony of *S. moniliformis,* composed of coccoid or coccobacillary units, is seldom more than 0.2 mm in diameter. It contains a dark brown center embedded in agar and surrounded by a delicate, translucent peripheral zone composed of large swollen bodies, amorphous material, and extracellular fatty droplets.

***Streptobacillus* Infections.** The human diseases produced by *S. moniliformis* include a milk-borne disease termed Haverhill fever, and rat-bite fever. Rat-bite fever is also caused by *Spirillum minor.* The source of *S. moniliformis* is usually the bite of a rodent, the initial wound healing without inflammation. The incubation period is usually 1 to 3 days but in some instances is as long as 3 weeks. The local wound becomes inflamed and indurated and there is lymphangitis and regional lymphadenitis. The onset of symptoms is sudden, with chills and fever, the subsequent course of which may be either relapsing or septic. A rash always develops, either at the first or later exacerbations of fever. In contrast to spirillar rat-bite fever, arthritis is a common complication in the bacillary disease; severe sore throat and congestion of the pharyngeal mucous membrane are also frequent complications. Mortality is about 15%. Penicillin or tetracycline are both effective in the treatment of streptobacillary infections. Treatment is complicated by persistence in the body of the L_1 form, which is resistant to penicillin.

The Bartonella Group

The family Bartonellaceae, a group of blood parasites, contains two genera, *Bartonella* and *Grahamella.* *Bartonella* contains a single species, *Bartonella bacilliformis,* which infects man but does not naturally infect animals. *Grahamella* species do not affect man. *B. bacilliformis* causes Oroya fever, a febrile hemolytic anemia, and verruga peruana, a benign skin eruption that is a continuing or secondary phase of Oroya fever. Collectively, this syndrome is known as bartonellosis or Carrion's disease.

Characteristics of *B. bacilliformis.* *B. bacilliformis* is a gram-negative, non-acid-fast, pleomorphic, flagellated, predominantly rod-shaped microorganism. In size, morphology, staining characteristics, intracellular parasitism, and spread by an anthropod vector, *B. bacilliformis* resembles the rickettsiae, to which it is related. In cultivability, flagellation, and possession of a cell wall, *B. bacilliformis* resembles typical bacteria. *Bartonella* species exhibit stages closely resembling the bizarre forms of the mycoplasmas.

Bartonellosis. *B. bacilliformis* is indigenous to certain mountainous regions of Peru, Ecuador, and Colombia. Man is the reservoir host and the organism is transmitted from person to person by the bite of sand flies (*Plebotomus* species).

The incubation period averages about 20 days but may range from 10 days to several months. Onset is abrupt, with fever as high as 104°F (40°C), intermittent chills, intense pain, and abundant sweating. Subsequent symptoms of Oroya fever are intense pain in bones, joints, and muscles, fever, sweating, petechiae, and dull red papules, extreme pallor of the skin and mucosa, and a rapidly progressive hemolysis resulting in anemia in which erythrocyte and hemoglobin values fall to 25% of normal. The duration of the disease is usually 4 to 5 weeks. Fatal, fulminating cases may terminate in 10 days but usually linger for a month. About 1 month following recovery from Oroya fever, a benign skin eruption (verruga peruana) develops, which was originally thought to be unrelated to Oroya fever. During this phase the microorganisms do not invade erythrocytes but are found in the cytoplasm of endothelial cells. The wartlike lesions persist for 1 month to several years. The most prominent symptoms are intermittent pain and fever, usually most severe during the eruption of the lesions.

Bartonellosis responds dramatically to treatment with penicillin, chloramphenicol, or tetracycline. Secondary infections with salmonellae are common and require a broad-spectrum antibiotic for effective treatment.

ADDITIONAL READING

Chanock, R. M. 1965. Mycoplasma Infections of Man. N Engl J Med, **273,** 1199, 1257.

Charache, P. 1970. Cell Wall-defective Bacterial Variants in Human Disease. Ann NY Acad Sci, **174,** 903.

Clyde, W. A., Jr. 1971. *Mycoplasma pneumoniae* Pneumonia. Milit Med, **136,** 20.

Foy, H. M., Kinney, G. E., McMahan, R., Kaiser, G., and Gray-ston, J. R. 1970. *Mycoplasma pneumoniae* in the Community. Am J Epidemiol, **93,** 55.

Foy, H. M., Nugent, C. G., Kenny, G. E., McMahan, R., and Grayston, J. R. 1971. Repeated *Mycoplasma pneumoniae* Pneumonia after 4½ Years. JAMA, **216,** 671.

Furness, G. 1973. T-Mycoplasmas: Some Factors Affecting Their Growth, Colonial Morphology, and Assay on Agar. J Infect Dis, **128,** 703.

Gupta, U., Oumachigui, A., and Hingorani, V. 1973. Microbial Flora of the Vagina with Special Reference to Anaerobic Bacteria and Mycoplasma. Indian J Med Res, **61,** 1600.

Hayflick, L. (ed.) 1967. Biology of the Mycoplasma. Ann NY Acad Sci, **143,** 1.

Klieneberger–Nobel, E. 1962. *Pleuropneumonia-like Organisms (PPLO) Mycoplasmataceae.* Academic Press, New York.

Mardh, P. A., and Taylor–Robinson, D. 1973. New Approaches to the Isolation of Mycoplasmas. Med Microbial Immunol, **158,** 259.

McCormack, W. M., Rosner, B., and Lee, Y. 1973. Colonization with Genital Mycoplasmas in Women. Am J Epidemiol, **97,** 240.

Mufson, M. A. 1970. *Mycoplasma hominis* I in Respiratory Tract Infections. Ann NY Acad Sci, **174,** 798.

Naftalin, J. M., Wellisch, G., Zahana, Z., and Diengott, D. 1974. *Mycoplasma pneumoniae* Septicemia. JAMA, **228,** 565.

Neiman, R. E., and Lorber, B. 1980. Listeriosis in Adults: A Changing Pattern. Report of Eight Cases and Review of the Literature, 1968–1978. Rev Infect Dis, **2,** 207.

Razin, S. 1978. The Mycoplasmas. Microbiol Rev, **42,** 414.

Reiler, J. P. 1979. Perinatal and Neonatal Infections: Listeriosis. J Antimicrob Chemother, **5,** 51.

Watanabe, T. 1975. Proteolytic Activity of *Mycoplasma salivarium* and *Mycoplasma orale:* I. Med Microbiol Immunol, **161,** 127.

Watanabe, T., Mishima, K., Fujita, O., Horikawa, T., Noguchi, T., Ishizu, T., and Kinoshita, S. 1972. Possible Role of Mycoplasmas in Periodontal Disease. Bull Tokyo Med Dent Univ, **19,** 93.

32

Rickettsial and Chlamydial Infections

George S. Schuster

Rickettsiae

Physiochemical Characteristics. The genus *Rickettsia*, family Rickettsiaceae, contains ten species, divided into spotted fever, typhus, and scrub typhus groups. Also included in the Rickettsiaceae are *Coxiella burnetii*, the cause of Q fever, and *Rochalimaea quintana*, the agent that causes trench fever. *C. burnetii* resembles the typical rickettsiae in many of its physiological aspects, while *R. quintana*, previously classified as a species of *Rickettsia*, resembles them in its route of transmission and in some features of the infection it produces. Members of the genus *Rickettsia* are small coccobacilli, 0.3 to 0.5 μm by 0.8 to 2.0 μm, that are similar to gram-negative bacteria in their fine structure and chemical composition. The cell walls of rickettsiae contain peptidoglycan and have an endotoxin-like lipopolysaccharide. The cells have a cytoplasmic membrane and contain both DNA and RNA. Members of the genera *Rickettsia* and *Coxiella* multiply by transverse fission. *R. prowazekii* possesses an amorphous capsule. All members of the genus *Rickettsia* are obligate intracellular parasites. Special stains are needed to demonstrate rickettsiae in cell preparations. Although most strains of the rickettsiae are rather unstable and fragile, *C. burnetii* is one of the more resistant non-spore-forming microorganisms.

Growth of Rickettsia. Rickettsiae are commonly cultured in embryonated eggs or in tissue cultures derived from laboratory animals. Laboratory animals are useful for primary isolation and virulence studies. *Rochalimaea quintana* differs from rickettsiae in that it can be cultivated on relatively simple bacteriological media. The natural hosts of the rickettsiae include a variety of mammals and arthropods. Mammals, including man, are infected by inoculation of the organisms into the skin during feeding of an infected arthropod; conversely, arthropods can become infected by feeding on infected mammals. Arthropods often serve as both a vector and a reservoir, because the rickettsiae can be transferred from arthropod to arthropod transovarially. In some instances, notably *R. prowazekii*, multiplication in the gut leads to death of the louse vector.

Pathogenesis. Rickettsiae have an affinity for the endothelial cells of small blood vessels, causing their hyperplasia. Perivascular infiltration and local thrombosis permit blood to leak into the surrounding tissues. Inflammation of the blood vessels, particularly in the skin and brain, causes the rash and terminal shock that are common clinical signs of a rickettsial infection. Although it has not been characterized, there appears to be a toxin that participates in the pathogenesis of rickettsial diseases. The rickettsial endotoxin-like lipopolysaccharide contributes at least in part to the fever, rash, and intravascular coagulation. Unlike typical endotoxins they elicit production of protective antibodies.

Rickettsiae adhere to the surface of cells and are taken up by endocytosis. They destroy the phagosomal membrane and multiply in the cytoplasm. Some host cells are killed, releasing organisms, but some organisms are also released from living cells by exocytosis.

Treatment. *Rickettsia* and *Rochalimaea* species are resistant to sulfonamides but are inhibited by *p*-aminobenzoic acid. Penicillin and streptomycin only slightly inhibit rickettsiae and are of no therapeutic value. Broad-spectrum antibiotics (e.g., oxytetracycline, chlortetracycline, deoxycycline, and chloramphenicol) are quite useful for rickettsial infections.

Diagnosis. Rickettsial infections can be diagnosed by identification of the causative organism, either by infection of laboratory animals or serologically. At best, however, isolation of rickettsiae is a hazardous and technically difficult procedure. If rickettsiae are isolated they can be identified by neutralization with specific antisera.

Serological procedures are most useful for the diagnosis of rickettsial infections. One of the most useful of such tests is the Weil–Felix test. Rickettsiae and strains of *Proteus,* referred to as OX strains, share common heat-stable antigens. The Weil–Felix test is based on the agglutination of *Proteus* strains by antibodies formed against these common antigens during some of the rickettsial infections. Antibodies to group-specific and type-specific antigens may be detected by complement-fixation tests. Immunofluorescence, ELISA, and agglutination reactions are also useful in the diagnosis of rickettsial infections, particularly if the Weil–Felix test is negative.

The principal human rickettsial infections, their causal agents, the arthropod vector, and their principal serological reactions are listed in Table 32.1.

Rickettsial Diseases

European Epidemic Louse-Borne Typhus.
European epidemic louse-borne typhus is caused by *Rickettsia prowazekii*, which is transmitted from person to person by body or head lice. The incubation period of typhus averages about 12 days and is divided into four phases, each characterized by definite symptoms, but there is fever in all stages. The first or invasive stage lasts 3 to 4 days. In addition to fever there is headache and myalgia. Conjunctivitis with photophobia often occurs. The second stage, which lasts for 4 days, is characterized by a rash that begins on the trunk and spreads to the extremities (Figs. 32.1 and 32.2). The third stage, characterized by prostration, delirium, and collapse, lasts until the 12th day after onset and terminates in a crisis in which the patient is desperately ill. If the patient survives the crisis and if there are no complications, he enters the fourth stage, in which there is usually satisfactory recovery. However, there is often a variety of complications, many of which are quite severe. Mortality of the disease is related to age, for death seldom occurs in children less than 5 years old, and the mortality rate increases with age so that after age 50 it may be as high as 60%. Treatment is principally symptomatic, but chloramphenicol and the tetracyclines have been used successfully to treat the disease. Recovery from an initial typhus infection confers resistance to a second attack. Several types of typhus vaccines have been used for active immunization. Their application has reduced the severity of the disease and perhaps reduced its incidence also.

Extrahuman reservoirs of *R. prowazekii* exist. In the eastern United States natural infection of flying squirrels and their ectoparasites is widespread. The strain appears identical to the human strains of *R. prowazekii*. Infection of humans with this strain can produce sylvan typhus. This form is more mild than classic epidemic typhus. It is characterized by fever and headache but the rash may not be present.

Brill's Disease. Brill's disease, also known as recrudescent epidemic typhus, is a rickettsial infection with symptoms similar if not identical to European epidemic louse-borne typhus. It was first described in New York in recent immigrants, particularly those from Eastern Europe, where epidemic typhus was common. The disease represents a recrudescence of a latent typhus infection acquired previously, for it is not acquired from lice in the usual way. Asymptomatic carriers may harbor the rickettsiae for many years and are probably the reservoir of classic typhus.

Endemic Murine Flea-Borne Typhus. This form of typhus is caused by *Rickettsia typhi,* which naturally infects several species of rats and occasionally cats, possums, or rabbits. *R. typhi* is transferred between rats by rat lice or rat fleas and from rats to humans by the fleas. The disease is characterized by the abrupt onset of fever, headache, nausea, malaise, and a maculopapular rash that begins on the trunk

Table 32.1: Rickettsial Diseases, Causal Agents, and Insect Vectors

Disease	Causal Agent	Insect Vector	Weil–Felix Reaction
1. European epidemic louse-borne typhus	*Rickettsia prowazekii*	Human body louse (*Pediculus corporis*); human head louse (*Pediculus capitis*)	Positive OX-19
2. Brill's disease (recrudescent epidemic typhus)	*R. prowazekii*	(Recrudescence of previous infection)	Usually negative
3. Endemic murine flea-borne typhus	*Rickettsia typhi*	Rat louse (*Polydax spinulosus*); rat flea (*Ceratophyllus fasciatus and anisus*); rat mite (*Liponyssus bacoti*); flea (*Xenopsylla cheopis*)	Positive OX-19
4. South African tick-bite fever	*Rickettsia conorii*	Common dog tick (*Haemaphysalis leachi*); hare tick (*Amblyomma hebraeum*)	Positive OX-19, OX-2
5. North Queensland tick typhus	*Rickettsia australis*	Tick (*Ixodes holocyclus*)	Positive OX-19, OX-2
6. North Asian tick-borne rickettsiosis	*Rickettsia sibiricus*	Ticks (*Dermacentor nuttalli; Dermacentor silvarium; Haemaphysalis concina*)	Positive OX-19, OX-2
7. Scrub typhus (Tsutsugamushi disease)	*Rickettsia tsutsugamushi*	Chigger mites (*Trombicula akamushi* and *Trombicula deliensis*)	Positive OX-K
8. Trench fever	*Rochalimaea quintana*	Human louse (*P. corporis*)	Negative
9. Rocky Mountain spotted fever	*Rickettsia rickettsii*	American dog tick (*Dermacentor variabilis*); Rocky Mountain wood tick (*Dermacentor andersoni*); Lone Star tick (*Amblyomma americanum*); South American tick (*Amblyomma cajennense*); brown dog tick (*Rhipicephalus sanguineus*); rabbit tick (*Haemaphysalis leporis palustris*)	Positive OX-19, OX-2
10. Fievre boutonneuse	*R. conorii*	Dog ticks (*Rhipicephalus sanguineus*)	Positive OX-19, OX-2
11. Q fever (Query fever)	*Coxiella burnetii*	Cattle ticks (*Boophilus annulatus microplus* and *Haemophysalis bispinosa*); Lone Star tick (*A. americanum*); Rocky Mountain wood tick (*Dermacentor andersoni*); North African ticks (*Hyalomma savignyi* and *Hyalomma dromedarii*)	Negative
12. Rickettsialpox	*Rickettsia akari*	House mouse mite (*Allodermanyssus sanguineus*)	Negative

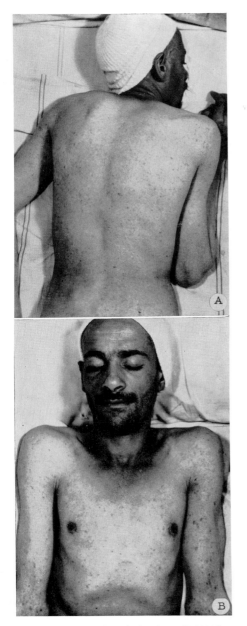

Figure 32.1: Typhus rash, 10th day. (AFIP 60-1001.)

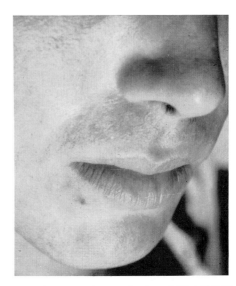

Figure 32.2: Primary lesion of typhus. (AFIP A44-256.)

mites. It is a very severe febrile illness, with the usual symptoms of typhus (Fig. 32.3). The disease lasts about 3 weeks and has a fatality rate of up to 50%. Broad-spectrum antibiotics are highly effective in suppressing growth of *R. tsutsugamushi,* but recrudescences are common and recovery ultimately depends on antibody formation.

Trench Fever.   More than 1 million cases of trench fever occurred during World War I and World War II. The causal organism is *Rochalimaea quintana,* which is transmitted to humans by the human body louse, *Pediculus corporis.* The incubation period of the disease, which in humans is from 2 weeks to 2 months, is followed by a febrile disease that normally lasts for no longer than a month. It has the characteristics of typhus. The mortality rate is low.

Rocky Mountain Spotted Fever.   Rocky Mountain spotted fever has been reported in 43 states of the United States and in Canada, Mexico, and South America. It is caused by *Rickettsia rickettsii.* A rickettsial reservoir is maintained in rabbits and small rodents and is transmitted among animals by ticks. In the western United States the organism is transmitted to man by the wood tick *Dermacentor andersoni,* in the eastern United States and Mexico by the dog tick *Dermacentor variabilis,* and in South America by other ticks. The incubation period of Rocky Mountain spotted fever is no longer than 2 weeks. The onset is sudden with headache, fever, and chills. Rash appears from the third and seventh day, and a temperature as high as 107°F (41°C) occurs that may continue for 2 or 3 weeks. The rash characteristically appears on the palms, soles, and other areas of the extremities as erythematous macules or maculopapules, and spreads to the trunk. It may become petechial or de-

and spreads to the extremities. Involvement of the face, palms, and soles is rare. There may be renal, pulmonary, and neurologic involvement. Untreated illness may last 10 to 14 days. Murine typhus is not as severe as epidemic typhus, having a mortality rate of less than 5%.

Scrub Typhus (Tsutsugamushi Disease). Scrub typhus, which occurs in India, Southeast Asia, the East Indies, Northern Australia, and many islands of the Southwest Pacific, is caused by *Rickettsia tsutsugamushi.* It is transmitted to man by trombiculid

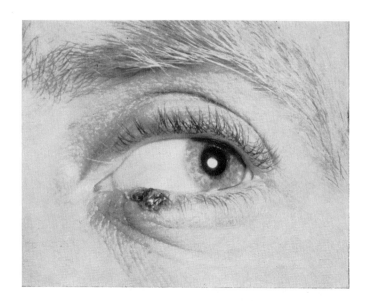

Figure 32.3: Scrub typhus showing eschar of eyelid. (AFIP 1st MFL 86-1.)

velop into large purpura. The widespread vasculitis that develops accounts for multisystem symptoms such as abdominal pain, vomiting, diarrhea, conjunctival suffusion, headache, lethargy, convulsions, coma, and various cardiovascular abnormalities. Maculopapular oral lesions have been occasionally seen as well. Convalescence is slow and complications are frequent. No lasting immunity results from a primary infection. Mortality has ranged from 40% in children to 80% in adults, although the mortality rate is much lower at the present time because of vaccination and antibiotic therapy. Initial diagnosis and treatment should be done on the basis of clinical findings. Laboratory diagnosis involving serologic tests is useful for confirmation of infection. Chloramphenicol and tetracycline are used for treatment with success. Nearly two thirds of all cases in the United States occur east of the Mississippi. The disease is not uncommon in the United States; the infection rate is around 0.5 cases per 100,000, many occurring in the mid-Atlantic and south-central regions. Foci of the disease have been reported in the Cape Cod area and in Virginia.

Q Fever (Query Fever). Q fever clinically resembles influenza and primary atypical pneumonia, and is unique among rickettsioses in three ways: transmission to man is usually not arthropod-borne, no skin rash develops, and patients do not develop agglutinins for *Proteus* strains. The causal rickettsia, *Coxiella burnetii,* is probably maintained in various rodents, among which it is spread by a number of species of ticks. They transmit it to domesticated animals, in which it produces mild disease and from which it is excreted in milk and feces. *C. burnetii* is somewhat different from other rickettsiae since it grows intracellularly within vacuoles or phagolyso-

somes rather than in the host cell cytoplasm. It has a cycle consisting of a vegetative and a spore-like differentiation. Thus, it is unusually resistant to heat and drying, and may survive pasteurization in milk. It also persists for long periods in the dried effluvia of infected animals, whence it is acquired directly or indirectly by susceptible cattle and man. Transfer from infected to susceptible persons is possible but not common. Very likely, Q fever is or will be globally distributed.

The incubation period of Q fever is about 3 weeks. Infection may be unapparent or produce a very mild illness. Clinically recognized Q fever has a sudden onset and resembles influenza. A severe febrile illness lasts about 2 weeks on the average, but fever may continue for several months. Pneumonitis is a common accompaniment. Mortality is very low. Differential diagnosis is quite difficult and is most readily established retrospectively when specific antibodies develop. Recovery is usually uncomplicated, although rather slow. Endocarditis may occur up to several years later and affect previously damaged heart valves. Such cases have a high fatality rate, 30% to 55%.

Rickettsialpox. Since rickettsialpox was first recognized in New York City in 1946 it has been reported in many major cities and in other countries. It is caused by *Rickettsia akari,* which is transmitted by the common house mouse mite vector *Allodermanyssus sanguineus.* Because of the mild nature of rickettsialpox, it may go unrecognized and may actually be more common and widespread than is currently reported.

The general pathology of rickettsialpox is unknown. The most distinctive of the lesions is the initial skin lesion, which develops about the bite of the in-

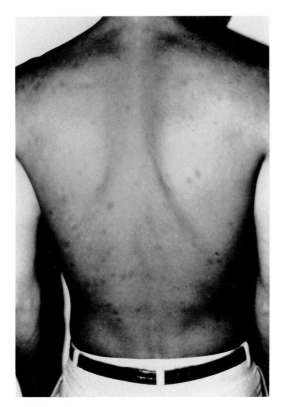

Figure 32.4: Rash of rickettsialpox in a 24-year-old man. The initial lesion was present on the forearm.

fected mite after about 24 to 48 hours. The lesion is a firm red papule, 1 to 2.5 cm in diameter, which vesiculates, then forms a black eschar that scabs and heals after 2 or 3 weeks, with some scarring. The systemic reactions that occur in rickettsialpox about 9 to 14 days after the bite are fever, chills, sweating, backache, sore throat, and muscular pain. Concurrent with or within a few days after onset of fever, a rash of wide distribution appears that has been described as maculopapular, discrete, and erythematous (Fig. 32.4). The lesions usually develop a small central vesicle or pustule, hence the name rickettsialpox. Vesicles develop after a few days and heal without scarring. Oral lesions of a transient nature have been reported in rickettsialpox. Although they have not been found consistently, vesicles do occur on the tongue and palate.

The diagnosis of rickettsialpox is based on clinical symptoms and on complement-fixation or fluorescent antibody tests. In many ways the disease resembles varicella (chickenpox), variola (smallpox), tick typhus, Rocky Mountain spotted fever, scrub typhus, and, to a lesser extent, tularemia and plague.

Control of Rickettsial Diseases. Rickettsial infections may be controlled by antibiotics, immunization, or by disrupting the transmission cycles of the causative rickettsiae. Epidemic typhus may be prevented by delousing humans with DDT. Elimination of rodents and their parasites helps control murine typhus, scrub typhus, and rickettsialpox. Clearing of infested land and the use of protective clothing will help prevent spotted fever. Avoiding infected animals and proper pasteurization of milk will help control Q fever. Proper disposal of garbage and control of mice will control rickettsialpox.

Chlamydiae

The genus *Chlamydia* contains two species, *Chlamydia trachomatis* and *Chlamydia psittaci,* which can be further divided into many different strains on the basis of their antigenic composition, host range, virulence, and pathogenic effects. The chlamydiae are obligate intracellular parasites and do not synthesize adenosine triphosphate (ATP), but in many ways they resemble bacteria. The chlamydiae have cell walls similar to those of gram-negative bacteria, they contain both DNA and RNA, they divide by binary fission, and they are susceptible to antibiotics. Their genome is relatively small, with a molecular weight of 6.6×10^8 daltons. Chlamydiae have a life cycle that involves two alternate forms, the elementary body and the reticulate body (Fig. 32.5). The elementary bodies, the infectious forms, adhere specifically to receptors on endothelial cells and are taken into the cells by endocytosis. These inhibit phagosome–lysosome fusion and remain in the former. Here they reorganize into the reproductive forms, the reticulate bodies. The events of the developmental cycle are not fully understood, but at the end of the logarithmic phase there is a mixture of elementary bodies and reticulate bodies. These fill the phagosome and are the inclusion bodies seen with Giemsa staining. In the course of reproduction some cells burst and die. However, others live and reproduce. Thus, new cells are infected by released organisms, while daughter cells may be infected during reproduction.

Chlamydiae have little or no ability to generate energy and depend on the host cell for this function. This contributes to host cell death because the host cell is unable to maintain itself.

All chlamydiae share a common genus-specific antigen. *C. trachomatis* strains also share species-specific and type-specific antigens to varying degrees. Antibodies can be detected in sera by complement-fixation, immunofluorescence, or neutralization tests.

Chlamydiae infect a wide range of animal hosts, including birds, mice, cats, dogs, and humans. The mechanism by which they cause disease is not known, but in general the chlamydiae are not very pathogenic. However, many of these diseases may have a latent stage that permits the disease to recur following treat-

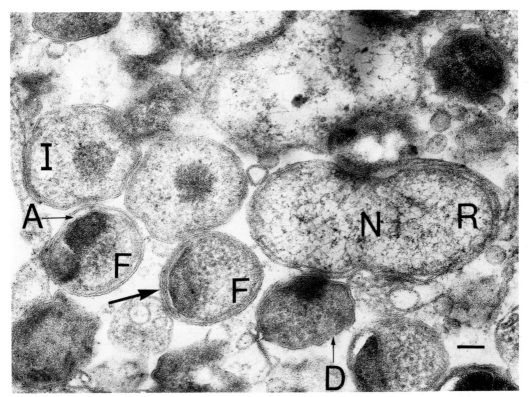

Figure 32.5: Electron micrograph of *Chlamydia psittaci* in an infected yolk sac cell showing various particulate forms of the organism: the early stage of the division (*N*) of a reticulate body (*R*); intermediate body (*I*); less condensed elementary bodies (*F*) whose membranes are closely apposed (*arrow*) except for a distention adjacent to the nucleoid (*A*) and irregularly shaped, highly condensed elementary bodies (*D*). (Courtesy of Dr. J. W. Costerton and reproduced by permission of the National Research Council of Canada: *Can J Microbiol,* **21,** 1433–1477, 1975.)

ment. Chlamydial infections are usually easily controlled or cured by chemotherapy. *C. trachomatis* is susceptible to sulfonamides, and both *C. trachomatis* and *C. psittaci* are susceptible to broad-spectrum antibiotics.

Chlamydial Infections

Trachoma. Trachoma, a disease of the eye caused by *C. trachomatis,* is found naturally only in man and is the greatest single cause of blindness. It is found in nearly every country and flourishes in areas with poor public sanitation and poor personal hygiene. It is transmitted primarily by hand to eye contact or by fomites. Flies may transmit the disease. Onset is sudden, with inflamed conjunctivae. Within a few weeks characteristic follicles form beneath the conjunctival surface, followed later by vascularization of the cornea and pannus. This may result in partial or complete blindness. The conjunctiva may become scarred and the normal flow of tears is disturbed, resulting in bacterial infections of the eyes.

The mechanisms of pathogenesis are not known. However, blindness may result from a variety of factors. Growth of organisms may lead to formation of hard lesions on the inner aspect of the eyelids. This results in repeated scratching of the cornea and repeated secondary infections. The scratching may also permit infecting organisms to infiltrate the cornea, causing excessive granulation tissue, vascularization, and blindness. In addition, pannus may represent an allergic response to chlamydial antigens.

Immunity may result from a combination of cell-mediated immunity and antibodies blocking adherence and inhibiting the mechanism that obstructs phagosome–lysosome fusion. Nevertheless, acquired immunity is low and short-lived, as evidenced by the frequency of latent disease and relapses.

Trachoma may be diagnosed from the clinical symptoms or by isolation of the causative organism from conjunctival scrapings in embryonated eggs or tissue cultures, by location of cytoplasmic inclusions in conjunctival cells with staining or fluorescent antibodies, or by detection of trachoma-specific antibodies in eye secretions.

Inclusion Conjunctivitis. Inclusion conjunctivitis is a prevalent inflammatory eye infection that is sometimes termed inclusion blenorrhea or swimming pool conjunctivitis. The causal organism is a strain of *C. trachomatis.* Disease in the adult likely results from contamination of the eyes by genitourinary or other exudates on the hands or fomites. The conjunctivitis resembles the early stages of trachoma but usually does not progress to a chronic disease. Inclusion conjunctivitis is often a disease of the newborn, acquired during birth from an infected maternal genital tract. The disease is difficult to diagnose clinically and final diagnosis depends on the demonstration of characteristic basophilic granular inclusions (Thygeson bodies) in the cytoplasm of epithelial cells from the affected area or by isolating the agent in cell cultures. Immunofluorescence studies have allowed differentiation of the causative organism of inclusion conjunctivitis from that of trachoma. Inclusion conjunctivitis is benign and self-limited and leaves no residual damage. It can be cured readily with sulfonamides, tetracyclines, or chloramphenicol.

Neonatal Pneumonia. *Chlamydia trachomatis* may cause infant pneumonitis: the children usually become ill at 1 to 4 months of age. They have prominent respiratory symptoms of cough and wheezing but lack fever. Chlamydial conjunctivitis may precede the onset of pneumonia.

Nongonococcal Urethritis. Chlamydiae are the leading identified cause of nongonococcal urethritis in males; perhaps 25% to 50% of cases are due to *C. trachomatis.* Many men with gonorrhea will have nongonococcal urethritis that manifests after treatment of gonorrhea, especially if the gonorrhea is treated with a penicillin, since the chlamydiae are not sensitive to these agents. The infection may be transmitted to females, producing symptomatic or asymptomatic infections, especially of the cervix.

Lymphogranuloma Venereum. Lymphogranuloma venereum (also known by a variety of other names) is a protean venereal disease of worldwide distribution, although it occurs most often in the tropics. The causative agent of lymphogranuloma venereum usually is a strain of *C. trachomatis.*

Lymphogranuloma venereum is usually transmitted by sexual contact either with those who have overt disease or with asymptomatic carriers. Incubation periods are variable, but they appear to be generally 10 and 30 days. Primary lesions appear most often in the genital or anorectal regions and the oral cavity, according to the site of contact (Fig. 32.6). Nonvenereal infection often involves the hands, particularly the fingers of dentists and other medical personnel. The primary lesion usually appears first as a distinct vesicle that later ruptures, leaving a shallow, grayish ulcer or chancre. It is not painful and heals without scarring.

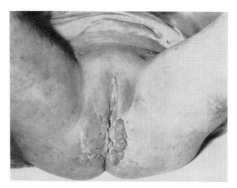

Figure 32.6: Perianal lesions of lymphogranuloma venereum. (AFIP D-45421.)

The initial stages of infection are not accompanied by systemic reactions.

In an initial oral infection, the tongue is most often affected with a painless, blister-like lesion. As the disease progresses, the tongue is enlarged, with zones of scarring and retraction. Such symptoms are sometimes mild, at other times severe. Deep grooves are often found on the dorsum of the tongue, with zones of intense red coloration and loss of superficial epithelium; or, alternatively, grayish opaque papules may develop. The dorsum of the tongue may be painful to salts or sour foods. When only the margins of the tongue are involved, the subjective symptoms are few. The lesions on the tongue are generally of long duration; sometimes the lesions subside spontaneously only to recover their original aspects.

Within 7 days to as long as 2 months after appearance of the initial lesion, a painful regional lymphadenitis occurs, with varying degrees of enlargement. In most cases the affected lymph nodes suppurate, forming abscesses and fistulas. Adenopathy may subside after several months but the fistulous tracts usually persist for years. During the intermediate stage of the disease the constitutional symptoms are variable but consist of headache, fever, vomiting, lassitude, and skin eruptions, indicating a generalized infection.

In the later stages of the disease, which may not be manifest in all those infected, the manifestations are esthiomene, the urethro-genital-perineal syndrome, penoscrotal elephantiasis, rectal stenosis, and/or plastic induration of the penis. During this stage the skin and sense organs and the cardiovascular, respiratory, digestive, genitourinary, and nervous systems may be affected. In general, the latter-day manifestations are accompanied by weakness, loss of weight, mental changes, and anemia.

Laboratory procedures useful in the diagnosis of lymphogranuloma venereum include examination of stained films of pus or tissue sections, including affected lymph nodes, for intracellular organisms. Perhaps the most common diagnostic aid, although not necessarily the most used, is the Frei test, in which antigen and control material are injected intradermally. The test is positive if the papule raised by the antigen is larger than the control papule. The Frei test becomes positive within 6 months after infection and remains so for many years. A false positive reaction sometimes is obtained, particularly in syphilis. Treatment with tetracyclines cures the acute signs and decreases complications.

Ornithosis and Psittacosis. Caused by *C. psittaci*, psittacosis is the term applied to infections of psittacine birds such as parrots and parakeets, while ornithosis refers to infection of nonpsittacine birds. Birds may have latent infections that become active with increased stress. The organisms may be transmitted to other birds by contact, droplets, or infected droppings. Once infected, the birds lose weight and have diarrhea and discharge from the eyes. The infection is usually fatal to the birds. Humans usually acquire the disease from birds by inhalation of infected material in which the organisms may persist for a prolonged period; direct human spread has been observed.

In man, the infection may be asymptomatic or may appear as a mild to moderately severe respiratory infection. The incubation period ranges from 6 to 15 days. The more severe forms are characterized by the sudden onset of signs and symptoms of bronchitis and bronchopneumonia. High fever may occur and a cough is common. Prior to treatment the patient is severely ill.

The clinical signs of these infections are not sufficiently characteristic to establish a diagnosis. Laboratory diagnosis of human infection is based on isolation of the organism from blood or sputum or from infected material, and identification by neutralization of infectivity, a complement-fixation test, or immunofluorescence.

Broad-spectrum antibiotics are useful for treating ornithosis and psittacosis.

ADDITIONAL READING

Baca, O. G., and Paretsky, D. 1983. Q Fever and *Coxiella burnetii:* A Model for Host-Parasite Interactions. Microbiol Rev, **47,** 127.

Brettman, L. R., Lewin, S., Holzman, R. S., et al. 1981. Rickettsialpox: Report of an Outbreak and Contemporary Review. Medicine, **60,** 363.

Dawson, C. 1973. Therapy of Diseases Caused by Chlamydia Organisms. Int Ophthalmol Clin, **13,** 93.

Duma, R. J., Sonenshine, D. E., Bozeman, F. M., et al. 1981. Epidemic Typhus in the United States Associated with Flying Squirrels. JAMA, **245,** 2319.

Dupont, H. C., Horneck, R. B., Dawkins, A. T., Heiner, G. G., Fabrikant, I. B., Wisseman, C. L., and Woodward, T. E. 1974. Rocky Mountain Spotted Fever: A Comparative Study of the Active Immunity Induced by Inactivated and Viable Pathogenic *Rickettsia rickettsii.* J Infect Dis, **128,** 340.

Grayston, J. T., Wang, S., Yeh, L., et al. 1985. Importance of Reinfection in the Pathogenesis of Trachoma. Rev Infect Dis, **7,** 717.

Hand, W. L., Miller, V. B., and Reinarz, J. A. 1970. Rocky Mountain Spotted Fever: A Vascular Disease. Arch Intern Med, **125,** 879.

Hattwick, M. A., Peters, A. H., O'Brien, R. J., and Hanson, B. 1976. Rocky Mountain Spotted Fever: Epidemiology of an Increasing Problem. Ann Intern Med, **84,** 732.

Kelsey, D. S. 1979. Rocky Mountain Spotted Fever. Pediatr Clin North Am, **26,** 367.

Lennette, E. H., and Schmidt, N. F. (Eds.) 1969. *Diagnostic Procedures for Viral and Rickettsial Diseases,* Ed. 4. American Public Health Association, New York.

Lumicao, G. G., and Heggie, A. D. 1979. Chlamydial Infections. Pediatr Clin North Am, **26,** 269.

Maulitz, R. M., and Imperato, P. J. 1974. Rocky Mountain Spotted Fever in an Urban Setting. NY State J Med, **74,** 1403.

Moulder, J. W. 1985. Comparative Biology of Intracellular Parasites. Microbiol Rev, **49,** 298.

North, E. 1980. Concerning the Epidemic of Spotted Fever in New England. Rev Infect Dis, **2,** 811.

Oriel, J. D., Powis, P. A., Reeve, P., Miller, A., and Nicol, C. S. 1974. Chlamydial Infections of the Cervix. Br J Vener Dis, **50,** 11.

Paovonen, J. 1979. Chlamydial Infections: Microbiological, Clinical, and Diagnostic Aspects. Med Biol, **57,** 135.

Rose, H. M. 1949. The Clinical Manifestations and Laboratory Diagnosis of Rickettsialpox. Ann Intern Med, **31,** 871.

Schachter, J. 1978. Chlamydial Infections. N Engl J Med, **298,** 428.

Schachter, J., and Grossman, M. 1981. Chlamydial Infections. Annu Rev Med, **32,** 45.

Stamm, W. E., Guinan, M. E., Johnson, C., et al. 1984. Effect of Treatment Regimens for *Neisseria gonorrheae* or Simultaneous Infection with *Chlamydia Trachomatis.* N Engl J Med, **310,** 545.

Weiss, E. 1973. Growth and Physiology of Rickettsiae. Bacteriol Rev, **37,** 259.

Part VI

Mycotic Infections

33

Mycotic Infections

George S. Schuster

The fungi are plantlike organisms that are widely distributed in water and soil and on living and dead and decaying plants. Of the 200,000 or so species, very few are human parasites or pathogens. Pathogenic fungi are restricted to yeasts and molds. They are generally immotile and have no leaves, stems, or roots. Since they are not photosynthetic, they must exist as parasites or saprophytes.

Although the fungi are much less differentiated than the usual plants, they are more differentiated and complex than bacteria. The yeasts exist as a single cell (i.e., they are monomorphic), while the molds exist either as single cells or as multicellular filamentous colonies (i.e., they are dimorphic). However, the uninucleated individual cells of fungi can differentiate into sexually distinct cells, single yeast cells, multinucleated filamentous strands, or bodies that produce spores.

Fungi are pathogenic for humans, other mammals, birds, and plants, often with serious consequences. However, they perform many useful functions as soil scavengers, as producers of antibiotics, organic acids,

hormones, and in the production of such foods as cheese, bread, and ethanol for beverages.

Morphology

The cells of fungi resemble those of higher plants in that they have a distinct nucleus, with a limiting membrane, nucleoli, an endoplasmic reticulum, mitochondria, and other organelles. Some have an external coating like a slime layer or a capsule. Yeasts usually exist as spherical or oval cells 2 to 15 μm in diameter. Occasionally, yeast cells form chains of individual cells that adhere together. Molds may exist in a yeast form, but their principal vegetative form is the hypha. Hyphae are tubules that range from 2 to 10 μm in diameter and grow by producing side branches or by elongation. As they grow, they form an intertwining mass termed a mycelium. As the mass increases in size it forms a colony or thallus. As the thallus forms, hyphae that penetrate the culture medium to absorb the nutrients are known collectively as the vegetative mycelium; the hyphae that project above the surface of the thallus form the aerial mycelium. If aerial mycelia bear reproductive cells or spores, such aerial hyphae are collectively known as the reproductive mycelium.

Hyphae may be either septate or nonseptate. The nonseptate hyphae are usually multinucleate (coenocytic); the septate hyphae usually contain only one nucleus in each compartment.

Candida

Organisms in the genus *Candida* appear both as yeast cells and with pseudohyphae. *C. albicans* also produces true hyphae. Pseudohyphae are chains of budding cells that fail to detach, so they appear as branching networks resembling true hyphae. In this form the colonies have a soft, white appearance, in contrast to the cottony growth of true mycelia. The yeast cells of *C. albicans* are gram-positive, oval, and range in size from 2 by 3 μm to 8.5 by 14 μm. In addition to the true mycelia and pseudomycelia, *C. albicans* may appear as blastospores and chlamydospores. Blastospores grow in round clusters at intervals along the pseudomycelia. Terminal chlamydospores grow at the end of the hyphae; they are rarely seen on any other species of *Candida*. Chlamydospores are large (8 to 12 μm), round, and have a thick wall composed of an outer layer, a β-1,3 glucan, and an inner protein layer.

The various species of *Candida* have been classified into six antigenic groups based on a series of ten antigens. All species share a common antigen. The important antigens appear to be surface polysaccharides. In *C. albicans* these are glucans and mannans, appearing as complexes of polysaccharide–protein linked by *N*-acetylglucosamine.

Eight species of *Candida* have been isolated from man: *C. albicans, C. tropicalis, C. pseudotropicalis, C. krusei, C. guilliermondi, C. parapsilosis, C. stellatoidea,* and *C. rugosa*. All species except *C. rugosa* are encountered in human disease. *C. albicans* is the most frequent pathogen, although *C. tropicalis* has become a serious cause of disseminated infection in immunocompromised patients.

Candidiasis

Candidiasis, caused by species of the genus *Candida,* may vary from a benign localized infection of skin or mucous membranes to an acute, disseminated infection of lung or intestine that often terminates fatally within a relatively short time, particularly when there is septicemia, endocarditis, or meningitis. Onset is generally related to factors that lower resistance either

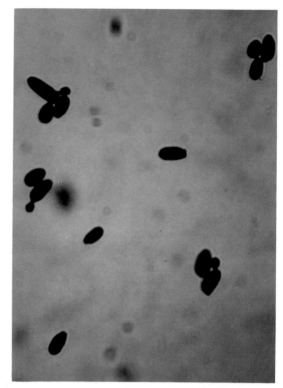

Figure 33.1: *Candida albicans* reproducing by budding.

locally or generally. Candidiasis is worldwide in distribution and occurs in all races and at all ages.

Candida albicans. *C. albicans* is an oval, thin-walled, budding, yeastlike cell 2 to 5 μm in diameter when it is first obtained from a lesion. Positive identification can best be made from the growth on cornmeal agar, which contains characteristic budding cells and chlamydospores (Figs. 33.1 and 33.2). *C. albicans* can also be differentiated from nonpathogenic species by the formation of germ tubes growing out from the cell after about 90 minutes in serum at 37°C. These are short filaments, about 1.5 by 15 μm. They may sometimes be seen in *C. stellatoidea*. This species also can produce blastospores, pseudohyphae, and, rarely, chlamydospores. *C. tropicalis* produces pseudohyphae, true mycelia, and chlamydospores rarely, but not germ tubes.

Candidal Infection. A number of clinical and pathological entities are attributable to *C. albicans* and are collectively referred to as candidiasis. They involve many structures. Some infections remain localized and benign; others are disseminated and acute. Candidiasis generally falls into three broad categories: cutaneous, systemic, and chronic mucocutaneous. Cutaneous candidiasis involves infection of the skin, mucous membranes, and nails by endogenous *Candida* and may result from chronic maceration of these areas, physiological changes in the host, or a compromised immune status. From the localized lesions, the organisms may disseminate directly or hematogenously. The initial infection is more likely to involve the skin or mucosa of the mouth or other portions of the gastrointestinal tract, the vagina, and the lungs. Systemic candidiasis follows dissemination directly in tissues, resulting in infection of the urinary and gastrointestinal tracts, the middle ear and mastoids, vagina, pleura, or diaphragm, depending on the location of the initial infection. Also from the initial infection, the yeast cells can invade blood vessels and disseminate to almost any area of the body.

Candidiasis in Infants. An acute and definitive infection of *C. albicans* is oral candidiasis of infants, commonly called thrush. The original lesions develop in otherwise healthy infants often within 8 or 9 days after passage through an infected birth canal. The disease is then usually transmitted to other infants in a ward or nursery by nipples, pacifiers, and contaminated utensils until it becomes epidemic. The lesions are characterized by whitish, flaky, loosely adherent membranes covering part or all of the tongue, lips, gingiva, or buccal mucous membrane. Less frequently the uvula, fauces, and soft palate are involved. Beneath the membrane, the mucosa is bright red and moist. The reported prevalence of oral candidiasis in newborns ranges from less than 1% to more than 18%. A realistic figure is less than 5%.

The gastrointestinal tract of infants also may be infected with *C. albicans*. The esophagus is the most frequent site, with lesions of the stomach and intestine being less common. Esophageal infections are characterized by the development of a whitish pseudomembrane sometimes of sufficient size to occlude the esophagus. Ulcerations may develop and sometimes cause fatal bleeding. As seen at autopsies, membrane formation may occur in gastric and intestinal infections, sometimes with ulceration and perforation.

Candidal infection of the respiratory tract occurs in infants but less often than intestinal tract infection. When the tonsils and larynx are involved, the disease resembles diphtheria. The pharynx may be involved, with the infection sometimes extending through the eustachian tube to involve the ear or mastoids.

After oral candidiasis, superficial cutaneous candidiasis of infants is most common. It usually begins in the perianal region and spreads to the thighs or abdomen, but rarely the back. Weeping lesions occur about the neck or axillary region, and almost the entire cutaneous surface may be involved.

Systemic candidiasis in infancy results from dissemination of the yeast in the blood, usually preceded by extensive cutaneous candidiasis. Clinical features are suggestive: anorexia, severe vomiting, progressive wasting, severe diarrhea, and sudden collapse.

Candidiasis in Adults. In the adult, oral candidiasis may be either subacute or chronic, or occasionally may take an acute course. Subacute candidiasis in adults is characterized by white, cream-colored, or grayish plaques surrounded by erythema and scattered over all or part of the oral mucous membranes. When a patch is removed, usually with difficulty, the remaining base appears brightly inflamed. In the chronic adult form of candidiasis, which may relate to the development of hypersensitivity, there is a dry red buccal mucosa with little or no covering membrane, sometimes in the form of patches. The tongue has a "raw beef," shiny appearance and is dry, fissured, cracked, and swollen. Since the entire mucous membrane is dry and burning, mastication of anything but bland foods is difficult, and nutritional deficiencies may complicate the situation if the disease continues for a long time.

Candidal infection of the lips, often called perleche, is a symmetrical erosion of the labial commissures. The upper layers of the epidermis are lost, while those beneath are red in appearance. Deep cracks, sometimes covered with a gray or white membrane, develop in the folds at the corner of the mouth. A somewhat similar lesion develops in riboflavin deficiency, which may be difficult to differentiate from candidiasis. It is probable that nutritional deficiency predisposes to candidal infection of the lips, and that perleche is the infection of vitamin deficiency lesions by *C. albicans*.

Candidal vulvovaginitis is often associated with diabetes, pregnancy, or the use of hormones, including birth control pills. Lesions appear as gray to white pseudomembranous patches on the vaginal mucosa. A yellowish discharge may also be present.

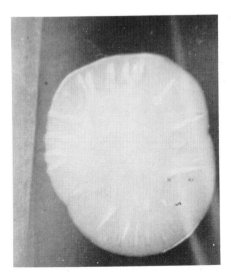

Figure 33.2: Colonial form of *Candida albicans*. (AFIP 218663-1-53.)

Cutaneous candidal lesions may be localized, generalized, and allergic (candidiids). Wetting of the skin and other factors that lower resistance predispose to this type of infection. The region about the fingernails is the most common site of cutaneous candidal infection (onychia and paronychia). Intertrigo, commonly involving the axillae, gluteal folds, and groin and occasionally the webs of the toes and the perianal region, is an example of a generalized cutaneous candidal infection. Generalized infection of the smooth skin may occur, usually related to oral or other localized grouped vesicular candidal lesions occurring over the hands, arms, or body surface.

Chronic Mucocutaneous Candidiasis. Chronic mucocutaneous candidiasis is a syndrome resulting from proliferation of *C. albicans* in which the cutaneous structures become chronically infected (Fig. 33.3). It is not a single entity but the final common pathway resulting when one or more of the defense mechanisms that normally restrict *C. albicans* proliferation are defective. Organisms apparently penetrate the membrane of viable epithelial cells and exist as intracellular parasites. The degree of involvement varies from patient to patient and in a single patient at different times. The classic lesions are verrucous, with tissue projections growing out from the skin. The lesions appear early and become chronic, with development of extensive epithelial hyperplasia. Most patients have deficiencies in cell-mediated immunity. Apparently, any of the T-cell–dependent immunodeficiencies may permit this condition to develop. Other abnormalities such as endocrinopathies, leukemias, and thymomas may contribute to the pathogenesis. Chronic mucocutaneous candidiasis can also occur in patients with no apparent immunological defects.

Immunity. Cell-mediated immunity appears to be more important than humoral immunity in resistance to *Candida* infections. In chronic skin infections there often are disturbances in T-cell function. There are suggestions that candidiasis occurs because T-cells cannot recognize the antigen or produce migration inhibition factor (MIF). There also are suggestions that macrophage chemotaxis is depressed. Although cell-mediated responses to *Candida* antigens occur in healthy individuals, those with chronic candidiasis are often anergic to its antigens, and transformation of their lymphocytes by *Candida* antigen may be depressed. B-lymphocytes and circulating antibodies are normal. Individuals with abnormalities in humoral immunity do not appear to have special susceptibility to *Candida*.

Healthy individuals likely develop a natural immunity to *Candida* early in life, during colonization with the organism. The surface glycoproteins are thought to stimulate both cellular and humoral immunity.

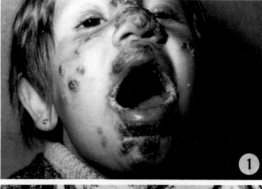
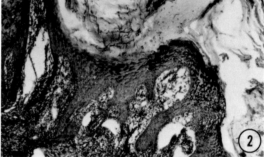
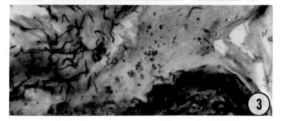

Figure 33.3: Chronic mucocutaneous candidiasis and disseminated histoplasmosis in a 14-year-old girl. The oral lesions show thick white scales alternating with eroded red areas. Histologically, there was hyperkeratosis and parakeratosis. Pseudohyphae were associated with leukocytes. (Courtesy of Dr. Leopoldo F. Montes and reproduced with permission from J. Kriner, et al.: Chronic Mucocutaneous Candidiasis and Disseminated Histoplasmosis. *J Cutan Pathol,* **7,** 58, 1980. © 1980, Munksgaard, Copenhagen, Denmark.)

Laboratory Diagnosis of Candidiasis. Laboratory methods useful in the diagnosis of candidiasis are microscopic examination of stained tissue sections, microscopic examination of a gram-stained film of hydroxide-cleared pus, sputum, or scrapings of suspected lesions, and direct culture. Sabouraud's glucose agar (with chloramphenicol or without this antibiotic) is most useful for initial isolation of *Candida* species.

A method for determining the presence of candidal infection is to examine under a microscope a portion of the membrane from a suspected lesion, treated with potassium hydroxide until it has cleared.

C. albicans appears in tissue as a fine, branching, nonsegmented mycelial net, sometimes with small, oval, budding, thin-walled cells, and clusters of microspores scattered about the microscopic field. The germ tube test is one of the more useful diagnostic tools for species identification. A presumptive diagnosis of *C. albicans* can be made in 2 to 4 hours with a final diagnosis based on the sucrose assimilation.

Treatment of Candidiasis. It is useful in the treatment of candidiasis to institute all measures that will improve the general health of the patient. The antibiotics available for the treatment of candidiasis are amphotericin B, nystatin, ketoconazole, and miconazole.

Geotrichosis

Geotrichosis is thought to be an uncommon chronic disease caused by one or more species of *Geotrichum,* a common fungal inhabitant of the upper respiratory and gastrointestinal tracts. As with candidiasis, infection with *Geotrichum* species is most often associated with lower resistance of the host.

Geotrichum **Species.** The various infective species of *Geotrichum,* particularly *G. candidum,* can be demonstrated from the lesions by direct examination or can be isolated by appropriate cultural techniques. In tissue, the organisms appear as oblong or rectangular cells. Microscopic examination of the growth in culture reveals hyphae that segment into rectangular arthrospores; spherical cells up to 10 to 12 μm in diameter can be seen that are also segmented from the hyphae.

Infection. Four clinical forms of geotrichosis occur: oral, intestinal, bronchial, and pulmonary. In geotrichosis of the oral cavity, white membranous patches are found that are difficult to distinguish from the lesions of candidiasis. Intestinal geotrichosis presents a more confusing picture since the clinical picture is variable and species of the fungus are often present in the intestine of normal individuals. Bronchial geotrichosis, a more common form, is characterized by bronchitis, coughing, and gelatinous blood-streaked sputum. Clinically it resembles acute tuberculosis, with extensive involvement of the lungs.

Diagnosis. Clinical symptoms, direct microscopic examination, and culture are appropriate methods for the diagnosis of geotrichosis. In specimens, fungal cells appear oblong, rectangular, or spherical. In culture, rectangular arthrospores and spherical cells up to 12 μm in diameter are characteristically produced.

Treatment of Geotrichosis. The prognosis of geotrichosis is good, especially if adequate treatment is instituted. Treatment of the pulmonary form is similar to that for tuberculosis. The polyene antibiotics are effective in treating oral and intestinal geotrichosis.

Histoplasmosis

Histoplasmosis is caused by *Histoplasma capsulatum.* Before 1935, histoplasmosis was considered to be uniformly fatal. However, later surveys indicated that a self-limited, clinically undetected chronic pulmonary infection with *H. capsulatum* is widespread, affecting an estimated 30 million people in at least 22 countries, whereas progressive histoplasmosis of either the acute pulmonary or disseminated type is relatively rare.

Histoplasma capsulatum. In the yeast form in tissues, *H. capsulatum* appears as small oval bodies. On Sabouraud's glucose agar this fungus grows slowly, producing white, cottony aerial mycelia with branching, septate hyphae bearing chlamydospores.

Clinical Course. Histoplasmosis is primarily a benign disease of man. Patients with a subclinical disease are asymptomatic, although the illness may be evident on radiographic examination.

The acute pulmonary form of the disease is characterized by the sudden onset of fever, malaise, cough, chest pains, and dyspnea. There is a focal granuloma and a lymphadenitis that heals, often with calcification, resembling tuberculosis radiographically. The illness may range from a subclinical form to a severe flulike illness. Recovery is usually rapid, with development of strong immunity, although progressive disease occurs in a fraction of a percentage of cases.

The chronic progressive pulmonary form may resemble acute pulmonary disease but with exaggerated symptoms. However, there is slow progression of the disease, with necrosis, caseation, and cavitation, resembling tuberculosis.

The disseminated type can occur at any age but is usually seen in severely debilitated older individuals, middle-aged men, or infants. It has a rapid, fatal course. Mucocutaneous lesions are characteristic of disseminated histoplasmosis. The oral lesions of histoplasmosis occur on the lips, buccal mucosa, palate, and tongue. They are granulomatous and may persist as nodules, or they may ulcerate. These lesions may simulate carcinoma or tuberculosis.

Epidemiology. *Histoplasma* has been isolated from animals, soil, and bird feces. It is usually acquired exogenously from contaminated dust and apparently is not transmitted from animal to animal. Pulmonary disease results when the individual inhales the organisms. Progressive disseminated disease may occur with spread of the fungus throughout the body after varying periods of time.

Diagnosis. The diagnosis of histoplasmosis depends to a great extent on the clinical manifestations, although it may be confused with tuberculosis, carcinoma, leukemia, and Hodgkin's disease. Also required for diagnosis is the detection of the organisms by microscopy, culture, and isolation.

H. capsulatum appears in tissues as small, oval, yeastlike cells that appear to have a capsule, although they do not possess such a structure. The organism is usually intracellular in mononuclear leukocytes in the peripheral blood and in macrophages elsewhere, particularly in the spleen and bone marrow. It may be cultivated from blood, biopsy material, or sputum.

Several immunological tests are available, including a skin test similar to the tuberculin test used for detection of hypersensitivity to *Mycobacterium tuberculosis*. This test uses a culture filtrate called histoplasmin for detecting hypersensitivity to the organism.

Treatment. Ketoconazole and amphotericin B are effective for treatment. Antifungal treatment may be combined with surgical removal of localized lesions for the treatment of chronic pulmonary histoplasmosis.

Sporotrichosis

Sporotrichosis, caused by *Sporothrix schenckii,* is a chronic granulomatous mycotic disease that has been reported from every continent. It is most prevalent in the north central United States and in Mexico.

Sporothrix schenckii. *S. schenckii* seldom can be found by direct microscopic examination of unstained human pus or tissue. The tissue phase in human beings, which is difficult to differentiate from normal cellular constituents, is polymorphic, assuming such shapes as rings and hollow spheres. In biopsy specimens, an asteroid body has been described that is somewhat analogous to the sulfur granule seen in actinomycosis (Fig. 33.4). In culture, *S. schenckii* is dimorphic, occurring in either a mycelial or a yeast phase.

Clinical Course and Appearance. There are five local types of sporotrichosis which relate to the area of tissue involved, including the lymphatics, skin, mucous membranes, skeleton, and viscera. The upper extremities are most often involved.

Sporotrichosis begins as an ulcer at the site at which the causative fungus enters the body, frequently at a site of trauma. The injury fails to heal, then ulcerates. This is followed by an infection that progresses along lymphatics to regional lymph nodes, where ulceration occurs. Infection seldom extends beyond regional lymph nodes, although sometimes a disseminated form occurs that involves no characteristic area or tissue. The lesions of cutaneous sporotrichosis occur as plaques, follicles, nodules, and papules and may represent a previous sensitization to the organ-

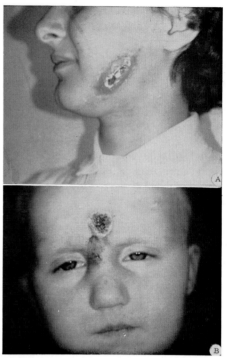

Figure 33.4: Sporotrichosis. (**A**) Cutaneous lesion of sporotrichosis resembling actinomycosis. (**B**) An uncommon localized lymphangitic type of cutaneous sporotrichosis. (Reproduced with permission from W. M. Mikkelsen, R. L. Brandt, and E. R. Harrell: Sporotrichosis. *Ann Intern Med,* **47,** 435, 1957.)

ism. Mucosal sporotrichosis more commonly involves the nose, mouth, or pharynx with erythematous, ulcerative, suppurative, or vegetative lesions. When the oral cavity is the site of the initial infection, the mucosal lymphatics may be involved locally. Oral lesions also may be derived from a hematogenous dissemination and may resemble those occurring on the skin.

Laboratory Diagnosis of Sporotrichosis. The microscopic examination of tissue fluid specimens, although sometimes useful, cannot be depended on for a positive diagnosis. More dependable is direct culture, which is easily accomplished on blood agar or Sabouraud's agar. Animal inoculation (mice, rats) is also useful in diagnosis, but direct culture is preferred.

Treatment. Potassium iodide is specifically curative and thus is the treatment of choice for sporotrichosis. It is administered for up to 4 to 6 weeks after apparent recovery. Amphotericin B, ketoconazole, stilbamidine, and dihydroxystilbamidine also have been reported to be successful.

North American Blastomycosis

North American blastomycosis is a chronic, infectious, granulomatous disease caused by *Blastomyces dermatitidis.* It often resembles tuberculosis, from which it may be difficult to distinguish. Blastomycosis is mostly restricted to the midwestern and southeastern United States but sporadic cases have been described from all the states.

Blastomyces dermatitidis. In tissues, *B. dermatitidis* appears as spherical or oval, thick-walled, yeastlike cells that reproduce by budding. When cultured at 37°C, *B. dermatitidis* retains its yeastlike characteristics, but at 25°C this organism grows in a mycelial form.

Clinical Course. Human infection with *B. dermatitidis* is apparently from exogenous sources and occurs by a pulmonary route. There is no person-to-person spread. Once lesions appear the regional lymphatics become involved, with resulting lymphadenopathy. Blastomycosis appears in a pulmonary, cutaneous, or systemic form. Although infection is by the pulmonary route, it may be asymptomatic and the first manifestations may be cutaneous. Skin lesions begin as small, firm papules with satellite lesions that coalesce (Fig. 33.5). The lesions break down and discharge pus that contains numbers of the organisms. There is a granulomatous inflammatory reaction and a mononuclear cell infiltration. As the disease progresses a mass of tissue forms that ulcerates and drains pus from multiple openings, simulating actinomycosis. The disease spreads slowly through subcutaneous tissues while healing and scar formation occur in the center of the lesion. Such lesions may be seen on any body surface or in the oral cavity. Pulmonary blastomycosis resembles histoplasmosis or tuberculosis. The systemic form results from dissemination from a pulmonary lesion and may appear in any organ system. Initial infection by *B. dermititidis* is not easily established, but once present, progresses steadily. Spontaneous resolution is rare.

Diagnosis. Laboratory diagnostic procedures are direct microscopic examination of tissue or exudates and cultural procedures and biopsy. Immunological procedures are skin and complement fixation tests. Cutaneous hypersensitivity is determined by the use of a culture fitrate, termed blastomycin, which is analogous to tuberculin. Consequently, the blastomycin skin test is quite similar to the tuberculin test.

Treatment of North American Blastomycosis. Success in treatment has been reported with the aromatic diamidines (stilbamidine, 2-hydroxystilbamidine), but the course of treatment is long and relapses are frequent. Amphotericin B and ketoconazole are also useful treatments.

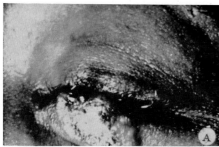

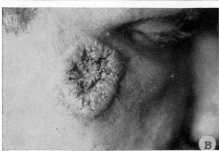

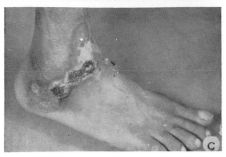

Figure 33.5: The cutaneous lesions of North American blastomycosis. (**A**) Eyelid, (**B**) face, and (**C**) ankle. (**A**, AFIP 57-10448; **B**, AFIP 53-2219; **C**, AFIP 55-15884.)

Paracoccidioidomycosis

Paracoccidioidomycosis is a mycotic disease limited to Central and South America. It is caused by *Paracoccidioides brasiliensis,* a fungus somewhat similar to *Blastomyces dermatitidis.*

Paracoccidioides brasiliensis. *P. brasiliensis* appears as two types of thick-walled, yeastlike cells. One type is a single-budding cell, the other a multiple-budding cell. The single-budding cells resemble *B. dermatitidis,* but the multiple-budding cells are differential and diagnostic for *P. brasiliensis.*

Clinical Appearance. South American blastomycosis has varying clinical manifestations which to a certain extent are mediated by the site of inoculation and the organ or tissue infected.

Primary infection often is pulmonary and inapparent. The organisms then are transported to the oral mucosa by macrophages. Occasionally initial infection occurs in the skin, producing ulceration and invasion of subcutaneous tissues. The infection then spreads locally, producing secondary lesions. Lymphatic dissemination may further spread the infection, and hematogenous dissemination may result in invasion of the lungs and brain.

Paracoccidioidomycosis is usually classified into

mucocutaneous, visceral, lymphatic, and mixed forms. The lesion common to the various clinical forms is an ulcerative granuloma. Almost any oral tissue may be involved in paracoccidioidomycosis, including the tongue, lips, gingiva, palate, tonsils, and buccal mucosa. Lesions in the throat or oral cavity are so painful during swallowing that they interfere with the intake of food. Ulcerative stomatitis and gingivitis are common to paracoccidioidomycosis. Lymphatic spread results in hard, painful nodes that adhere to the skin, soften, then ulcerate. Visceral involvement results in lesions in the spleen, liver, pancreas, intestines, and kidneys.

Treatment.   Paracoccidioidomycosis is chronic and eventually almost always fatal unless some form of treatment is instituted. Sulfonamide therapy has been effective in some cases. Amphotericin B and ketoconazole are the only drugs that are very useful for treatment of the disseminated disease. Miconazole is a useful secondary agent in the treatment of paracoccidioidomycosis.

Coccidioidomycosis

Coccidioidomycosis occurs in North America, especially the southwestern United States, and central South America. It is caused by *Coccidioides immitis*, a fungus that is widely distributed in soils and dust. In some areas of the southwestern United States as much as 80% of the population reacts to coccidioidin skin tests, which suggests that a great number of cases are asymptomatic or are not distinguished from other respiratory infections. Coccidioidomycosis also may present with various clinical manifestations, including a nondisseminated and a disseminated form.

Coccidioides immitis.   *C. immitis* occurs in distinct phases in tissue and in culture. From an arthrospore it develops in tissue and body fluids and exudates into a nonbudding spherule packed with endospores. In reproduction the spherules rupture, and the endospores are set free and develop into full-sized spherules. In culture, mycelia grow from either spherules or arthrospores. Spherules do not form during cultivation in vitro but can be produced in the yolk sac of embryonated eggs.

Clinical Appearance.   Coccidioidomycosis is primarily a respiratory infection. The organisms usually enter the human body by inhalation of spores in contaminated dust, initiating the respiratory infection. There is no known person-to-person or animal-to-animal transmission of the disease.

Nondisseminated coccidioidomycosis is characterized by upper respiratory involvement with nasopharyngitis. It is self-limiting. Pleural pain, chills, and a nonproductive cough are common. A pulmonary form may develop with symptoms of acute pneumo-

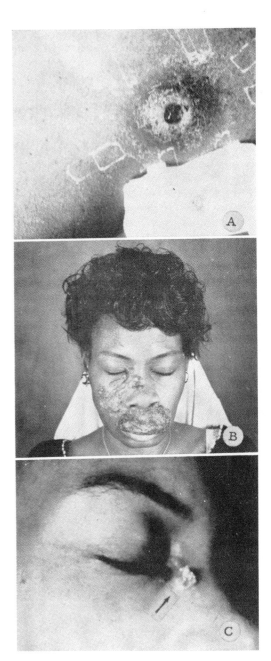

Figure 33.6: Cutaneous lesions of coccidioidomycosis. (**A**, AFIP 57-11831; **B**, AFIP; **C**, AFIP 56-7603-32.)

nia. Complications are not common, although dissemination sometimes occurs. Less commonly, patients develop erythematous skin lesions within 2 to 20 days after onset of the disease (Fig. 33.6). Primary skin lesions are rare.

In the disseminated form of coccidioidomycosis that develops in severe cases of primary disease, there is also a respiratory infection and progressive debilitation that usually takes a rapid course. It is characterized by fever, production of mucopurulent sputum, and weight loss. Lesions appear in subcutaneous tissues, bones, and internal organs. This form is usually fatal within a year. The oral manifestations appear as purple nodules of several weeks' duration. Other oral manifestations are erythema exudativum multiforme and erythema nodosum.

Diagnosis. The diagnosis of coccidioidomycosis is based on clinical symptoms and laboratory findings. The symptoms are likely to be confused with those of tuberculosis. North American blastomycosis, histoplasmosis, influenza, upper respiratory infections, and neoplastic diseases. Laboratory procedures include animal inoculation (mice or guinea pigs), microscopic detection of the causative organisms in sputum or body fluids, skin testing, and serological tests.

A culture filtrate of medium in which the organisms have been grown, known as coccidioidin, comparable to tuberculin or histoplasmin, may be used as a skin test material for the detection of hypersensitivity.

Treatment. The treatment of coccidioidomycosis is mostly symptomatic. Amphotericin B and ketoconazole are useful, with miconazole as a secondary treatment agent.

Cryptococcosis

Cryptococcosis is caused by the inhalation of dust and bird droppings contamined by a yeastlike organism, *Cryptococcus neoformans*. The disease may be chronic, wasting, and highly fatal, although there are many subclinical cases, especially in the United States. It involves the respiratory tract and has a predilection for the central nervous system, being the most common cause of mycotic meningitis.

Cryptococcus neoformans. *C. neoformans* occurs as a thick-walled, heavily encapsulated oval yeast. The cells reproduce only by budding, usually by a single bud. *C. neoformans* can be grown on all the usual media.

Pathogenesis of *C. neoformans*. Cryptococcosis commonly occurs in the respiratory tract, where it has the characteristics of a chronic lung infection, with few evident or distinctive symptoms. The pulmonary disease per se seldom progresses sufficiently to cause death, but in a considerable fraction of cases it disseminates to the central nervous system or other organs. Following dissemination it may produce ulcers or granulomas, particularly in the spleen, kidneys, liver, and mesenteric lymph nodes. Bone abscesses also may occur. Clinically evident disease has a high fatality rate.

C. neoformans is only weakly antigenic and the immunological response plays little or no part in the course of the disease. Some degree of hypersensitivity to *C. neoformans* develops but this has not been useful in diagnosis. Laboratory diagnostic procedures entail direct examination of tissue fluid or exudates, culturing, and animal inoculation.

Treatment of Cryptococcosis. Treatment of cryptococcosis is by amphotericin B.

Mucormycosis

The organisms involved in mucormycosis (phycomycosis) are in the order Mucocales, particularly *Absidia, Mucor,* and *Rhizopus* species. These are ordinarily nonpathogenic saprophytes found in soil and starchy foods (the common bread molds are phycomycetes) which can, under proper conditions, produce disease. Mucormycosis is an opportunistic fungal disease that occurs in the setting of severely depressed resistance. Affected patients may have debilitating conditions such as diabetes with acidosis, renal failure, leukemia, cirrhosis, severe burns, or even infections such as tuberculosis, syphilis, or amebic colitis. They are often being treated with therapeutic agents such as antibiotics, antineoplastic drugs, steroids, or other immunosuppressive drugs.

Clinical Course and Appearance. The classic picture of mucormycosis is orbital cellulitis and meningoencephalitis in an acidotic diabetic. In acidotic patients primary infection often occurs in the nose due to *Rhizopus oryzae* or *Rhizopus arrezus*. These species are the most common causes of this type of infection because they possess the enzyme ketoreductase, and acidotic patients generally have ketone bodies in their serum.

In pulmonary disease seen in patients with malignancies such as leukemia or lymphoma, primary infection occurs. Growth on the bronchial mucosa penetrates the wall. The causative organisms have an affinity for blood vessels and lymphatics and may be found in the vessel walls. They can penetrate into the lumen to produce thrombosis. Ulceration due to ischemia and local invasion may be present, and the lungs show necrosis and cavitation. Organisms are regularly found in the margins of the ulcer craters, and there is a polymorphonuclear leukocyte infiltrate around the margin. Gastrointestinal mucormycosis may occur in which the intestinal or gastric mucosa is invaded, and there have been reports of disseminated disease.

In cervicofacial disease the organisms enter by way of the nose or mouth, then by direct extension reach the paranasal sinuses, orbit, and cranial cavity. Discrete ulcerations of varying size may occur. The organisms invade the walls of blood vessels and proliferate, causing thrombosis and subsequent necrosis. Symptoms may include unilateral headache, facial pain, periorbital numbness, swelling of the eyelid, eye irritation, lacrimation, and blurring of the vision (Fig. 33.7).

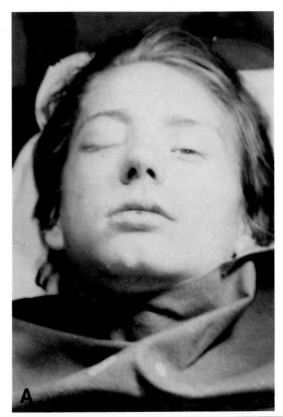

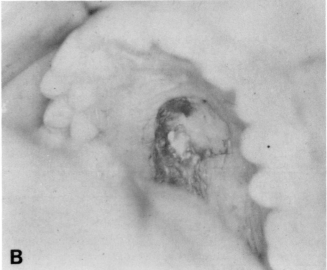

Figure 33.7: Rhinomaxillary phycomycosis in 16-year-old male diabetic. (**A**) Appearance at time of admission to hospital. There is edema in the right perinasal and periorbital areas, anesthesia of the right infraorbital region, loss of corneal reflex, and ptosis of the upper right eyelid. (**B**) Palatal ulcer. Note black necrotic tissue at margin. (Courtesy of Dr. Thomas D. Moye, Jr., and reproduced with permission from T. D. Moye and R. J. Caudill: Rhinomaxillary Phycomycosis: Report of a Case. *J Oral Surg,* **38,** 132, 1980. Copyright by the American Dental Association. Reprinted by permission.)

Involvement of the nasal cavity results in rhinorrhea, epistaxis, nasal stuffiness, a dark, blood-stained discharge, and a reddish black necrotic appearance of the septum and turbinates. A dull steady pain over the sinus is a common finding. Necrotic lesions of the hard and soft palate may be present as sharply demarcated areas of black-gray eschar covering the surface mucosa.

Mucormycosis does not usually occur in patients with normal immunity to infection. Uncontrolled diabetes is often an underlying problem. The hyperglycemia may stimulate the growth of the fungus and perhaps at the same time impair phagocytosis. In experimental diabetes, polymorphonuclear leukocytes respond to *Rhizopus* but the leukocytes show nuclear pyknosis. Also, high glucose levels may impair phagocytosis of other organisms. Thus if leukocytes and other immune factors cannot restrain the organism, it invades vessels and causes infarcts in the tissues supplied by those vessels.

Diagnosis. Although the majority of cases have been diagnosed at necropsy, phycomycosis may be diagnosed from clinical manifestations, usually coupled with a history of debilitating disease. Detection of the fungi in tissue and exudates by microscopic observation is useful. In tissues the fungi appear as broad, nonseptate hyphae. Culturing may be helpful in diagnosis, but since these organisms are common laboratory contaminants, it is not definitive.

Treatment. Treatment involves control of the underlying debilitating condition to the extent possible, coupled with chemotherapy and possibly surgical excision of localized septic areas. Desensitization with autogenous vaccines and administration of iodides are used in the treatment, but amphotericin B also is beneficial.

Maduromycosis

Maduromycosis is a distinct clinical entity caused by 13 or more fungal species. Mycetoma is a term applied to localized granulomatous and suppurative lesions that affect the skin, subcutaneous tissues, bone, and fascia of feet and hands. The causative agents are either actinomycetes or several species of fungi. The fungi commonly involved are *Aspergillus jeanselmi, Allescheria boydii, Madurella grisea,* and *Madurella mycetomi.* The initial lesions are papules, nodules, or vesicles, which are first characterized by remission and recurrence. As the disease progresses, abscesses and fistulas develop and the infection spreads to bone and other deep tissues, until the foot or leg becomes club-shaped and enlarged to several times its normal size. The primary mycosis usually is not systemic, but secondary bacterial infections occur with systemic manifestations.

Laboratory Diagnosis of Maduromycosis. Laboratory diagnosis may be made by direct microscopic examination of pus or fluid from lesions or fistulas. Isolation of the causal organism by culturing is useful in diagnosis; animal inoculation is not.

Treatment of Maduromycosis. Maduromycosis is slowly and surely progressive and the prognosis is poor unless the affected limb is amputated. Death usually results from secondary bacterial infection rather than from direct action of the causal fungus. Polyene antibiotics may be useful in some cases.

Rhinosporidiosis

Rhinosporidiosis, caused by *Rhinosporidium seeberi,* is a chronic disease affecting principally the mucous membranes of the nasopharynx but sometimes also affects the upper respiratory tract. It is rare in humans, but the causal organism is apparently widespread in nature and infects both man and domestic animals such as horses, mules, and cattle.

Rhinosporidium seeberi. *R. seeberi* has not as yet been definitely cultured. Its life cycle in tissues begins as a thin-walled, round corpuscle. As it enlarges the corpuscle becomes double-walled. The nucleus but not the cytoplasm of the corpuscle then divides repeatedly until some 2,000 to 4,000 nuclei are produced; the cytoplasm then divides, enveloping each nucleus to form numerous individual mature spores.

Pathogenesis of Rhinosporidiosis. The regions most often affected by rhinosporidiosis are the nostrils and nasopharynx and the soft palate. Except for the upper respiratory tract, other areas of the body are rarely involved. The principal lesions of the disease are sessile but sometimes pedunculated polyps, which are red, bleed easily, and sometimes enlarge sufficiently to obscure the passageway, interfering with breathing.

Treatment of Rhinosporidiosis. Though many drugs have been tested, none has proved definitely effective. Surgical intervention seems to be the most useful measure, but recurrence is likely unless extensive amounts of unaffected tissue are removed.

Chromoblastomycosis

Chromoblastomycosis is an uncommon, noncontagious disease of mixed fungal origin that results in chronic cutaneous granulomatous nodular growths on the head, neck, and trunk. The fungal species most often involved are *Fonsecaea pedrosoi, Fonsecaea compacta, Phialophora verrucosa,* and other *Fonsecaea* species.

Mycotic Agents of Chromoblastomycosis. *F. pedrosoi* is somewhat variable as to the type and color of its colonies. Usually it is slow-growing and forms dark brown to black colonies. *F. compacta* also grows slowly, producing a characteristic heaped, brittle colony, black in color. *P. verrucosa* is slow-growing and forms greenish brown colonies. It produces conidia from cuplike structures that are situated either laterally or terminally on aerial hyphae. In either unstained or stained sections of infected tissues, the organisms are seen as spherical or oval, thick-walled, sometimes septate bodies.

Pathogenesis of Chromoblastomycosis. The various causative agents of chromoblastomycosis exist saprophytically in the environment, in some instances in soils, and accidentally gain entrance into the body through some abrasion or wound. Most cases have occurred in tropical and subtropical areas but are by no means restricted to them.

Chromoblastomycosis is slow in developing, chronic, and usually involves the skin of the face or trunk with a granulomatous, inflammatory reaction. Occasionally an extremity will be affected. The initial lesion resembles that of ringworm. After some time, new lesions develop peripherally along superficial lymph channels. The affected areas have a raised cauliflower appearance. Such lesions are ordinarily painless unless secondarily infected. In diagnosis, clinical observations should be supplemented by microscopy of the exudates, histological examination of tissue, cultural studies, and animal inoculation.

Treatment of Chromoblastomycosis. There is no specific therapy for chromoblastomycosis. The treatment of choice has been surgical excision of the cutaneous lesion, unless it is extensive, supplemented by iodide or polyene antibiotic therapy.

Aspergillosis

Many species of *Aspergillus* are widespread in the environment. Certain of these species, particularly *Aspergillus fumigatus,* are occasional pathogens for man, causing a disease known as aspergillosis.

Aspergillus Species. Species of *Aspergillus* appear as fragmented mycelia and characteristic spore heads and spores.

Pathogenesis of Aspergillosis. Human aspergillosis is largely an occupational disease affecting agricultural or industrial workers who must handle or come into close contact with material contaminated with aspergillus spores, although not infrequently severe burns become infected with these organisms.

Aspergillosis is essentially an inflammatory granulomatous reaction involving most commonly the ear, bronchi and lungs, bones, nasal and maxillary sinuses, genitalia, and the integument, either primarily or secondarily. Pulmonary infection may closely simulate tuberculosis, bronchopneumonia, tracheitis, or bronchitis, and the differential diagnosis may be difficult.

Treatment of Aspergillosis. Antibiotic treatment has not only been generally useless but in some instances seems to favor the development and spread of the aspergilli and contributes to a fatal outcome. However, amphotericin B is sometimes useful for treatment.

The Dermatomycoses

A number of fungi infect the superficial skin, rarely invade the deeper tissues, and never cause systemic infections. These superficial skin infections are known as the dermatomycoses. Species of the three genera, *Microsporum, Trichophyton,* and *Epidermophyton* are

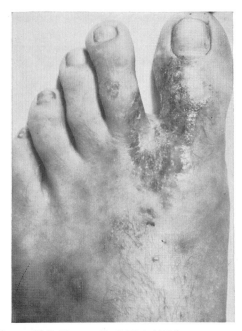

Figure 33.8: Tinea pedis. (AFIP A-44904).

the most common etiological agents, although yeasts or other fungi causing systemic infections, such as *Candida albicans,* may be involved. Since several species can cause identical lesions in the same area of the body, and since a single species can cause different lesions in different areas of the skin, considerable confusion has arisen over the classification and naming of the various manifestations. The dermatomycoses are usually classified according to the area of body affected, regardless of the responsible fungus, using a binomial system. The generic name for such a disease is tinea (literally, a gnawing worm; colloquially ringworm), followed by a term describing its location, such as pedis (foot) (Fig. 33.8), capitis (head), barbae (beard), unguium (nail), corporis (body), favosa (scalp), cruris (groin), and imbricata (scaly skin). Other names sometimes used are tinea versicolor (changeable in color), tinea nigra (dark or black), and tinea albigena (white or without color). Sometimes all mycoses of smooth skin are classified as tinea glabrosa.

The clinical features of mycotic infections are quite variable and may resemble those of neoplastic or bacterial diseases. In most instances, therefore, identification of the causal organism is essential to the specific diagnosis of the disease. The morphological and cultural characteristics of the dermatophytes are the principal basis for their identification; and in some instances physiological properties are used as well. Certain properties are generally common to the dermatophytes: asexual spore formation, simple nutritional requirements, growth at room temperature, and growth in media either sufficiently acid or alkaline to suppress bacterial growth. Other characteristics serve for differentiation.

ADDITIONAL READING

Abernathy, R. S. 1973. Treatment of Systemic Mycoses. Medicine, **52,** 385.

Allen, C. M., and Beck, F. M. 1983. Strain-Related Differences in Pathogenicity of *Candida albicans* for Oral Mucosa. J Infect Dis, **147,** 1036.

Allen, A. M., and Taplin, D. 1973. Epidemic *Trichophyton mentagrophytes* Infections in Servicemen. JAMA, **226,** 864.

Armstrong, C. W., Jenkins, S. R., Kaufman, L., et al. 1987. Common-Source Outbreak of Blastomycosis in Hunters and Their Dogs. J Infect Dis, **155,** 568.

Aufdemorte, T. B., and McPherson, M. A. 1978. Refractory Oral Candidiasis. Oral Surg, **46,** 776.

Baker, R. D. 1970. The Phycomycoses. Ann NY Acad Sci, **174,** 592.

Bardana, E. J., Jr., Gerber, J. D., Craig, S., and Cianciulli, F. D. 1975. The General and Specific Humoral Immune Response to Pulmonary Aspergillosis. Ann Rev Respir Dis, **112,** 799.

Bayer, A. S., Yoshikawa, T. T., Galpin, J. E., and Guze, L. B. 1976. Unusual Syndromes of Coccidioidomycosis: Diagnostic and Therapeutic Considerations. A Report of 10 Cases and Review of the English Literature. Medicine, **55,** 131.

Bodenhoff, J. 1965. Some Important Mycotic Infections with Oral Manifestations. Tandlacgebladet, **69,** 77.

Bradford, L. G., and Montes, L. F. 1972. Perioral Dermatitis and *Candida albicans*. Arch Dermatol, **105,** 892.

Chmel, H., Grieco, M. H., and Zickel, R. 1973. Candida Osteomyelitis: Report of a Case. Am J Med Sci, **266,** 299.

Ciegler, A. 1975. Mycotoxins: Occurrence, Chemistry, Biological Activity. Lloydia, **38,** 21.

Cohen, S. G., and Greenberg, M. S. 1980. Rhinomaxillary Mucormycosis in a Kidney Transplant Patient. Oral Surg, **50,** 33.

Couch, L., Theilen, F., and Mader, J. T. 1988. Rhinocerebral Mucormycosis With Cerebral Extension Successfully Treated With Adjunctive Hyperbaric Oxygen Therapy. Arch Otolaryngeal Head Neck Surg, **114,** 79.

Cruickshank, G., Vincent, R. D., Cherrick, H. M., and Derby, K. 1977. Rhinocerebral Mucormycosis. J Am Dent Assoc, **95,** 164.

Cush, R., Light, R. W., and George, R. B. 1976. Clinical and Roentgenographic Manifestations of Acute and Chronic Blastomycosis. Chest, **69,** 345.

Davenport, J. C., and Wilton, J. M. A. 1971. Incidence of Immediate and Delayed Hypersensitivity to *Candida albicans* in Denture Stomatitis. J Dent Res, **50,** 892.

Davies, R. R., and Denning, T. J. V. 1972. Growth and Form in *Candida albicans*. Sabouraudia, **10,** 180.

Davis, C. M., Garcia, R. L., and Riordon, J. P. 1972. Dermatophytes in Military Recruits. Arch Dermatol, **105,** 558.

Diamond, R. D., Root, R. K., and Bennett, J. E. 1972. Factors Influencing Killing of *Cryptococcus neoformans* by Human Leukocytes In Vitro. J Infect Dis, **125,** 367.

Drake, T. E., and Maiback, H. I. 1973. *Candida* and Candidiasis. Postgrad Med, **83,** 120.

Dwyer, J. M. 1981. Chronic Mucocutaneous Candidiasis. Annu Rev Med, **32,** 491.

Echols, R. M., Selinger, D. S., Hallowell, C., Goodwin, J. S., Duncan, M. H., and Cushing, A. H. 1979. Rhizopus Osteomyelitis. Am J Med, **66,** 141.

Edwards, J. E., Jr., Foos, R. Y., Montgomerie, J. Z., and Guze, L. B. 1974. Ocular Manifestations of Candida Septicemia: Review of Seventy-Six Cases of Hematogenous Candida Endophthalmitis. Medicine, **53,** 47.

Edwards, L. B., Acquaviva, F. A., and Livesay, V. T. 1973. Further Observations on Histoplasmin Sensitivity in the United States. Am J Epidemiol, **98,** 315.

Epstein, J. B., Truelove, E. L., and Izutzu, K. T. 1984. Oral Candidiasis: Pathogenesis and Host Defense. Rev Infect Dis, **6,** 96.

Erdos, M. S., Butt, K., and Weinstein, L. 1972. Mucormycotic Endocarditis of the Pulmonary Valve. JAMA, **222,** 951.

Evers, R. H., and Whereatt, R. R. 1974. Pulmonary Sporotrichosis. Chest, **66,** 91.

Feigin, R. D., Shackelford, P. G., Eisen, S., Spitler, L. E., Pickering, L. K., and Anderson, D. C. 1974. Treatment of Mucocutaneous Candidiasis with Transfer Factor. Pediatrics, **53,** 63.

Felton, F. G., Muchmore, H. G., McCarthy, M. A., Monroe, P. W., and Rhoades, E. R. 1974. Epidemiology of Cryptococcosis: II. Evaluation of a Patient's Environment. Health Lab Sci, **11,** 205.

Fischer, J. B., and Kane, J. 1974. The Laboratory Diagnosis of Dermatophytosis Complicated with *Candida albicans*. Can J Microbiol, **20,** 167.

Fishbach, R. S., White, M. L., and Finegold, S. M. 1973. Bronchopulmonary Geotrichosis. Am Rev Respir Dis, **108,** 1388.

Fitzgerald, E., Lloyd-Still, J., and Gordon, S. L. 1975. Candida Arthritis: A Case Report and Review of the Literature. Clin Orthop, **106,** 143.

Forrest, J. V. 1973. Common Fungal Diseases of the Lungs: II. Histoplasmosis. Radiol Clin North Am, **11,** 163.

Gaines, J. D. 1973. Diagnosis of Deep Infection with Candida. Arch Intern Med, **132,** 699.

Gartenberg, G., Bottone, E. J., Keusch, G. T., and Wertzman, I. 1978. Hospital-acquired Mucormycosis (*Rhizopus rhizopodiformis*) of Skin and Subcutaneous Tissue. N Engl J Med, **299,** 1115.

Gold, J. W. M. 1984. Opportunistic Fungal Infection in Patients with Neoplastic Disease. Am J Med, **76,** 458.

Grappel, S. F., Bishop, C. T., and Blank, F. 1974. Immunology of Dermatophytes and Dermatophytosis. Bacteriol Rev, **38,** 222.

Green, R. 1976. Blastomycosis of the Lung and Parotid Gland: Case Report. Milit Med, **141,** 100.

Habte-Gsbr, E., and Smith, I. M. 1973. North American Blastomycosis in Iowa: Review of 34 Cases. J Chronic Dis, **26,** 585.

Hofforth, G. A., Joseph, D. L., and Shumrick, D. A. 1973. Deep Mycoses. Arch Otolaryngol, **97,** 475.

Holbrook, W. P., and Keppax, R. 1979. Sensitivity of *Candida albicans* from Patients with Chronic Oral Candidiasis. Postgrad Med J, **55,** 692.

Jacobs, P. H. 1978. Fungal Infection in Childhood. Pediatr Clin North Am, **25,** 357.

Jenkins, W. M. M., Thomas, H. C., and Mason, D. K. 1973. Oral Infections with *Candida albicans*. Scott Med J, **18,** 192.

Kammer, R. B., and Utz, J. P. 1974. Aspergillus Species Endocarditis: The New Face of a Not So Rare Disease. Am J Med, **56,** 506.

Kannan-Kutty, M., and Teh, E. C. 1974. *Rhinosporidium seeberi*: An Electron Microscopic Study of Its Life Cycle. Pathology, **6,** 63.

Kaplan, W. 1973. Epidemiology of the Principal Systemic

Mycoses of Man and Lower Animals and the Ecology of Their Etiologic Agents. J Am Vet Med Assoc, **163,** 1043.

Kirkpatrick, C. H., and Smith, T. K. 1974. Chronic Mucocutaneous Candidiasis: Immunologic and Antibiotic Therapy. Ann Intern Med, **80,** 310.

Klein, B. S., Harris, C. A., Small, C. B., et al. 1984. Oral Candidiasis in High Risk Patients as the Initial Manifestation of the Acquired Immunodeficiency Syndrome. N Engl J Med, **311,** 354.

Klein, B. S., Vergeront, J. M., Weeks, R. J., et al. 1986. Isolation of *Blastomyces dermatitidis* in Soil Associated with a Large Outbreak of Blastomycosis in Wisconsin. N Engl J Med, **314,** 529.

Lewis, J. L., and Rabinovich, S. 1972. The Wide Spectrum of Cryptococcal Infections. Am J Med, **53,** 315.

Londero, A. T., and Ramos, C. D. 1972. Paracoccidioidomycosis: A Clinical and Mycologic Study of Forty-One Cases Observed in Santa Maria, RS, Brazil. Am J Med, **52,** 771.

Marshall, J. 1973. Tropical Dermatoses. Practitioner, **211,** 620.

McCornick, W. F., Schochet, S. S., Jr., Weaver, P. R., and McCrary, J. A. III. 1975. Disseminated Aspergillosis. Arch Pathol, **99,** 353.

Melbye, M., Schonheyder, H., Kestens, L., et al. 1985. Carriage of Oral *Candida albicans* Associated with a High Number of Circulating Suppressor T-Lymphocytes. J Infect Dis, **152,** 1356.

Meyer, R. D., and Kaplan, M. H. 1973. Cutaneous Lesions in Disseminated Mucormycosis. JAMA, **325,** 737.

Meyers, B. R., Worriser, G., Hirschman, S. Z., and Blitzer, A. 1979. Rhinocerebral Mucormycosis: Postmortem Diagnosis and Therapy. Arch Intern Med, **139,** 557.

Montes, L. F. 1971. Oral Amphotericin B in Superficial Candidiasis. Clin Med, **78,** 14.

Montes, L. F., Carter, R. E., Moreland, N., and Ceballos, R. 1968. Generalized Cutaneous Candidiasis Associated with Diffuse Myopathy and Thymoma. JAMA, **204,** 351.

Montes, L. F., Krumdieck, C., and Cornwell, P. E. 1973. Hypovitaminosis A in Patients with Mucocutaneous Candidiasis. J Infect Dis, **128,** 227.

Morduchowicz, G., Shmueli, D., Shapira, Z., et al. 1986. Rhinocerebral Mucormycosis in Renal Transplant Recipients: Report of Three Cases and Review of the Literature. Rev Infect Dis, **8,** 441.

Moye, T. D., and Caudill, R. J. 1980. Rhinocerebral Phycomycosis: Report of Case. J Oral Surg, **38,** 132.

Murray, H. W., Littman, M. L., and Roberts, R. B. 1974. Disseminated Paracoccidioidomycosis (South American Blastomycosis) in the United States. Am J Med, **56,** 209.

Nudtz–Jorgensen, E. 1973. Cellular Immunity in Acquired Candidiasis of the Palate. Scand J Dent Res, **81,** 360.

Ozato, K., and Uesaka, I. 1974. The Role of Macrophages in *Candida albicans* Infection in Vitro. Jpn J Microbiol, **18,** 29.

Pickard, R. E., and Kotzen, S. 1973. Histoplasmosis of the Larynx. South Med J, **66,** 1311.

Powell, K. E., Dahl, B. A., Weeks, R. J., and Tosh, F. E. 1972. Airborne *Cryptococcus neoformans.* J Infect Dis, **125,** 412.

Ray, T. L., Digse, K. B., and Payne, C. D. 1984. Adherence of Candida Species to Human Epidermal Corneocytes and Buccal Mucosal Cells: Correlation with Cutaneous Pathogenicity. J Invest Dermatol, **83,** 37.

Rayner, C. R. W. 1973. Disseminated Candidiasis in a Severely Burned Patient. Plast Reconstr Surg, **51,** 461.

Rebell, G., and Taplin, D. 1970. *Dermatophytes: Their Recognition and Identification,* Ed. 2. University of Miami Press, Coral Gables, Fla.

Reese, M. C., and Colclasure, J. B. 1975. Cryptococcosis of the Larynx. Arch Otolaryngol, **101,** 698.

Renner, R. P., Lee, M., Andors, L., and Namara, T. F. 1979. The Role of *C. albicans* in Denture Stomatitis. Oral Surg, **47,** 323.

Renstrup, G. 1970. Occurrence of Candida in Oral Leukoplakias. Acta Pathol Microbiol Scand, **78,** 421.

Restrepo, A., and de Uribe, L. 1976. Isolation of Fungi Belonging to the Genera *Geotrichum* and *Trichosporum* from Human Dental Lesions. Mycopathologia, **59,** 3.

Rist, T. E., and Caves, J. M. 1973. Fluorescent Technique for Identification of *Candida albicans* from Skin Scrapings. Arch Dermatol, **108,** 426.

Roberts, G. D. 1976. Laboratory Diagnosis of Fungal Infections. Hum Pathol, **7,** 161.

Robinson, E. D. 1974. The Diagnosis and Treatment of Fungal Infections. JAMA, **229,** 709.

Sagel, S. S. 1973. Common Fungal Disease of the Lungs: I. Coccidioidomycosis. Radiol Clin North Am, **11,** 153.

Sakula, A. 1974. Fungous Infection of the Lung. Practitioner, **212,** 335.

Sales, J. L., and Mundy, H. B. 1973. Renal Candidiasis: Diagnosis and Management. Can J Surg, **16,** 139.

Sarosi, G. A., Hammerman, K. J., Tosh, F. E., and Kronenberg, R. S. 1974. Clinical Features of Acute Pulmonary Blastomycosis. N Engl J Med, **290,** 540.

Sauer, G. C. 1974. Monilial Vaginitis. JAMA, **227,** 941.

Schubert, M. M., Peterson, D. E., Meyers, J. D., et al. 1986. Head and Neck Aspergillosis in Patients Undergoing Bone Marrow Transplantation. Cancer, **57,** 1092.

Shorne, S. K., Sirkar, D. K., and Gugnani, H. C. 1973. Changing Spectrum of Cryptococcosis in Dehli. Indian J Med Res, **61,** 23.

Sievers, M. K. 1974. Disseminated Coccidioidomycosis among Southwestern American Indians. Am Rev Respir Dis, **109,** 602.

Simpson, J. R. 1974. Tinea Barbae Caused by *Trichophyton erinacei.* Br J Dermatol, **90,** 697.

Smith, J. D., Murtishaw, W. A., and McBride, M. E. 1973. White Piedra (Trichosporosis). Arch Dermatol, **107,** 439.

Swatek, F. E. 1970. Ecology of *Coccidioides immitis.* Mycopathol Mycol Appl, **40,** 3.

Taschdjian, C. L. 1970. Opportunistic Yeast Infections, with Special Reference to Candidiasis. Ann NY Acad Sci, **174,** 606.

Theologides, A. 1970. Opportunistic Infections in Neoplastic Diseases. Geriatrics, **25,** 126.

Utz, J. P., and Shadomy, S. 1974. Fungal Infections. Clin Pharmacol Ther, **16,** 912.

Warder, F. R., Chikes, P. G., and Hudson, W. R. 1975. Aspergillosis of the Paranasal Sinuses. Arch Otolaryngol, **101,** 683.

Warnock, M. L., Fennessy, J., and Rippon, J. 1974. Chronic Eosinophilic Pneumonia, a Manifestation of Allergic Aspergillosis. Am J Clin Pathol, **62,** 73.

Whiting, D. A., and Bisset, E. A. 1974. The Investigation of Superficial Fungal Infections by Skin Surface Biopsy. Br J Dermatol, **91,** 57.

Young, L. L., Dolan, C. T., Sheridan, P. J., and Reeve, C. M. 1972. Oral Manifestations of Histoplasmosis. Oral Surg, **33,** 191.

Part VII

Virology

34

General Principles of Virology I

Gretchen B. Caughman

Historical Overview

Toward the end of the 19th century it was discovered that some agents that cause disease are smaller than bacteria. These entities, which passed through bacteriological filters, were referred to as *contagium vivum fluidum,* since such infectious filtrates could cause disease in susceptible hosts. This phenomenon, first described in plants, was followed shortly by the discovery of similar "viruses or poisons" in animals, bacteria, and finally fungi.

During the early years animal viruses could only be identified by the pathologic changes they produced in infected cells, since no instrument was available that had the capability to further distinguish them. However, various types of virus-induced intracellular structures termed inclusions were recognized, which aided in the pathodiagnosis of certain viral diseases, for example, the intracytoplasmic Guarnieri bodies of smallpox and the Negri bodies of rabies.

In many ways viruses did not act like living entities since they could be manipulated chemically to the point of being crystallized, were absolutely dependent on an intracellular environment (obligate intracellular parasitism), contained only one type of nucleic acid, DNA or RNA, and often had only one other component, a protein coat. Furthermore, it was difficult to assay them in animals, since host responses could be complex and variable. By using the tissues of the embryonated chicken egg, it was possible to circumvent the problems of studying infections in the adult animal, and in the early 1930s definitive studies with animal viruses began. For example, it was soon found that the poxviruses and herpes simplex viruses could elicit discrete lesions on the surface of the chorioallantoic membrane of eggs. Other viruses such as influenza could be propagated in cells lining the allantoic and amniotic cavities, and virus-containing allantoic fluid served as the source of material for study.

When bacterial viruses (bacteriophages) were first discovered during World War I, it was presumed that they could be used to control bacterial diseases, but it was soon realized that this was not feasible. Thus, studies with them were essentially abandoned and not resumed until after World War II, when it became apparent that bacteriophages were valuable tools in understanding the biology of viruses themselves. When studies on the fundamental biology of bacterial viruses were resumed, particularly with those infecting *Escherichia coli* and other members of Enterobacteriaceae, the roles of protein and nucleoprotein were elucidated and the complexities of virulent and latent replicative cycles unraveled. Also, temperate phages that had the ability to integrate into the host genome were found to participate in a number of genetic phenomena. For example, in lysogenic conversion, the presence of the integrated prophage changes the genome so that new antigens or toxins are manifest (e.g., diphtheria toxin), and in transduction, the bacteriophage acts as the vector for the interchange of bacterial genes between host bacteria.

When it became possible to visualize virus particles because of advances in electron microscopy, recognition of viral components and distinctive morphological features permitted their use in classification schemes. With the advent of practical tissue culture procedures, animal viruses that had eluded culture in the fertile hen's egg could be studied. At first only viruses that caused total cell destruction or cytopathogenic effect were isolated from tissue culture; however, as new types of cell cultures were developed and techniques to detect viral effects such as hemadsorption, cell fusion, and interference were employed, more elusive viruses were discovered. The golden era of medical virology had arrived, and in the 1960s and 1970s many of the viruses known to cause human disease were isolated and a number of vaccines were developed to control infections.

Development of more sophisticated biochemical techniques permitted definition of the replicative cycles of animal viruses. These data have been used in conjunction with morphological and biochemical criteria for purposes of classification and for the study of antiviral chemotherapeutic agents. In these studies it also became evident that, like bacteriophages, certain animal viruses could replicate in a virulent fashion or integrate into the host genome. Some of these integrated viruses were found to have the ability to transform normal cells into those with malignant characteristics, leading to new insights on tumorigenesis.

Virus Structure and Classification

Definition of a Virus

Viruses are small infectious agents that range in size from 20 to 300 nm. They are differentiated from higher organisms by their simple organization, nucleic acid content, mode of replication, their dependence on living cells for replication, and their lack of energy-producing enzymes. Some of the distinguishing characteristics of viruses compared to other infectious microorganisms are shown in Table 34.1. Viruses do not divide and grow as bacteria do but instead have the ability to direct the synthesis of their component parts and assemble them in the cells they parasitize. Thus, they are considered alive, although extracellularly they are metabolically inert.

Structure and Composition of Viruses

The virus particle, or virion, is composed of a protein coat or capsid that surrounds a nucleic acid core; together these structures are referred to as a nucleocapsid. In some viruses certain enzymes needed for viral replication may be associated with the nu-

Table 34.1: Comparison of Properties of Infectious Microorganisms*

Characteristic	Microorganism				
	Mycoplasmas	**Bacteria**	***Chlamydia***	**Rickettsiae**	**Viruses**
Growth outside host cell	Yes	Yes	No	No	No
Independent protein synthesis	Yes	Yes	Yes	Yes	No
Generation of metabolic energy	Yes	Yes	No	Yes	No
Rigid envelope	No	Yes	Variable	Yes	Variable
Antibiotic susceptibility	Yes	Yes	Yes	Yes	No
Mode of reproduction	Fission	Fission	Fission	Fission	Host cell synthesis of subunits; then assembly of virion
Nucleic acids	DNA and RNA	DNA and RNA	DNA and RNA	DNA and RNA	DNA or RNA, not both

*Reproduced with permission from the publisher and F. Rapp: Nature and Classification of Viruses. In *Virology*, edited by D. A. Stringfellow. The Upjohn Co., Kalamazoo, Mich., 1983.

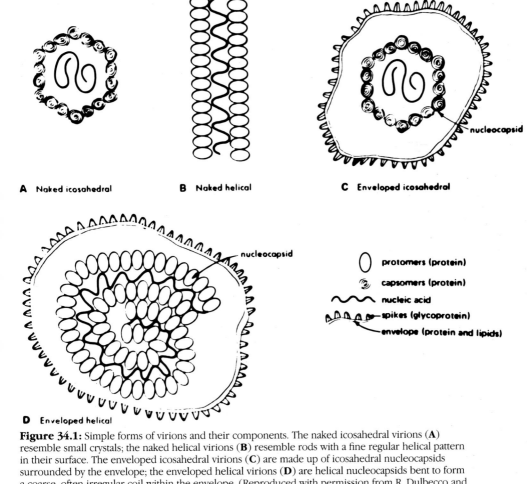

A Naked icosahedral   **B** Naked helical   **C** Enveloped icosahedral

nucleocapsid

nucleocapsid

protomers (protein)
capsomers (protein)
nucleic acid
spikes (glycoprotein)
envelope (protein and lipids)

D Enveloped helical

Figure 34.1: Simple forms of virions and their components. The naked icosahedral virions (**A**) resemble small crystals; the naked helical virions (**B**) resemble rods with a fine regular helical pattern in their surface. The enveloped icosahedral virions (**C**) are made up of icosahedral nucleocapsids surrounded by the envelope; the enveloped helical virions (**D**) are helical nucleocapsids bent to form a coarse, often irregular coil within the envelope. (Reproduced with permission from R. Dulbecco and H. S. Ginsberg: *Virology,* Ed. 2. J. B. Lippincott Co., Philadelphia, 1988. Copyright 1988, Harper & Row.)

cleocapsid. For certain virus families, such as the picornaviruses, the naked nucleocapsid is the complete infectious virion, but for many viruses the nucleocapsids are surrounded by various types of envelopes that are derived in part from host cell membrane structures and contain proteins, carbohydrates and lipids. Glycoprotein spikes or peplomers may protrude from this envelope and often function in the virus's attachment to a host cell, mediate cell–cell fusion, and aid in the release of progeny virus particles (Fig. 34.1).

Viral Nucleic Acids. Nucleic acids function as the viral genome and may be associated with neutral proteins or histones. The amount of genetic information per virion varies for different viruses. Small viruses may possess only three or four genes while large viruses may contain several hundred. With the exception of the retroviruses, the virions contain only a single copy of the genomic sequence.

Double-stranded DNA genomes may be linear, as in the herpesviruses, or circular, as in the papovaviruses. The linear DNA molecules may have repetitive sequences at the end (terminal redundancy) which can be several hundred basepairs long. In some viruses, the DNAs are terminally redundant, but the repeated sequences are inverted or reversed relative to each other.

Single-stranded DNA genomes also may be circular, as in some bacteriophages, or linear, as in the parvoviruses. In the bacteriophages, the base sequence of the strand is the same in all virions. In some of the parvoviruses, such as adeno-associated viruses, some viral particles contain DNA strands that are complementary to those in other virions within the same virus population.

Most of the RNA viruses have genomes that are single-stranded. These single-stranded genomes may be in a single piece of RNA, as in picornaviruses, or segmented into several unique pieces, as in ortho-myxoviruses. All have considerable secondary structure that may have important functions in gene expression and replication. The retroviruses contain two genetically identical, single-stranded RNA molecules held together near one end by a dimer linkage. Thus, the retroviruses are considered diploid, rather than haploid, as are most viruses. Unlike the other RNA viruses, the reoviruses have genomes that are double-stranded RNA. Also, the genome is segmented into ten to twelve unique pieces.

Capsid.   The capsid is a protein coat that protects the nucleic acid genome. In naked (nonenveloped) viruses, the capsid serves as the external surface of the virion, and as such it participates in virus attachment to cells and determines the antigenicity of the virus. Viral capsids are highly organized architecturally. There are several types of capsid symmetry and these variations determine virus morphology. Individual proteins are termed protomers. Depending on the virus, there may be one or several types of protomers making up the capsid. The protomers aggregate during viral assembly into clusters called capsomers, which are discernible as morphological units by electron microscopy.

Helical Viruses.   In helical viruses, the protomers are of a single type and are bound together by identical bonds to form a ribbon-like helical structure. The viral genome is coiled between the turns of this helix. Although the diameter of helical viruses is determined by the nature of the protomers, their length is dependent on the size of the nucleic acid genome. Helical viruses that possess an envelope are less rigid than naked viruses since the former have to coil within the envelope. This flexibility accounts for the variety of shapes (pleiomorphism) of some enveloped helical viruses.

Icosahedral or Cubical Viruses.   The capsids of icosahedral viruses are composed of capsomers that, depending on the virus, may be formed from identical protomers or from protomers of several different types. The simplest icosahedron is a regular solid with 12 vertices and 20 triangular faces. In the smallest viruses, the icosahedron is made up of 60 protomers, three on each of the 20 faces and each one located at one of the 12 vertices. The five protomers at each vertex form a capsomer termed a penton. In order to create larger icosahedrons, the faces must enlarge, and this occurs by adding more capsomers to the structure. Thus, in larger viruses, the pentons are linked to other protomers arranged in groups of six (hexons) to make up the capsid structure. The number, arrangement, and morphology of these capsomers are distinctive taxonomic criteria. In the icosahedral viruses, the presence of histones or histone-like compounds associated with the nucleic acid allows it

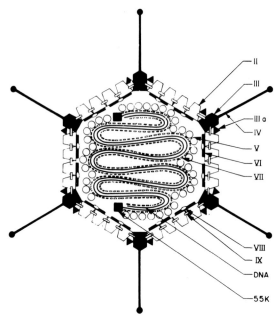

Figure 34.2: Model of an adenovirus particle showing the apparent architectural interrelationships of the structural proteins (*roman numerals*) and the nucleoprotein core. The capsid is composed of the hexon (*II*), the penton base (*III*) and fiber (*IV*), and the hexon-associated proteins (*IIIa, VI, VIII* and *IX*). Proteins *V* and *VII* are core proteins associated with viral DNA. The 55k protein is covalently linked to the 5′ end of the DNA. (Reproduced with permission from B. D. Davis, et al.: *Microbiology,* Ed. 3. Harper & Row, Hagerstown, Md., 1980.)

to be looped and tightly packed in the central core of the virion. The icosahedral capsid is very rigid and its size limits the amount of nucleic acid that can fit into it. By the same token, capsids that contain no nucleic acid are the same size and shape as those that are full. The association of structural proteins and the nucleic acid is diagramed for an adenovirus in Figure 34.2.

Complex Viruses.   Some large DNA bacteriophages have what is termed binal symmetry: their heads are icosahedral and their tails are helical in structure. With regard to animal viruses, poxviruses also are structurally complex, although in a different way. They are brick-shaped and are covered with a layer of coarse fibrils. The DNA genome is enclosed in a biconcave disk-shaped nucleoid. Thus, a precise symmetry is not defined.

Enzymes.   Enzymes are an integral part of some viruses. Most function in the replication of the virion, such as RNA-dependent RNA polymerases, which transcribe RNA genomes into mRNA; reverse transcriptase, which copies virion RNA into DNA; and enzymes that add specific terminal groups to viral mRNA or replicate or process the nucleic acid. Other enzymes of host origin, either constitutive or induced early in infection, include nucleases, nucleotide phosphorylases, protein kinases and mRNA-capping enzymes. Some viral enzymes that affect interaction of virions with host cells are an integral part of the envelope and are discussed below.

Envelopes. The nucleocapsids of many viruses are surrounded by an envelope. With the exception of the poxviruses's outer membrane, which is synthesized by the virus de novo, viral envelopes are derived from specific host cell membranes modified during infection and are acquired during the final stage of assembly. The proteins, carbohydrates, and lipids that the envelope contains confer on the virion various distinctive characteristics. For example, the shape of enveloped viruses often depends on the physical state of the complex mixture of neutral lipids, phospholipids, and glycolipids, or the presence or absence of connections between envelope proteins. A nonglycosylated viral-encoded matrix (M) protein sometimes is found on the inner aspect of the envelope surface. M proteins reinforce the envelope, form a bridge between the nucleocapsid and the envelope, and play a critical role in the formation of virions. Glycoprotein spikes, or peplomers, function as attachment sites for specific host tissue receptors and often for certain erythrocytes as well, in which case they are referred to as hemagglutinins. Some viral peplomers have neuraminidase activity, which facilitates virus release from cells, and fusion activity, which imparts both hemolytic capabilities and the ability to form multinucleate syncytia. The envelope contains antigenic glycoproteins that stimulate the immune response and subsequently bind specific antibodies. If such binding occurs it may neutralize or block viral infectivity. Viral envelopes are readily lysed by cell membrane–lysing disinfectants such as phenol and lipid solvents. Since the integrity of the envelope is critical to the virus's infectivity, such disinfectants are very effective at inactivating enveloped viruses.

Virus Classification and Nomenclature

Historically, viruses were informally classified on the basis of epidemiological and pathological characteristics. For instance, enteric viruses were those that entered the body and multiplied primarily in the enteric tract; arboviruses were *ar*thropod-*bo*rne viruses. This type of classification can be convenient at times but leads to the grouping together of many viruses with very different physicochemical and biological properties. Thus, as more became known about these properties, the criteria used for classifying viruses came to include the nature of the nucleic acid (type, strandedness, linear, segmented, or circular); the virus size (in nanometers) and shape (symmetry); the presence or absence of an envelope; the site of assembly; and the physical and chemical nature of the virion (Table 34.2 and Fig. 34.3). Further differentiation may be made on the basis of distinctive physical and chemical properties (e.g., low pH lability, ether sensitivity), the form of intracellular replication, or antigenic differences. More recently, nucleic acid sequences and genetic homology to known viruses have become important considerations in classifying new viruses and, in some instances, reclassifying known viruses.

Classification of viruses into families and genera has been well accepted, but the further subdivisions into species versus strains, subtypes, and variants remains controversial, since the requirements for such designations are not absolutely defined and the classification varies among the viral families. In terms of nomenclature, families are named with the suffix *-viridae,* as in Herpesviridae. Subfamilies have the suffix *-virinae,* as in Alphaherpesvirinae, and genera the suffix *-virus.* Vernacular terms are used for viral species and strains, as in poliovirus and mumps virus.

Viral Replication

Viral replication can be divided into several phases: adsorption (attachment), penetration, uncoating, transcription, translation, synthesis of nucleic acid, assembly or maturation of new viral particles, and egress. The first three phases are similar for all the DNA and RNA viruses, while the latter stages vary greatly depending on the virus family. The events of each phase are described here in general terms; more details are provided in the chapters on individual virus families.

During primary infection of cells, virus adsorption occurs through electromagnetic forces and chemical affinities between the virus and specific cell receptors on the cell surface. The initial attachment is reversible and temperature independent. The presence of receptors accounts to some extent for specific cell or tissue tropisms. Whether or not receptors for a particular virus are present on a cell depends on the species and tissue from which the cell is derived and on its physiological state.

After adsorption, the virus may penetrate the host cell membrane by invagination of the membrane into phagocytic vesicles (viropexis). Nonenveloped viruses may penetrate morphologically intact through the plasma membrane into the cytoplasm, while some enveloped viruses enter after fusion of the viral envelope and host cell membrane. Following penetration, uncoating, the opening of the protein capsid to free the viral genome, occurs. Uncoating is complex and varies with the particular virus–cell system studied. It is mediated by the action of cellular enzymes for all animal viruses except poxviruses, although the nature of the enzymes may be different.

Table 34.2: Properties of Virus Families of Human Interest

	Capsid Symmetry	Envelope	Shape	Virion Diameter (nm)	Genome Molecular Weight (×10⁶)	Genome Nature*
DNA Viruses						
Parvoviridae	Icosahedral	−	Icosahedral	18–26	1.5–2	ss, linear
Papovaviridae	Icosahedral	−	Icosahedral	40–45	3–5	ds, circular
Adenoviridae	Icosahedral	−	Icosahedral	60–90	20–25	ds, linear
Herpetoviridae	Icosahedral	+	Spherical	120–200	100–150	ds, linear
Poxviridae	Complex	Complex coats	Brick shaped	300 × 240 × 100	85–140	ds, linear
Hepadnaviridae	Spherical	+	Spherical	42	1.8	partial ds, circular
RNA Viruses						
Picornaviridae	Icosahedral	−	Icosahedral	22–30	2.3	ss, +, 1
Orthomyxoviridae	Helical	+	Spherical	90–100	5	ss, −, 8
Paramyxoviridae	Helical	+	Spherical	125–250	5–7	ss, −, 1
Rhabdoviridae	Helical	+	Bullet shaped	180 × 75	4	ss, −, 1
Filoviridae	Helical	+	Filamentous	800 × 80	4	ss, −, 1
Coronaviridae	Helical	+	Spherical	80–200	6	ss, +, 1
Togaviridae	Icosahedral	+	Spherical	60–70	4	ss, +, 1
Flaviviridae	Icosahedral	+	Spherical	40–50	4	ss, +, 1
Bunyaviridae	Helical	+	Spherical	90–100	4–7	ss, − or +/−, 3
Arenaviridae	Beaded, circular	+	Spherical	110–130	3–5	ss, +/−, 2
Caliciviridae	Icosahedral	−	Icosahedral	31–35	2.6	ss, +, 1
Retroviridae	Helical (?)	+	Spherical	80–110	2 × (2–3)†	ss, +, 1
Reoviridae	Icosahedral	−	Icosahedral	70–80	11–15	ds, 10–12

*Key: ss, single-stranded; ds, double-stranded; + or −, polarity of single-stranded nucleic acid; 1 to 12, number of molecules in genome. DNA genomes are each a single molecule. All RNA genomes are linear.
†Genome is diploid; two identical molecules are linked together at the 5′ ends.

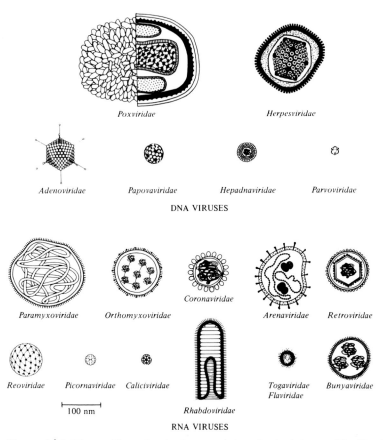

Poxviridae

Herpesviridae

Adenoviridae   Papovaviridae   Hepadnaviridae   Parvoviridae

DNA VIRUSES

Coronaviridae

Paramyxoviridae   Orthomyxoviridae   Arenaviridae   Retroviridae

Reoviridae   Picornaviridae   Caliciviridae   Togaviridae   Bunyaviridae
                                                                        Flaviridae

100 nm   Rhabdoviridae

RNA VIRUSES

Figure 34.3: Diagram illustrating the shapes and sizes of animal viruses of families that include human pathogens. The virions are drawn to scale, but artistic license has been used in representing their structure. In some, the cross-sectional structures of capsid and envelope are shown, with a diagrammatic representation of the genome; with the very small viruses, only their size and symmetry; in the largest, both. (Reproduced with permission from D. O. White and F. J. Fenner (Eds.): *Medical Virology,* Ed. 3. Academic Press, Orlando, Fla., 1986.)

For example, poliovirus, a small nonenveloped virus, is easily stripped of its protein coat by the host cell's proteolytic enzymes, releasing the RNA into the cytoplasm. A complex virus such as the poxvirus, vaccinia, has a more involved uncoating process. The outer membrane of this virus, located in a vesicle within the cell cytoplasm, is broken down by cellular hydrolytic enzymes. Following this an RNA polymerase, carried by the virus in its core, transcribes a portion of the viral genome into mRNA which codes for a protein that directs the release of viral DNA from the core. Uncoating marks the onset of the eclipse phase, which is characterized by the inability to detect or recover infectious virus.

Once the virus is uncoated, the synthetic phase of the virus replication begins. This encompasses synthesis of viral mRNA and proteins and replication of viral genome. Transcription into appropriate mRNAs occurs via the action of viral or host enzymes and the mRNAs subsequently are translated on host ribo-

somes into proteins. In some RNA viruses, the genome itself serves as messenger so that this first transcription stage is eliminated and translation of protein occurs directly on the genomic RNA. For most RNA viruses, the genetic information is expressed soon after uncoating, and synthesis of progeny genomes begins shortly thereafter. In the case of double-stranded DNA viruses, gene expression can be divided into early and late phases. The early period of the synthetic phase is devoted mainly to the synthesis of regulatory proteins and gene products necessary for initiating viral genome replication. This may involve inhibition of host metabolic steps such as DNA, RNA and protein synthesis, and enzyme formation, especially RNA and DNA polymerases. For some viruses the early phase is further subdivided into an immediate early phase and an early phase. Onset of viral DNA replication marks the beginning of the late period, during which the formation of structural proteins destined to become components of the progeny viral particles occurs, as well as the synthesis of some enzymes and other nonstructural proteins that function during viral morphogenesis. The late viral mRNAs are transcribed from different sequences of the viral genome than the early ones, and furthermore are transcribed from progeny genomes. The various genomic replication strategies are described below and in more detail in the chapters on specific viruses.

After progeny genomes and capsid proteins are formed, they are assembled into progeny virus particles. Assembly is a spontaneous process and most of the necessary information resides in the amino acid sequences of the capsid polypeptides; nucleic acid performs no essential function during morphogenesis of most animal viruses.

Release, or egress, of the newly formed progeny virus particles varies with the nature of the virus and its site of maturation, i.e., nuclear versus cytoplasmic. Cell lysis is the simplest method of release and is generally the method of egress for nonenveloped viruses. Replication of the virus proceeds until it fatally impairs the cell, the cell undergoes lysis, and the progeny virions are released into the extracellular milieu as the cell membranes disintegrate. Alternatively, some viruses are extruded from the cells without lysis. Other viruses are released slowly, by budding or reverse phagocytosis from the host cell. These viruses direct alterations in the structure and/or composition of host cell membrane, in a nonrandom fashion, necessary for their release. The viral envelope is formed by aggregation of viral glycoproteins and cell lipids in the host membrane. The virions are then slowly extruded from the cell, acquiring the altered-membrane envelope in the process. Some viruses that replicate in the nucleus acquire their envelopes from the nuclear membrane. Viruses that bud into cytoplasmic vacuoles are released when the vacuoles fuse with the plasma membrane. Those viruses that bud from the nuclear membrane into the cytoplasm may reach the outside through cytoplasmic channels.

Molecular Events of Viral Replication

Viral replication is a fascinating set of events that are extremely diverse and often unique to a particular virus family. Some of the mechanisms are similar or identical to those used by cells for their own gene expression and nucleic acid synthesis, while others are unique activities never found in uninfected cells. Elucidation of the replication strategies of various animal viruses has led to an enormous expansion in our knowledge not only of virus–cell interactions but also of the fundamental molecular biology of eukaryotic cells.

DNA-Containing Viruses

Replication of the DNA viruses relies on many of the same strategies used in cellular gene expression and DNA replication. The early phases of transcription of most DNA viruses are accomplished by cellular enzymes. Except for the poxviruses, transcription takes place in the cell nucleus and the resulting mRNAs usually are processed and translated much like cellular mRNA. The mode of DNA replication is semiconservative, but the methods used to achieve complete replication vary considerably among the virus families.

Adenovirus DNA replication occurs asymmetrically by initiating at the 3' end of one of the strands and proceeding by a strand displacement mechanism wherein the synthesized strand displaces the preexisting strand of the same polarity. The displaced parental strand then replicates in a similar fashion after terminal inverted repeat sequences form a panhandle structure. The circular genome of papovaviruses is replicated bidirectionally and symmetrically via cyclic intermediates. The herpesvirus genome is linear, but it is replicated via circular intermediates. First the linear DNA undergoes limited exonucleolytic digestion, which allows the ends to join and form circular structures. These are replicated to form tandem head-to-tail concatemers, which are subsequently processed to unit-length molecules during maturation. The single-stranded parvovirus DNA genome has an unusual structure with terminal palindromes capable of forming hairpins. Replication occurs through a complicated process that yields both viral DNA and DNA molecules that are complementary in sequence to viral DNA. Poxviruses have a large genome whose double strands are joined at each end. The replicative intermediates are concatemers containing pairs of genomes in either head-to-head or tail-to-tail configurations. Genome-length molecules are generated by staggered cuts and ligation. Hepadnavirus (human hepatitis B virus) genomes are partially double-stranded circular DNA molecules with a complete negative strand and an incomplete positive strand. After uncoating, the partial positive strand is completed to yield a covalently closed, circular structure which is then transcribed. The RNA transcripts are then reverse transcribed into DNA by the viral enzyme, reverse transcriptase. The hepatitis B virus reverse transcriptase is very similar in activity to that of the retroviruses, and the model by which the enzyme reverse transcribes the RNA template to produce progeny DNA genomes includes many of the same features, including a jump during synthesis from one direct repeat sequence to the other.

RNA-Containing Viruses

The genomes of RNA viruses are composed of widely diverse types of RNA, and because of this their replication strategies also are extremely varied. An RNA genome may be single- or double-stranded; it may exist as one single molecule or be segmented into several pieces. If single-stranded, the genome may be able to serve as mRNA, in which case it is considered to be of positive polarity, or it may be complementary in sequence to mRNA, in which case it is considered negative sense.

Replication of an RNA molecule, whether to produce mRNAs or progeny RNA genomes, requires an enzyme activity not present in uninfected animal cells: RNA-dependent RNA polymerase. Thus, the virus must provide this enzyme, which is also referred to as the viral transcriptase; the virus cannot commandeer it from the host cell's repertoire. In the case of positive-sense RNA viruses, whose genome will act as message and will be translated on cellular ribosomes immediately after uncoating, the RNA-dependent RNA polymerase protein(s) is one of the translation products generated. Thus, it is sufficient for the positive-sense virus to carry only the polymerase gene (rather than some of the protein as well), since translation is the first step in its replication after uncoating. In contrast, the negative-sense virus cannot use its genome as mRNA; instead, it must be able to transcribe mRNA from its RNA genome as the first replicative step after uncoating. Therefore, it must bring the RNA-dependent RNA polymerase protein molecule(s) into the cell as part of the virion particle so that the enzyme is available immediately to begin synthesis of viral mRNA. During latter steps in replication, new molecules of the polymerase are synthesized from the polymerase gene(s) contained in the virus genome, and some of these polymerase proteins will be packaged into the progeny viral particles so that they can function in the next round of infection. As discussed below, the positive-sense and negative-sense RNA viruses can be further subdivided according to variations in replication strategy. Replication of the double-stranded RNA genomes of the reoviruses also occurs via a viral transcriptase but in a unique manner which is unlike either that of the other RNA viruses or the strategy by which double-stranded DNA is replicated. The retroviruses also have a totally different method of replication that requires another enzymatic activity unique to viruses: RNA-dependent DNA polymerase, or reverse transcriptase. This enzyme transcribes the RNA genome into double-stranded DNA that be-

comes integrated into host cell genome; viral mRNAs are transcribed from these integrated DNA sequences.

RNA virus gene expression to produce viral proteins occurs via three main strategies. In some (positive-sense) viruses, the virion RNA, acting as messenger, is translated monocistronically into a large polyprotein, which is then cleaved to yield individual viral proteins. In other (negative-sense) viruses, the virion RNA is transcribed to produce monocistronic mRNAs by initiating transcription at different locations on the genome. In still others, the genome itself consists of separate RNA molecules, each of which is transcribed into monocistronic mRNA.

The RNA-containing animal viruses can be divided into seven different classes based on the nature of the viral RNA and its replication strategy. Viruses in classes I and II have genomes that are positive-sense. In **class I viruses,** the genomic RNA acts first as messenger from which polyprotein is translated. It then also serves as the replication template to synthesize a complementary negative-strand intermediate from which progeny genomic RNA molecules (positive-sense) can be transcribed. The picornaviruses are an example of class I viruses.

In **class II viruses,** the genome is partially translated to yield the viral transcriptase that transcribes a full-length negative strand. This strand then is used as a template to transcribe a 3′-coterminal nested set of subgenomic mRNAs, each of which is translated into a unique protein. The negative strand also serves as template for the synthesis of full-length progeny genomes. The coronaviruses are an example of class II viruses.

In **class III and IV viruses,** the genomes are negative-sense. Class III viruses contain a virion transcriptase that transcribes separate, monocistronic mRNAs initiating at a single promoter. In the second phase of transcription, a full-length positive strand is synthesized to act as template for genomic RNA production. Examples of class III viruses are the paramyxoviruses.

The genome of class IV viruses (orthomyxoviruses) consists of nonoverlapping, segmented pieces of RNA. Each is transcribed by the virion transcriptase into mRNA. Unlike most of the RNA viruses, which replicate in the cytoplasm, the orthomyxoviruses have a nuclear phase wherein messengers from two genomic segments undergo splicing. Also, the virus utilizes the capped 5′ fragments of cellular mRNAs obtained by endonucleolytic cleavage as primers in synthesizing the viral mRNAs, which are also polyadenylated. Positive-sense strands synthesized without polyadenylation are used as templates for genomic RNA production.

Class V viruses have genomes which are different from any of the other RNA genomes. They are said to have an *ambisense* genome, because about half of it is negative-sense and is transcribed by a virion transcriptase, while the other half is positive-sense. The latter half is transcribed twice: a full-length transcript is produced first which then is used to transcribe mRNA. Thus, the genetic information is encoded in opposite directions in the same molecule, an unusual occurrence for an RNA virus. Arenaviruses are an example of class V viruses.

In **class VI viruses** (reoviruses), the genome consists of nonoverlapping, segmented pieces of double-stranded RNA. During infection, only partial uncoating of the core occurs and the genomic segments are not released free into the cytoplasm. Initially, early mRNAs are synthesized from only some of the genomic segments by the virion transcriptase. This stage is followed by late gene expression in which all genomic segments are transcribed and translated. Unlike the semiconservative replication of double-stranded DNA, replication of the reovirus double-stranded RNA genome occurs via a conservative mechanism such that neither strand of the parental RNA is present in any daughter RNA segment.

The RNA genome of **class VII viruses** (retroviruses) is transcribed by a complex mechanism into double-stranded DNA by the viral enzyme, reverse transcriptase. The DNA molecule moves to the nucleus and integrates into the host cell DNA as a provirus. The provirus DNA is transcribed back to RNA by cellular DNA-dependent RNA polymerase II. Some of the RNA molecules become progeny viral genomes while others are processed to mRNAs.

Virus-Related Agents

Several other infectious agents have been reported that do not fit into the categories of the conventional viruses. Viroids, which cause serious diseases in many different plants, each consist of a small, cyclic, single-stranded RNA molecule. The viroid particle does not contain any proteins nor does it code for any. The RNA molecule bears some striking resemblances to some of the small nuclear RNAs involved in splicing of introns in cells, and it is thought that some of the viroid's pathogenicity may be due to interference with normal splicing events. Virusoids, another type of related agent, are satellites of some plant viruses and are encapsidated along with the viral RNA into particles. Although these agents are pathogens of plants, it has been postulated that the delta agent associated with some hepatitis B infections is a virusoid-like agent.

Another novel class of infectious agents appears to comprise those that cause the diseases termed subacute spongiform encephalopathies. This group includes scrapie, a disease of sheep, and two diseases of man, kuru and Creutzfeldt–Jakob disease. No virus has been isolated from infected tissues, but a characteristic protein has been observed which led to the postulation that a proteinaceous agent completely devoid of nucleic acid may be responsible. However, the existence of this controversial agent, termed a prion, has not been firmly established.

ADDITIONAL READING

Dulbecco, R. 1988. Multiplication and genetics of animal viruses. In *Virology,* Ed. 2, p. 77, R. Dulbecco and H. S. Ginsberg. J. B. Lippincott Co., Philadelphia.

Matthews, R. E. F. 1985. Viral taxonomy for the nonvirologist. Annu Rev Microbiol, **39,** 451.

Rapp, F. 1983. Nature and classification of viruses. In *Virology,* p. 9. The Upjohn Co., Kalamazoo, Mich.

Rapp, F. 1983. Virus Replication. In *Virology,* p. 21. The Upjohn Co., Kalamazoo, Mich.

35

General Principles of Virology II

Virginia A. Merchant

Pathogenesis of Viral Infections

The outcome of a viral infection depends on properties of the virus, the host cell, and the environment in which the virus–host cell interaction occurs. Viruses must have the ability to spread from one cell to another and, if virulent, must also have the capacity to cause functional alterations in the cells they infect. Virus–cell interactions that lead to pathology in the host fall into one of three categories: cytocidal infection, steady-state infection, or transformation.

Cell lysis is the final outcome of most virus–cell interactions. In a cytocidal infection cytopathic changes occur, virus is produced, and the cell dies. Steady-state infections are seen with several RNA viruses. The cells survive, continuing to grow and divide for long periods and producing viable virions that are released by budding. Viruses that are oncogenic may transform cells to a malignant state. The viral genome is usually integrated into the host cell genome. Infectious virions are not produced in cells transformed by DNA viruses. The only RNA viruses that are onco-

genic are the retroviruses. In these viruses, DNA is reverse transcribed from the genomic RNA, becomes integrated into the host cell genome, and viral replication continues with the production of infectious virions.

In the host, viral infections usually present as either an asymptomatic (inapparent, subclinical) infection, a localized infection, or a disseminated infection. Asymptomatic infections occur when the host defense mechanisms are effective in preventing virus spread or when the virus has reduced virulence. The majority of viral infections are inapparent. An immune response with seroconversion occurs, but with no evidence of disease, or, in the case of some infections, with a very mild disease. Asymptomatic infections may be either localized or disseminated (systemic) in regard to viral replication within the host, virus shedding, and the immune response. Figure 35.1 compares characteristics of localized and disseminated (systemic) infections.

Localized infections occur at the site of entry into the body with little or no invasion of underlying tis-

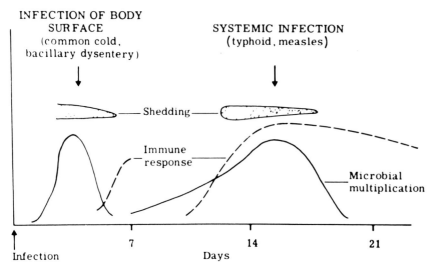

INFECTION OF BODY
SURFACE
(common cold,
bacillary dysentery)

SYSTEMIC INFECTION
(typhoid, measles)

Shedding

Immune
response

Microbial
multiplication

7   14   21

Infection   Days

Figure 35.1: Localized vs. systemic infections. (Reproduced with permission from C. A. Mims: *The Pathogenesis of Infectious Disease,* Ed. 3. Academic Press, London, 1987.)

sues. Localized infections may occur on a skin surface, on a mucous membrane surface, or within the respiratory or gastrointestinal tract. These infections tend to have short incubation periods. The immune response is primarily localized, and although the viruses usually do gain access to the lymphatics, stimulating a systemic immune response, viremia does not occur. Immunity to reinfection is usually short-lived.

Systemic infections are infections that disseminate throughout the body via the lymphatics and the bloodstream and ultimately cause disease at some site distant from the initial site of entry into the body (Fig. 35.2). Viruses that cause systemic infections initially replicate at the site of entry, but further replication occurs within the lymphatics and other organs. Systemic viral diseases have long incubation periods, viremic phases, and a more pronounced immune response that usually conveys a lifelong immunity.

Viral Immunology

Viruses are generally potent immunogens and infection usually produces a strong host immune response. This response is of two types: a humoral response, leading to the production of virus-specific antibodies, and a cellular response, resulting in the generation of several different subpopulations of sensitized T-lymphocytes. The purpose of the immune response is to protect the host from injury and eliminate the virus from the body. However, in some instances the immune responses to viral infections are more pathogenic than the virus itself; in mice, for instance, infection with lymphocytic choriomeningitis virus results in immune complex disease due to accumulation of antigen–antibody complexes in the kid-

neys. Certain viral infections may suppress rather than stimulate components of the host immune response. This suppression is usually due to the fact that the virus is replicating in cells and thus impairing the function of cells that are critical to host immunity. This phenomenon occurs to a moderate degree in cytomegalovirus infections, in which the virus infects mononuclear cells, preventing their synthesis of interleukin-1, and to an extreme degree in human immunodeficiency virus infections, where helper T-cells (T4) as well as other immune cells are infected and destroyed, ultimately leading to AIDS.

As discussed in Chapter 10, the two types of immune responses are triggered by different antigenic stimuli. B-cells recognize free antigens, while T-cells recognize foreign antigens in the context of host cell membrane proteins. Thus, antibodies can be produced against free viral particles (either intact or disrupted) or soluble viral antigens, while cytotoxic T-lymphocytes (CTLs) are sensitized against virus-infected cells. CTLs and antibodies produced against the same virus usually recognize different viral epitopes (antigenic determinants) because of their different requirements for antigen presentation. Once produced, they act in different ways to alter the course of viral infection. Antibodies neutralize viral particles by blocking infectivity, thus preventing cells from being infected. CTLs destroy virus-infected cells, preventing cell-to-cell virus spread. Infected cells also may be destroyed by macrophages and other cells activated by antibodies in antibody-dependent cell cytotoxicity reactions or by complement (complement-dependent cell cytotoxicity). In general, antibodies are more important in preventing viral infection (hence the efficacy of viral vaccines in eliciting spe-

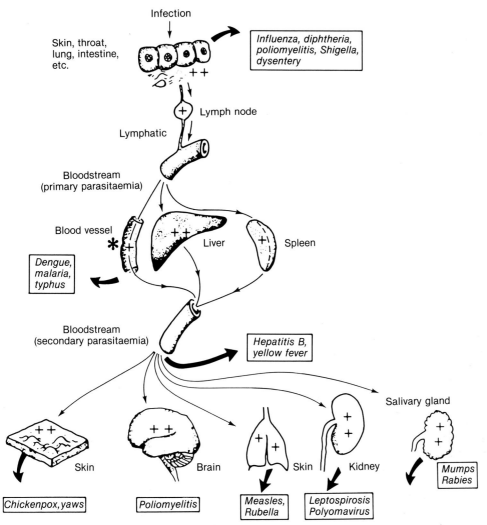

Figure 35.2: Spread of infection through the body. *Plus sign* denotes sites of possible multiplication; *large arrows* indicate sites of possible shedding to the exterior; *asterisk* indicates multiplication within the bloodstream or vascular epithelium rather than in visceral organs. (Reproduced with permission from C. A. Mims: *The Pathogenesis of Infectious Disease,* Ed. 3. Academic Press, London, 1987.)

cific antibodies and preventing primary infection), whereas once an infection is established, the cellular responses are critical to confining and eliminating it.

Persistent Viral Infections

In most types of viral infections, whether asymptomatic, localized, or systemic, the host defense mechanisms successfully eliminate the virus. These infections are referred to as acute infections. Some viral infections, however, are persistent. These infections are particularly important epidemiologically because infectious virus can be transmitted for prolonged periods by seemingly healthy individuals. There are three major types of persistent infections: latent, chronic, and slow.

In latent infections, the virus persists as DNA integrated into the host cell genome and is usually not demonstrable. Virus may be shed periodically, but disease is generally absent, and the individual is noninfectious except during periods of reactivation. This type of infection is characteristic of the herpesviruses. Chronic infections occur when infectious virus continues to be produced for very long periods. Disease may or may not be apparent and often has an immunopathological basis. Hepatitis B virus sometimes causes chronic infection. Slow infections are slowly progressive, lethal diseases with prolonged incubation periods. This term was originally applied to the subacute spongiform encephalopathies: scrapie of sheep and goats, mink encephalopathy, and kuru and Creutzfeldt–Jakob disease in man. Lentiviruses, including the AIDS virus, are now also designated as slow virus infections. Virus is shed throughout the course of the infection, although disease manifestations are inapparent until years later.

Kuru and Creutzfeldt–Jakob disease (CJD) are now thought to be caused by a class of unconventional agents referred to as prions (see Chap. 34). These degenerative diseases of the human brain progress slowly, ultimately resulting in death. Kuru, which has only been seen in New Guinea, is apparently related to cannibalism and is almost extinct. CJD occurs worldwide, affects middle-aged individuals, and has been transmitted via corneal transplants and neurosurgical procedures. The infectious agents of CJD are particularly resistant to inactivation. Prolonged autoclaving cycles (121°C, 15 psi for 60 to 90 minutes) or exposure to sodium hypochlorite solutions has been shown to inactivate these agents.

Diagnosis of Viral Infections

Most viral infections are diagnosed by clinical criteria; however, laboratory diagnosis is increasingly available and is used almost routinely when an infection occurs that has the potential to be of more than trivial significance to the individual or community. Until recent years, laboratory diagnosis of viral infections was largely an academic exercise, since specific treatment was not available for any viral infection. Patients either recovered on their own or with supportive therapy, or they died. Diagnosis was important only from a public health or epidemiological viewpoint in most cases and had little direct impact on the affected individual. Today, with a growing number of antiviral agents and more effective supportive treatments, at least some of the morbidity and mortality associated with many viral infections can be reduced if a specific diagnosis is made.

Laboratory diagnosis of viral infections can be accomplished by 1) isolation of the infecting virus, 2) direct assays for viral antigen, 3) electron microscopic observation of viral particles, or 4) serological diagnosis via identification of specific viral antibodies. Viable virus for isolation is most likely to be recovered early in the illness from secretions, from feces in enteric infections, or from vesicular fluid in diseases associated with vesicular skin lesions. Depending on the infection, virus can also often be recovered from blood, urine, cerebrospinal fluid, or tissue biopsies.

Cultivation of Viruses

Virus isolation in tissue culture is still considered the reference standard for the laboratory diagnosis of an infection, although this method is hampered by the

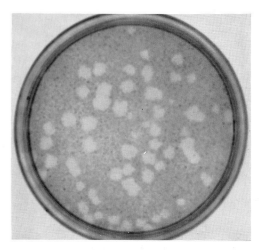

Figure 35.3: Plaques formed by herpes simplex virus on a monolayer culture of rabbit kidney cells grown in a plastic tissue culture dish. This illustrates the use of agar overlays to limit the spread of viruses growing in cell culture monolayers, thus localizing the areas of cell destruction or plaques. By counting the number of plaques produced by various dilutions of virus, the number of infectious virus units can be determined. (Courtesy of W. K. Ashe.)

time required and is rapidly being replaced by immunological assays, many of which are now available as commercial test kits. The methodology is not yet available for isolation of certain viruses in tissue culture, and alternative host systems such as suckling mice, adult mice, or embryonated eggs are required if viral isolation is needed, as in the case of influenza viruses for vaccine production.

Specimens for tissue culture must be properly preserved in a suitable transport medium. If holding is required, they should be stored at −60°C or below.

Virus susceptibility of cells in tissue culture depends on such factors as compatible receptor sites on the virus and host cell surface and the metabolic potential of the cell to allow replication to proceed. In infected cell monolayers, viruses can be detected by the specific cell destruction they cause, known as cytopathic effect (Fig. 35.3), or their ability to interfere with indicator viruses that do cause cell destruction (e.g., rubella virus interferes with the cytopathic effect of some enteric viruses). In addition to cytolysis, cytopathic effect includes other changes visible under the light microscope: swelling or shrinking of cells, the formation of multinucleated giant cells, the production of nuclear or cytoplasmic inclusions, changes in the nucleus, and vacuolation of the cytoplasm. Light microscopic examinations of stained scrapings from viral lesions have been used to aid in the clinical diagnosis of certain infections by looking for cytopathic effects on cells. In addition, certain viruses change the cytoplasmic membrane of cells, causing them to adsorb specific erythrocytes (hemadsorption) in the same manner as the infecting hemagglutinating virion (e.g., paramyxoviruses), and this characteristic can be used as an indication of infection by these viruses.

In most cases following the isolation of a virus in tissue culture, definitive identification must be accomplished by further testing. This is usually done by reacting specific antibodies with the unknown virus. The standard methods for definitive identification include viral neutralization, complement fixation, and hemagglutination inhibition. Viral neutralization involves the reaction of virus with specific neutralizing antibodies that render the virus noninfectious and thus prevent the cytopathic effect when the virus is incubated with susceptible cells. The complement fixation test involves the reaction of specific antiserum with an unknown antigen; if antigen–antibody complexes are formed, complement will be fixed, activated, and depleted, preventing lysis of sheep erythrocytes added to the test system. In the hemagglutination inhibition assay, virus is mixed with dilutions of antisera; if the antibody reacts with the virus, the virus will fail to agglutinate red blood cells added to the system. Although these assays are specific, the traditional methods require skill and accuracy of performance and are being increasingly replaced by quicker, less tedious tests that are available commercially. Additionally, infected cells grown on slides or coverslips can be used in assaying for specific viral antigens using fluorescent dyes or enzymes conjugated to specific viral antibodies.

Direct Assays for Viral Antigen

A variety of immunological techniques have evolved for the detection of viral antigens directly in patient specimens. These assays may involve the addition of specific antisera directly to slide smears prepared from lesions or from smears of tissue specimens, secretions, sputum, urine, etc. Specific fluorescein-labeled antibodies are widely employed in several methodologies for detection of a variety of viral antigens. Immunoperoxidase staining, based on the same principle as fluorescent antibody testing, is a newer and often better methodology for antigen detection.

The detection of viral antigens in clinical samples can also be accomplished via an enzyme-linked immunosorbent assay (ELISA) or a radioimmunoassay (RIA). These assays are based on reacting antibody-coated beads with clinical specimens, washing the beads to remove unbound specimen, adding (in the case of the ELISA) enzyme-conjugated antiviral antibodies, which in turn bind to the bound antigen, and following this with a substrate that reacts with the enzyme, producing a color change that can be mea-

sured. ELISAs continue to be developed for the detection of viral antigens, and there is an increasing number of commercially available kits. RIAs are rarely used except for the detection of hepatitis B surface antigen, anti-HBs, and hepatitis Be antigen; ELISA kits are now available for the detection of these antigens as well as the corresponding hepatitis antibodies.

Electron Microscopy

Clinical applications of electron microscopy include the detection of poxviruses in vesicular fluid, herpes simplex virus in brain biopsy tissue, cytomegalovirus in urine, and rotavirus as well as other enteric viruses in fecal specimens. Immunological techniques are sometimes employed to enhance the recovery of virus from specimens for electron microscopy. Electron microscopy is especially useful in detecting viruses such as rotaviruses that are difficult to culture by conventional methods.

Serological Diagnosis

Detection of specific antibody in the serum of the infected individual can be used for diagnosis. Current or recent infection can be confirmed by an increase, traditionally fourfold or greater, in the level of serum antibodies. This determination requires at least two serum samples, one obtained early in the acute phase of illness and the second collected at least 10 to 14 days after the first. The first sample should be seronegative (no antibodies to the virus) and the second should show a fourfold or greater increase in the antibody titer. Specific assays that detect IgM rather than IgG antibodies can also be used to confirm active infections since IgM is only present early in most infections. (Herpesvirus infections are an exception, since reactivation of latent infections can stimulate IgM production as well as primary infections.)

The presence of viral antibodies is also used to evaluate an individual's past history of viral infections. With the exception of persistent viral infections, the possession of antibodies to a particular virus (seropositivity) usually prevents the development of a second episode of clinical disease caused by that virus in the individual, although subclinical reinfections do sometimes occur, boosting the immune response.

A number of serological methods have been used for detection of viral antibodies. These include immunofluorescence assays, immunoperoxidase staining, ELISAs, RIAs, hemagglutination inhibition, neutralization, complement fixation, immune adherence hemagglutination, passive agglutination, passive hemagglutination, and counter immunoelectrophoresis. Many of these assays are available as commercial kits and can be used without any special skills in almost any diagnostic laboratory. The reader is referred to Chapter 11 on serology or publications on diagnostic assays for further information.

Control of Viral Infections

Immunization

There are three categories of viral vaccines: incomplete or component vaccines, killed or inactivated virus vaccines, and live or attenuated virus vaccines. Table 10.2 lists viral vaccines currently licensed for administration in the United States.

Incomplete or component vaccines reduce the potential for infectivity due to incomplete inactivation of the virions (hepatitis B) or toxicity related to the virion itself (influenza A and B). The vaccine consists of a purified preparation of immunogenic viral antigens. No intact virions, either killed or viable, remain; therefore, component vaccines cannot themselves cause the disease that they are produced to prevent.

Killed or inactivated vaccines contain intact virions that have been treated, usually with formalin or other chemical agents, to render the virus noninfectious. These vaccines, like component vaccines, induce antibody formation to antigenic components found on the surface of the inactivated virions.

Live, attenuated virus vaccines are composed of viable virus that has lost its pathogenicity for humans. Following immunization, the vaccine virus replicates in the host, inducing an immune response very similar to that seen following natural infection. The protection conferred by replicative vaccines is longer lasting and more complete than that conferred by killed or component virus vaccines. Since the vaccine virus has been selected to be nonpathogenic, disease manifestations are rare, but reversion to virulence is occasionally seen with the development of disease. Paralytic poliomyelitis due to reemergence of virulent vaccine virus strains has occurred infrequently, but the risk is minimal in healthy individuals and is certainly overshadowed by the benefits of immunization within the population.

Generally speaking, live virus vaccines should not be given to immunocompromised individuals since their ability to limit the infection is reduced. Varicella vaccine, however, has been successfully administered to leukemic children without adverse effects. In most cases, live vaccines should not be administered to pregnant women since there is a theoretical risk to the developing fetus.

Immune globulins, obtained from blood plasma from donor pools preselected for a high antibody content against a specific antigen, can be used to provide passive protection to individuals with defective immune responses or who have not been adequately immunized against infection. Immune globulins can modify the severity of measles and chickenpox and can prevent the development of clinical symptoms of hepatitis A and B.

Viral Inhibition

Most commercially available disinfecting solutions will readily inactivate enveloped viruses. Nonenveloped viruses are more difficult to render noninfectious since their outer coat is protein in nature, and in clinical settings they are usually associated with organic materials, which may further limit the contact of disinfectant with these relatively resistant viral particles. Chlorine compounds, iodophors, synthetic phenols, formaldehyde, and the glutaraldehydes when used appropriately can effectively inactivate all conventional viral agents.

Interferons

Interferons are a group of low molecular weight glycoproteins that make cells inhospitable for virus replication. The term *interferon* was coined after it was discovered that the supernatants of virus-infected cells contained a substance(s) which, when used to treat other cells, interfered with subsequent virus infection of these cells. Interferon (IFN) was found to be produced and secreted by cells infected with almost any RNA or DNA virus, but unlike antiviral antibodies, interferon is not specific for a particular virus. Rather, it confers on the cell a state in which virus replication is inhibited. Interferons are somewhat species-specific, however, as they are coded for by the host cell genome, and interferons produced in cells of one animal species will not necessarily be effective against viral infection of cells of a different species.

Two types of interferons have been distinguished: type I interferons, which are produced by leukocytes and fibroblasts in response not only to viral infection but also to a variety of chemical stimuli, and type II interferon, or IFN-γ, which is a lymphokine produced by T-cells stimulated by antigen or mitogen. Type I interferons are classified antigenically into two groups, IFN-α (formerly known as leukocyte interferon) and IFN-β (formerly known as fibroblast interferon).

Interferons do not inhibit viral replication directly. Instead, they bind to cell membranes via specific receptors; this binding triggers the activation of cellular genes encoding antiviral proteins. There are multiple activities induced by interferons, and they probably vary among different virus–cell systems. A major target for interferon-induced inhibition is protein translation, which is blocked by at least two mechanisms. One mechanism involves a protein kinase that

Table 35.1: Antiviral Chemotherapeutic Agents

Antiviral	Mechanism of Action	Active Against*
Agents Approved by the U.S. Food and Drug Administration		
Amantadine	Blocks assembly	**Influenza A** Rubella Parainfluenza viruses
Ribavirin	Interferes with synthesis of GMP/ Inhibits RNA and DNA synthesis	**Respiratory syncytial virus** RNA viruses DNA viruses
Methisazone	Inhibits synthesis of late poxvirus proteins	**Poxviruses**
Vidarabine	Inhibits DNA synthesis (phosphory- lated by cellular enzymes)	**Herpesviruses** **Vaccinia virus**
Acyclovir	Inhibits DNA synthesis (phosphory- lated by viral enzymes)	**Herpes simplex virus** **Varicella zoster virus** **Epstein–Barr virus** Hepatitis B
Idoxuridine and Trifluridine	Inhibits DNA synthesis (phosphory- lated by both cellular and viral enzymes)	**Herpesviruses**
Zidovudine	Inhibits reverse transcriptase (phos- phorylated by cellular enzymes)	**Human immunodeficiency virus**
Interferon	Blocks viral protein synthesis	RNA viruses DNA viruses **Hepatitis B** **Papillomaviruses** **Herpesviruses**
Other Agents That Are Effective But Not Yet Approved by the U.S. Food and Drug Administration		
Foscarnet (phosphono- formic acid)	Inhibits viral DNA polymerase	**Herpes simplex viruses** **Cytomegalovirus**
	Inhibits reverse transcriptase	Retroviruses
Ganciclovir†	Inhibits DNA synthesis (phosphory- lated by viral enzymes?)	**Cytomegalovirus**

*The viruses in boldface are those usually targeted for treatment with the antiviral listed.
†Approval pending.

phosphorylates and inactivates initiation factor eIF-2. The other translation block is due to a multistep induction of a nuclease that degrades mRNA. The induction of these two mechanisms depends not only on interferon but also on the presence of double-stranded (ds) RNA in the cell. Only minute quantities of dsRNA are necessary, and its presence seems to signal to the cell that a viral infection is under way.

The discovery of interferons was met with great enthusiasm for their therapeutic potential, and it was hoped that purified interferon preparations might eventually be used as effective antiviral drugs. However, such hopes have not been realized, and the therapeutic use of interferon has met with limited success. This is at least partly due to the fact that interferons are effective for only relatively short times after administration, they have no effect on viral synthesis in cells already infected, and the high doses required to produce antiviral effects also have serious toxic effects on the host. However, the results of clinical trials using recombinant IFN-α for certain viral conditions, particularly genital warts and laryngeal papillomatosis (both

caused by papillomaviruses), have been encouraging, and the idea of therapeutic interferon use has not been abandoned.

Antiviral Chemotherapy

Significant advances have been made in antiviral chemotherapy in the past decade. Because viruses depend on host cells for their replication, many of the agents that might prevent viral replication also interfere with the host cell's replication and thus would eliminate not only the virus but the host as well. Safer, less toxic compounds that selectively inhibit virus-coded enzymes or proteins needed for assembly, or that prevent attachment of the virus particle, its disassembly, or release continue to be investigated and provide a slowly growing arsenal of antiviral agents. Only a small number of antiviral chemotherapeutic agents have been found to be both safe and effective, and have been approved for use by the Food and Drug Administration (FDA). These are listed in Table 35.1 along with several other drugs that have proved effective in clinical trials but have not yet received FDA approval. Other potential antivirals, particularly for the treatment of herpesviral and retroviral infections, continue to be investigated.

The potential for toxicity and the development of resistant viral strains limits indiscriminate use of even approved antivirals. Acyclovir, the least toxic of the nucleoside analogues, has been compared with penicillin as a "magic bullet." However, it can still precipitate in the renal tubules, resulting in renal failure when administered in large doses, and can also affect the central nervous system, causing confusion. Its derivative, ganciclovir, causes bone marrow suppression. Although the development of resistant viruses was postulated by virologists, clinical isolates have rarely been seen until recently. So far, those acyclovir-resistant strains of herpes simplex virus (HSV) that have been isolated have generally been less neurovirulent and less efficient in establishing ganglionic latency. (Clinical isolates of resistant HSV strains have a marked decrease in viral thymidine kinase activity, thus preventing phosphorylation of acyclovir.) However, with the long-term use of antivirals in immunocompromised patients, resistant strains are being increasingly isolated. Whether or not these resistant viruses will become widespread and cause disease in others remains to be determined.

The future promises new advances in antiviral chemotherapy. It is anticipated that an antiviral will be approved for treatment of oral herpetic infections in nonimmunocompromised patients within the next decade. (Acyclovir has only received FDA approval for treatment of oral herpetic infections in immunocompromised patients.) Topical antivirals have limited use due to their low penetrability, and the systemic administration of currently recognized antivirals has the potential for toxic side effects and the possibility of selecting for resistant strains. Dentists must carefully weigh the potential disadvantages against the benefits when considering an antiviral in the treatment of a patient with mild disease. In immunocompromised patients or patients with severe disease, the benefits usually overshadow any potential side effects that might arise.

ADDITIONAL READING

Advisory Committee on Immunization Practices. 1984. Adult Immunization: Recommendations of the Immunization Practices Advisory Committee. MMWR, **33,** 1S.

Advisory Committee on Immunization Practices. 1986. New Recommended Schedule for Active Immunization of Normal Infants and Children. MMWR, **35,** 577.

Advisory Committee on Immunization Practices. 1989. General Recommendations on Immunization. MMWR, **38,** 205.

Crumpacker, C. S. II. 1989. Molecular Targets of Antiviral Therapy. N Engl J Med, **321,** 163.

Ginsberg, H. S. 1988. Pathogenesis of Viral Infections. In *Virology,* Ed. 2, p. 131, R. Dulbecco and H. S. Ginsberg. J. B. Lippincott Co., Philadelphia.

Hirsch, M. S., and Schooley, R. T. 1989. Resistance to Antiviral Drugs: The End of Innocence. N Engl J Med, **320,** 313.

Lennette, E. H. (Ed.). 1985. *Laboratory Diagnosis of Viral Infections.* Marcel Dekker, New York.

Lennette, E. H., Balows, A., Hausler, W. J., Jr., and Shadomy, H. J. 1985. *Manual of Clinical Microbiology,* Ed. 4. American Society for Microbiology, Washington, D.C.

Mims, C. A. 1987. *The Pathogenesis of Infectious Disease,* Ed. 3. Academic Press, London.

Prusiner, S. B. 1987. Prions and Neurodegenerative Diseases. N Engl J Med, **317,** 1571.

Rothschild, H., and Cohen, J. C. (Eds.). 1986. *Virology in Medicine.* Oxford University Press, New York.

White, D. O., and Fenner, F. J. 1986. *Medical Virology,* Ed. 3. Academic Press, New York.

36

Adenoviruses and Parvoviruses

Gretchen B. Caughman and Virginia A. Merchant

Adenoviridae

In the early 1950s, scientists noted that explant cultures of human adenoid tissue spontaneously degenerated during prolonged incubations. The cytopathic changes were found to be due to infectious agents emerging from latency in the adenoid tissues; these agents were termed adenoviruses. Soon it was realized that adenoviruses not only persisted in many individuals as latent infections of adenoids and tonsils but also caused clinical disease in a variety of locations, including the respiratory tract, the eye, and the gastrointestinal tract. The family Adenoviridae is divided into two genera, *Aviadenovirus*, which infects birds, and *Mastadenovirus*, which, in addition to numerous species specific for other mammalian hosts, currently includes 41 human adenoviruses divided into six subgenera. Several of these cause cancer when experimentally inoculated into baby rodents, but there is no evidence that adenoviruses are associated with any malignancies in man.

Properties. The adenovirus virions are nonenveloped icosahedrons that range in size from 60 to 90 nm. The capsid is composed of 252 capsomers arranged as 240 hexons and 12 pentons. Each penton consists of a base structure with an attached fiber and also is termed a toxin since it can cause cells in culture to clump, round up, and detach from the growth surface. The isolated fiber portion, which is present in infected cells as a soluble protein as well as in pentons, impairs the cells' biosynthetic processes so that they are incapable of supporting replication of related or unrelated viruses. The genome, consisting of a single linear molecule of double-stranded DNA of molecular weight 20 to 25×10^6 with inverted terminal repetitions, is associated with several viral proteins to form the core structure.

Adenoviruses enter the cell by pinocytosis, and the DNA core is uncoated in the cytoplasm and transported to the nucleus for replication. With the aid of cellular RNA polymerase II, immediate early and early mRNAs are transcribed from five separate regions of the genome in a coordinately and sequentially regulated manner. Viral DNA-binding proteins and DNA

Table 36.1: Diseases Caused by the Adenoviruses*

Age Group Affected	Syndromes	Common Causal Adenovirus Serotypes
Infants	Coryza, pharyngitis (most asymptomatic)	1, 2, 5
Children	Upper respiratory disease	1, 2, 4–6
	Pharyngoconjunctival fever	3, 7
	Hemorrhagic cystitis	11, 21
	Diarrhea	2, 3, 5, 40, 41
	Intussusception	1, 2, 4, 5
	Meningoencephalitis	2, 6, 7, 12
Young adults	Acute respiratory disease and pneumonia	3, 4, 7
Adults	Epidemic keratoconjunctivitis	8, 19, 37
Immunocompromised	Pneumonia with dissemination, urinary tract infection	5, 34, 35, 39
	CNS disease, including encephalitis	7, 12, 32

*Reproduced with permission from G. L. Mandell, R. G. Douglas, Jr., and J. E. Bennett: *Principles and Practice of Infectious Diseases,* Ed. 3. Churchill Livingstone, New York, 1990.

polymerase synthesized during this phase then initiate DNA replication, which proceeds asymmetrically by a strand displacement mechanism. As progeny DNA molecules are formed, a polycistronic late mRNA is transcribed that is processed into monocistronic messages to be translated into structural proteins. Adenovirus assembly is very inefficient and the characteristic nuclear lesions represent accumulations of excess viral DNA and structural proteins as well as crystalline arrays of viral particles.

Pathogenesis and Clinical Manifestations. Lack of good animal models has made the study of pathogenesis difficult. In cell culture, adenoviruses have profound effects on cell metabolism. Host cell DNA synthesis is inhibited within a few hours of infection, followed shortly by inhibition of cellular RNA and protein production. The basophilic nuclear inclusion bodies seen in culture in infected cells also have been observed in bronchiolar epithelial cells from the pulmonary lesions of individuals with adenoviral pneumonia.

Adenoviral infections are frequently asymptomatic, and the virus often is isolated in the absence of symptoms. However, a variety of syndromes can be caused by adenoviruses, and a single serotype may be associated with different clinical presentations. Some of the syndromes and the serotypes of adenoviruses most commonly associated are listed in Table 36.1. The virus frequently becomes latent in the lymphoid tissues following symptomatic or asymptomatic primary infection. Latent persistent infections apparently are made possible by the fact that the infected cells are not lysed and the viral particles or genomes are sequestered in their nuclei. Recurrent illness due to reactivation of the latent virus apparently does not

occur readily in healthy individuals but may occur in immunocompromised patients.

Adenoviruses cause 5% to 10% of acute respiratory infections in young children. The illness often presents as a mild pharyngitis with coryza, but may present as a pharyngitis with exudative tonsillitis which can be confused with β-hemolytic streptococcal pharyngitis. In the more severe form, this infection is frequently accompanied by conjunctivitis, nasal congestion, cough, fever, myalgia, and headache. Adenoviruses can also cause laryngotracheobronchitis (croup) and are responsible for approximately 10% of pneumonias in young children.

Several adenovirus serotypes, particularly Ad4, Ad7, and Ad21, may cause a tracheobronchitis known as acute respiratory disease (ARD) in young adults. This syndrome, characterized by pharyngitis, rales, cough, fever, sore throat, and rhinorrhea, lasts for 3 to 5 days. It is seen most commonly in young adults under conditions of crowding and has been responsible for outbreaks among military recruits.

Pharyngoconjunctival fever, commonly caused by serotypes Ad3 and Ad7, occurs in small epidemics among children, particularly those residing in groups such as in summer camps. It is characterized by an acute onset with symptoms of conjunctivitis, pharyngitis, rhinitis, and cervical adenitis with a mild fever of 38°C that lasts for 3 to 5 days.

Epidemic keratoconjunctivitis was once referred to as shipyard workers' conjunctivitis because of its prevalence among these workers. Ocular trauma predisposed the workers to infection by virus, which in at least one outbreak was transmitted by roller towels used for drying hands and faces. After an incubation period of 4 to 24 days, the onset of conjunctivitis is

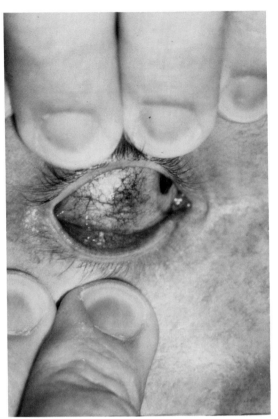

Figure 36.1: Adenovirus infection of the eye manifested as acute follicular conjunctivitis.

insidious and frequently bilateral. Preauricular adenopathy is commonly seen and is accompanied by excessive lacrimation, periorbital edema, and serous exudation. Keratitis develops and may lead to superficial corneal opacities and visual disturbances lasting for several months. Ulceration does not occur and recovery is usually complete, although temporary visual disturbances may last for months or even years. Sporadic cases of acute follicular conjunctivitis (Fig. 36.1) are often seen. These are usually caused by Ad3 and Ad7, with symptoms, as above, lasting from 1 to 4 weeks.

Serotypes Ad11 and Ad21 may cause a hemorrhagic cystitis in children. The condition, more common in boys than in girls, is characterized by a gross hematuria that persists for about 3 days. Associated symptoms of dysuria and increased urinary frequency may continue somewhat longer.

Adenoviruses are second only to rotaviruses as the etiological agent of viral gastroenteritis in infants. Adenoviral gastroenteritis is a milder disease than that caused by rotaviruses. Diarrhea is the predominant symptom, with or without vomiting. Respiratory symptoms may accompany the gastrointestinal symp-

toms. Serotypes Ad40 and Ad41 have been most commonly associated with gastroenteritis.

Adenoviruses may cause more serious manifestations in immunocompromised patients. Pneumonia with dissemination and neurological disease have been attributed to several adenovirus types.

Diagnosis. Adenoviral infections often can be diagnosed solely on the basis of their distinctive symptoms, particularly when these are associated with an outbreak of cases. Immunofluorescence assays can be used to detect the presence of group-specific hexon antigen, and specific neutralizing antisera are available for virus typing. Serological diagnosis is made by either microneutralization, hemagglutination inhibition, or complement fixation tests.

Epidemiology. Adenoviruses are ubiquitous and usually are acquired by contact with infected respiratory secretions. Since they often establish asymptomatic latent infections of the tonsils and adenoids, latently infected individuals may serve as a source for contagion to susceptible individuals. Serotypes associated with acute respiratory disease are readily transmitted under crowded living conditions. Those that cause respiratory or eye infections are quite contagious and may be transmitted by direct contact; by contact with contaminated fomites, such as ophthalmic solutions; or by aerosols, including those generated during dental treatment.

Prevention and Treatment. Good personal hygiene is the best protection against respiratory or ocular adenoviral infection. The use of protective eyewear and masks in dentistry reduces potential mucous membrane exposure to adenoviruses.

An oral vaccine in the form of enteric capsules containing live Ad4 and Ad7 is currently administered to military recruits by the U.S. military in an effort to prevent outbreaks of ARD. These strains have proved to be excellent immunogens when given by this alternate route and do not cause respiratory symptoms. This practice has markedly decreased the number of cases of ARD in the military in recent years. The vaccine is not recommended for other populations.

Treatment is symptomatic. There are no specific drugs utilized in the treatment of adenoviral infections.

Parvoviridae

Small, icosahedral viruses that belong to the family now known as Parvoviridae were observed first in association with adenoviruses. It soon was discovered that these viruses are defective in that their replication in a cell depends on coinfection by a helper virus, particularly an adenovirus, to provide some essential replicative functions. Hence, they became known as adeno-associated viruses (AAVs). Subsequently other viruses were identified that were similar to the AAVs in size and structure but were autonomously replicating, i.e., they did not require the presence of a helper virus in order to replicate. The AAVs now comprise the *Dependovirus* genus of the family Parvoviridae, and the autonomously replicating viruses from various higher animal species are members of the *Parvovirus* genus. The members of a third genus, *Densovirus*, infect only arthropods. Five human AAVs have been identified so far, but although infection appears common, none has been associated with a specific disease. One presumably nondefective human parvovirus, B19, causes at least two very different clinical syndromes, erythema infectiosum (fifth disease) and aplastic crisis in hemolytic anemia. A putative parvovirus, RA-1, has been isolated from the joint tissues of rheumatoid arthritis patients, but the virus's role, if any, in that disease process is not yet known.

Properties. The paroviruses are the smallest of all viruses (*L. parvus*, small); the virion consists of a nonenveloped icosahedral capsid, 18 to 26 nm in diameter, surrounding a single-stranded DNA molecule. The DNA molecule within any one virion may be either positive- or negative-sense, although only the negative-sense strand directs the transcription of mRNA. Because of its small size (MW = 1.5 to 2.0 × 10^6), the genome has a very limited coding potential that is used mainly to specify three viral proteins. Viral replication occurs only in actively dividing cells and apparently depends on one or more cellular functions generated during the late S or early G_2 phases of the mitotic cycle. The viral DNA is replicated in the nucleus by a complicated process utilizing cellular DNA polymerase. In the case of the *Dependovirus* genus, the viral genome can integrate into the infected cell's DNA in the absence of helper virus and remain there in a stable, nonproductive state. Recent evidence suggests that the distinctions between the replication of the dependoviruses and the autonomously replicating paroviruses may not be as clearcut as was originally thought, since under certain conditions the dependoviruses can be induced to replicate without co-infecting helper virus.

Pathogenesis and Clinical Manifestations. The parvoviruses's predilection for actively dividing cells in differentiating tissues and their cytolytic potential are reflected in the diseases they cause in various animal species; these syndromes include fetal death, malformations, dwarfism, panleukopenia, immunological disorders, and craniofacial and dental anomalies. In human parvovirus B19, these characteristics are evident in its affinity for erythroid progenitor cells, a property which can result in aplastic crisis in individuals with underlying blood disorders. B19 was

first related to aplastic crisis in patients with hemolytic anemia in 1981. The virus infects and destroys actively dividing immature red blood cells (RBCs) in the bone marrow, consequently causing a decrease in the number of RBCs in the blood. This decrease goes unnoticed in people without preexisting anemia but can precipitate a crisis in patients with hemolytic anemias such as sickle cell disease.

Erythema infectiosum, commonly known as fifth disease, has been recognized for at least 100 years, but its etiological agent, parvovirus B19, was not recognized until 1983. Infections present as a mild rash disease or may be asymptomatic. Symptoms are generally milder in children than in adults. The incubation period is usually 14 to 18 days. Infected adults often experience a low-grade prodromal fever accompanied by malaise, myalgia, chills, and pruritus approximately a week after infection. These prodromal symptoms coincide with viremia and, shortly thereafter, the appearance of circulating IgM–parvovirus immune complexes. The viremia subsides prior to the appearance of the rash, a finding that supports the idea that the exanthem is an immune reaction rather than directly virus induced. When it is present, the rash occurs in three stages. First, an erythematous rash described as "slapped cheek" appears on the face (Fig. 36.2). This is followed, either concurrently or up

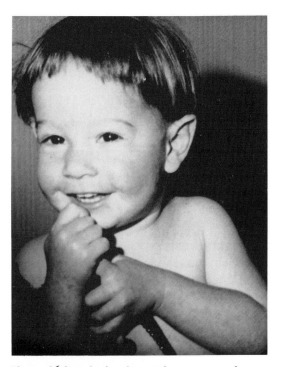

Figure 36.2: Rash of erythema infectiosum. Note forearm rash and "slapped cheek" appearance.

to 4 days later, by a morbilliform rash on the extremities. In the third stage, which lasts a week or two, the rash may remit and recur. As many as 81% of adults experience mild arthritis/arthralgia, particularly of the hands, wrists, and knees, which may be long-term and chronic. Joint symptoms frequently occur in the absence of rash in infected adults.

Parvoviruses that infect animals frequently cause severe birth defects if infection occurs during pregnancy. Studies to identify a possible association of parvovirus B19 infection with adverse fetal outcome in humans have resulted in mixed findings. Currently available evidence, however, suggests that there may be some association of maternal parvovirus B19 infection with stillbirth or hydrops fetalis.

Epidemiology. Parvovirus B19 was first discovered in human blood in 1975. Transmission is primarily by respiratory secretions and occurs prior to the appearance of the rash. Whole blood and factor VIII have also served as sources for virus transfer. School-aged children are most commonly infected, and outbreaks have been seen in primary schools in a number of communities in recent years. Studies have indicated that as many as 60% of adults are seropositive.

Diagnosis. Differential diagnosis of erythema infectiosum includes all illnesses with erythematous, maculopapular rashes. Allergies, scarlet fever, rubella, rubeola, and enterovirus infections must be considered. There is particular difficulty in distinguishing rubella and erythema infectiosum since the symptoms are often identical.

Immunoassays can be used for diagnosis and for detection of serum antibodies. Techniques for countercurrent immunoelectrophoresis, enzyme-linked immunosorbent assay, and radioimmunoassay have been developed.

Prevention and Treatment. Since transmission of virus by respiratory secretions occurs during the incubation period prior to the appearance of the rash, isolation of infected children cannot be used to prevent infection. However, because of the possible association of B19 and hydrops fetalis, it is recommended that pregnant women avoid exposure to the virus, e.g., from patients with erythema infectiosum.

There is no specific treatment for erythema infectiosum, and even symptomatic treatment is rarely necessary. Anemic individuals who develop aplastic crises may require red cell transfusions.

ADDITIONAL READING

Anderson, M. J. 1987. Human Parvoviruses. In *Principles and Practice of Clinical Virology,* p. 507, edited by A. J. Zuckerman, J. E. Banatvala, and J. R. Pattison. John Wiley, New York.

Baum, S. G. 1990. Adenovirus. In *Principles and Practice of Infectious Diseases,* Ed. 3, p. 1185, edited by G. L. Mandell, R. G. Douglas, Jr., and J. E. Bennett. Churchill Livingstone, New York.

Centers for Disease Control. 1989. Risks Associated with Human Parvovirus B19 Infection. MMWR, **38,** 81.

Cohen, B. J., Mortimer, P. P., and Pereira, M. S. 1983. Diagnostic assays with monoclonal antibodies for the human serum parvovirus-like virus (SPLV). J Hygiene, **91,** 113.

Marx, J. L. 1984. First Parvovirus Linked to Human Disease. Science, **223,** 152.

Siegl, G., and Tratschin, J.-D. 1987. Parvoviruses: Agents of distinct pathogenic and molecular potential. FEMS Micro Rev **46,** 433.

Thurn, J. 1988. Human Parvovirus B19: Historical and Clinical Review. Rev Infect Dis, **10,** 1005.

White, D. O., and Fenner, F. J. 1986. Adenoviruses. In *Medical Virology,* Ed. 3, p. 389. Academic Press, New York.

37

Papovaviruses

Virginia A. Merchant and Gretchen B. Caughman

The family Papovaviridae is named as an abbreviated combination of its first three member viruses: *pa*pilloma virus, *po*lyoma virus, and simian *va*cuolating 40 virus. Viruses of two genera, *Papillomavirus* and *Polyomavirus,* have been isolated in man and animals. The papillomaviruses cause warts in humans and papillomatoses in a number of animals. Some of the polyomaviruses are known to have oncogenic potential in animals, and those isolated from man have been associated with a slow virus infection, progressive multifocal leukoencephalopathy (PML), with Wiscott–Aldrich syndrome, and with a viruria in immunosuppressed individuals. Because of some members' capacity to induce malignant transformation, the papovaviruses, particularly polyomaviruses, are referred to as oncogenic DNA viruses or DNA tumor viruses.

Properties of Papovaviruses

The papovaviruses are small, naked icosahedrons 45 to 55 nm in diameter which contain circular, double-stranded DNA enclosed in a capsid with 72 capsomers. Members of this family are very resistant to heat and formalin inactivation, which explains why in earlier years the potentially oncogenic virus of monkeys, simian vacuolating virus 40 (SV40), survived in what were thought to be formalin-inactivated vaccines against various viral infections such as polio.

Much of our knowledge of papovavirus replication comes from studies of SV40 and other animal polyomaviruses because, unlike the papillomaviruses, these viruses can be cultivated routinely in tissue culture. In a productive SV40 infection, after adsorption and penetration of the virus particle, the capsid is translocated to the infected cell's nucleus where viral replication occurs in two phases, early and late. Early transcription produces a large primary transcript that is spliced and processed into several early mRNAs. These direct the synthesis of a family of related polypeptides called T (tumor) antigens. The T antigens are multifunctional viral proteins that regulate viral and cellular gene expression during productive infection of permissive cells and function in transformation of nonpermissive cells. The late phase of viral replication begins with the onset of viral DNA synthesis, which is initiated at a specific origin and proceeds bidirectionally around the circular genome. At the same time, late mRNAs are produced, processed, and translated into structural proteins that, together with the daughter DNA, ultimately assemble into progeny virions. In contrast, in cellular transformation, early but not late viral gene expression occurs. The cell's transformation to an abnormal phenotype may be transient (abortive transformation) or permanent; in the latter instance the viral genome, or at least the early gene region, becomes permanently integrated into the host cell DNA. The papillomaviruses are assumed to replicate in generally the same manner, but the precise events are not yet known.

Papillomaviruses

The human papillomaviruses (HPVs) can infect the skin and mucous membranes at various sites and may induce the small, flesh-colored hyperplastic papules known as warts. At least 57 HPV types have been identified on the basis of serology and/or DNA homology; some of the types are much more common than others and tend to be found at specific locations on the body. While by far the majority of warts are benign lesions that often spontaneously regress, there is growing evidence that genital infections with certain HPV types are strongly associated with cancer of the uterine cervix, vagina, penis, and anus. Recent research findings have also linked HPVs to oral and pharyngeal cancers.

Pathogenesis and Clinical Manifestations. Warts are a common infection, primarily of childhood, acquired through direct contact. Papillomaviruses gain entrance to the keratinized layers of the skin through minor abrasions where they infect single epidermal cells, which are stimulated to divide to form a well-delineated hyperplastic papule that extends to the depth of the basal layer. Acanthosis, parakeratosis, and hyperkeratosis are evident in the lesion. Warts may be found on the fingers (Fig. 37.1), the palms (palmar), the soles of the feet (plantar), or other exposed flat surfaces of the body. Oral warts in the form of focal epithelial hyperplasia have been described primarily in children, although it is not a common infection. In adults, genital warts, referred to as condylomata acuminata, are transmitted sexually. Oral warts, generally in the form of condylomata acuminata, are seen with increasing frequency and may be the result of oral–genital contact. Laryngeal papillomas seen in young children are apparently acquired at birth from virus in the mother's genital secretions.

Clinical evidence of infection usually does not ap-

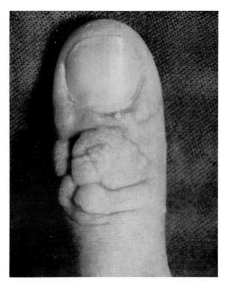

Figure 37.1: Common warts (verruca vulgaris) in a child. (AFIP AMH 10737-B.)

pear until the virus has replicated for 1 to 20 months. The hyperplastic lesions of the skin are usually flesh-colored to brown and may be flat, rounded, or filiform in shape. Condylomata acuminata, which are most commonly seen on mucosal surfaces, generally appear as soft, pink, cauliflower-like growths (Figs. 37.2 and 37.3). Lesions of oral focal epithelial hyperplasia occur on the lips or buccal mucosa as soft, multiple, 1- to 5-mm nodular lesions of the same color as the adjacent mucosa.

Human warts can be divided into seven categories according to their clinical presentation. These are listed by site of infection in Table 37.1, along with the commonly associated HPV types. Verrucae vulgaris, plana, and plantaris are primarily nuisances, although plantar warts are often painful. The HPV types associated with epidermodysplasia verruciformis (EV), condyloma acuminatum, and laryngeal papillomas have

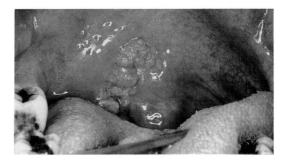

Figure 37.2: Large papillomatous lesion of the right soft palate. (Courtesy of Dr. J. A. Molinari.)

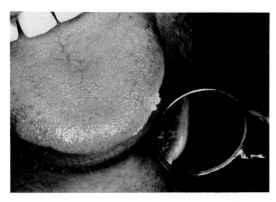

Figure 37.3: Small condyloma on the lateral border of the tongue. (Courtesy of Dr. J. A. Molinari.)

been associated with malignant changes. Recent evidence suggests that HPV-16, 18, and 33 may play a role, perhaps the primary causative role, in the development of cervical dysplasia and cervical carcinoma.

Epidemiology. Papillomas occur in humans worldwide. Skin warts occur most frequently in older children. The incidence of genital warts has increased significantly in recent years, making this infection one of the major sexually transmitted diseases of the 1980s. Evidence of HPV-infected cells has been noted in up to 2% of all routine uterine cervical smears and in up to 10% of young women screened. Approximately 70% of the sexual partners of symptomatically infected patients develop lesions.

Diagnosis. Warts are usually diagnosed on clinical appearance alone; however, histology of biopsy specimens can verify the clinical impression. Immunodiagnosis is limited to detection of an antigen common to all members of the *Papillomavirus* genus by immunofluorescence or immunoperoxidase staining of fixed sections. HPV typing by DNA hybridization is available only in certain research laboratories.

Prevention and Treatment. There are no specific preventive measures for papillomavirus infection. In terms of treatment, almost any procedure might be regarded as a "cure" if it is performed long enough, since warts spontaneously disappear in many cases after variable periods of time. This disappearing act has provided credence to many home remedies. Regression is most likely due to a stimulation of both the cell-mediated and the humoral immune responses. When multiple warts are present, they all tend to regress at the same time. However, in other individuals, the lesions persist and may spread or recur if removed.

Human warts of the forms that have been associated with malignant changes should be removed surgically or by the use of caustic chemicals. Other types of warts that are in areas likely to be traumatized or to pose problems of aesthetics may also be removed. Cryosurgery is probably the most popular mode of treatment. Topical podophyllin has long been a treatment of choice for anogenital warts but should not be used orally due to associated toxicity. The topical application of lactic or salicylic acid is an inexpensive yet effective treatment commonly recommended for skin warts. Recent research studies have shown that interferon therapy may be efficacious in treatment of refractory cases of genital warts.

Polyomaviruses

Two human polyomaviruses have been identified, JC virus and BK virus, so named for the initials of the individuals from which they were first isolated. SV40, which normally infects monkeys, can also cause disease in man.

Pathogenesis and Clinical Manifestations. The increasing prevalence of antibodies to JC virus and BK virus with age suggests that initial infection commonly occurs in childhood as an inapparent in-

Table 37.1: Sites of Infection, Clinical Presentations, and Commonly Associated HPV Types

Site of Infection	Clinical Presentation	HPV Types
Skin	Common warts (verruca vulgaris)	2, 7, 27, 29
	Flat warts (verruca plana)	3, 10, 26, 28
	Epidermodysplasia verruciformis	5, 8, 9, 12, 14, 15, 17, 19–25
Soles and palms	Plantar and palmar warts (verruca plantaris)	1, 4
Genitalia, oral cavity	Condyloma acuminatum	6, 11, 16, 18, 30, 31, 33, 35
Larynx, pharynx	Laryngeal papillomatosis	6, 11
Oral mucosa	Focal epithelial hyperplasia	13

fection. Persistent infection results, but clinical disease is only seen under conditions of chronic immunosuppression. No disease in man has yet been associated with BK virus, and although it is oncogenic in vitro, there is no evidence that it plays a role in human malignancies.

Progressive multifocal leukoencephalopathy is the result of infection of the brain by the JC virus, although at least two cases have been attributed to SV40 infection. The clinical syndrome is characterized by multiple, progressively evolving demyelinative lesions in the brain and is now recognized as an opportunistic infection occurring in patients with impaired cell-mediated immune responses. Neurological deterioration is rapid and remissions are rare. Death usually occurs within 4 to 6 months of initial neurological symptoms.

Epidemiology. Infection with JC virus and BK virus is apparently quite common, given the high prevalence of antibodies in the population. Approximately 70% of adults have antibodies to JC virus and 60% to 70% have antibodies to BK virus. SV40 antibodies are less common now that monkey kidney cultures are no longer used for vaccine production. Progressive multifocal leukoencephalopathy is generally only seen in immunodeficient patients. Previously diagnosed only rarely, its incidence is increasing as a well-recognized complication of acquired immunodeficiency syndrome (AIDS).

Diagnosis. Progressive multifocal leukoencephalopathy should be considered when an immunodeficient patient develops a rapidly progressive neurological illness. Diagnosis by serology is not possible since most normal adults have antibodies to JC virus. Computed tomography or magnetic resonance imaging shows the demyelinative lesions.

Prevention and Treatment. There are no specific preventive measures against infection. Treatment of progressive multifocal leukoencephalopathy generally has been unsuccessful. Some cases have gone into remission after the use of adenine or cytosine arabinoside, but there are no controlled studies to establish their efficacy.

ADDITIONAL READING

Bender, M. E., Ostrow, R. S., Watts, S., Zachow, K., Faras, A., and Pass, F. 1983. Immunology of Human Papillomavirus: Warts. Pediatric Dermatol, **1,** 121.

Butler, S., Molinari, J. A., Plezia, R. A., Chandrasekar, P., and Venkat, H. 1988. Condyloma Acuminatum in the Oral Cavity: Four Cases and a Review. Rev Infect Dis, **10,** 544.

Howley, P. M., and Schlegel, R. 1988. The Human Papillomaviruses. Am J Med, **85** (Suppl), 155.

Norkin, L. C. 1982. Papoviral Persistent Infections. Microbiol Rev, **46,** 384.

Reichman, R. C., and Bonncz, W. 1990. Papillomavirus. In *Principles and Practice of Infectious Diseases,* Ed. 3, p. 1191, edited by G. L. Mandell, R. G. Douglas, Jr., and J. E. Bennett. Churchill Livingstone, New York.

Richardson, E. P., Jr. 1988. Progressive Multifocal Leukoencephalopathy 30 Years Later. N Engl J Med, **318,** 315.

Weck, P. K., Buddin, D. A., and Whisnant, J. K. 1988. Interferons in the Treatment of Genital Human Papillomavirus Infections. Am J Med, **85** (Suppl), 159.

White, D. O., and Fenner, F. J. 1986. Papovaviruses. In *Medical Virology,* Ed. 3, p. 381. Academic Press, New York.

38

Herpesviruses

Gretchen B. Caughman and Virginia A. Merchant

Herpesviruses (family Herpesviridae) are enveloped, icosahedral, DNA-containing viruses with dermatotropic, neurotropic, and lymphotropic predilections. They have the remarkable ability to persist indefinitely in an infected individual. This persistence takes the form of a latent state, from which the virus may emerge (reactivate) periodically to cause recurrent active disease. In addition, some herpesviruses have teratogenic and/or oncogenic potential. Herpesviruses are widespread in the animal kingdom, and numerous animal species ranging from oysters to chickens to horses to man have been found to be infected with their own particular herpesviruses. The human herpesviruses are extremely important pathogens whose impact continues to increase. They, along with the herpesviruses of other animals, are grouped into three subfamilies. The Alphaherpesvirinae subfamily (herpes simplex virus group) includes herpes simplex virus types 1 and 2 (HSV-1, 2), which cause primary and recurrent orofacial and genital lesions; varicella–zoster virus (VZV), which causes chickenpox and may recur as shingles; and herpes B virus of monkeys, which is not a natural pathogen of humans but can cause serious and often fatal disease when accidentally acquired. The Betaherpesvirinae (cytomegalovirus group) includes human cytomegalovirus (CMV), which generally produces asymptomatic infection in healthy individuals but can cause severe disease in immunosuppressed patients and is responsible for a spectrum of physical and mental developmental defects in children who were infected in utero. The Gammaherpesvirinae (lymphoproliferative virus group) includes Epstein–Barr virus (EBV), which is the etiological agent of infectious mononucleosis and also is associated with two neoplasias, Burkitt's lymphoma and nasopharyngeal carcinoma. A comparison of some of the clinical characteristics of these viruses is given in Table 38.1. A sixth human herpesvirus has been discovered recently and is designated simply human herpesvirus type six (HHV-6). While HHV-6's properties and pathogenic potential are not yet as clearly defined as those of the other human herpesviruses, it has been implicated as the cause of one of the childhood rashes, exanthem subitum.

356

Table 38.1: Characteristics of the Human Herpesviruses*†

Property	Herpes Simplex Viruses 1 and 2	Varicella–Zoster Virus	Cytomegalovirus	Epstein–Barr Virus
Common clinical manifestations‡	Skin and mucous membrane lesions	Skin and mucous membrane lesions	Mononucleosis syndrome (negative heterophile antibody test)	Mononucleosis syndrome (positive heterophile antibody test)
Transmission	Contact with lesions or secretions	Contact; saliva	Saliva, urine, breast milk, transplants, semen	Saliva; blood transfusion
Oral	Yes	Yes	Yes	Yes
Sexual	Yes	No	Yes	No
Blood transfusion	No	No	Yes	Yes
Fomites	Yes	?	Yes	Yes
Establishes latent infection	Yes	Yes	Yes	Yes
Site of latent virus	Sensory and autonomic nervous ganglia	Sensory ganglia (dorsal root ganglia)	Monocytes and lymphocytes (?)	B-lymphocytes, epithelial cells
Asymptomatic virus shedding	Common	?Possible, rare§	Common	Common
Frequency of recurrence	Frequent (as often as once per month)	Usually only one recurrence‖	Not usually symptomatic	Usually no clinical manifestations
Reinfection	Yes	Yes	Yes	Yes
Congenital or perinatal infection	Congenital—rare; Perinatal—yes	Yes, if primary infection in mother during pregnancy	Major cause of birth defects: Congenital—0.5%–2% of live births; Perinatal—1%–13% of healthy newborns	No evidence
Disseminated infection, occurrence	Neonates; also malnourished, immunocompromised, or burn patients	Immunocompromised patients	Immunocompromised patients (renal and bone transplant patients)	B-cell lymphomas; immunocompromised patients

*From J. A. Molinari and V. A. Merchant: Herpesviruses: Manifestations and Transmission. *J Calif Dent Assoc,* **17,** 24, 1989. Reprinted with permission of the *Journal of the California Dental Association.*

†Human herpesvirus 6 is not included here; see text for information.

‡With the exception of VZV infection, the majority of infections are asymptomatic.

§Virus in respiratory secretions near end of incubation period.

‖May have reactivation without clinical symptoms.

Properties of Herpesviruses

Herpesviruses are relatively large (180 to 200 nm diameter), enveloped viruses with icosahedral capsid symmetry. The envelope is derived from the infected cell's nuclear membrane into which viral glycoproteins have been inserted. A granular zone (tegument) of globular proteins fills the space between the envelope and the capsid. The icosahedral capsid is composed of 162 elongated capsomers, each with a small central hole. The capsid encloses a dense, torus-shaped core structure which consists of one linear molecule of double-stranded DNA genome wrapped around a fibrous spool of proteins. Like other enveloped viruses, herpesviruses are relatively unstable at room temperature and are readily inactivated by lipid solvents.

HSV-1 and 2 are the prototypes in the study of herpesvirus molecular biology. During infection, the virion enters the cells by either pinocytosis or fusion of the envelope with the cell membrane, and the nucleocapsid is released into the cytoplasm. The DNA-containing core moves into the nucleus, and transcription of some of the viral genes by cellular DNA-dependent RNA polymerase II begins. Herpesviral gene expression is a complex and intricately regulated process in which various genes are transcribed only at certain times in the replication cycle. Three major phases of gene expression have been defined: immediate early, early, and late. The immediate early genes code for regulatory proteins that are required to "turn on" subsequent phases of gene expression. The early proteins that are synthesized next include viral enzymes such as DNA polymerase and thymidine kinase needed for viral DNA replication, as well as some of the viral glycoproteins. After the necessary enzymes are produced during the early phase, viral DNA replication begins, along with the onset of the last (late) phase of gene expression. The late proteins are mostly structural proteins, which then are used as architectural components in the assembly of daughter virions. Intranuclear inclusions referred to as Cowdry type A inclusions are the sites of initial virus assembly. However, the mature inclusion does not contain virions, since envelopment and budding occur at the nuclear membrane and the virions then traverse the cytoplasm through the endoplasmic reticulum or vacuoles to be released at the cell surface (Fig. 38.1).

Viral Latency

Primary herpesvirus infection, whether it is symptomatic or inapparent, results in the establishment of viral latency. In the latent state, although there is no infectious virus production, the viral genome persists

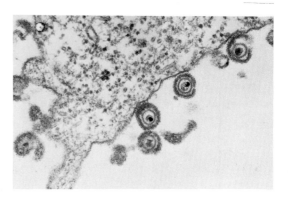

Figure 38.1: Herpes simplex virus type 1 in extracellular space. The nucleocapsid is surrounded by an envelope at least partly derived from host cell membranes (× 80,000). (Reproduced with permission from H. D. Mayor, S. Drake, and L. Jordan: The Replication of Adeno-Associated Satellite Virus: The Three-Component System, Satellite, Herpes Virus, and Adenovirus. *J Ultrastruc Res,* **52,** 52, 1975.)

in certain host cells and, when appropriately stimulated, is capable of reactivation. During reactivation, the lytic replication cycle is reinitiated, infectious viral particles are produced, and an active, recurrent disease episode ensues. Reactivation episodes may be months, years, or decades after the primary infection and may occur seldom or with great frequency. The site of latency within the host—that is, the location of the cells that continue to harbor the viral genome—depends on the virus and, in some cases, the location of the primary infection. For HSV-1 and HSV-2, the latent infection is harbored in sensory nerve ganglia that innervate the site of primary infection. Thus, in orofacial infections, it is usually the trigeminal nerve ganglion that becomes latently infected; in genital infections, the thoracic, lumbar, and sacral dorsal root ganglia are frequent sites of latency. VZV primary infection (chickenpox) is more disseminated and thus latency may be established in the sensory ganglia of the vagal, spinal, or cranial nerves (Fig. 38.2). EBV establishes latency in B-lymphocytes and in some epithelial cells. The site(s) of CMV latency is not clear but may include peripheral blood mononuclear cells.

The mechanisms controlling the establishment and maintenance of latency as well as the factors governing reactivation are poorly understood and are the focus of much of the current research on herpesviruses. In the case of HSV, recent evidence indicates that during latency the viral genome is maintained in a nonintegrated (extrachromosomal) circular state and is associated with nucleosomes in a chromatin-like structure. Also, although very little viral gene expression can be detected in latently infected ganglia, the genome is not completely silent; several latency-associated RNA transcripts have been detected that originate from viral DNA sequences not usually ex-

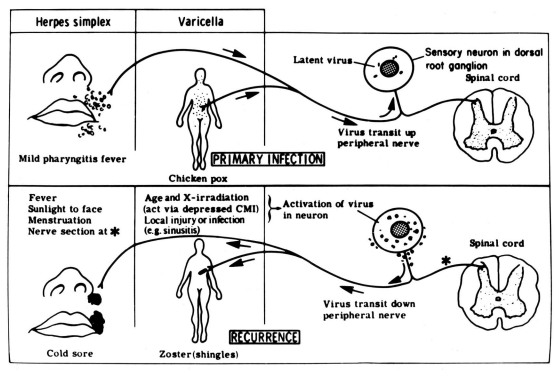

Herpes simplex	Varicella

Figure 38.2: Mechanisms of latency in herpes simplex and zoster infections. Primary infection occurs in childhood or adolescence; latent virus is harbored in cerebral or spinal ganglia; later activation causes recurrent herpes simplex or zoster. (Reproduced with permission from C. A. Mims: *The Pathogenesis of Infectious Disease,* Ed. 3. Academic Press, London, 1987.)

pressed (or expressed in very low amounts) during lytic infection. The significance and possible functions of these transcripts are not yet known. Reactivation can be induced by a wide variety of factors, including sunlight, heat, cold, fever, menstruation, and emotional or physical stress. Exactly how these inducers trigger new virion production and recurrent disease is not known.

Herpes Simplex Virus Types 1 and 2

Herpes simplex infections are caused by two virus types, 1 and 2, which are closely related serologically; in fact their genomes have about 50% genetic homology. The diseases caused by HSV include vesicular eruptions of the skin and mucous membranes that are often characterized by recurrent episodes, and disseminated infections involving the viscera or nervous system. Since the viruses have in vitro oncogenic potential, they have been implicated in cervical carcinomas and, to a lesser degree, in oral carcinomas. However, the idea that HSV has a pivotal role in these or any other malignancies has not been borne out.

An individual only experiences one primary infec-

tion with HSV, whether it is with HSV-1 or HSV-2. By convention, the first infection with the other virus type, or another (exogenous) strain of the same virus type, is referred to as an initial infection. Reactivation of a latent (endogenous) virus infection is referred to as a recurrent infection.

Pathogenesis and Clinical Manifestations. Herpes simplex virus gains access to the parabasal and intermediate epithelial cells of the mucous membranes of the oral cavity, genitalia, or eye, or through traumatic inoculation into the skin, where it initiates infection. It has been estimated that up to 90% of primary oral infections and about 50% of primary genital infections are inapparent and asymptomatic. In clinically symptomatic infections, multinucleated cells that contain the typical inclusions are formed, and these show ballooning degeneration. As these cells are lysed, a local inflammatory response develops that appears first as a small patch of erythema and then evolves into a vesicle filled with a clear fluid. Virus is more likely to be recovered from this vesicle fluid than from the crusts that develop as it heals. Additional virus replication may result in a viremia and dissemination to the viscera such as the lungs and liver or through peripheral nerves to the central nervous system. Individuals with impaired cellular immune responses are likely to develop more severe disease than normal individuals, and in fact, viremias are rare in immunocompetent individuals. The development of neutralizing antibodies, sensitized T-cells, and interferon all play a role in the resolution of primary herpes simplex infections. During the initial infection of the epithelium, virus gains access to the adjacent nerve endings and travels rapidly in the axons to the ganglia, where it persists in a latent state. During reactivation, the latent virus is stimulated to reinitiate viral replication. In a healthy individual, the presence of neutralizing antibodies and cellular immunity limits the dissemination of the reactivated virus, but the virus does migrate from the ganglion back along the axon to contiguous cells and there produces the characteristic localized lesions of recurrent herpetic infection.

Oral Infection

Oral primary infection with HSV, if symptomatic, most often presents as herpetic gingivostomatitis (Fig. 38.3). The disease may range from mild to severe. In the classic form, it presents as soreness of the mouth with excessive salivation accompanied by cervical lymphadenopathy and systemic symptoms of fever and malaise. Oral lesions, which initially appear as vesicles but rapidly ulcerate, typically develop throughout the oral cavity. They may occur on the buccal mucosa, tongue, gingival tissues, hard and soft palate, and the tonsillar pillars. Lesions may extend extraorally and are readily spread via contact with virus-containing saliva (see Fig. 38.3). Mild primary infections may mimic the less severe recurrent infection commonly referred to as a fever blister or cold sore. Primary oral infections sometimes present as herpetic pharyngitis, particularly in adolescents or

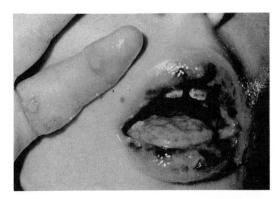

Figure 38.3: Primary herpetic gingivostomatitis with auto-inoculation of fingers. Reproduced with permission from the *Southern Medical Journal:* R. E. Haynes, *South Med J,* **69,** 1069, 1976.

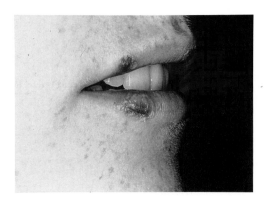

Figure 38.4: Recurrent herpes labialis.

young adults, and may be associated with concomitant genital infection. Symptoms occur after an incubation period of 1 to 26 days (median of 6 to 8 days) and generally last from 10 to 14 days before complete resolution. Complications, which are rare, include disseminated skin and visceral infections and encephalitis.

Recurrent oral disease may manifest as herpes labialis (fever blisters or cold sores), perioral lesions, or recurrent intraoral herpes simplex infection. Approximately one third of individuals who have been infected orally with HSV will experience recurrent lesions. Recurrences are due to reactivation of virus latent in the trigeminal ganglion. Herpes labialis is usually a mild disease that presents as a single lesion or cluster of lesions on or adjacent to the vermilion border of the lips (Fig. 38.4). Vesicles appear after a prodromal period of 6 to 24 hours in which symptoms of burning, itching, warmth, or some other sensation alert the individual that a recurrence is imminent. Lesions may occur around the nose, on the chin, cheek, or forehead, or any area innervated by the trigeminal nerve. Progression from vesicle to crust occurs over a period of 24 to 48 hours. Recurrent infections in immunocompetent individuals are characteristically of short duration with complete resolution within 7 to 10 days. More extensive disease is seen in immunocompromised patients and may persist for prolonged periods.

Recurrent intraoral herpes simplex infection (RIHS) is less commonly recognized than the extraoral lesions of herpes labialis but is probably no less frequent. The lesions occur on attached mucosa, i.e., attached gingiva and the hard palate (Fig. 38.5) They occur initially as vesicles that rapidly coalesce to form ulcerative lesions. Typically the lesions appear as a cluster of small white to gray or yellow ulcers with an erythematous halo. The lesions may be painful but discomfort is generally mild and patients may be completely unaware of their presence. A single individual may experience oral recurrences as RIHS or herpes

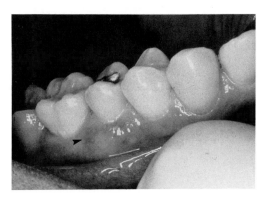

Figure 38.5: Recurrent intraoral herpes simplex infection on the attached gingiva.

labialis or both, but lesions are almost never expressed simultaneously in both forms. Minor aphthous lesions are often confused with lesions of RIHS; however, their distribution differs since aphthae are normally only found on movable mucosal surfaces such as the buccal or labial mucosa, soft palate, or tongue.

Ocular Infection

Ocular HSV infections in adults and children are most commonly caused by HSV-1 and may be due to primary infection or autoinoculation or extension from an oral infection. Infants may acquire infection during passage through an HSV-infected (commonly HSV-2) birth canal. Infection is usually unilateral and may occur as a blepharitis, conjunctivitis, keratitis, or chorioretinitis. Regional lymphadenopathy is often seen in primary infections. If the cornea is involved, dendritic ulcerative lesions develop that are pathognomonic. Corneal involvement often leads to scarring and loss of vision, making HSV infection a frequent cause of blindness in the United States and other developed nations. Recurrences following primary/initial infection apparently occur in about one third of affected individuals and can lead to further loss of visual acuity.

Genital Infection

Genital herpes is almost always acquired sexually and is most often due to HSV-2, although the incidence of HSV-1 genital infection continues to increase. As in oral HSV infections, primary disease is characteristically more severe than recurrent disease. Patients who have previously experienced an HSV infection, frequently an oral HSV-1 infection, tend to have less severe initial genital infections, indicating some protective cross-immunity.

Like primary oral infections, first-episode genital infections often have associated systemic symptoms of fever, malaise, and anorexia. Local symptoms include pain, itching, dysuria, vaginal or urethral discharge, tender inguinal lymphadenopathy, and lesions of the external genitalia. Most lesions in males occur on the penis but can extend into the urethra. Urethral involvement may result in dysuria, urinary retention, and associated neuralgias. In females, lesions commonly are seen on both the external and internal genitalia. It has been estimated that approximately 50% of primary/initial genital herpetic infections are asymptomatic.

Recurrence rates vary greatly; however, recurrences are more frequently seen in individuals infected genitally with HSV-2 than with HSV-1 (80% vs. 55%). Recurrent infections are usually milder, with less systemic involvement and fewer genital lesions. Reactivation of latent infection may also present as shedding of HSV in genital secretions in the absence of clinical lesions.

The prevalence of genital HSV infections continues to increase in the United States, and visits to physicians prompted by genital HSV rose significantly in the 1970s and 1980s. Rectal and perianal HSV infections, usually the result of anorectal intercourse with an infected partner, are also being diagnosed more frequently, particularly among homosexual men.

Herpetic Whitlow and Other Skin Infections

Herpetic whitlow, an HSV infection of the finger, has been most frequently seen in health care providers, especially those coming in contact with oral secretions, but contact with lesions or virus-containing secretions can precipitate the infection in anyone. The virus enters through a break in the skin or as the result of trauma and causes a localized infection (Fig. 38.6). HSV-1 is the usual cause of herpetic whitlow in health care providers, whereas HSV-2 is the

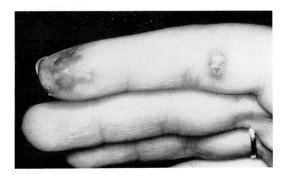

Figure 38.6: Recurrent herpetic whitlow in a dental hygienist.

more frequent cause of finger infections in the general population.

Usually within a few days following infection, itching in the affected area precedes the appearance of vesicular lesions. Lesions most often occur on the distal phalanx and are often around the nail, where breaks in the epithelial integrity allow the virus to gain access to the underlying basal cells. If the lesions extend under the nail, intense pain develops and may necessitate perforation of the nail to relieve the pressure. Regional neuralgia and axillary lymphadenopathy are common. If the infection is not mistaken for a pyogenic paronychia and excised, it will resolve in 2 to 3 weeks. Surgical excision causes extension of the infection into the underlying and surrounding tissues, delays healing, and is often associated with secondary bacterial infection. Following initial infection, the virus remains latent in the sensory ganglia of C6, C7, C8, or T1. The incidence of recurrences of herpetic whitlow is unestablished, but multiple recurrences with loss of sensation in the affected finger have been reported.

If the virus gains access to other areas of the skin through a cut or abrasion, HSV infection may result. The prolonged unprotected skin contact engaged in during athletic competitions such as wrestling can lead to herpetic infection and has been seen frequently enough that it has been designated herpes gladiatorum. Individuals with eczema may develop severe infections following exposure to HSV. These can be fatal if bacterial superinfection occurs in individuals whose immune response is compromised. Burn patients are particularly susceptible to HSV infection and can develop disseminated skin or visceral disease.

Nervous System Infections

HSV is the most common cause of viral encephalitis in the United States, with an incidence of approximately 2.3 cases per 1 million population per year, and accounts for 10% to 20% of all cases of viral encephalitis. HSV-1 is the primary causative agent, being responsible for more than 95% of cases. There is a biphasic age distribution with peaks between 5 and 30 years of age and again above 50 years of age. HSV encephalitis may follow primary infection, reactivation of latent virus, or reinfection with an exogenous virus strain.

The virus primarily infects the temporal lobes, and a necrotizing hemorrhagic encephalitis results. Onset may be sudden or follow a brief flu-like illness. Symptoms include headache, fever, behavioral disorders, speech difficulties, and focal seizures. Diagnosis is difficult since cerebrospinal fluid usually does not contain infectious virus or show any changes that specifically indicate an HSV infection. Biopsy of the temporal lobe with histological and cultural examination remains the most appropriate and reliable method for definitive diagnosis.

If untreated, HSV encephalitis is fatal in 80% of cases. Intravenous vidarabine or acyclovir (the latter is more effective) have been shown to significantly reduce the mortality and morbidity of the disease. However, neurological sequelae are frequent even with therapy.

HSV meningitis is an acute, self-limited disease often associated with primary genital HSV-2 infection. Symptoms include headache, fever, and mild photophobia and last from 2 to 7 days. HSV meningitis accounts for 0.5% to 3% of hospital-diagnosed cases of aseptic meningitis. Complete recovery is the norm.

Autonomic nervous system dysfunction may be associated with HSV infection, particularly in the sacral region. Peripheral nervous system involvement is sometimes associated with HSV reactivation and in the facial area can manifest as Bell's palsy.

Visceral Infections

Viremia may lead to multiple organ involvement but is rare in immunocompetent patients. Esophagitis, pneumonitis, and hepatitis are the most common clinical manifestations of disseminated HSV infection. In immunocompromised patients, dissemination to other visceral organs, such as the adrenal glands, pancreas, intestine, and bone marrow, occasionally occurs.

Neonatal Infections

Although transplacental infection of the fetus occasionally occurs as the result of viremic spread following a primary HSV infection during pregnancy, contact with virus-containing genital secretions during parturition is the most common cause of neonatal HSV disease. Approximately 70% of neonatal HSV infections have been attributed to infection with HSV-2. The majority of neonatal HSV-1 infections are acquired postnatally via contact with a symptomatic or asymptomatic family member having oral–genital disease or via nosocomial transmission. Untreated neonatal disease results in disseminated or central nervous system involvement in more than 70% of infections and has a mortality rate of 65%. Antiviral chemotherapy has reduced the mortality rate to approximately 25%, but morbidity is still high.

HSV in the Immunocompromised Host

Patients who are immunosuppressed or immunocompromised are at risk of severe HSV infections. Although there is the potential for severe primary or initial infections, reactivation of latent virus is the most frequent cause of morbidity in these patients. Transplant recipients on immunosuppressive therapy to prevent rejection commonly shed virus in secretions and may develop severe persistent lesions that last weeks to months. Various studies have reported an oral lesion prevalence of 50% to 90% in seropositive bone marrow transplant patients. Reactivation of latent HSV may lead to severe chronic or progressive mucocutaneous infections in patients being treated with cancer chemotherapeutic agents. Oral HSV lesions have been reported in 40% to 70% of these patients. With the AIDS epidemic and its associated mushrooming numbers of immunocompromised individuals, severe HSV infections are becoming much more common as one of the most frequent causes of opportunistic disease in patients infected with human immunodeficiency virus (HIV).

Epidemiology, Diagnosis, and Treatment

Epidemiology. Herpes simplex infections are worldwide in distribution and are acquired by direct contact with infected secretions such as saliva or lesion exudates from active cases, or from individuals shedding virus in secretions in the absence of clinical lesions. Although there is no marked sexual or seasonal variation, rates of infection have been related to socioeconomic status, and, in the case of genital infections, to the degree of promiscuity. Surveys have shown that up to 90% of individuals in a lower socioeconomic status show evidence of HSV-1 infection, whereas only 30% to 50% of those from higher strata are infected. The incidence of HSV-2 is somewhat less but increasing. Moreover, there is an expected age difference in the acquisition of both types. For example, neonates are more likely to acquire HSV-2 infections of the eye or central nervous system during birth, whereas other HSV-2 infections occur after puberty, following the initiation of sexual activity, and are usually confined to the genitalia. HSV-1 infections can be easily transmitted by casual contact. Young children readily acquire oral infection from contact with parents, siblings, or playmates. As the number of potential contacts increases, either with crowded living conditions or through contacts in play groups or daycare, the incidence of infection increases. The old axiom that HSV-1 infections are found primarily from the waist up and HSV-2 infections from the waist down no longer holds, since changes in sexual practices also have changed the pattern of serotypes found at the sites of primary/initial infection.

Herpetic whitlow has been an occupational hazard of dentists, physicians, and auxiliary medical or dental personnel who come in contact with saliva and other secretions that may contain HSV in the absence of obvious lesions. Although never very prevalent, considering the frequency of asymptomatic oral shedding of HSV, the use of gloves in respiratory therapy and dentistry has made this hazard much less significant. Adherence to universal precautions in the treatment of all patients when dealing with body fluids should virtually eliminate any occupational risk of infection with HSV. Nosocomial infections with HSV have occasionally occurred in neonatal nurseries, but the practice of restricting nurses with recurrent herpes labialis from working in the nursery has been discontinued since transmission can be prevented with good hygienic practices. In fact, transmission is probably more likely from an individual who is asymptomatically shedding virus in oral secretions since the need for precautions is not as apparent.

Transmission of HSV in the dental office has been assumed to occur but has rarely been documented. An outbreak of infection has been documented in which a dental hygienist, after apparently acquiring an HSV infection of her hands from a patient, transmitted infections resulting in herpetic gingivostomatitis to 20 of 46 patients treated over a 4-day period. One of the 20 patients who developed clinical symptoms had had recurrent oral infections prior to the reinfection.

Asymptomatic excretion of HSV in oral and genital secretions is not uncommon. Studies have revealed the presence of HSV-1 in the saliva of 2% to 9% of asymptomatic seropositive adults and 5% to 8% of children. HSV-2 has been isolated from genital secretions of less than 1% to 15% of individuals with histories of genital herpes during periods in which lesions did not occur. Asymptomatic shedding may also occur following trauma. A recently published study reported asymptomatic shedding of HSV-1 in the saliva of 41% of seropositive oral surgery patients at some time during the month following the surgical procedure.

HSV, often considered to be very labile, can survive for a number of hours outside the body. Several studies have investigated HSV survival on a variety of surfaces, with a maximum time span for recovery of viable virus ranging from 45 minutes to 88 hours after inoculation or contamination. In one study, virus was isolated from the hands of six of nine adults with virus-positive herpes labialis and a survival time of 2 hours on skin was determined. In another study, virus suspended in blood was isolated from dental charts up to 4 hours after inoculation.

The mechanisms of reactivation of latent infection remain to be elucidated. Certain factors have been shown to stimulate reactivation in some individuals. Stress, whether of daily living or associated with major life events, has been recognized as a trigger of HSV recurrences for many years. Students typically develop recurrent lesions during final examination week. Exposure to sunlight or other ultraviolet light sources stimulates recurrences (particularly oral) in many individuals. Respiratory infections, such as the common cold, and hormonal changes associated with the menstrual cycle are also frequently reported as inciting the development of lesions. Trauma to mucocutaneous tissues may trigger a recurrence. Oral reactivation of latent HSV is commonly observed in dental patients following even mildly traumatic procedures. These reactivations are typically manifested as RIHS, although some patients experience labial lesions.

Diagnosis. Laboratory confirmation of a clinical diagnosis of herpes simplex infection can be made by viral culture, direct examination, or immunoassay. Viral culture is widely used but requires time and the availability of a virology laboratory and usually does not distinguish HSV from other herpesviruses. Likewise, direct examination techniques by electron or light microscopy are not specific and cannot distinguish HSV from the other herpesviruses. Once the only diagnostic procedure routinely available, light microscopic evaluation of infected cells for characteristic changes (ballooning degeneration of cells, ground-glass nuclei containing a basophilic inclusion and marginated chromatin, eosinophilic intranuclear inclusions, and multinucleated giant cells) is rarely used today. Immunofluorescence assays using fluorescein isothiocyanate-labeled antibodies to HSV antigens is the most commonly used technique for rapid diagnosis of HSV infections, although it is less sensitive than viral culture early in the course of disease. Enzyme-linked immunosorbent assays (EIA) are now commercially available for HSV antigen detection and are more useful for typing, i.e., discriminating between HSV-1 and HSV-2 infections, since they are more type specific.

Demonstration of a fourfold or greater rise in antibody titers during the course of illness can confirm a primary HSV-1 or HSV-2 infection. Demonstration of IgM antibodies may be indicative of a primary infection, although extensive recurrent disease or reinfections can precipitate an IgM antibody response as well. HSV serodiagnosis, which was traditionally accomplished either by complement fixation or viral neutralization assays, is now more commonly performed by EIA. Quantification of viral-specific IgG and IgM antibodies can be accomplished by using peroxidase-conjugated antibodies specific for human IgG or IgM.

Prevention and Treatment. The widespread prevalence of herpes simplex viruses makes it impossible to completely avoid the acquisition of this disease; however, certain precautions can be taken. Direct contact with herpetic lesions or associated secretions should be avoided by others as well as by the individual affected, since autoinoculation of other sites can occur. Since virus shedding in the absence of symptoms occurs periodically in most individuals with histories of active recurrent disease, special precautions should be taken when feasible to prevent transmission. Particular care should be taken to avoid transmission of infection to infants or to individuals whose cell-mediated immune response is impaired by disease or immunosuppressive agents. The use of protective barriers—i.e., gloves, masks, and protective eyewear—in the treatment of all dental patients is effective in preventing transmission of virus from the oral cavity of a patient to the practitioner's hands or mucous membranes of the oral cavity, nose, or eyes. Condom use can reduce the risk of acquiring genital herpetic infections.

Neonatal transmission at birth usually can be avoided by cesarean section prior to membrane rupture, if virus is present in the vaginal tract at the time of delivery. Monitoring of virus shedding by culture during the latter part of pregnancy in women who have, or whose sexual partners have, a history of genital herpes infection is now routine in major metropolitan areas. If cultures are negative just prior to delivery and there is no evidence of clinical lesions, a vaginal delivery is usually safe.

Since 1962, when topical idoxuridine was shown to be effective for the treatment of HSV keratitis, a number of antiviral agents have been evaluated and found to have varying degrees of efficacy and safety in the treatment of HSV infections. The most efficacious and least toxic of the antivirals evaluated to date is acyclovir. Acyclovir is a nucleoside analogue that requires phosphorylation by virus-specific thymidine kinase (TK) for its activation as a potent inhibitor of viral DNA polymerase. It is not effectively phosphorylated by cellular TK and thus has minimal effects on uninfected cells.

Acyclovir, available commercially as a topical ointment, an oral capsule, and an intravenous preparation, has been shown to be effective in the management of some HSV infections. Topical treatment with any of the antivirals is relatively ineffective except in ocular infections and in the management of severe skin infections in immunocompromised patients. Oral preparations decrease the time of viral shedding and accelerate healing in genital infections and have shown promise in the management of primary oral infections, although they are not yet approved for this use. Less benefit is seen when they are used in the treatment of recurrent infections in immunocompetent patients. The prophylactic use of oral preparations to suppress reactivation of latent infection and prevent recurrences has been somewhat successful, but long-term effects of drug use are not known, and routine suppressive therapy is not recommended.

Prolonged or indiscriminant use of acyclovir in healthy individuals with mild or moderate disease is inadvisable as there is the very real possibility of the development of acyclovir-resistant strains of HSV. Resistant strains are being recognized with increasing frequency in immunocompromised patients undergoing extended antiviral treatment to manage HSV infections or to prevent their reactivation.

Both primary and recurrent ocular HSV infections should be treated with topical trifluorothymidine or vidarabine to prevent progressive disease and possible loss of vision. Corticosteroids should never be used in ocular herpetic infections as they can cause progression of HSV disease. Central nervous system or disseminated HSV disease is usually managed with intravenous acyclovir or vidarabine.

Foscarnet (trisodium phosphonoformate), a pyrophosphate analogue that inhibits DNA polymerase, has been shown to be effective in management of acyclovir-resistant mucocutaneous HSV infections in patients with AIDS. This drug is still experimental and does not have FDA approval.

No antiviral is approved at present by the FDA for the treatment of oral HSV infections in immunocompetent patients. A number of over-the-counter palliative agents are available that may reduce the discomfort associated with labial herpetic lesions but have no effect on healing. Topical anesthetic suspensions are useful in reducing the discomfort of eating when extensive intraoral lesions are present.

Several laboratories are investigating possible vaccines for prevention of HSV infection. There is considerable reluctance to use a live vaccine virus, since it would be likely to establish life-long latency in the inoculated individual and could have unforeseen consequences. However, as more information is gathered about the initiation and maintenance of the latent state, it may be possible to construct virus strains that are specifically engineered so as to be unable to establish latency. Another promising approach is through the development of subunit vaccines that would contain only certain viral polypeptides capable of inducing a protective immune response.

Varicella–Zoster Virus

The primary infection with VZV is varicella, more commonly known as chickenpox, and unlike other herpesvirus infections, almost always results in clinical disease. The virus establishes latent infection in the sensory ganglia of the peripheral or cranial nerves. Reactivation of the endogenous virus may lead to zoster (shingles). Although similar to HSV in morphology, ability to produce Cowdry type A inclusions, and ability to elicit a disease with vesicular, latent, and neurotropic characteristics, VZV differs from HSV-1 and 2 in its larger size (180 to 200 nm), inability to cause disease in animals or chick embryos, higher cell association in culture, and different antigenicity.

Pathogenesis and Clinical Manifestations. Although the exact route of invasion of VZV is uncertain, it is presumed that the virus enters the body through the respiratory tract, where it multiplies and invades the bloodstream to be carried to the skin or other organs. Lesions are similar to those of herpes simplex in that ballooning degeneration in cells of the epidermis, and to a lesser degree of the corium, occurs with focal cellular destruction. Vesicle fluid is predominantly polymorphonuclear leukocytic. Multinucleated giant cells are formed that contain Cowdry type A intranuclear inclusions. Following primary infection, a latent state develops in the dorsal ganglia and is probably maintained by cellular immunity. Upon reactivation in the zoster syndrome, the initial cutaneous lesions are similar to those of varicella, but dorsal root ganglia also show cellular infiltration, focal hemorrhages and degeneration. Nerve destruction may extend back to the posterior column of the cord and forward to the skin.

Varicella is a highly contagious exanthematous-enanthematous disease that is characterized by successive crops of lesions (Fig. 38.7). Usually a relatively mild disease of childhood, it tends to be a much more extensive and serious infection when it occurs in older teenagers and adults. Also, varicella can be potentially life-threatening to children who are immunocompromised and who develop progressive disease. After an incubation period of 14 to 15 days,

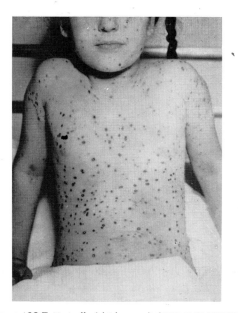

Figure 38.7: Varicella (chickenpox). (AFIP AMH 10529E.)

vesicles having a characteristic teardrop shape begin to appear. The eruption may be preceded by a prodrome of flu-like symptoms lasting several days. The eruption usually begins on the head or trunk and spreads centrifugally. Intraoral lesions are common and may be the first sign of infection. Conjunctival lesions also may occur. The skin vesicles rapidly crust, and all stages of lesions from macule to crust can be found during the period of eruption. Mucous membrane lesions rapidly ulcerate and are most often seen in this stage. Since lesions are limited to the epithelium, scarring is not a characteristic of the infection. Pruritus and scratching, however, can lead to secondary bacterial infections with subsequent scarring.

Complications are uncommon, especially in healthy children. Pneumonia and encephalopathies are among the more common serious sequelae. Reye's syndrome, a serious noninflammatory encephalopathy accompanied by fatty changes in the liver, has been seen following varicella in healthy children and is associated with a high rate of morbidity and mortality. The syndrome usually develops within several days of apparent recovery. Evidence linking ingestion of salicylates during viral infections to the development of Reye's syndrome has led to the printing of statements on aspirin labels warning against use of the medication during respiratory infections or chickenpox in children or teenagers.

Congenital varicella syndrome with cutaneous scarring, limb hypoplasia, and eye abnormalities may develop if fetal infection occurs during the first or second trimester of pregnancy, making varicella a very serious infection for the pregnant woman. Disseminated disease with a high degree of mortality may develop in infants whose mothers are infected just prior to birth or in infants without passive immunity who are exposed to VZV at an early age.

Unlike other herpesvirus infections of man, VZV usually results in symptomatic disease, although in very mild cases the infection may go undiagnosed. Reinfections are apparently common, but second cases of chickenpox rarely occur and appear to be linked to failure to develop an adequate immune response following primary infection.

Zoster, popularly referred to as shingles, is the recurrent manifestation of latent VZV infection. With reactivation, a vesicular eruption may occur on the skin or mucous membrane supplied by the affected sensory ganglion. The eruption is characteristically unilateral, involving one to three dermatomes. Lesions are most frequently seen in the area supplied by the thoracic or lumbar ganglia, although facial and cervical lesions are also common (Fig. 38.8). The lesions are similar to those of chickenpox, and new lesions may appear for several days. Constant or intermittent pain, described as stabbing, burning, or ach-

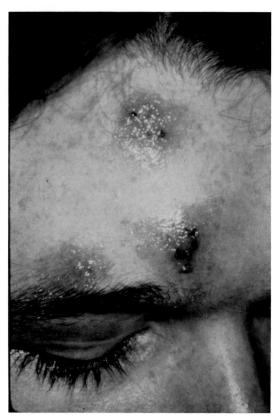

Figure 38.8: Herpes zoster involving the ophthalmic branch of the trigeminal nerve. Note that the lesions do not cross the midline.

ing, is characteristic of zoster and may appear during the prodromal period, during the acute stage, during healing, or even after the lesions disappear. Oral zoster from latent infection established in the trigeminal ganglion is sometimes seen. Unless lesions are present at the midline where an obvious delineation occurs, it may be confused with the more common RIHS. Dental pathosis, an infrequent complication of oral zoster, may manifest as osteonecrosis of the jaw, tooth exfoliation, severe periodontitis, scarring of the skin, and root resorption.

Zoster can occur at any age, including during infancy, but it is most common in older individuals or those who are immunosuppressed or immunocompromised. Immunocompetent patients rarely have more than a single episode of zoster. Patients whose immune systems are compromised often develop severe disease and are subject to multiple and frequent recurrences. Zoster is a frequent cause of both morbidity and mortality in posttransplant patients and patients with malignant disease or AIDS.

Epidemiology.   Varicella is primarily a disease of childhood and is common throughout the world.

It has been estimated that most adults in the United States have acquired either a clinical or subclinical infection by the time they reach middle age. In temperate regions, chickenpox has a higher incidence of occurrence in the winter and spring. Infection is acquired through contact with infected secretions from patients with varicella or zoster, but unlike variola (smallpox), scabs are relatively uninfective. It is generally accepted that once the lesions are fully scabbed, the individual is no longer contagious; however, this is not proven, and contact with individuals at high risk of infection should be avoided. Since infectious virus may be present in respiratory secretions for several days before eruption of the lesions of chickenpox, children are likely to transmit infection to susceptible contacts during this period. This probably accounts in large part for the high rate of contagion seen with varicella.

The risk of zoster increases sharply with increasing age in individuals over 50. The individual with zoster is infectious and can transmit virus to susceptible contacts. Grandparents are often the source of infection for a child who becomes the index case for an outbreak of chickenpox.

Diagnosis. The distinctive symptoms of varicella and zoster facilitate their diagnosis on a clinical basis. Laboratory confirmation is required only when confusion exists or the illness is atypical. Laboratory diagnosis can be made most effectively by identification of viral antigen in vesicular fluid. Two methods are available: direct immunofluorescence and countercurrent immunoelectrophoresis. Serodiagnosis is still done by complement fixation techniques, although newer methods such as EIA are also available.

Prevention and Treatment. Since VZV is shed in respiratory secretions prior to the appearance of varicella lesions, preventing the spread of infection among children is difficult. A live attenuated virus vaccine to the Oka strain of VZV has been developed and tested extensively in both normal and immunocompromised children in the United States as well as Europe and Japan. This vaccine is licensed in Japan and in Europe but has not yet been approved for use in the United States. The vaccine has been shown to be effective in preventing disease in healthy children and reducing the severity if not preventing the disease in children with leukemia. One obstacle to licensure is the vaccine's potential for causing zoster after successful immunization; however, studies of immunized children have shown zoster due to vaccine virus to be mild and to occur at what is probably a lower rate than that following natural varicella infection. It is expected that the vaccine will initially be recommended for children at risk of severe disease, particularly those undergoing chemotherapy for leukemia.

Treatment of varicella and zoster is usually symp-tomatic. Pruritus may be treated with topical calamine solutions or by the administration of trimeprazine. Pain associated with zoster may be treated with analgesics. Zoster immune globulin (ZIG) is effective in reducing the severity of varicella in immunocompromised children and adults. Both acyclovir and interferon are somewhat effective in the management of VZV disease. Interferon may be effective in reducing postherpetic neuralgia associated with zoster. Treatment is warranted in immunocompromised patients and in patients with severe primary or recurrent disease.

Cytomegalovirus

Human cytomegalovirus (CMV) infections cause a variety of illnesses ranging from inapparent to devastating and life-threatening. There are several closely related strains of this virus which are antigenically distinct from the other herpesviruses and, like VZV, remain primarily cell associated. The virion is about 180 to 250 nm in diameter. In cell culture, it replicates very slowly and only in diploid fibroblast cells, where it produces characteristic plaque-like cytopathic effects.

Pathogenesis and Clinical Manifestations. Infections are most often asymptomatic; however, CMV also causes clinical disease in the form of congenital birth defects, a mononucleosis syndrome in healthy children and adults, and a variety of opportunistic infections in immunosuppressed or immunocompromised patients. The pathologic lesion involves necrosis and pathognomonic cellular alterations. The infected cells become very large (*cytomegalo*) and have nuclei that contain huge eosinophilic inclusion bodies; the cytoplasm also may be swollen and vacuolated. Whether or not clinical manifestations are present, latent infection is established with the potential for reactivation at a later time. The exact site of CMV latency is still to be determined, but evidence now implicates T-lymphocytes and monocytes.

CMV congenital infection occurs when the mother has a primary CMV infection, reactivation of a latent infection, or reinfection with another CMV strain during pregnancy. Infection of the fetus may range from asymptomatic to severe viscerotropic or neurotropic disease, sometimes resulting in death or a variety of neurologic sequelae in survivors. Table 38.2 lists possible manifestations of congenital, natal, and postnatal CMV infection. Risk of severe disease is greatest in infants whose mothers have a primary CMV infection during pregnancy. Evidence suggests that the most apparent developmental defects are seen in infants infected during the third trimester of pregnancy. Manifestations of intrauterine infection may not be appar-

Table 38.2: Manifestations of Congenital or Perinatal Cytomegalovirus Infection*

Congenital	Natal
Low birth weight	Failure to thrive
Hepatomegaly	Hepatomegaly
Splenomegaly	Splenomegaly
Jaundice	Pneumonitis
Petechiae, purpura	Anemia
Pneumonitis	Chronic gastroenteritis
Microcephaly	
Hydrocephalus	*Postnatal*
Cerebral calcification	Pneumonitis
Deafness	Hepatomegaly
Blindness	Gray pallor
Chorioretinitis	Splenomegaly

*Adapted with permission of the publisher from L. R. Stanberry and L. A. Glasgow: Viral Infections of the Fetus and Newborn. In *Virology,* edited by D. A. Stringfellow. Upjohn Co., Kalamazoo, Mich., 1983.

ent until early childhood, when neuromuscular disturbances, progressive auditory damage, impairment of vision, and defects of amelogenesis may become evident. Infants may also be infected perinatally, usually from contact with CMV in breast milk or in vaginal secretions during birth. Perinatal infection is almost always asymptomatic, although it occasionally may result in clinical disease. However, like congenital infection, it is associated with prolonged viral shedding in saliva and urine.

CMV mononucleosis is manifested as malaise with fever, often accompanied by a mild hepatitis. It is the most common form of heterophile antibody-negative mononucleosis and is usually associated with primary infection. Table 38.3 contrasts the signs and symptoms of CMV and EBV mononucleosis. CMV hepatitis is usually a mild disease but may be severe with icterus.

Reactivation of latent CMV infection with associated virus shedding is common but rarely leads to symptomatic disease except in individuals with depressed cell-mediated immune responses. These patients may develop a variety of opportunistic CMV infections, including chorioretinitis, pneumonia, gastrointestinal disease, and meningoencephalitis. Ninety percent of patients with AIDS develop active CMV infections at some point, and up to one fourth develop either sight- or life-threatening disease. Posttransplant patients who are immunosuppressed to prevent transplant rejection are also at risk of disease from reactivation of latent CMV infection or from a primary infection acquired by seronegative recipients of seropositive tissues. Efforts aimed at avoiding the transplanting of seropositive tissues to seronegative individuals has significantly reduced the incidence of such infections.

Epidemiology. Human CMV has a worldwide distribution, and most people become infected at some time during their life. Individuals of higher socioeconomic background are more likely to reach adulthood without exposure, and in some populations 30% to 50% of adults are seronegative. There are multiple strains of CMV, and a single individual may be infected repeatedly, and apparently becomes persistently infected by each strain. Acquisition of infection is age-related and normally occurs either within the first 2 years of life or in early adulthood. The majority of infections are asymptomatic, but the infected individual sheds virus in secretions for several months to several years following infection. Periodic reactivation of the latent virus can also result in shedding and possible transmission. Reactivation is most

Table 38.3: Comparison of EBV and CMV Mononucleosis

	EBV Mononucleosis	CMV Mononucleosis
Symptoms	Malaise Sore throat	Malaise
Signs	Fever Cervical lymphadenopathy Pharyngitis	Fever
Hematologic findings	Mononuclear lymphocytosis >50% mononuclear cells >10% atypical lymphocytes	Lymphocytosis (commonly occurs) 12%–55% atypical lymphocytes
Heterophile antibodies	Transient appearance	Negative
Specific antibodies for diagnosis	IgM anti-VCA IgG anti-VCA Anti-EA/D Anti-EA/R Anti-EBNA	IgM anti-CMV IgG anti-CMV
Age range	10–30 years	18–66 years

Note: VCA = viral capsid antigen, EA = early antigen, EBNA = Epstein–Barr nuclear antigen.

likely in individuals whose immune systems are suppressed, although other factors may precipitate the reappearance of the latent virus. CMV has been isolated from saliva, urine, breast milk, blood, semen, and vaginal secretions. The infection is commonly transmitted in oral secretions, sexually, and from mother to infant.

CMV is the major cause of congenital viral infection in the United States and other developed countries. It is estimated that between 30,000 and 44,000 infants are born in the United States each year with congenital CMV infection. Of these infants, 3,000 to 4,000 are born with symptomatic disease and, if they survive, are usually severely debilitated (see Table 38.2). Of those who appear healthy at birth, approximately 15% later develop significant handicaps, including deafness or neurological problems. Fetal infection is likely to result if the mother experiences a primary CMV infection, reactivation of latent virus infection, or reinfection during pregnancy. Although reactivation of latent CMV or maternal reinfection can lead to fetal infection, symptomatic disease rarely develops. The infant at greatest risk of developing severe CMV disease is one whose mother has a primary CMV infection during pregnancy. CMV infection of the infant during or after birth rarely results in symptomatic disease but may on occasion.

Because so many young children are infected with CMV, day care centers are prime spots for transmission of this virus. Saliva-contaminated toys and urine-soiled diapers are major sources of virus. Toddler-aged children are particularly susceptible to infection as they explore their surroundings and interact with their peers. Serological studies have documented seroconversion of children in day care centers, day care workers, and the parents of children who acquired CMV infection while in day care.

The rise in CMV seroprevalence in young adults can be attributed to sexual transmission or to infection acquired from young children. In these individuals, the virus is recovered more frequently from semen and cervical secretions than from urine and other secretions. CMV has also been transmitted via blood transfusions and kidney transplants.

Diagnosis. Virus can be isolated from urine, saliva, and other secretions, and viral culture is the most sensitive method for detecting the presence of virus in secretions. The detection of CMV IgM antibody is suggestive of primary CMV infection, although anti-CMV IgM persists for as long as 6 months following infection and may be produced following recurrent infection as well. The major use for serological assay is to document prior infection with CMV (seropositivity) or susceptibility to CMV (seronegativity). A variety of methods are available, including complement fixation and indirect hemagglutination techniques. Commercial kits for EIA are also available and often are employed in diagnostic laboratories.

Prevention and Treatment. The individuals who are at high risk of serious CMV infection are seronegative women of childbearing age and immunocompromised patients. A live attenuated vaccine has been developed and has undergone preliminary testing, but a number of unanswered questions regarding latency, reinfection, and oncogenicity make it unlikely that it or any other CMV vaccine will be licensed within the near future.

Seronegative women who anticipate a pregnancy are at significant risk of developing primary CMV infection and possibly transmitting that infection to their infants. Good personal hygiene, including hand washing, has been shown to be effective in preventing infection in nurses caring for CMV-infected infants or renal transplant or dialysis patients. Since CMV is transmitted sexually, a seronegative woman should avoid a pregnancy if her spouse develops a primary CMV infection, until she seroconverts or her spouse is no longer shedding virus.

Since CMV is present in saliva, there is a risk of CMV transmission in the dental office. However, if infection control protocols are followed, particularly the use of masks and protective eyewear, it is highly unlikely that CMV infection would result. Primary CMV disease following transfusions and organ transplantations can be avoided if seronegative recipients are not given blood or transplants from seropositive donors.

Interferon has not been shown to be effective in the treatment of CMV disease. Likewise, acyclovir is relatively ineffective in blocking CMV replication. A derivative of acyclovir, ganciclovir, is an effective inhibitor of CMV and is the most potent antiviral agent for treatment of CMV disease. It has been shown to be efficacious in treating CMV retinitis and gastroenteritis in AIDS patients, but relapse frequently occurs once the medication is discontinued. Neutropenia and bone marrow suppression are associated toxic side effects complicating its use.

Epstein–Barr Virus

Epstein–Barr virus (EBV) is 180 to 200 nm in diameter and is characterized by its transforming and lymphoproliferative effects and the ability to cause abnormal lymphocytes in infected individuals.

Pathogenesis and Clinical Manifestations. EBV is usually acquired via the oral route and the virus replicates initially in the oropharyngeal epithelium and the epithelium of the salivary gland ducts. From these tissues the infection progresses to include the B-lymphocytes in the adjacent lymphoid tissues and ultimately in the circulation. EBV infections may be subclinical or may manifest in a variety of acute or malignant illnesses, depending on the age, health, and national origin of the individual. Children most often develop asymptomatic infections but may present with tonsillitis or occasionally infectious mononucleosis. Approximately half of primary EBV infections in adolescents and young adults present as infectious mononucleosis (IM). EBV is being associated increasingly with malignant and lymphoproliferative disease. It has been linked with the development of both Burkitt's lymphoma, seen in African children, and nasopharyngeal carcinoma, most commonly seen in Oriental males. Although EBV is implicated as the causative agent of these disorders, this relationship has not been confirmed. Some cases of thymic carcinoma also have been associated with EBV. An increasing number of lymphomas in both immunocompromised and apparently immunologically competent individuals are being attributed to EBV infections. The lymphoproliferative lesions of hairy leukoplakia seen in many HIV-infected patients contain EBV antigens and may be the result of EBV infection (see Chap. 47).

EBV infectious mononucleosis typically manifests with headache, fever, cervical lymphadenopathy, mild to severe pharyngitis with or without exudate, and malaise (see Table 38.3 for a comparison of EBV IM and CMV mononucleosis). Onset is usually insidious and follows an incubation period of a few weeks to several months. Lymphadenopathy is an outstanding characteristic of the disease and involves the anterior and posterior cervical chains as well as the axillary, epitrochlear, inguinal, mediastinal, and mesenteric nodes. Splenomegaly develops in half of the patients, with 10% to 15% showing signs of hepatomegaly and approximately 5% jaundice. Hepatocellular enzymes are elevated in 80% to 90% of the patients. A rash may occur, but almost invariably develops in patients treated with ampicillin. Palatal petechiae are more common, although not diagnostic, and are seen as multiple lesions at the junction of the hard and soft palate. The illness is usually self-limiting and resolves over a period of 2 to 3 weeks although symptoms may recur following apparent recovery. The sore throat persists 3 to 5 days and then diminishes, but the fever is more prolonged and usually lingers 10 to 14 days.

Mononuclear lymphocytosis is common in EBV IM, and atypical lymphocytes are considered a hematologic hallmark of the disease. Approximately 90% of patients will be heterophile antibody positive at some point during the clinical illness, and these nonspecific antibodies have traditionally been used for diagnosing EBV IM (see Diagnosis).

Complications of EBV IM are relatively rare but include autoimmune hemolytic anemia, thrombocytopenia, and neurological complications. Splenic rupture, a potentially fatal complication, is rare. Since it is most often seen following trauma, participation in contact sports is to be avoided following the diagnosis of EBV IM.

A chronic form of mononucleosis became increasingly prevalent in the 1980s, and EBV was implicated as the cause due to the associated elevation of EBV-specific antibodies characteristic of acute EBV disease. Whether EBV, HHV-6, or an as yet unidentified or unrelated agent is responsible for this chronic syndrome remains to be elucidated. It is quite possible that the elevation of EBV-specific serologic markers is due to a nonspecific immunological response. The most notable symptom of the syndrome is an unexplained chronic fatigue, lasting for a year or more. Other symptoms are variable and may be cyclical. Regardless of the relationship between EBV and the syndrome recognized as "chronic mononucleosis," severe, chronic EBV infections do occur. These either begin as proven primary EBV infections or are associated with grossly abnormal EBV antibody titers; they have histological evidence of major organ involvement and have EBV proteins or nucleic acid in affected tissues.

Reactivation of EBV infection with viral shedding apparently occurs quite frequently in most if not all seropositive individuals, but this virus production is rarely associated with any symptoms. Lymphoproliferative lesions linked to EBV infection are being diagnosed more frequently and are likely to be a manifestation of reactivated latent infection.

Epidemiology.   EBV has a worldwide distribution, with 80% to 95% of adults in most populations being seropositive. The virus is shed in saliva and is transmitted primarily by oral secretions, as suggested by its designation as the "kissing disease." Infection occurs before 5 years of age in populations where hygiene is poor or socioeconomic factors increase the opportunity for exposure to EBV-containing saliva. In other populations, the first exposure to virus usually occurs in adolescence or young adulthood. Infection in young children is typically asymptomatic or very mild. Teenagers and young adults are more likely to manifest symptomatic disease, although only about half of the infections at this age are clinically evident.

While transmission of infection generally requires fairly intimate oral contact, saliva-contaminated fomites such as shared drinking glasses or dental aerosols can disseminate the virus. However, studies of college students in the '50s, '60s, and early '70s showed that susceptible roommates of index cases were no more likely to develop infection than other susceptibles on the campus. In families, about 10% of exposed susceptibles develop EBV infection. Although oral transmission is the major mode of spread, EBV has also been transmitted by blood transfusions.

Table 38.4: Interpretation of EBV Antibody Profiles

Indicative of:	Detection of Antibodies to:					
	HA	VCA, IgM	VCA, IgG	EA/D*	EA/R†	EBNA
Acute primary infection	+	+	+	+/0	+/0	0
Recent primary infection	0	0	+	+/0	+/0	+/0‡
Prior infection (seropositive)	0	0	+	0	0	+
Reactivation of infection	0	0	+	+/0	+/0	+
Susceptibility, EBV seronegative	0	0	0	0	0	0

*Anti-EA/D appears at 3 to 4 weeks after the onset of IM and persists for 3 to 6 months.

†Anti-EA/R appears 2 weeks to several months after onset and persists for 2 months to more than 3 years.

‡Anti-EBNA appears 3 to 4 weeks after onset and persists for life.

The high incidence of asymptomatic infection as well as the prolonged oropharyngeal shedding following infection allows this virus of low contagiousness to spread unsuspected within a population. It is rare to be able to identify the source of infection, particularly in the case of a socially active teenager or young adult. EBV continues to be shed in oropharyngeal secretions for 5 to 18 months following infection. Although EBV IM patients commonly curb their social activities for 4 to 6 weeks, they remain contagious for months. In addition, 10% to 25% of normal healthy seropositive adults can be expected to be shedding EBV in their saliva at any point in time. The frequency of excretion is even greater in transplant patients or patients with leukemia or lymphomas.

Diagnosis. Diagnosis of EBV IM is usually made by a combination of clinical, hematological, and serological criteria. The frequency of this infection in adolescents and college students suggests the diagnosis when the typical clinical manifestations appear in individuals in this age group. A presumptive diagnosis can then be made if Paul–Bunnell heterophile antibodies and atypical lymphocytes are detected. If a more definitive diagnosis is required, antibodies to specific EBV antigens, such as Epstein–Barr nuclear antigen (EBNA), viral capsid antigen (VCA) and early antigen (EA), can be determined via indirect immunofluorescence or EIA. Table 38.4 presents an interpretation of EBV antibody profiles. The syndrome designated as "chronic mono" has been diagnosed in part based on the presence of antibodies to EA which once were thought to be relatively short lived; however, data now suggest that these antibodies may persist for 3 years or longer following EBV IM in apparently healthy individuals.

Prevention and Treatment. Infection with EBV probably cannot be avoided given the customary social interactions of life. Transmission in the dental office can be avoided, however, by using recommended barriers to prevent inoculation of mucous membranes with virus-containing aerosols. Given the oncogenic potential of this virus, a live, attenuated vaccine likely would be associated with too much risk, but a component vaccine is a future possibility.

Supportive and symptomatic treatment is usually all that is required in EBV IM. Acyclovir has been used successfully in treating EBV infections including hairy leukoplakia in HIV patients. It has also been effective in management of patients with other severe or chronic EBV disease.

Human Herpesvirus Type 6

First reported in 1986, HHV-6 is the newest member of the herpesvirus family recognized to infect humans. It was isolated initially from six patients with lymphoproliferative disorders. HHV-6 appears to be typical of the herpesviruses in size, morphology, and overall polypeptide content. The DNA genome of HHV-6 is unique but has been reported to share some homology with human CMV. Although at first a virus without a disease, seroepidemiologic evidence strongly suggests that HHV-6 is the causative agent of exanthem subitum, and the virus has been isolated from infants with this disease. Additionally, serologic evidence has linked a mild, nonspecific, afebrile illness in adults with HHV-6 infection.

Exanthem subitum, commonly known as roseola infantum, is an acute febrile exanthematous disease of early childhood. It most frequently occurs in infants and children between 6 months and 3 years, and although apparently contagious, usually occurs sporadically without evidence of exposure. The incubation period appears to be 9 to 15 days. The disease begins with a fever of 104°F or higher which persists for 3 to 5 days. As the fever dissipates, a maculopapular rash appears and lasts from a few hours to a few days. The sequence of rash following fever is clinically diagnostic. Other symptoms are unusual although mild, non-specific respiratory symptoms may precede the fever. Complications other than febrile convulsions are rarely seen.

Seroepidemiological studies in Japan have indicated that almost all infants seroconvert, with or without evidence of roseola, prior to 1 year of age, and that approximately 80% of adults have antibody to the virus. A study in the United States indicated seropositivity of 56% to 79% of adults tested, depending on the assay used.

ADDITIONAL READING

Baichwal, V. R., and Sugden, B. 1988. Latency Comes of Age for Herpesviruses. Cell, **52,** 787.

Corey, L., and Spear, P. G. 1986. Infections with Herpes Simplex Viruses. N Engl J Med, **314,** 686.

Forbes, B. A. 1989. Acquisition of Cytomegalovirus Infection: An Update. Clin Microbiol Rev, **2,** 204.

Ginsberg, H. S. 1988. Herpesviruses. In *Virology,* Ed. 2, p. 161, R. Dulbecco and H. S. Ginsberg. J. B. Lippincott Co., Philadelphia.

Kieff, E., Dambaugh, T., Heller, M., et al. 1982. The Biology and Chemistry of Epstein–Barr Virus. J Infect Dis, **146,** 506.

Manzella, J. P., McConville, J. H., Valenti, W., et al. 1984. An Outbreak of Herpes Simplex Virus Type I Gingivostomatitis in a Dental Hygiene Practice. JAMA, **252,** 2019.

Niederman, J. C. 1982. Infectious Mononucleosis: Observations on Transmission. Yale J Biol Med, **55,** 259.

Reed, E. C., and Meyers, J. D. 1987. Treatment of Cytomegalovirus Infection. Clin Lab Med, **7,** 831.

Stagno, S., Pass, R. F., Cloud, G., et al. 1986. Primary Cytomegalovirus Infection in Pregnancy: Incidence, Transmission to Fetus, and Clinical Outcome. JAMA, **256,** 1904.

Straus, S. E. 1988. The Chronic Mononucleosis Syndrome. J Infect Dis, **157,** 405.

Weller, T. H. 1983. Varicella and Herpes Zoster. N Engl J Med, **309,** 1362.

Yow, M. D. 1989. Congenital Cytomegalovirus Disease: A NOW Problem. J Infect Dis, **159,** 163.

39

Poxviruses

Virginia A. Merchant and Gretchen B. Caughman

Poxviruses (family Poxviridae) are large, complex DNA viruses that produce diseases characterized by vesicular skin lesions in man and animals. Members of this virus family share a common internal antigen and are divided into specific genera and species by differences in morphology, specific antigens, and natural hosts.

Poxviruses that cause disease in man belong to the *Orthopoxvirus* and *Parapoxvirus* genera or remain unclassified. Among those with primary human hosts are the unclassified poxvirus, molluscum contagiosum virus; and the orthopoxviruses, variola (smallpox) and vaccinia, the vaccine strain (perhaps a human strain of cowpox). Animal poxviruses that are sometimes transmitted to man include the unclassified monkey poxviruses, Yaba and Tanapox; the orthopoxvirus, cowpox; and the parapoxviruses: paravaccinia virus of cattle, which causes milker's nodules, and the orf virus of sheep and goats, which causes contagious pustular dermatitis.

Properties of Poxviruses

The virions are brick-shaped and asymmetrical, measure $300 \times 240 \times 100$ nm, and have a whorled surface. An outer membrane composed of tubular lipoprotein subunits encloses an internal dumbbell-shaped core of DNA and protein, and there are two lateral (elliptical) bodies of unknown nature (Fig. 39.1). Unlike the envelopes of other viruses, which are acquired by budding of some modified cell membrane, the poxvirus's outer membrane is totally viral in origin and arises by de novo synthesis.

Poxvirus replication occurs entirely within the cytoplasm of the infected cell and begins with attachment and phagocytic engulfment of the virus particles. The virus is uncoated in a two-stage process and viral gene expression occurs in three phases: immediate early, delayed early, and late. In the first phase, a virion RNA polymerase present in the core interacts with the encased viral DNA to transcribe immediate early

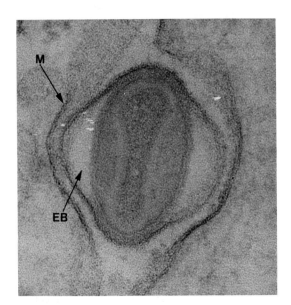

Figure 39.1: Thin section of intact vaccinia virus particle showing the inner nucleic acid core and surrounding membranes. The elliptical body (*EB*) on either side of the nucleoid causes a prominent central bulging of the virion. The particle is located between two cells (*M*) (× 120,000). (Reproduced with permission from S. Dales: The Uptake and Development of Vaccinia Virus in Strain L Cells Followed with Labeled Deoxyribonucleic Acid. *J Cell Biol,* **18,** 51, 1963.)

mRNAs which direct the synthesis of proteins necessary for the release of viral DNA from the core. After these final uncoating events, delayed early gene expression ensues, resulting in the synthesis of enzymes necessary for viral DNA replication and some structural proteins. After viral DNA replication has begun, late mRNAs are synthesized and translated to produce structural proteins and enzymes that will be incorporated into the progeny virions.

Poxvirus virions are generally resistant to drying and thus can remain viable on fomites for long periods of time, an important factor in the epidemiology of many poxvirus diseases. They have been shown to be inactivated by autoclaving, heating for 10 minutes at 60°C, or exposure to quaternary ammonium compounds, iodophors, chlorine, and formaldehyde.

Smallpox

Throughout history, smallpox was one of the great plagues of mankind and as such had tremendous medical, cultural, and political impact. Due to the success of a worldwide confinement and immunization effort, the World Health Organization declared the world free of smallpox in May 1980.

Epidemiology. Prior to its global eradication, smallpox was readily transmitted from one patient to another by contaminated fomites, via respiratory secretions, and by the exudates from lesions of the skin and mucous membranes. The virus is particularly resistant to drying and could persist for months in contaminated bedding and clothing, thus facilitating its transmission.

Pathogenesis and Clinical Manifestations. Two clinical forms of smallpox are recognized: variola major and variola minor, or alastrim. Variola major is an acute exanthematous–enanthematous disease with a case-fatality rate of 10% to 25%. Virus is readily transmitted from patient to patient by vesicle fluid, contaminated fomites, or respiratory secretions. It enters the body via the respiratory tract, where it replicates in the mucosa and regional lymph nodes. This is followed by a transient viremia that disseminates virus to the internal organs. The incubation period of 12 to 14 days ends in a second viremia and the onset of a prodromal phase lasting 3 to 6 days and characterized by fever, chills, vomiting, severe backache, and prostration. At the end of the prodrome, a generalized, centrifugally spreading rash begins on the back. The single crop of lesions progresses through stages from papule to vesicle, pustule, scab, and scar over a period of 2 to 4 weeks (Fig. 39.2). The scars, referred to as pocks, remain since the corium is involved and actually necroses. Patients who survived severe cases were disfigured by these pocks, particularly on the face, where the density of lesions was often greatest. Lesions occur intraorally and are most commonly seen on the buccal mucosa, tongue, and soft palate.

Alastrim, or variola minor, follows the same pattern of symptoms but is less severe and has a case-fatality rate below 1%. The skin lesions are more superficial and of shorter duration. Although epidemiological evidence indicates that the two disease

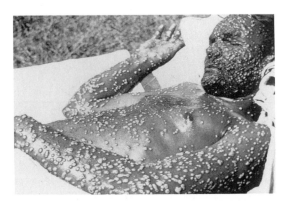

Figure 39.2: Distribution of smallpox rash on the trunk, head, and arms. (Reproduced with permission from R. T. D. Emond: *A Colour Atlas of Infectious Diseases.* Wolfe Publishing, London, 1974.)

forms are distinct entities, it has not been possible to distinguish the differences in the viruses responsible for them. Natural infection in either clinical form normally results in lifelong immunity for those who survive the disease.

Vaccinia

Vaccinia virus is an orthopoxvirus whose origin is unknown but which has been successfully used for immunization against smallpox. In its present form, it differs both from cowpoxvirus, originally used for vaccination against smallpox, and from variola virus. However, due to the presence of shared antigens, all orthopoxviruses are serologically similar, and the development of immunity following infection with any of these viruses provides protection against infection with the other orthopoxviruses.

Variolation and Vaccination. The inoculation of susceptible individuals with material taken from smallpox lesions, referred to as variolation, was originally practiced hundreds of years ago in Asia and Africa and found its way to Europe in the 1700s. This practice generally produced a milder disease than natural smallpox infection but was risky. In 1796 Dr. Edward Jenner, who is recognized for developing the first viral vaccine, performed the first vaccination by a physician of a nonrelative or nonservant. After years of observing the protection against smallpox acquired by dairymaids and farmers who had been infected with cowpox, as well as the successful immunization of his own son, Dr. Jenner successfully immunized a young boy against smallpox with material from a cowpox lesion.

The vaccination technique requires the introduction of the vaccine into the skin by scratching or by intradermal injection. Following primary vaccination, a papule develops in about 3 days, followed by a vesicle, then a pustule, a scab, and finally a scar about 1 cm in diameter. Both humoral and cellular immunity develop within 5 days of immunization, but the level of protection wanes over a period of 3 to 10 years. As long as immunity remains, revaccination produces an accelerated reaction with a response varying from a small papule to a vesicle.

Routine vaccination of children in the United States was discontinued in 1971 and is now no longer practiced anywhere in the world. In the United States, the vaccine is available only for immunization of laboratory workers exposed to orthopoxviruses and of military personnel. The Department of Defense continues to vaccinate all active duty personnel as a preventive measure against the employment of orthopoxviruses as a biological warfare agent.

Complications from Vaccination. Complications of smallpox vaccination are not uncommon and approached 1 per 1,000 as a serious complication, with the risk of death 1 per million. The type of complication that develops often depends on the age of the recipient, his/her immune status, or the presence of dermatological disease.

Progressive vaccinia, or vaccinia necrosum, is a very serious complication that is most commonly seen in patients with impaired immunity. Viral multiplication is not terminated by the host response, and the infection spreads, causing a progressive cellular necrosis. Treatment with methisazone coupled with vaccinia immune globulin has proved effective.

Postvaccinal encephalitis is apparently a hypersensitivity reaction associated with primary vaccinations and occasionally with revaccination. It is fatal in 10% to 30% of cases and causes permanent neurological sequelae in survivors.

Eczema vaccinatum is a common complication seen in infants or in eczematous contacts of vaccinees. When raw or broken skin is exposed to vaccinia, a condition similar to smallpox infection occurs, resulting in multiple lesions and scarring (Fig. 39.3).

Congenital vaccinia of the fetus has been reported following vaccination of pregnant women. Less severe complications are more commonly seen in vaccinees and include generalized vaccinia, frequent exanthematous reactions, and accidental autoinoculation of other body sites (Fig. 39.4). In addition, infection can be transmitted to nonimmune contacts of vaccinees.

At one time, smallpox vaccination was sometimes recommended as a "prophylactic treatment" for individuals who experienced frequent recurrences of herpes simplex viral infection. The rationale was that the vaccination stimulated the immune response and prevented further recurrences. There is no validity to

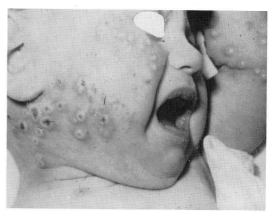

Figure 39.3: Eczema vaccinatum in a child. (AFIP 53-728 10).

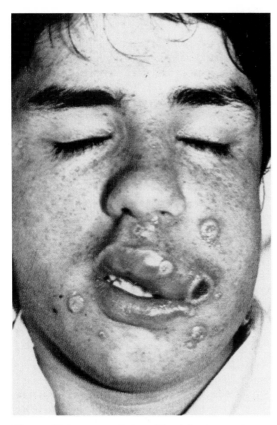

Figure 39.4: Autoinoculation of face following vaccination. (Reproduced with permission from R. T. D. Emond: *A Colour Atlas of Infectious Diseases.* Wolfe Publishing, London, 1974.)

this hypothesis, and smallpox vaccination is only effective in preventing infection with the orthopoxviruses.

Global Eradication of Smallpox. The Smallpox Eradication Program for the global elimination of smallpox was initiated by the World Health Organization (WHO) in January 1967. In October 1977 the last naturally acquired case of smallpox occurred, in Somalia, Africa, and in May 1980 WHO declared the world free of smallpox. Smallpox is the first important disease of man to be completely eradicated.

The success of this program was in large part due to certain biological features of variola virus, which Fenner has listed as follows. First, smallpox is a severe disease and was easily recognized. Second, subclinical infection does not occur. Third, smallpox is much less contagious than many other viral diseases, requiring direct or at least face-to-face contact with infected individuals or their secretions on fomites. The infected individual is not infectious prior to the development of the rash, and viral shedding is proportional to rash severity. Fourth, unlike many other viral diseases, there is no carrier state in smallpox, and recurrence of

clinical disease does not occur. Fifth, there is only one serotype of variola virus, and the development of immunity following infection with any of the orthopoxviruses protects against infection with all others. Sixth, the availability of a heat-stable vaccine allowed more effective immunization of susceptible individuals in remote areas where refrigeration was unavailable or unreliable. Seventh, smallpox had a pronounced seasonal fluctuation, allowing efforts to control outbreaks with mass immunizations during periods when the disease was least prevalent. Finally, variola virus only causes disease in man; therefore, no animal reservoir of smallpox virus exists with the potential for reintroduction to the human population.

Today, variola virus only exists as laboratory smallpox virus stocks in two laboratories, one at the United States Public Health Service Centers for Disease Control in Atlanta, Georgia, and the other at the Research Institute for Viral Preparations, Moscow, U.S.S.R.

Vaccinia as an Immunization Vector. Recent studies have shown that foreign genes can be inserted into the large vaccinia genome in such a way that their presence does not interfere with the virus's subsequent infectivity and replication. Moreover, the proteins coded for by the foreign genes are expressed along with the vaccinia viral proteins in infected cells. Hybrid viruses containing the genes for major antigens from unrelated pathogens such as herpes simplex virus, hepatitis B virus, and *Plasmodium* sp. have been constructed and vaccination with these hybrids has induced immune responses against the nonvaccinial proteins in experimental animals. Thus, there may be considerable potential for the use of vaccinia as an immunization vector for a variety of human and animal diseases. However, in view of the rare but serious complications of vaccination, it is likely that new attenuated vaccinia strains will need to be developed for such purposes.

Treatment. When smallpox was a clinical problem, patients and their contacts were given methisazone to reduce the severity or prevent infection. Administration of vaccinia immune globulin was also effective in further reducing the severity of symptoms. In some cases, rifampin was found to be useful.

Molluscum Contagiosum

Molluscum contagiosum is caused by an unclassified poxvirus, the molluscum contagiosum virus. It is usually seen as a benign, chronic infection of the skin or mucous membranes.

Epidemiology. Molluscum contagiosum infection is worldwide in distribution but is not commonly seen in immunocompetent individuals in developed countries. When the disease occurs, it is most fre-

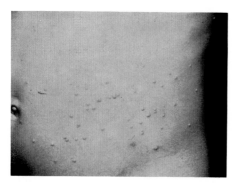

Figure 39.5: Cutaneous manifestations of molluscum contagiosum (AFIP 7757-37).

quently seen in children. Although it is an occupational hazard of athletes, barbers, beauticians, and masseurs, the infection is more commonly seen as a sexually transmitted disease in adults. The virus is transmitted via direct skin contact as well as by fomites.

Pathogenesis and Clinical Manifestations. Following an incubation period of 14 to 50 days, characteristic papular lesions appear (Fig. 39.5). These are typically smooth-surfaced, firm, spherical, and umbilicated. The lesions, ranging from 2 to 5 mm in diameter, may be flesh-colored, white, pearly gray, or yellow. A milky exudate may be expressed from the central depression. The lesions are characterized by a markedly abnormal epidermis with extensive downgrowth of infected cells bearing large eosinophilic cytoplasmic inclusion bodies, Henderson–Paterson inclusions. Inflammation is usually not seen. The papules frequently occur without other symptoms, although some patients complain of tenderness, pain, or pruritus.

Lesions may be single or multiple and generally number under 20, although hundreds of lesions sometimes occur. Patients with impaired immune function often experience multiple lesions and widespread infection. Disseminated molluscum contagiosum is frequently seen in AIDS patients. Since the disease in adults is often transmitted sexually, it is commonly manifested on the lower abdominal wall, inner thighs, and genitalia but can occur on any skin or mucous membrane surface. Oral mucous membrane lesions are occasionally seen. In children, the lesions are most often present on the face, trunk, and proximal extremities.

The lesions heal without scarring in about 2 months if secondary infection is absent. However, since spread to adjacent areas is common, the disease may persist from 6 months to 3 years. Antibodies against the virus are never produced in approximately one third of patients, and second outbreaks are common.

Diagnosis. The lesions are most often confused with common warts. Clinical diagnosis can be confirmed by microscopic examination of scrapings or the exudate of lesions. The cytoplasmic inclusions of molluscum contagiosum can be detected by staining smears with Wright's, Giemsa, or gram stain. Biopsy sections stained with hematoxylin–eosin also readily demonstrate the inclusion bodies. Fluorescent antibody techniques to demonstrate the presence of viral antigen are sometimes used.

Prevention and Treatment. Avoidance of contact is the most effective method of prevention. The use of barriers in dentistry prevents exposure if lesions are present intraorally or on the face.

Spontaneous resolution of lesions usually occurs, but treatment may shorten duration and decrease transmission to others or via autoinoculation. Surgical curettage or cryotherapy is the recommended treatment. Corrosive chemicals such as podophyllin or phenol may cause scarring.

Animal Poxviruses Contagious to Man

Two orthopoxviruses of animals are recognized as contagious to man. These are cowpox and monkeypox. Cowpox is normally acquired by milking infected cows. It usually appears on the hands and resembles primary vaccinia. Monkeypox causes an infection in man that is clinically indistinguishable from smallpox but is much less contagious. Human cases seen in Africa are probably acquired from contact with infected wild animals, particularly monkeys. The infection has been seen in monkeys in captivity but never in the wild.

Another poxvirus transmitted from cows to man is paravaccinia virus of cattle, which belongs to the genus *Parapoxvirus* and causes milker's nodules. This virus causes lesions on exposed surfaces, manifested initially as watery, painless small papules that grow over a period of a week into red to brown or purplish nodules 1 to 2 inches in diameter. Usually the primary lesions are not painful and subside within 4 to 8 weeks. Immunization with vaccinia protects against cowpox but not against infection with paravaccinia virus.

Orf virus of sheep and goats also is a parapoxvirus that sometimes infects man. In sheep, it causes a contagious papulovesicular eruption confined to the lips and surrounding skin, referred to as "scabby mouth." The disease in man acquired by contact with infected animals occurs as a single lesion that eventually heals without scarring. Human-to-human transmission has not been documented.

Two unidentified poxviruses that cause infection primarily in African monkeys also may be transmitted to man. Yaba monkey tumor virus causes benign histiocytomas in monkeys and in man. Tanapox virus has been associated with papulovesicular lesions accompanied by an acute fever in man. It is thought to be transmitted via an arthropod to man.

ADDITIONAL READING

Behbehani, A. M. 1983. The smallpox story: Life and death of an old disease. Microbiol Rev, **47,** 455.

Brown, S. T. 1984. Molluscum contagiosum. In *Sexually Transmitted Diseases,* p. 507, edited by K. K. Holmes, P-A. Mardh, P. F. Sparling, and P. J. Wesner. McGraw-Hill, New York.

Fenner, F. 1982. Global eradication of smallpox. Rev Infect Dis, **4,** 916.

Jawetz, E., Melnick, J. L., and Abelberg, E. A. 1989. Poxvirus Family. In *Review of Medical Microbiology,* Ed. 18, p. 409. Lange Medical Publications, Los Altos, Calif.

Laskaris, G., and Sklavounou, A. 1984. Molluscum contagiosum of the oral mucosa. Oral Surg, **58,** 688.

Mackett, M., and Smith, G. L. 1986. Vaccinia virus expression vectors. J Gen Virol, **67,** 2067.

White, D. O., and Fenner, F. J. 1986. Poxviruses. In *Medical Virology,* Ed. 3, p. 433. Academic Press, New York.

40

Picornaviruses and Coronaviruses

Gretchen B. Caughman and Virginia A. Merchant

Picornaviridae

The family Picornaviridae is one of the largest of all virus families; almost 200 host-specific picornaviruses have been associated with infections in humans, and numerous others cause disease in a variety of animals. There are four genera of picornaviruses: *Enterovirus, Rhinovirus, Aphthovirus,* and *Cardiovirus.* Only the first two are significant causes of disease in man. The *Enterovirus* genus currently consists of 69 member viruses, including the polioviruses, coxsackieviruses, and hepatitis A virus. Despite the name, enteroviruses are not major causes of gastrointestinal disease. Rather, they tend to cause asymptomatic or mild infections of the enteric tract but may disseminate to other organs and in some instances cause serious disease. The *Rhinovirus* genus has over 100 members which cause the common cold. In contrast to the enteroviruses, which are stable at pH 3 and thus can withstand the acidity of the stomach, the rhinoviruses are acid labile and do not survive ingestion. Also, the rhinoviruses replicate more efficiently at the slightly cooler temperatures of the nasal mucosa rather than at core body temperature, a fact that helps to explain their confinement to the nose and upper respiratory tract.

Properties of Picornaviruses

The name picornavirus reflects the fact that the viruses in this family are physically the smallest (*pico* = small) RNA viruses. The typical virion consists of a naked icosahedral capsid, 22 to 30 nm in diameter, which contains one molecule of single-stranded, positive-sense RNA with a protein, VPg, covalently linked to its 5' end. The capsid is composed of 32 capsomers made up of molecules of three proteins, VP1, VP2, and VP3; another protein, VP4, is associated internally with the inner surface of the capsid and the viral RNA.

Picornaviruses initiate infection by attachment to specific host cell surface receptors that are found in much greater number in susceptible than in nonsusceptible tissues. After penetration, the virion is uncoated to release its single molecule of positive-sense RNA into the cytoplasm. This RNA is monocistronic in

379

that it is translated into one large polyprotein which is subsequently cleaved to form proteins with RNA-dependent RNA polymerase activity for nucleic acid replication and the virion structural proteins. RNA replication first involves the synthesis of negative-sense complementary copies of the genomic RNA, which then serve as templates for transcription of positive-sense RNA. The small viral protein, VPg, is covalently linked to the 5′ terminus of each RNA produced and apparently acts as a primer for the replication complexes. VPg is cleaved from about half of the positive RNA molecules, and only those RNAs retaining VPg are encapsidated in the progeny viral particles. Picornavirus replication is quite rapid and several hundred viral particles are produced per infected cell. Most of these particles are released from the cell in a burst that is accompanied by death and lysis of the cell. Most species of picornaviruses readily cause cytopathologic effect (CPE) in cell cultures which include intranuclear alterations, small intranuclear inclusion bodies, formation of a large eosinophilic mass in the cytoplasm, nuclear pyknosis, and cell rounding.

Enteroviruses

There are 69 viruses (serotypes or species) of the genus *Enterovirus* known to infect man. Historically they were divided into three groups: polioviruses, coxsackieviruses, and echoviruses. Although these names are being retained for the original viruses, more recently identified enteroviruses are designated simply by "enterovirus" and a number. One such virus, enterovirus 72, is more commonly known as hepatitis A virus and is discussed in Chapter 48.

Pathogenesis. Enteroviruses have been associated with the full spectrum of viral diseases. Table 40.1 lists the syndromes associated with some of the more common enteroviruses. Many enteroviruses cause similar disease manifestations, although the majority of enteroviral infections are asymptomatic. After ingestion, the virus undergoes replication in the epithelial or lymphoid cells of the alimentary tract. Virus drains into the local lymphatics and from there into the blood. This transient viremia serves to transport the virus to other susceptible tissues and organs. Clinical symptoms, when they occur, usually are referable to infection of these secondary target organs; enteroviruses are not responsible for serious gastrointestinal disease. Viral replication in these secondary target tissues may provide another source of virus to be fed back into the bloodstream, resulting in a more prolonged viremia. However, it should be emphasized that most enteroviral infections do not progress

Table 40.1: Diseases Caused by Enteroviruses

Syndrome	Common Causative Viruses
Rashes	
Maculopapular exanthem	Echoviruses 2, 4, 9, 11, 16, 19, 25 Coxsackieviruses B1, 5
Hand-foot-and-mouth disease	Coxsackieviruses A4, 5, 7, 9, 10, 16 Coxsackieviruses B2, 5
Herpangina	Coxsackieviruses A1–6, 8, 10, 16, 22 Coxsackieviruses B1–5 Echoviruses 3, 6, 9, 17, 25, 30
Respiratory	
Colds	Coxsackieviruses A21, 24 Echoviruses 11, 20
Conjunctivitis	Enterovirus 70 Coxsackievirus A24
Myocarditis	All coxsackieviruses B Coxsackieviruses A4, 16 Echoviruses 9, 22
Epidemic pleurodynia	Coxsackieviruses B
Meningitis	Many enteroviruses
Paralysis or encephalitis	Polioviruses 1, 2, 3 Enteroviruses 70, 71 Coxsackieviruses A7, 9 Coxsackieviruses B1–5 Echoviruses 6, 9
Hepatitis A	Enterovirus 72
Pancreatitis	Coxsackieviruses B

through this entire sequence of events, and asymptomatic or very mild disease usually results.

Epidemiology. Enteroviruses have a worldwide distribution. Children are the prime targets of infection since they have not been previously exposed. Outbreaks are common among young children and may occur as overt epidemics, since many infections are asymptomatic. Immunity following natural infection is permanent but monotypic, and since multiple serotypes can produce similar syndromes, a single individual may have repeated episodes of a particular syndrome. Reinfection with the same serotype occurs, but circulating antibodies normally prevent a second episode of disease manifestations. Natural immunity is acquired with increasing age, assuming exposure to the various serotypes occurs. Enteroviral infections are endemic year round in the tropics and semitropics but are most prevalent during the summer and autumn in temperate climates.

Transmission of most enteroviral infections is by the fecal–oral route, making these infections more prevalent in areas where crowding, poor hygiene, and other opportunities for fecal contamination exist. Those infections which have a respiratory component also are spread by this route, although fecal shedding tends to be more prolonged. Viruses that cause conjunctivitis are primarily spread by fingers, fomites, and ophthalmological instruments.

Susceptibility patterns for poliovirus infections (q.v.) have changed markedly since the advent of the polio vaccines. In the prevaccine era, almost all children were infected in early childhood without paralysis. As the standard of living and hygiene improved, infection was often delayed until later childhood or adulthood, when the development of paralytic disease is more frequent. Following the introduction of the attenuated trivalent oral vaccine (Sabin), the disease virtually disappeared in developed countries except in isolated communities, where inadequate immunization usually can be proven. Since the vaccine virus is a live virus, it replicates in the gastrointestinal tract and is shed in feces. Rarely, these attenuated strains revert to a neurovirulent form and can cause paralysis, but the incidence is much less than what would occur in the absence of immunization for poliovirus infection.

Diagnosis. It is often difficult to establish the diagnosis of an enteroviral infection in an isolated case. During an epidemic, diagnosis can usually be made presumptively, based on knowledge that a particular virus is circulating in the community.

Specific enteroviral diagnosis requires special procedures and is available only in a limited number of laboratories. The method of choice for diagnosis is by isolation of the virus in tissue culture. Since there are so many serotypes, serodiagnosis is costly and laborious, and in most cases is only important from an epidemiological standpoint.

If an enteroviral infection is presumed, confirming the diagnosis can prevent the unnecessary use of antibiotics and provide reassurance during an epidemic. If the presentation is of a more serious nature, i.e., affecting the nervous, respiratory, or cardiovascular system, the need for a specific diagnosis is more critical.

Prevention and Treatment. There are no specific antiviral agents available for treatment of enteroviral infections (q.v.). Management is supportive and symptomatic. In the case of paralysis of respiratory muscles, respirators are necessary to maintain breathing. Heat is usually helpful in relieving pain from myalgias.

There are two vaccines available for immunization against infection with the three polioviruses. The original vaccine, the inactivated poliovaccine (IPV) or Salk vaccine, was introduced in 1955. In 1962, an improved live-virus (attenuated) vaccine, the oral poliovaccine (OPV) or Sabin vaccine, was introduced in the United States. The trivalent OPV, producing immunity against all three poliovirus serotypes, is the currently recommended vaccine. This vaccine is preferred in most cases to the IPV, since the former elicits both a secretory and humoral immune response and induces an immunity that is more long-lasting. OPV is recommended for infants in four doses (at 2 months, 4 months, 6 months, and 18 months). At present, boosters are not recommended except for certain health care workers exposed to virus, those traveling to highly endemic foreign areas, or in the event of an epidemic. OPV is not routinely recommended for previously unimmunized adults or for anyone who is immunodeficient or immunosuppressed.

Enteroviruses: Poliovirus

There are three poliovirus types (types 1, 2, and 3) that have the potential to cause illness ranging from subclinical to an acute form involving the central nervous system and producing symptoms of aseptic meningitis, encephalitis, or paralysis (designated poliomyelitis, polio, or infantile paralysis).

Pathogenesis and Clinical Manifestations. As was described generally for enteroviruses, following ingestion the virus first replicates in lymphatic tissue such as tonsils and the lymphoid tissues of the gut, and after spreading to the deeper lymph nodes it initiates viremia when it reaches cells of the reticuloendothelial system. In subclinical infection, it may remain there to elicit a primary antibody response, or replicate and give rise to a second viremia that corresponds to the clinical symptoms known as abortive poliomyelitis. Virus may be excreted in the stool and nasopharynx at this point. With a persistent viremia, virus may pass through capillary walls and enter the central nervous system. The virus also may spread to the central nervous system from peripheral ganglia by transmission along nerve fibers. Destruction of neurons, especially in the anterior horn cells of the spinal cord and motor nuclei of the pons and medulla, results in paralysis. In the medulla and brain stem (bulbar polio) this reaction can be fatal since respiratory or cardiac failure can result. In fatal cases, necrosis of a number of visceral organs and lymph nodes is apparent, in addition to involvement of cerebellar nuclei, the hypothalamus, the thalamus, and cerebral hemispheres. Also, edema and lymphocytic and neutrophilic infiltration are pronounced in the perivascular spaces.

The incubation period of poliomyelitis can vary from 1 to 7 weeks, but most clinical cases develop within the second week. The disease may proceed through several stages or terminate at any point. It is important to realize that paralysis is a relatively infrequent complication of poliovirus infection. A profile

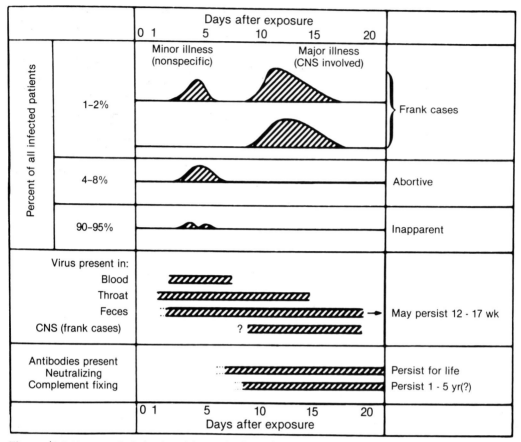

Figure 40.1: Times at which the clinical forms of poliomyelitis appear, correlated with the times at which virus is present in various sites and with development and persistence of antibodies. The high incidence of subclinical poliovirus infection is also noted. (Reproduced with permission from D. M. Horstmann: *Yale J Biol Med,* **36,** 5, 1963.)

of the clinical forms of poliovirus infection is shown in Figure 40.1. The majority of infections (90% to 95%) are actually subclinical. Another 4% to 8% are manifested as a minor illness, sometimes referred to as "abortive poliomyelitis." This presentation was referred to as the "summer grippe" in polio's heyday. It is characterized by fever, headache, sore throat, inflammation of the pharynx, listlessness, anorexia, vomiting, and pain in the muscles of the abdomen. The illness occurs following an incubation period of several days and may last only a few hours to as long as 48 hours.

Approximately 1% of cases proceed to neurological manifestations 1 to 2 weeks after exposure. Aseptic meningitis is more common and has as its primary symptom stiffness of the neck and back. Frank paralysis occurs in about 0.1% of all poliovirus infections. Paralytic poliomyelitis may present as a biphasic course, with the "major" illness following the "minor" illness. This is more common in children, with the two phases being separated by a symptom-free period

of several days. Paralysis is flaccid, and loss of motor function is characteristically asymmetric and noncontiguous. Breathing may be impaired when the diaphragm and intercostal muscles are involved. Paralytic poliomyelitis is rarely fatal unless the respiratory muscles are affected. Progression of paralysis usually halts after several days to a week and coincides with the patient becoming afebrile. Recovery of function then begins and is generally related to the degree of paralysis. Most reversible damage disappears within a month.

Bulbar paralysis occurs when muscle groups innervated by the cranial nerves are affected. The ninth and tenth cranial nerves are most frequently involved, with resulting pharyngeal paralysis, but any of the cranial nerves can be affected. Although rarely affected, involvement of the fifth nerve causes difficulties with swallowing. The facial nerve is affected in approximately 50% of cases. Bulbar paralysis is most common in adults and occasionally occurs in the absence of spinal involvement. Patients who have had tonsillectomies, even in the remote past, are more susceptible to the development of bulbar paralysis.

Complications include encephalitis with seizures, respiratory failure, aspiration pneumonia, pulmonary embolism, myocarditis, gastrointestinal hemorrhage, paralytic ileus, and gastric dilatation.

Other Enteroviral Infections

The enteroviruses cause a variety of clinical manifestations. Most infections are asymptomatic or subclinical, which explains the apparent sporadic disease often seen in young children. Rashes, upper respiratory tract infections, and undifferentiated febrile illnesses with or without respiratory symptoms are common manifestations of enteroviral infections.

Exanthems and Enanthems

Enteroviral exanthems are usually mild diseases with little morbidity, but they may be confused with other rash diseases having more serious implications. Exanthems may be rubelliform, roseoliform, herpetiform, or petechial.

Rubelliform rashes caused by various echoviruses are most commonly seen in the summer months. Echovirus 9 causes a rash that occurs simultaneously with fever. It begins on the face and may spread down the body. It is sometimes difficult to distinguish from rubella; however, there is no pruritus or lymphadenopathy. Other echoviruses have also been associated with rubelliform rashes. Coxsackievirus A9 usually causes a herpetiform rash but sometimes presents as a maculopapular eruption that begins on the face and trunk. Lesions are most numerous on the distal portions of the limbs. Fever, malaise, and lymphadenopathy may also occur, making the symptomatology very similar to that of rubella.

Roseoliform exanthems mimic roseola in that the rash appears as the fever resolves. Echovirus 16 is the most common cause of this infection. The fever lasts 24 to 36 hours and is followed by salmon-pink macules on the face and upper chest. The rash lasts 1 to 5 days and sometimes occurs simultaneously with the fever rather than after defervescence.

Herpetiform rashes include the enanthems of herpangina and hand-foot-and-mouth disease, which will be discussed below. Sometimes coxsackievirus A9 or echovirus 11 will cause a generalized vesicular eruption on the head, trunk, and extremities. Unlike other generalized vesicular diseases such as chickenpox, the lesions do not form scabs but regress after the vesicular stage. Intraoral vesicular lesions such as those shown in Figure 40.2 are sometimes seen alone or in conjunction with an exanthem.

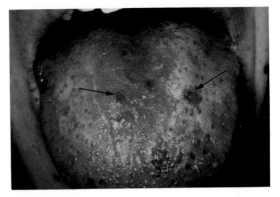

Figure 40.2: Vesicular lesions of the tongue caused by coxsackievirus.

Herpangina is a vesicular enanthem of the fauces and soft palate. Following a 2- to 10-day incubation period, there is a sudden onset of fever (37 to 40°C), which may be accompanied by vomiting, myalgia, and headache. Sore throat and pain on swallowing are the most prominent symptoms. Initially there is erythema and possibly a tonsillar exudate. The enanthem begins as macules, progresses to form vesicles, and then ulcerates (Fig. 40.3). The lesions, usually two to six in number, most commonly occur on the free-hanging margin of the soft palate but may be located anywhere in the posterior oral cavity. The fever and other systemic symptoms subside within a few days, although the ulcers may persist for up to a week. Most cases are caused by coxsackieviruses A1 to 6, 8, 10, 16, and 22 and less commonly by coxsackieviruses B1 to 5 or echoviruses 3, 6, 9, 17, 25, and 30.

Acute lymphonodular pharyngitis is a variant of herpangina. The lesions appear as tiny nodules of packed lymphocytes which recede without vesiculation or ulceration, unlike typical herpangina. This presentation is usually attributed to coxsackievirus A10.

Hand-foot-and-mouth disease is caused by a va-

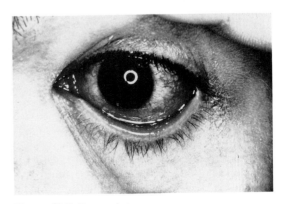

Figure 40.3: Herpangina.

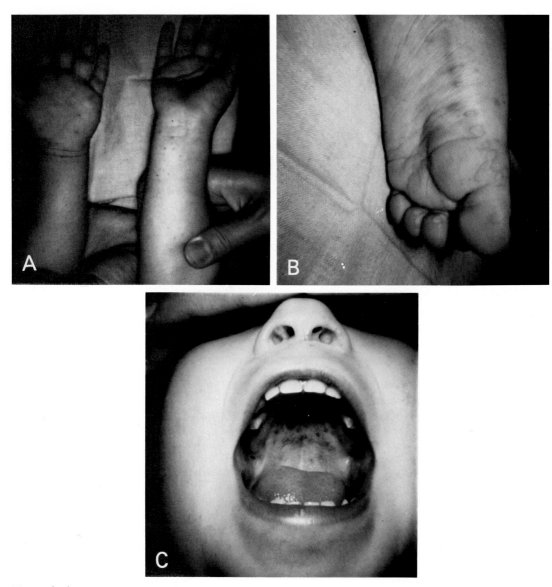

Figure 40.4: (**A**) Ventral surface of hands and forearms of a child with hand-foot-and-mouth disease. Note multiple vesicular lesions, some of which have ulcerated. (**B**) Foot of child with hand-foot-and-mouth disease. Vesicular lesions are present along the plantar surface of the foot and toes. (**C**) Palate of child showing initial lesions of hand-foot-and-mouth disease. Some vesicular lesions have ruptured, leaving painful ulcerated areas that are surrounded with erythematous halos. Note the exudative rhinitis in the nares. This occurred at the same time as the onset of the lesions. (Photos courtesy of Dr. R. V. McKinney. Reproduced with permission from R. V. McKinney: Hand, Foot, and Mouth Disease: A Viral Disease of Importance to Dentists. *J Am Dent Assoc,* **91,** 122, 1975. Copyright by the American Dental Association. Reprinted by permission.)

riety of coxsackieviruses (A5, A7, A9, A10, A16, B2, B5) but is most frequently due to A16. It is characterized by lesions occurring in the oral cavity and on the hands and feet (Fig. 40.4). The vesicular oral lesions are located primarily on the buccal mucosa and tongue but sometimes occur on the hard palate and may occur anywhere in the oral cavity. These fre-

quently ulcerate. Although the oral lesions are almost always present, hand and foot lesions only occur in approximately 75% of patients. These cutaneous lesions are located on the extensor surfaces as well as the palms and soles and frequently are painful. These lesions are vesicular and do not scab. Lesions may occur more proximally, i.e., on the buttocks of small children. The infection has an incubation period of 3 to 6 days, is mild, and lasts for a week or less. Initially there may be a low-grade fever. Children complain of a sore mouth or throat. Complications are extremely rare.

Petechial and purpuric rashes may be caused by echovirus 9 or coxsackievirus A9. These hemorrhagic exanthems may be confused with meningococcemia, particularly if there are also symptoms of meningitis.

Respiratory Syndromes

Acute respiratory disease may be caused by most enteroviral subtypes. Sore throat, cough, or coryza are characteristic, making these illnesses difficult to differentiate from other upper respiratory tract infections caused by viruses. Coxsackieviruses A21 and A24 are often associated with symptoms of the common cold but with an accompanying fever. Echovirus 11 produces an infection characterized by sore throat, coryza, cough, and sometimes fever.

Conjunctivitis

Acute hemorrhagic conjunctivitis has been associated with both enterovirus 70 and coxsackievirus A24. Epidemics caused by either or both of these viruses have occurred primarily in the Far East but have been seen throughout the world. Sporadic cases also occur and may be confused with adenoviral conjunctivitis. The conjunctivitis begins abruptly, is usually bilateral, and reaches its peak on the first day (Fig. 40.5). The symptoms are burning, a foreign body sensation, and ocular pain, with hemorrhages, photophobia, swelling of the eyelids, and a watery discharge. Recovery usually begins on the second or third day with complete resolution within 10 days.

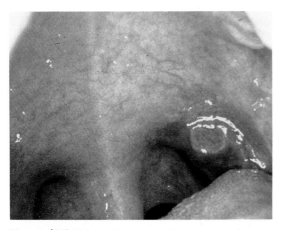

Figure 40.5: Echoviral conjunctivitis.

Epidemic Pleurodynia

This is an acute febrile illness characterized by sharp, spasmodic pain in the chest or upper abdomen. It is most often due to group B coxsackieviruses and probably results from muscle invasion by the viruses following viremia. The intensity of pain varies but resembles a "stitch" in the side. Most individuals are ill for 4 to 6 days. Children usually have less severe symptoms than adults.

Myocarditis and Pericarditis

Infection of the pericardium and/or myocardium varies in severity from asymptomatic to fulminant disease with intractable heart failure and death. Infections tend to be particularly severe in the neonate, who usually acquires the infection from an infected mother, although nosocomial infections have occurred. Older children and adults usually recover uneventfully, although permanent myocardial injury sometimes occurs. The disease frequently occurs 1 to 2 weeks following an upper respiratory tract illness. Symptoms include dyspnea, precordial pain, fever, and malaise. All group B coxsackieviruses, coxsackieviruses A4 and 16, and echoviruses 9 and 22 have been associated with myocarditis and pericarditis.

Meningitis, Encephalitis, and Paralytic Disease

Enteroviruses cause approximately 70% of the cases of aseptic meningitis in which the etiological agent is identified. Most, although not all, enteroviral serotypes have been associated with meningitis. Children under 1 year of age are at greatest risk of enteroviral meningitis and are more likely to have permanent neurologic sequelae. Although infection also occurs in older children and adults, their recovery is usually uneventful and without sequelae.

Encephalitis is not a usual manifestation of enteroviral infection but does occur and accounts for 11% to 22% of cases of viral encephalitis. Coxsackievirus types A9, B2, B5, and echovirus types 6 and 9 have been most often associated with encephalitis. Older children and young adults usually recover completely.

A mild flaccid motor paralysis occasionally results from infection by enteroviruses other than polioviruses. Paralysis is rarely permanent, and in fact muscle weakness is a more common manifestation.

Hepatitis and Pancreatitis

Hepatitis A caused by enterovirus 72 is discussed in Chapter 48. Group B coxsackieviruses have been associated with pancreatitis and have been implicated as a precipitating agent, if not actually the cause, of at least some cases of type I diabetes mellitus.

Rhinoviruses

The 100+ members of the genus *Rhinovirus*, along with viruses from several other families, are responsible for one of the most frequent disease syndromes of man: acute afebrile upper respiratory disease, or the common cold. Although common colds are almost never serious or life-threatening diseases, they nonetheless account for a tremendous amount of discomfort as well as school and work absenteeism.

Pathogenesis and Clinical Manifestations. Viral infection and replication is confined to the ciliated columnar epithelium of the nose; virus can be isolated from the nasopharyngeal secretion but not from other secretions or body fluids. The common cold caused by rhinoviruses typically presents as rhinorrhea with nasal obstruction and a sore, scratchy throat. Fever is uncommon. Cough and hoarseness may occur and are more pronounced in individuals who smoke. The symptoms appear to be related to inflammatory responses to the infection rather than to direct viral-induced pathology. The incubation period is 24 to 48 hours, and symptoms rarely last more than a week, peaking on the third or fourth day. Complications are rare and include sinusitis, otitis media, and precipitation of asthmatic attacks.

Epidemiology. Rhinoviruses are worldwide in distribution and are one of the most frequent causes of disease in man. Rhinovirus colds are most common in the early fall and late spring in temperate climates. Transmission is primarily via autoinoculation after hand-to-hand contact or contact with fomites and is common among members of a family or others who share objects that become contaminated by handling.

Diagnosis. Rhinovirus infections usually are diagnosed as a common cold on the basis of clinical presentation. They generally are not differentiated from colds caused by other viruses, such as coronaviruses.

Prevention and Treatment. The only treatment for colds is symptomatic. Nasal decongestants and cough suppressants when needed are appropriate in managing the infection. Aspirin or acetaminophen will ameliorate any associated systemic symptoms. Antibiotics, on the other hand, are not appropriate except in cases of secondary bacterial sinusitis or otitis media.

The prospect for a vaccine to prevent rhinoviral colds is limited. Experimental vaccines have been shown to be effective in reducing symptoms following exposure; however, the multiplicity of rhinoviral serotypes precludes developing a single vaccine to prevent what is actually a rather innocuous disease. Frequent hand washing and the use of disinfectants on contaminated objects are the most effective methods to prevent transmission of infection.

Picornaviruses of Animals That May Infect Man

Foot-and-mouth disease of cattle is caused by *Aphthovirus*. This is primarily a zoonotic infection and is rare in man; however, the infection may be transmitted to man via contact with infected cattle or their byproducts. The disease is characteristically biphasic and follows an incubation period of 2 to 18 days. Lesions initially appear at the site of contact on the skin or mucous membranes, ulcerate, and heal without scarring. Following a period of quiescence, fever occurs and is followed by a more generalized outbreak of vesicles, particularly on the soles, palms, digits, and interdigital areas. Lesions in the oral cavity may be seen on the tongue, pharynx, and lips, and are usually painful. The virus can be isolated in tissue culture, or diagnosis can be confirmed by serology.

Encephalomyocarditis virus of mice, a *Cardiovirus*, has occasionally been implicated in aseptic meningitis in man. It is probably contracted through contact with contaminated mouse feces.

Coronaviridae

Members of the family Coronaviridae are associated with diseases of the respiratory tract, enteric tract, and liver in a variety of mammals and birds. Coronaviruses have not been convincingly linked with serious disease in these organ systems in man, but they are an important cause of the common cold syndrome and may be the etiological agent of some cases of viral gastroenteritis.

Properties. The coronaviruses are enveloped, helical viruses, approximately 100 nm in diameter, with a genome consisting of a single linear molecule of positive-sense, single-stranded RNA. The envelope is covered with unusually large, club-shaped peplomers which give the appearance of a solar corona.

The coronavirus genome is expressed in a unique manner. The genomic RNA is translated directly and one of the products is an RNA-dependent RNA polymerase, which then transcribes a full-length complementary RNA. This full-length RNA is then used as a template to transcribe a 3'-coterminal nested set of subgenomic mRNAs, each of which is translated into a unique protein. Replication takes place in the cytoplasm and the envelope is acquired as the particle buds through the membranes of the endoplasmic reticulum and Golgi apparatus.

Pathogenesis and Clinical Manifestations. The virus enters the upper respiratory tract and remains confined to the epithelium there. The symptoms are those of the typical cold with a profuse nasal discharge. Adult volunteers inoculated intranasally with coronaviruses most commonly develop coryza, nasal congestion, sneezing, and sore throat. Less frequent symptoms include headache, cough, muscular or general aches, chills, and fever. Colds caused by coronaviruses are of shorter duration (6 to 7 days) than those caused by rhinoviruses, but the incubation period is longer (about 3 days). Coronaviruses are less often associated with symptomatic respiratory infections in children than in adults, unlike many other respiratory viral infections. Asymptomatic infections are apparently common, and children as well as adults have neutralizing antibodies to coronaviruses. Lower respiratory tract disease, especially in infants, has occasionally been attributed to coronavirus infection.

Coronaviruses have been associated with diarrheal diseases in mammals, and they may be a cause of viral gastroenteritis in man. Coronavirus-like particles have been seen via electron microscopy in stool specimens of patients with acute nonbacterial gastroenteritis and necrotizing enterocolitis. Enteric coronaviruses may be responsible for some cases of acute nonbacterial gastroenteritis and necrotizing enterocolitis in infants.

Epidemiology. Coronavirus infections occur primarily in the winter and early spring, and large outbreaks occur every few years in adults as well as children. It has been estimated that 10% to 30% of all colds are due to coronaviruses. Neutralizing antibodies to coronaviruses have been detected in up to 50% of children aged 5 to 9 years and in 70% of adults.

Diagnosis and Treatment. Specific diagnosis is generally not necessary. Diagnostic assays via complement fixation, hemagglutination inhibition, and EIA are available for epidemiological purposes.

No specific treatment is available. The use of decongestants, antihistamines, or analgesics may relieve some of the symptoms and make the affected individual more comfortable.

ADDITIONAL READING

Ginsberg, H. S. 1988. Coronaviruses. In *Virology*, Ed. 2, p. 216, R. Dulbecco and H. S. Ginsberg. J. B. Lippincott Co., Philadelphia.

Ginsberg, H. S. 1988. Picornaviruses. In *Virology*, Ed. 2, p. 193, R. Dulbecco and H. S. Ginsberg. J. B. Lippincott Co., Philadelphia.

Gwaltney, J. M. 1982. Rhinovirus. In *Viral Infection of Humans: Epidemiology and Control*, p. 491, edited by A. S. Evans. Plenum, New York.

Modlin, J. F. 1990. Coxsackievirus and Echovirus and Newer Enteroviruses. In *Principles and Practice of Infectious Diseases*, Ed. 3, p. 1367, edited by G. L. Mandell, R. G. Douglas, Jr., and J. E. Bennett. Churchill Livingstone, New York.

Modlin, J. F. 1990. Poliovirus. In *Principles and Practice of Infectious Diseases*, Ed. 3, p. 1359, edited by G. L. Mandell, R. G. Douglas, Jr., and J. E. Bennett. Churchill Livingstone, New York.

White, D. O., and Fenner, F. J. 1986. Coronaviruses. In *Medical Virology*, Ed. 3, p. 541. Academic Press, Inc., Orlando, Fla.

41

Orthomyxoviruses

Virginia A. Merchant and Gretchen B. Caughman

Members of the family Orthomyxoviridae are the etiological agents of influenza, an acute infectious respiratory disease that has occurred for centuries in epidemic and pandemic forms. There are three influenza virus types: types A, B, and C. Infections with type A or B result in the classic flu syndrome; type C generally causes a very mild cold-like disease. Influenza (caused by A or B) is characterized by the sudden onset of fever, malaise, headache and myalgia. In uncomplicated cases, disease is self-limiting and recovery occurs within a week. However, severe morbidity and mortality can occur in elderly or medically compromised patients. Influenza type A is further divided into a number of subtypes based on the antigenicity of the glycoprotein peplomers. Type A subtypes have been isolated from a variety of animals and birds as well as man.

Properties of Influenza Viruses

Influenza viruses are 90 to 100 nm in diameter, enveloped viruses with segmented, negative-sense RNA genomes enclosed in helical capsids. They are roughly spherical (Fig. 41.1), although filamentous forms are often observed in fresh clinical isolates. Types A and B have eight discrete RNA segments, type C has seven segments. The envelope is studded with glycoprotein peplomers which have hemagglutinin (HA or H) and neuraminidase (NA or N) activities. In types A and B, these activities are on separate peplomers, while in type C a single type of peplomer has both functions. The HA and NA peplomers play very important roles in the epidemiology of influenza virus infections and are discussed further below. The inner aspect of the viral envelope is coated with molecules of matrix (M) protein, and several internal proteins, particularly the RNA-dependent RNA polymerases are associated with the nucleocapsid.

Influenza viruses attach to cell receptors by their hemagglutinin peplomers, enter into phagocytic vesicles, and are uncoated. Transcription of the viral genome takes place in the nucleus in a unique manner. A viral endonuclease cleaves the 5′-terminus (or "cap") from existing cellular mRNAs and these act

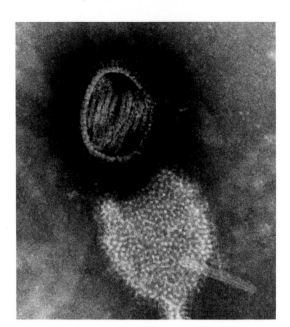

Figure 41.1: Influenzavirus A2. The nucleocapsid is loosely coiled inside an envelope that consists of protein and lipid, and to which glycoprotein spikes are attached. (Courtesy of M. V. Nermut; reproduced with permission from *Zinsser Microbiology,* Ed. 17, edited by W. K. Joklik, H. P. Willett and D. B. Amos. Appleton–Century–Crofts, New York, 1980.)

as primers for viral mRNA synthesis by the RNA-dependent RNA polymerase which was associated with the infecting virion. Six of the eight RNA segments of types A and B each code for a single protein. The other two segments produce complementary RNAs that are spliced, each yielding two mRNAs that are translated in different reading frames. During the second phase of RNA synthesis, full-length daughter genomic RNA segments are transcribed and subsequently encapsidated by nucleoprotein (NP). Viral assembly occurs at the cell membrane, where the nucleocapsids associate with the layer of M protein underlying areas of peplomer-coated cytoplasmic membrane. In order to be infectious, each daughter virus particle must have at least one of each of the eight RNA segments; how this directed assembly is accomplished is not understood. The assembly process is imperfect in that many defective viral particles are produced that do not contain all of the required RNA segments. The virions are enveloped and released by budding.

The antigenic characteristics of influenza viruses have particular epidemiological significance and warrant detailed discussion. A particularly distinctive feature of influenza is the frequency with which antigenic changes due to mutation occur, particularly in type A and less so in type B. Mutations occur in all the RNA segments, but the effects are most dramatic in the segments coding for the peplomers, the hemagglutinin and the neuraminidase, since changes in these segments may alter the peplomers' antigenicities and thus alter the host's immune response and susceptibility to viral infection. Antibodies produced during infection against these two peplomers are subsequently protective, since the hemagglutinin is utilized by the virion for attachment to host cells during infection and the neuraminidase is utilized for the release of the virus from the infected cell. Thus, antihemagglutinin antibodies prevent attachment to host cells and antineuraminidase antibodies decrease infectious virus release and also shorten the duration of illness. However, when sufficient antigenic changes occur in the neuraminidase and particularly in the hemagglutinin, individuals previously infected are not immune because their antibodies no longer recognize the peplomer structures. Two types of antigenic change have been documented for influenza virus. The first, known as antigenic drift, is due to point mutations in the nucleotides of the RNA segments and occurs in both types A and B. The resulting changes in antigenicity may be sufficient to render a portion of the population susceptible to new infection; if that portion is large enough, an epidemic can result. The second type of change, antigenic shift, is a major change in the antigenicity of type A viruses and is actually due to acquisition of a new (different) subtype of hemagglutinin or neuraminidase RNA segment. The subtypes of influenza type A hemagglutinin and neuraminidase are designated by number, i.e., H1, H2, N1, N2, etc. Twelve hemagglutinin and nine neuraminidase subtypes have been recognized. Antigenic shift occurs via genetic reassortment when two different type A subtypes infect one host cell, and, in the assembly and budding process, a daughter virion acquires, for instance, seven RNA segments from one subtype but the hemagglutinin gene segment from the other subtype. This is particularly devastating if the new hemagglutinin subtype is one that previously had been primarily in animal populations rather than in man. Such antigenic shifts result in epidemics, or, as occurred in 1918 and 1957, can cause worldwide pandemics, since very few individuals are immune. Therefore, antigenic patterns of the virions are important factors in the spread of influenza.

Influenza

Pathogenesis and Clinical Manifestations. Infection is transmitted mainly by respiratory droplets. In uncomplicated influenza the virus spreads directly in the mucous membranes of the respiratory tract; viremia is not common. During influenza there may be sufficient cell damage to the ciliated respiratory epithelium that breakdown products of dying cells are absorbed into the bloodstream, producing a toxic effect. This may explain why the symptoms are more severe than would be expected from a local infection of the respiratory tract. Immune mechanisms such as interferon production may also contribute to the general body aches and fever. Also, during the regeneration process there is a transitional stratified squamous epithelium that results in edema, hyperemia, congestion, and increased secretions.

The development of influenza follows an incubation period of 1 to 2 days. The illness due to influenza A or influenza B is characterized by an abrupt onset, fever of 102 to 104°F, malaise, myalgia, chills, headache, and anorexia. Respiratory symptoms are common but are overshadowed by the systemic symptoms. Dry cough, coryza, pharyngitis, nasal obstruction, and hoarseness are often seen; conjunctivitis and photophobia may occur. Systemic symptoms including fever last about 3 days; respiratory symptoms persist for another 3 to 4 days. Symptoms of cough and malaise may last an additional week or more. Nausea and vomiting are not characteristics of influenza except possibly in small children as reactions to the high fever, and the maladies generally described as "intestinal flu" are not due to influenza virus infections.

Influenza C infections are much milder than infections with types A or B and resemble the common cold. They occur most commonly in children.

Complications of Influenza. Pulmonary complications most commonly include primary influenza viral pneumonia or secondary bacterial pneumonia. These usually occur in elderly and debilitated individuals, but viral pneumonia may be seen in young healthy adults, particularly during outbreaks. Treatment is supportive, and mortality is high. Secondary bacterial pneumonia, on the other hand, can be effectively treated with antibiotics. The predominant bacterial pathogens responsible for this opportunistic infection are *Streptococcus pneumoniae, Staphylococcus aureus,* and *Haemophilus influenzae.*

Nonpulmonary complications include myositis, myocarditis, pericarditis, Guillain–Barré syndrome, and Reye's syndrome. Reye's syndrome is a very serious hepatic-CNS complication with a high mortality rate that has been seen following a number of viral infections. It is seen most commonly in children and teenagers after upper respiratory tract infections, but also after varicella and gastrointestinal infections. Reye's syndrome has often been associated with epidemics of influenza B. Recent evidence indicates that the administration of salicylates during the antecedent illness predisposes the child to the development of

Reye's syndrome and has led to warnings on aspirin labels.

Epidemiology. Influenza is a highly contagious disease transmitted by exposure to virus-containing respiratory secretions. The incidence of illness in a community from one year to the next is directly related to the immune status of the population for the virus strains currently in circulation. The "flu season" runs from late autumn to early spring of each year. The attack rate may be particularly high in the 5- to 14-year-old age group but rarely causes complications. Complications are most common in the elderly and debilitated.

Immune responses following infection lead to the development of both secretory and serum antibodies that offer protection against reinfection with the same or closely related virus strains. As the level of secretory antibodies decreases, this protection wanes and may not prevent reinfection but will likely reduce the severity of illness.

Epidemics occur when antigenic changes are sufficient to permit infection of a number of susceptible individuals in a population. These antigenic changes are usually the result of variations within the antigenic subtypes of hemagglutinin and neuraminidase and are referred to as antigenic drift. Major antigenic changes, referred to as antigenic shifts, result in the appearance or reappearance of new subtypes and produce widespread epidemics or pandemics (Table 41.1, Fig. 41.2). Generally speaking, epidemics of influenza A occur every 2 to 4 years and epidemics of influenza B every 4 to 6 years. Pandemics are less common and have occurred at intervals of 9 to 39 years in the 20th century.

Worldwide influenza virus surveillance occurs annually so that antigenic changes in hemagglutinin and neuraminidase subtypes can be detected. Changes that arise in virus strains can be followed, and the progress of a new strain's spread through the population can be monitored. This surveillance allows the development of influenza virus vaccines that contain killed virus of the most likely strains to circulate in the population in the upcoming season. Vaccines are produced during one season for the following season and normally contain two strains of influenza A virus and one strain of influenza B virus. For example, the trivalent vaccine developed for the 1986–1987 season contained the antigens A/Chile/1/83(H1N1), A/Mississippi/1/85(H3N2), and B/Ann Arbor/1/86. However, during the latter part of the 1985–1986 season, a new A(H1N1) strain arose in Asia that was poorly inhibited by antibody induced by A/Chile/1/83 (H1N1). Thus, for the 1986–1987 season, a supplemental monovalent vaccine against this new variant A/Taiwan/1/86(H1N1) was recommended in addition to the trivalent vaccine, and a probable epidemic was

Table 41.1: Antigenic Subtypes of Influenza A Virus Associated with Pandemic Influenza*

Year	Interval (Years)	Designation	Extent of Antigenic Change in Indicated Surface Protein†	Severity of Pandemic
1889	—	H3N2	?	Moderate
1918	29	H1N1‡	H + + + N + + +	Severe
1957	39	H2N2	H + + + N + + +	Severe
1968	11	H3N2	H + + + N −	Moderate
1977	9	H1N1	H + + + N + + +	Mild

*Reproduced with permission from R. F. Betts and R. G. Douglas, Jr.: Influenza Virus. In *Principles and Practice of Infectious Diseases,* Ed. 3, edited by G. L. Mandell, R. G. Douglas, Jr., and J. E. Bennett. Churchill Livingstone, New York, 1990.

† + = minor change; + + = moderate change; + + + = major change; − = no change.

‡Former designation was Hsw1N1.

prevented. The 1987–1988 vaccine was modified to contain A/Taiwan/1/86(H1N1), A/Leningrad/360/86 (H3N2), and B/Ann Arbor/1/86; and for the 1988–1989 season, in addition to A/Taiwan/1/86(H1N1), the vaccine contained two new isolates from the previous season: A/Sichuan/2/87(H3N2) and B/Victoria/2/87.

Diagnosis. Clinical symptoms in the setting of epidemiological spread of influenza are usually sufficient for diagnosis. For epidemiological purposes, virus can be isolated from respiratory secretions

via cell culture and identified as to serotype. The currently recommended assays for routine serodiagnosis are hemagglutination inhibition and complement fixation assays.

Prevention and Treatment. Immunization against influenza utilizes an inactivated vaccine containing antigens of influenza virus that are expected to be prevalent in the coming season. Annual vaccination is required since virus strains vary from year to year and immunity is of limited duration. Immunization is recommended for 1) high-risk persons more

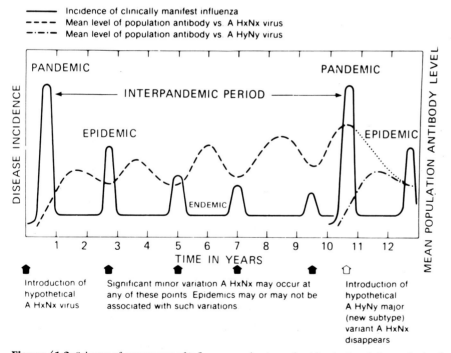

Figure 41.2: Schema of occurrence of influenza pandemics and epidemics in relation to the level of immunity in the population. *AHxNx* and *AHyNy* represent influenza viruses with completely different hemagglutinins and neuraminidases. (Courtesy of Dr. R. G. Douglas, Jr.; reproduced with permission from G. J. Glasso, T. C. Merigan, and R. A. Buchanan (Eds.): *Antiviral Agents and Viral Diseases of Man.* Raven Press, New York, 1979.)

than 6 months old and their medical-care providers or household contacts; 2) children and teenagers receiving long-term aspirin therapy, since they may be at increased risk of developing Reye's syndrome; and 3) other persons who wish to reduce their chances of developing influenza. Adults and children with chronic disorders of the pulmonary or cardiovascular systems, residents of nursing or other extended care facilities, persons over the age of 65, and individuals who are medically compromised by metabolic or immunosuppressive disorders are considered to be at greatest risk of complications. Dentists and other dental personnel should be immunized against influenza since exposure to aerosolized respiratory secretions increases their risk of infection.

The antiviral drug amantadine is effective in reducing the severity and duration of influenza A illness, but not that caused by influenza B. Amantadine is recommended for control of outbreaks of influenza A in institutions housing high-risk individuals. It is generally not recommended for the population at large since prophylaxis is required for the duration of influenza activity in the community and vaccination is much more efficacious.

Supportive therapy including bed rest, antipyretics, and analgesics is useful. Increased fluid intake should be encouraged to compensate for loss through fever. Antibiotics may be given to prevent the development of secondary bacterial pneumonia in individuals at risk.

ADDITIONAL READING

Betts, R. F., and Douglas, R. G., Jr. 1990. Influenza Virus. In *Principles and Practice of Infectious Diseases.* Ed. 3, p. 1306, edited by G. L. Mandell, R. G. Douglas, Jr., and J. E. Bennett. Churchill Livingstone, New York.

Centers for Disease Control. 1980. Influenza Nomenclature. MMWR, **29,** 514.

Centers for Disease Control. 1988. Prevention and Control of Influenza. MMWR, **37,** 361.

Ginsberg, H. S. 1988. Orthomyxoviruses. In *Virology,* Ed. 2, p. 217, R. Dulbecco and H. S. Ginsberg. J. B. Lippincott, Philadelphia.

Kendal, A. P. 1985. Influenza Viruses. In *Laboratory Diagnosis of Viral Infections,* p. 341, edited by E. H. Lennette. Marcel Dekker, New York.

White, D. O., and Fenner, F. J. 1986. Orthomyxoviruses. In *Medical Virology,* Ed. 3, p. 509. Academic Press, New York.

42

Paramyxoviruses

Gretchen B. Caughman and Virginia A. Merchant

Paramyxoviridae is a family of viruses that cause diverse illnesses affecting various organ systems. The member viruses have been differentiated into three genera: *Paramyxovirus, Morbillivirus,* and *Pneumovirus* (Table 42.1). All of the viruses initially infect and replicate in the respiratory tract. For some of the viruses, infection is confined to this tissue and therefore it is the only site of clinical disease. For others, the respiratory tract is a transient and often inapparent site of infection prior to viral dissemination to other major target organs. The human diseases caused by the paramyxoviruses are acute respiratory infections, including croup (parainfluenza virus) and bronchiolitis (respiratory syncytial virus); the morbilliform exanthem, measles; and infectious parotitis, mumps.

Properties of Paramyxoviruses

Paramyxoviruses are relatively large in size (125 to 250 nm in diameter). The virion consists of a helical nucleocapsid containing one large molecule of single-stranded RNA of negative polarity and surrounded by a protein and lipid envelope derived from the infected cell's plasma membrane. The envelope contains two distinctive, viral-encoded glycoprotein peplomers, one (HN) which possesses hemagglutinin and neuramidase activities and the other (F) which has hemolytic and cell fusion functions. Not all member viruses have all four biological activities; see Table 42.1 for a summary of the viruses' common properties and distinguishing characteristics. The virus enters a cell by fusing with the cell membrane and is uncoated in the cytoplasm, where five to eight separate regions of the RNA are transcribed by virion-associated RNA polymerase into monocistronic mRNAs that are translated into the proteins required for nucleic acid replication, structural proteins and peplomers. The peplomers are translocated through the endoplasmic reticulum, where they are glycosylated, and inserted into the cytoplasmic membrane. Specific proteolytic cleavage of the inserted peplomers by cellular enzymes must then occur in order for the peplomers to acquire biological activity. The entire negative-

Table 42.1: Characteristics of Human Paramyxoviruses*

Common Properties

Average size: 125–250 nm (range, 100–800 nm)
Nucleocapsid diameter: 18 nm (except RSV = 14 nm)
Viral genome: 5 × 10⁶ daltons (17–20 kb); single negative-strand molecules
Virion RNA polymerase: +
Reaction with lipid solvents: Disrupts
Syncytial formation: +
Cytoplasmic inclusion bodies: + (measles virus nuclear)
Site of multiplication: Cytoplasm

	Distinguishing Properties			
	Parainfluenza	Mumps	Measles	RSV
Hemagglutinin†:	+	+	+	–
Hemadsorption‡:	+	+	+	–
Hemolysin:	+	+	+	–
Neuraminidase:	+	+	+	–
Antigenic types:	5	1	1	1
Antigenic relationships:	Mumps	Parainfluenza	–	–
Genus:	Paramyxovirus	Paramyxovirus	Morbillivirus	Pneumovirus

Note: + = present, – = absent.
*Reproduced with permission from R. Dulbecco and H. S. Ginsberg: *Virology*, Ed. 2. J. B. Lippincott Co., Philadelphia, 1988.
†Chicken and guinea pig RBCs.
‡Infected cells absorb guinea pig RBCs.

sense genome is then transcribed to produce full-length positive-sense RNA, which serves as a template for the synthesis of daughter genomes. The daughter genomes associate with nucleoprotein (NP) molecules to form nucleocapsids. Virion assembly occurs as molecules of viral M protein form a bridge between the nucleocapsid and a plasma membrane site containing clustered viral peplomers; the virus particle acquires this altered membrane as its envelope by budding from the infected cell.

Paramyxovirus Genus

Parainfluenza Virus

There are five known serotypes of parainfluenza virus which are distinguished by antigenic differences in their HN and F peplomers and their internal nucleocapsid protein (NP). The serotypes differ somewhat in the types of acute respiratory disease they cause in children, the age of individuals they infect and the length of time the virus is shed. Types 1, 2, and 3 are major respiratory pathogens and have been estimated to cause at least 20% of all acute respiratory diseases in children. Type 4 infections are quite common but are often inapparent or very mild. Type 5 has been discovered only recently and little is known about its role in human disease.

Pathogenesis and Clinical Manifestations. The parainfluenza viruses most commonly cause relatively harmless upper respiratory tract infections in young children. The pathogenesis of parainfluenza virus infections is ill-defined. It is known that the virus infects the ciliated columnar epithelium of the respiratory tract; however, it causes no distinctive pathology in the lungs, nor is the mechanism for subglottic involvement known. Infection is confined to the respiratory tract and there is no viral dissemination to other organ systems. More serious disease is seen in 2% to 3% of primary infections, which manifest as croup (laryngotracheobronchitis), bronchiolitis, or pneumonia. The usual presentation with all serotypes, but particularly with type 4 virus, is that of a bad cold with a low-grade fever, coryza, and pharyngitis. Parainfluenza type 3 is often associated with bronchiolitis or pneumonia in infants under 6 months of age. Croup, generally seen in children 6 months to 5 years, is most commonly caused by infection with parainfluenza type 1, and less frequently type 2 or 3. The percentage of lower respiratory tract infections caused by parainfluenza types 1 to 3 is presented in Table 42.2.

The incubation period varies and is not well established but generally ranges from 3 to 6 days. Illness usually lasts only a few days. Asymptomatic infections

Table 42.2: Percentage of Lower Respiratory Tract Illnesses in Children Due to Parainfluenza Viruses*

Virus Type	Illness		
	Croup	Pneumonia	Bronchiolitis
1	18–21	3	1–3
2	4–8	1	1
3	9–13	3–13	5–14
Total	31–42	7–17	7–18

*Reproduced with permission from J. O. Hendley: Parainfluenza virus. In *Principles and Practice of Infectious Diseases,* Ed. 3, edited by G. L. Mandell, R. G. Douglas, Jr., and J. E. Bennett. Churchill Livingstone, New York, 1990.

may also occur. Clinical disease in older children and adults, whose infections are almost always reinfections, generally resembles the common cold.

Epidemiology. Most children are infected at least once prior to 5 years of age with each of serotypes 1 to 4 of parainfluenza virus. By 6 years of age, 75% of children have antibodies to type 1, 60% to type 2, 90% to 100% to type 3, and 50% to type 4. Reinfections are common, but disease is usually mild.

The parainfluenza viruses are worldwide in distribution. Types 1 and 2 are more likely to cause epidemic disease in the fall of alternating years, whereas types 3 and 4 are endemic, with infections apparently occurring throughout the year. Maternal antibody is believed to offer some protection to the newborn from infection with types 1 and 2; therefore, it is uncommon to see severe infection in infants under the age of 4 months due to these viruses. Boys seem to be more susceptible to croup caused by types 1 and 2, although antibody acquisition is the same in girls and boys. No sex differences are seen in the other parainfluenza virus types.

Transmission is via respiratory droplets. Virus is shed for a week or more after the incubation period. Protective immunity, imparted primarily by secretory IgA, is short-lived, and reinfection may occur within 3 months of the primary infection.

Diagnosis. The differential diagnosis of acute respiratory disease is difficult since numerous nonbacterial agents may produce identical clinical pictures. If the patient is an infant or young child, parainfluenza viruses and respiratory syncytial virus must be considered. The serological test of choice is the hemagglutination inhibition assay, which detects specific antibodies in the patient's serum that can block the virus's ability to clump red blood cells. Immunofluorescence assays of nasal secretions have also been used for rapid and accurate diagnosis.

Prevention and Treatment. Since reinfection with the parainfluenza viruses is common and the manifestations are usually mild, it is unlikely that disease can be completely prevented. A vaccine that offered even partial protection would be beneficial in that it might prevent the more severe forms of lower respiratory tract disease, providing it could be made effective in the age group at highest risk: very young infants. Several multivalent and monovalent vaccines are in the developmental stages, but none is available for routine administration as yet.

There is no specific antiviral treatment for parainfluenza virus infections. Upper respiratory tract infections require only palliative treatment of symptoms. Croup may be treated by humidification to prevent drying of secretions and to soothe the inflamed glottis. More severe cases may require hospitalization with oxygen therapy and on occasion the insertion of an endotracheal tube or a tracheostomy to maintain a patent airway.

Mumps Virus

Mumps is an acute infection that generally manifests as parotitis but may affect other organ systems, especially the central nervous system, the testes, the ovaries, and the pancreas. The mumps virus exists as a single serotype. Man is its only natural host.

Pathogenesis and Clinical Manifestations. The virus enters the respiratory tract and replicates in the epithelium and local lymph nodes. The incubation period of mumps is usually 16 to 18 days but may range from 12 to 25 days. During this time there is a generalized viremia that results in spread of the virus to the salivary glands and in some cases to other organs. The end of the incubation period is marked by the development of nonspecific prodromal symptoms of myalgia, anorexia, malaise, headache, and low-grade fever. Within a day, earache and tenderness over the infected parotid gland suggest mumps. The involved gland begins to enlarge, reaching its maximum size in 2 to 3 days (Fig. 42.1). The orifices of Wharton's and Stenson's ducts are often red and swollen. The parotid glands are most often infected, but both the submaxillary and submandibular glands may also be involved. Salivary gland swelling may be single or bilateral, with swelling in one gland preceding that of the other side by 1 to 5 days. Pain is most pronounced during the period of gland enlargement and begins to disappear once the swelling reaches its peak. Usually both swelling and other constitutional signs and symptoms resolve within a week. Complications of parotitis are rare but may be seen as acute or recurrent sialadenitis. An estimated 30% to 50% of mumps infections are subclinical and show none of the characteristic symptoms. However, such infected individuals do shed virus and may serve as sources of contagion.

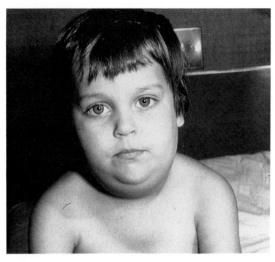

Figure 42.1: Mumps with diffuse lymphedema of anterior neck. (Centers for Disease Control, No. 59037.)

The most common glandular complication of mumps occurs in adult males. Epididymoorchitis develops in 20% to 30% of postpubertal males who are infected with mumps virus. Infection is unilateral in the majority of cases, and thus although pressure necrosis and atrophy of the testis may occur, sterility is rare. Oophoritis in postpubertal females is less common, affecting approximately 5%.

Central nervous system involvement is quite common during mumps infection and occurs in about half of all patients, although clinical meningitis is seen in less than 10% of patients. Mumps meningitis is benign, and complete recovery occurs without apparent sequelae. Encephalitis has been reported in 1 in 6,000 to 1 in 400 cases of mumps. Mumps encephalitis is fatal in about 1.3% of cases. Prior to the introduction of the mumps vaccine in the mid-1960s, mumps was the leading cause of viral encephalitis in the United States.

Other complications include hearing loss, pancreatitis, migratory polyarthritis or arthralgia, myocarditis, pericarditis, and impairment of renal function. A variety of other manifestations can occur but are extremely rare. The effect of mumps on the fetus is a subject of controversy; low birth weight in infants infected during the first trimester is the most likely sequela to in utero infection.

Epidemiology. The mumps virus is distributed throughout the world. It exists as a single serotype and man is its only natural host. Immunity is permanent after a single infection or immunization. Prior to the introduction of the mumps vaccine, epidemics occurred every 2 to 5 years in the United States. The virus is endemic and the highest prevalence of infection is in the late winter and early spring. The virus is transmitted by saliva and respiratory droplets, and virus shedding occurs from a few days before the onset of symptoms until about 2 weeks after onset. During this time, virus also may be found in the urine. Since asymptomatic infections are common, the disease may be spread by viral shedding from individuals with subclinical cases.

Diagnosis. A classic case of mumps parotitis can usually be identified from clinical manifestations. However, at least 30% of infections are subclinical or misdiagnosed. The differential diagnosis of clinical mumps includes parotid tumor, sialolithiasis, and sialectasis.

Prevention and Treatment. A live attenuated mumps vaccine was licensed in the United States in 1967, and the incidence of mumps has since declined by more than 95%. The vaccine is recommended for routine administration to infants between 12 and 15 months of age and usually is given in combination with measles and rubella vaccine. Immunization of adolescent and adult males who are seronegative is also recommended.

Management of infection is purely symptomatic. Treatment with an analgesic–antipyretic combination relieves the pain and reduces fever. Mumps immune globulin administered to adult males with mumps has been shown to reduce the incidence of orchitis.

Morbillivirus Genus

Measles Virus

Measles, also known as rubeola, is an extremely contagious disease with frequent complications, some of which can be very serious. Measles has been a major pathogen throughout the world for centuries and even today is responsible for many deaths in developing countries. There is only one serotype of the measles virus and man is its natural host, although measles is highly infectious for both humans and monkeys.

Pathogenesis and Clinical Manifestations. The measles virus enters the upper respiratory tract and, during the incubation period, replicates asymptomatically in the epithelium of the upper respiratory tract, the regional lymph nodes, and the conjunctivae, and ultimately disseminates to the bloodstream. At 9 to 12 days after infection a prodrome consisting of fever, malaise, anorexia, conjunctivitis, cough, and coryza occurs. These symptoms persist for several days. Toward the end of the prodrome, a characteristic enanthem, termed Koplik spots, appears. Koplik spots are small, irregular, white to blue-gray lesions with an erythematous base that appear on the mucosa of the lower lip and on the buccal mucosa opposite

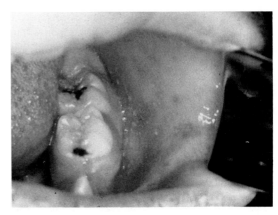

Figure 42.2: Koplik spots of rubeola, 3 days prior to eruption of exanthem. (Centers for Disease Control, No. 54393).

the premolars (Fig. 42.2). These lesions are pathognomonic of measles and disappear as the ensuing skin rash (the exanthem) reaches its peak. The exanthem, which develops 10 to 14 days after infection, follows an intense viremia during which the virus is spread to and replicates in the capillaries of the deep connective tissue and the skin. The rash itself is due more to immune responses to viral antigens than to viral replication. It appears first at the hairline and behind the ears. It becomes maculopapular and spreads rapidly downward over the face, neck, trunk, and extremities during the next 3 days (Fig. 42.3). The patient is most ill during the first or second day of the rash, after

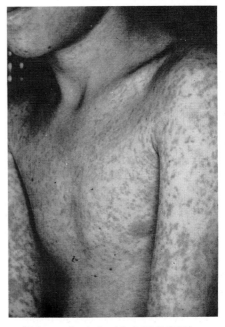

Figure 42.3: Measles (rubeola). (AFIP B 5037.)

which the fever abates and the patient begins to feel better. The rash becomes confluent, especially on the face and neck, and lasts about 5 days. As the rash fades, it becomes brown and desquamates. The uncomplicated illness lasts 7 to 10 days.

Complications include otitis media, viral or bacterial pneumonia, and encephalitis. Viral invasion of the CNS is common, but only 1 in 1,000 to 1 in 2,000 patients develop clinical signs of encephalitis. Acute measles encephalitis may be mild to severe, and survivors are often left with neurological sequelae.

Chronic measles infection of the CNS is thought to be the etiology of subacute sclerosing panencephalitis (SSPE). Patients with SSPE have unusually high titers of measles antibody both in their serum and cerebrospinal fluid, and a measles-like virus has been isolated from the brain and lymph nodes of patients with SSPE. The chronic infection is extremely rare (about one case per million) and is manifested 1 to 10 years following recovery from measles. It has been seen most often in children who had measles before the age of 2 years. SSPE has declined significantly since the introduction of the measles vaccine.

Hemorrhagic measles, also known as black measles, is a severe, rare form of the disease. It is characterized by a sudden high fever, convulsions, severe respiratory distress, and hemorrhages into the skin and from the mucous membranes.

Atypical measles may develop following exposure to wild measles virus, either after recovery from natural disease or more often following exposure in individuals immunized with killed measles vaccine. The rash begins peripherally and is accompanied by high fever, edema of the extremities, myalgia, abdominal pains, and prostration. It is believed that this syndrome represents a hypersensitivity reaction in a partially immune host.

Patients with compromised or deficient cellular immunity may develop severe measles. Giant cell pneumonia may develop without evidence of rash. Such children should not be immunized since the attenuated vaccine virus strain can cause severe infection in these individuals. Malnourishment has also been associated with severe measles and is thought to be due to inadequate cell-mediated immune responses secondary to malnutrition.

Unlike rubella (German measles), measles has not been associated with congenital anomalies. Spontaneous abortions and premature delivery, however, have been seen in pregnant women.

Epidemiology. Measles is an extremely infectious disease and is readily transmitted by respiratory secretions. Patients are most infectious during the later part of the prodrome when cough and coryza are most pronounced. Virus persists in respiratory secretions up to 48 hours after the onset of the skin rash. Asymptomatic cases of measles are quite rare, al-

though mild disease sometimes occurs, especially in infants under 12 months who retain some passively acquired maternal immunity, or in individuals given gamma globulin following exposure to measles.

Measles occurs worldwide and continues to cause many deaths in developing countries, where hundreds of thousands of malnourished infants die annually with measles. In countries in which immunization is practiced, there has been a marked decrease in measles cases. The incidence of measles in the United States has dropped from 200,000 to 500,000 reported cases per year to about 14,800 reported cases in 1989. Measles is now most common in adolescents and young adults who were not immunized and who reached adulthood without exposure. Mini-epidemics have occurred on a number of college and university campuses in recent years.

Diagnosis. Diagnosis is most often made on the basis of clinical presentation, but milder cases of measles can be confused with rubella or other viral exanthems, particularly in the small proportion of cases that do not present with Koplik spots. Evidence of giant cells in nasal smears and urine sediment may be used for diagnosis, as can the demonstration by immunofluorescence assays of measles antigens in these cells.

Prevention and Treatment. Both live and killed measles vaccines were licensed in 1963 for use in the United States. The killed vaccine was withdrawn from the market in 1968 after its association with atypical measles. Live measles vaccine is recommended for administration to healthy children at age 15 months and is usually given in combination with mumps and rubella vaccines. Measles vaccine should not be given to infants less than 12 months of age since failure to develop an adequate immune response has been documented in infants vaccinated before their first birthday. Passive immunization with gamma globulin is recommended for individuals at high risk of severe infection following exposure.

No specific treatment for measles is available. Antipyretics and fluids are recommended. Bacterial superinfections should be treated promptly, but prophylactic antibiotics do not prevent superinfection and are not recommended.

Pneumovirus Genus

Respiratory Syncytial Virus

Respiratory syncytial virus (RSV) infections, like parainfluenza virus infections, are primarily localized to the respiratory tract. RSV disease is most severe in young infants and is considered by many to be the major respiratory pathogen of childhood.

Pathogenesis and Clinical Manifestations. RSV is the major cause of lower respiratory tract dis-

Table 42.3: Proportion of Respiratory Illnesses Caused by Respiratory Syncytial Virus in Children*

Syndrome	% Caused by RSV
Bronchiolitis	43–90
Pneumonia	5–40
Tracheobronchitis	10–30
Croup	3–10
Asymptomatic	0.3

*Reproduced with permission from C. B. Hall: Respiratory syncytial virus. In *Principles and Practice of Infectious Diseases,* Ed. 3, edited by G. L. Mandell, R. G. Douglas, Jr., and J. E. Bennett. Churchill Livingstone, New York, 1990.

ease, including pneumonia, bronchiolitis, and croup, in young children. Primary infection results in pneumonia (most frequently) or bronchiolitis in 40% to 70% of young children. The percentages of lower respiratory tract infections caused by RSV are listed in Table 42.3. Lower respiratory tract disease is usually preceded by an upper respiratory tract infection with cough, nasal congestion, and often pharyngitis. Fever lasting 3 to 4 days occurs in almost all children and may resolve prior to development of lower respiratory tract disease. Otitis media, a common complication of RSV infection, may be solely due to RSV, or RSV may be isolated in conjunction with a bacterial pathogen.

RSV also causes upper respiratory tract infections, particularly in older children and adults. These most likely are due to reinfection. Upper respiratory tract infection due to RSV usually is more prolonged and more severe than that caused by other viruses. Illness generally manifests as fever, conjunctivitis, nasal congestion, cough, and earache. Symptoms last an average of 9 days, with a range of 1 to 32 days. Viral shedding in upper respiratory tract secretions averages 3 to 6 days. Asymptomatic infection is rare. Lower respiratory tract disease due to RSV can occur in adults and is seen more often in the elderly or in individuals with underlying disease.

Acute complications of RSV infection in infants include apnea, respiratory failure, and secondary bacterial infection. Fatal infections may occur in infants with cardiopulmonary or congenital disorders. Immunosuppressed patients of all ages are at risk of sometimes fatal RSV infection.

RSV has occasionally been associated with central nervous system infection (meningitis, myelitis, ataxia, hemiplegia) and a variety of exanthems, but in the great majority of cases it remains confined to the respiratory tract.

Epidemiology. RSV infection is quite common among children, and outbreaks occur annually, particularly during the winter and spring. Often it is the only, or the clearly predominant, infection in the community. Acquisition of infection occurs early, and 25% to 50% of children have specific antibody as the result of natural infection by 1 year of age. Almost all children acquire specific antibody by 4 to 5 years of age. Antibodies, however, do not prevent infection. Reinfections are common, and infections occur routinely in infants with abundant maternal antibody.

Transmission is via respiratory secretions, and the virus usually gains entry via the nose or eye. The incubation period averages 5 days, with a range of 2 to 8 days. Nosocomial infections, particularly in hospital nurseries, is common. Adult caretakers, who are frequently infected themselves, apparently spread the infection by contact and via contaminated fomites.

Diagnosis. Diagnosis of RSV infection in an infant is important, since it can cause severe morbidity and significant mortality and since specific antiviral therapy is available. Immunofluorescence assays to detect viral antigens in cells recovered from nasal or lung secretions provide rapid and specific diagnosis.

Prevention and Treatment. Attempts to produce a vaccine that prevents infection so far have been unsuccessful, although research is ongoing in this area. Efforts to interrupt transmission of infection in hospitals center on isolation of infected infants and careful hand washing by all personnel.

Supportive care is very important in managing severely ill infants. Specific therapy with the antiviral agent ribavirin ameliorates the symptoms of severe RSV infection in both adults and infants. The drug should be administered by aerosol continuously for a minimum of 3 days and should be used only after a specific diagnosis of RSV has been made.

ADDITIONAL READING

Baum, S. G., and Litman, N. 1990. Mumps virus. In *Principles and Practice of Infectious Diseases,* Ed. 3, p. 1260, edited by G. L. Mandell, R. G. Douglas, Jr., and J. E. Bennett. Churchill Livingstone, New York.

De Silva, L. M., and Hanlon, M. G. 1986. Respiratory Syncytial Virus: A Report of a 5-Year Study at a Children's Hospital. J Med Vir, **19,** 299.

Dulbecco, R., and Ginsberg, H. S. 1988. Paramyxoviruses. In *Virology,* Ed. 2, p. 239. J. B. Lippincott Co., Philadelphia.

Gershon, A. A. 1990. Measles Virus (Rubeola). In *Principles and Practice of Infectious Diseases,* Ed. 3, p. 1279, edited by G. L. Mandell, R. G. Douglas, Jr., and J. E. Bennett. Churchill Livingstone, New York.

Hall, C. B. 1990. Respiratory Syncytial Virus. In *Principles and Practice of Infectious Diseases,* Ed. 3, p. 1265, edited by G. L. Mandell, R. G. Douglas, Jr., and J. E. Bennett. Churchill Livingstone, New York.

Hendley, J. O. 1990. Parainfluenza virus. In *Principles and Practice of Infectious Diseases,* Ed. 3, p. 1255, edited by G. L. Mandell, R. G. Douglas, Jr., and J. E. Bennett. Churchill Livingstone, New York.

Marks, M. I. 1981. Mumps. In *Medical Microbiology and Infectious Disease,* Vol. II, p. 887, edited by A. I. Braude. W. B. Saunders, Philadelphia.

43

Rhabdoviruses and Filoviruses

Virginia A. Merchant and Gretchen B. Caughman

Rhabdoviridae

The family Rhabdoviridae includes over 60 member viruses that infect vertebrates, invertebrates, and plants. The most important member virus to man, rabies virus, belongs to the *Lyssavirus* genus.

Properties. Rabies virions, like other members of this family, are characteristically bullet-shaped, enveloped, helical nucleocapsids. The envelope consists of a lipid bilayer derived from the host cell's plasma membrane and contains proteins and knoblike glycoprotein peplomers. The helical nucleocapsid contains a single, negative strand of RNA, several proteins, and an RNA-dependent RNA transcriptase. Viral replication occurs in the cytoplasm in a fashion somewhat similar to that of the paramyxoviruses: five separate regions of the negative-sense genome are transcribed into monocistronic mRNAs, which are translated into structural and nonstructural proteins; full-length positive-sense RNA is transcribed from the genomic RNA and serves as the template for synthesis of daughter genomes. Assembly of the viral envelope begins with

insertion of the processed viral glycoprotein peplomers (G proteins) into the cell's plasma membrane. Virion assembly occurs as molecules of the viral M protein form a bridge between the nucleocapsid and a plasma membrane site containing clustered viral peplomers; the virus particle then acquires this altered membrane as its envelope by budding from the infected cell.

Pathogenesis and Clinical Manifestations. Rabies is an acute encephalitis, almost always fatal, that is usually acquired through the bite of a rabid animal. After a bite the virus remains localized in the connective tissue and muscle for days to months before it reaches the central nervous system (CNS) by traveling along the axoplasm of the peripheral nerves to the ganglia and eventually to the CNS, where it has a predilection for Purkinje cells. It has been suggested that the virus causes interference with neuronal function rather than overt neuronal destruction. Pathognomonic intracytoplasmic inclusions, termed Negri bodies, are prominent in ganglion cells of the hippocampus and cerebellum. The pons and medulla of the brain are edematous, hemorrhagic, and congested, and perivascular cuffing is evident.

The incubation period for rabies is long, usually ranging from 20 to 90 days, although longer periods have been reported, and appears to be directly related to the distance of the site of inoculation from the CNS as well as the size of the viral inoculum and the wound severity. Initial, or prodromal, symptoms are nonspecific, although one third to two thirds of cases experience pain or paresthesia at the site of the bite. Other symptoms include fever, headache, malaise, fatigue, and anorexia. Cough, chills, sore throat, abdominal pain, nausea, vomiting, or diarrhea are also common symptoms. The presence of neurological involvement is suggested by the onset of apprehension, anxiety, agitation, irritability, nervousness, insomnia, or depression. Following this prodromal period, which lasts 2 to 10 days, objective signs of neurologic involvement develop. This period is characterized by hyperactivity. Attempts to swallow can precipitate severe, painful spasms of the pharynx and larynx, leading to the designation of "fear of water" or hydrophobia. After this period of hyperactivity, flaccid paralysis develops, followed by coma and death. In approximately 20% of patients, the period of hyperactivity is absent and paralysis develops after the initial nonspecific symptoms.

Three cases of recovery from clinical rabies have been documented. In each of these cases the individual received preexposure or postexposure prophylaxis prior to the onset of symptoms and required extensive intervention and supportive measures during the illness. In all other known cases, infection has resulted in death. If not prevented by prophylactic immunization, infection invariably results in disease; there is no indication of asymptomatic infection with the rabies virus.

Epidemiology. Rabies continues to occur in the United States as a zoonotic infection, although cases of human rabies are now rare. A total of 24 cases of human rabies have been reported to the Centers for Disease Control (CDC) since 1975, although 42% of these were acquired outside the United States. In 1986, 5,551 cases of animal rabies were reported with a distribution among wild and domestic animals as shown in Figure 43.1. Vaccination of dogs and cats in the United States has had a major impact on reducing the incidence of cases of human rabies in this country.

Rabies is most commonly transmitted by the bite of an infected dog or, more frequently in the United States, a wild animal. The virus is shed in saliva. Virus can also enter the body via intact mucous membranes, and aerosolized virus in caves frequented by bats has been documented as causing rabies in man. The only documented cases of human-to-human transmission have been five cases of rabies that developed in the

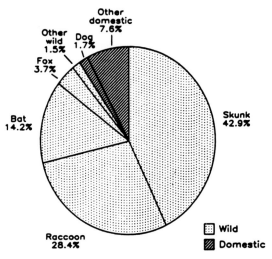

Figure 43.1: Distribution of reported cases of animal rabies in the United States in 1986. (Reproduced from Centers for Disease Control: Rabies Surveillance 1986. *MMWR,* **36** (3S), 1S, 1987.)

recipients of corneal transplants. Although human rabies in the United States and other industrialized countries is now rare, it is still seen in many parts of the world, particularly in the tropics.

Diagnosis. Diagnosis can be made by demonstrating rabies-specific Negri bodies in histopathological sections of fresh brain tissue or by the more specific and more sensitive immunofluorescence staining technique using brain tissue impression slides. The standard test for assay of rabies-neutralizing antibody is the virus neutralization test in mice. Other serological assays have been developed, including the more rapid methods, the fluorescent focus inhibition test and the indirect immunofluorescence antibody test.

Prevention and Treatment. Avoiding contact with animals that may harbor the virus is the most effective preventive measure. The CDC has advised against keeping wild animals as pets, and domestic dogs and cats should be vaccinated to prevent rabies.

Individuals at risk of contact with virus should be immunized prior to exposure. High-risk groups include rabies research workers, veterinarians, animal control personnel, speleologists, spelunkers, and wildlife control personnel. The vaccine may also be recommended for certain travelers to areas where rabies is endemic. Immunization with the current rabies vaccines is both safe and efficacious. The human diploid cell vaccine (HDCV) consists of virus propagated in human diploid cells and inactivated by either tri-(n)-butyl phosphate or β-propiolactone.

Postexposure treatment of persons not previously immunized should include prompt and aggressive cleansing of the wound to physically remove and/

or inactivate as much of the virus as possible, and administration of both HDCV and rabies immune globulin (RIG). Clinical rabies has occurred in some cases when only HDCV was given. RIG is given along with the initial dose of HDCV. Four additional doses of HDCV are given intramuscularly in the deltoid muscle on days 3, 7, 14, and 28.

Filoviridae

The newly classified family Filoviridae comprises two viruses, Marburg virus and Ebola virus, which were isolated during outbreaks of acute hemorrhagic fevers in 1967 and 1976, respectively. Several additional outbreaks of each have occurred since then, and, although infections with these viruses are rare, they are very serious since they are associated with a high mortality rate.

Properties. The filoviruses are long pleomorphic filaments that are 80 nm in diameter but vary in length from about 0.5 to 1.4 μm and may be branched, circular or U-shaped. The helical nucleocapsid is surrounded by an envelope studded with surface projections. The genome is a single molecule of single-stranded, negative-sense RNA. Viral multiplication occurs in the cytoplasm, and viruses bud from the plasma membrane.

Pathogenesis and Clinical Manifestations. Marburg virus and Ebola virus cause viral hemorrhagic fevers with similar clinical and pathological pictures. The incubation period is about a week, but in the case of Ebola virus infection may range from 2 to 21 days. There is a sudden onset of influenza-like symptoms, including fever, malaise, headache, myalgia, and sore throat. Additional signs and symptoms include diarrhea, abdominal pain, nausea, vomiting, conjunctivitis, proteinuria, and elevation of liver enzymes. Between days 5 and 7 after onset, a maculopapular rash appears and subsequently desquamates. Hemorrhagic manifestations commonly include both petechiae and frank bleeding. Bleeding throughout the gastrointestinal tract, including the gingival tissues, is characteristic. Necrotic foci occur in many organs, including the brain, the liver, and the lymphatic tissues. Severe viral hemorrhagic fever leads to shock and ultimately death.

Epidemiology. Marburg virus and Ebola virus are endemic to Central and East Africa, but their reservoir in nature is still unknown. The original outbreak of Marburg virus infection was linked to workers handling kidneys from African monkeys, but subsequent studies indicated that these animals were not the virus's natural hosts. The mode of acquiring natural infection with either virus remains to be determined, but person-to-person transmission does occur with close personal contact or contact with blood or body fluids.

The case-fatality rate for the initial outbreak of Marburg hemorrhagic fever was 23% for primary cases. Mortality rates are higher with Ebola virus infection and have ranged from 53% to 88%.

Diagnosis.   Specific diagnosis of both infections requires isolation of the virus from blood, or the demonstration of IgM antibody or a fourfold rise in IgG serum antibody. Because of the high risk associated with handling material infected with these devastating pathogens, clinical samples must be obtained with great care and usually are sent to one of the highest containment facilities for analyses.

Prevention and Treatment.   Since the source of the viruses is not known, no recommendations can be made regarding the prevention of primary acquisition of infection. The Centers for Disease Control have published guidelines for management of patients with viral hemorrhagic fever which include precautions to prevent secondary transmission.

Treatment for both Marburg and Ebola hemorrhagic fevers is supportive. There is limited information on the efficacy of antiviral drugs for treatment of these infections; neither ribavirin nor interferon has been shown to be effective against the viruses in vitro.

ADDITIONAL READING

Advisory Committee on Immunization Practices. 1984. Rabies Prevention—United States, 1984. MMWR, **33**, 393.

Centers for Disease Control. 1988. Management of Patients with Suspected Viral Hemorrhagic Fever. MMWR, **37**, S-3.

Centers for Disease Control. 1988. Rabies Surveillance 1987. MMWR, **37**, SS-4.

Howard, C. R., Simpson, D. I. H., and Ellis, D. S. 1987. Viral Haemorrhagic Fevers. In *Principles and Practice of Clinical Virology,* p. 433, edited by A. J. Zuckerman, J. E. Banatvala, and J. R. Pattison. Wiley/Liss, New York.

Johnson, H. N., and Emmons, R. W. 1985. Rabies Virus. In *Laboratory Diagnosis of Viral Infections,* p. 425, edited by E. H. Lennette. Marcel Dekker, New York.

Warrell, D. A., and Warrell, M. J. 1988. Human Rabies and Its Prevention: An Overview. Rev Infect Dis, **10**, S726.

44

Togaviruses, Flaviviruses, Bunyaviruses, and Arenaviruses

Gretchen B. Caughman and Virginia A. Merchant

Arboviruses

Historically, a large number of viruses have been termed arboviruses because they are *ar*thropod-*borne*; that is, they multiply in both vertebrate and arthropod hosts and are transmitted primarily by an arthropod's bite and subsequent blood meal. The viruses often cause disease in the vertebrate host but do not adversely affect the arthropod. The arbovirus group actually is comprised of viruses from several families that differ greatly in chemical and physical characteristics. Furthermore, not all of the viruses in these families are transmitted by arthropods.

Until recently, the flaviviruses were considered one of the four genera of the family Togaviridae. However, the flaviviruses differ enough from the togaviruses to warrant their reclassification as a separate family, Flaviviridae. Therefore, there are now only three gen-

era of togaviruses: *Alphavirus,* which includes several encephalitis-producing viruses indigenous to the United States, *Rubivirus* (rubella virus, which is not arthropod-borne), and *Pestivirus,* whose members infect only animals. The family Bunyaviridae not only includes the largest number of arthropod-borne viruses, but with more than 200 members is also the largest family of RNA-containing viruses. Members of the family Arenaviridae, although originally placed in the arbovirus group, do not require an arthropod vector. Their natural hosts appear to be rodents, in which they often produce chronic infections.

Properties. Some of the physical and biochemical properties of these four very different virus families are summarized in Table 44.1. In addition to the marked structural differences, the families vary in the strategy by which gene expression and replication of their RNA genomes occurs. Flavivirus protein syn-

Table 44.1: Properties of Togaviruses, Flaviviruses, Bunyaviruses and Arenaviruses

Property	Togaviruses	Flaviviruses	Bunyaviruses	Arenaviruses
Virion size	60–70 nm	40–50 nm	90–100 nm	110–130 nm
Nucleocapsid	Icosahedral	Icosahedral	Helical	Beaded, circular
Envelope	+	+	+	+
RNA	Single-stranded	Single-stranded	Single-stranded	Single-stranded
Polarity	Positive	Positive	Negative or ambisense	Ambisense
No. of segments	1	1	3	2

thesis and RNA replication is similar to that of picornaviruses in that the positive-sense genome is directly translated to a polyprotein that undergoes cotranslational and posttranslational processing to produce structural and nonstructural proteins. A full-length negative RNA is then transcribed and serves as the template for synthesis of daughter genomic RNA.

In alphavirus (Togaviridae) replication, a polyprotein also is translated, but only from the 5′ portion of the positive-sense genomic RNA. Next, a full-length, negative-sense complementary RNA is synthesized, and it serves not only as the template for replication of full-length daughter genomic RNA molecules but also for the transcription of a smaller messenger RNA that corresponds in sequence to the 3′ portion of the genomic RNA. This mRNA encodes a second polyprotein, which is subsequently processed to yield structural proteins.

Most of the bunyaviruses replicate much as the orthomyxoviruses do (see Chap. 41), except for the phlebovirus group. These viruses are not well characterized but appear to have unusual genomes, in that part of each genomic segment directly codes for a protein and is therefore positive-sense RNA, whereas sequences in the remaining portion of the genome segment behave as negative-sense RNA which is transcribed to an mRNA to be used in protein synthesis. Thus, the phleboviruses are said to have ambisense polarity.

The arenaviruses also display ambisense polarity and the biochemical events in their replication are similar to that of the phleboviruses. Morphologically, the arenaviruses have the unusual feature of granular structures (L., *arena,* sand) within the virions that are host cell ribosomes. Their presence in the viral particle is not required for infectivity and their significance is unknown.

Pathogenesis and Clinical Manifestations. A summary of the classification, distribution, and disease manifestations of the arthropod-borne viruses and clinically related viruses is given in Table 44.2. In general, four distinctive syndromes are caused by the arboviruses infecting man: undifferentiated fever, denguelike fever, hemorrhagic fever, and encephalitis. Undifferentiated fever is a mild, self-limiting febrile illness with no distinguishing signs or symptoms. Headache, myalgia, coryza, cough, nausea, vomiting, diarrhea, or lymphadenomegaly accompany the fever. Denguelike fever is characterized by the signs and symptoms of undifferentiated fever as well as the presence of a maculopapular or scarlatiniform rash and/or polyarthritis. Hemorrhagic fevers are febrile illnesses with associated bleeding ranging from the presence of a positive tourniquet test to the acute vascular permeability syndrome.

Yellow fever caused by a flavivirus presents as a variation of the typical hemorrhagic fevers in that liver involvement and jaundice may occur, hence the name. It is a febrile illness that varies in intensity from asymptomatic to severe bleeding resulting from impaired clotting factor production by a diseased liver. Following a 3- to 6-day incubation period, symptoms of undifferentiated fever may be manifested and last 1 to 7 days. Jaundice may be seen around the third day. Mortality is usually about 5%.

Lassa fever caused by an arenavirus, Lassa virus, is a serious febrile illness with a variable presentation. Early symptoms are not specific. Characteristics of the disease are fever, severe generalized myalgia, marked malaise, and pharyngitis. Chills, vomiting, and diarrhea are often among the early symptoms. Myocarditis, pneumonia with pleural effusion, encephalopathy, and hemorrhagic lesions develop in fatal cases. Cardiovascular collapse results in the death of 15% to 25% of hospitalized patients, although the infection is apparently only fatal in about 2% of infected patients. The incubation period is usually 7 to 12 days.

Encephalitides caused by togavirus and flavivirus infections are fairly common in the United States. Following percutaneous deposition, the virus replicates in lymphatic tissue and various organs before it elicits a viremia that results in viral involvement of the CNS. During the period of primary viremia, fever and other constitutional symptoms may be evident. Once the

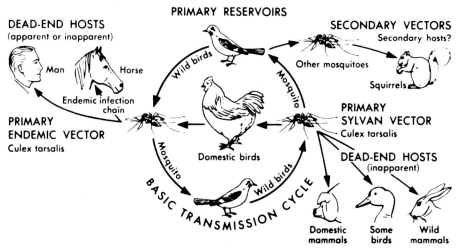

PRIMARY RESERVOIRS

DEAD-END HOSTS
(apparent or inapparent)

Man   Horse

Endemic infection chain

PRIMARY ENDEMIC VECTOR
Culex tarsalis

Wild birds

Mosquito

Domestic birds

Mosquito   Wild birds

BASIC TRANSMISSION CYCLE

Other mosquitoes

SECONDARY VECTORS
Secondary hosts?

Squirrels

PRIMARY SYLVAN VECTOR
Culex tarsalis

DEAD-END HOSTS
(inapparent)

Domestic mammals   Some birds   Wild mammals

Figure 44.1: Epidemiology pattern for western equine encephalitis (WEE) virus infections. The chains for rural St. Louis encephalitis are similar, except that horses are inapparent, rather than apparent, hosts. Eastern equine encephalitis (EEE) infections also have a similar summer infection chain, but a few significant differences exist: 1) the identity of the vector infecting man is unknown, 2) domestic birds do not appear to be a significant link in the chain, and 3) in pheasants it has a bird-to-bird secondary cycle whose role is unclear. (Reproduced with permission from A. D. Hess and P. Holden: *Ann NY Acad Sci,* **70,** 294, 1958.)

virus enters the brain, infection can be widespread and causes neuronal destruction, glial cell infiltration, and perivascular cuffing. Lesions in the basal nuclei may occur with eastern equine encephalitis (EEE) and in the cortex with western equine encephalitis (WEE). Clinically, arboviral encephalitis has four typical stages: a prodromal illness, an acute stage, a subacute stage, and convalescence. Incubation periods vary from 1 to 3 weeks. The prodromal stage lasts 2 or 3 days and is characterized by headache, anorexia, nausea, vomiting, abdominal pain, and sensory changes that may include psychotic episodes. This is followed by the acute stage, which extends for a period of 3 or 4 days during which the mental status of the patient may range from confusion and disorientation to coma. During the subsequent 7 to 10 days (the subacute stage), the CNS involvement lessens but neurological deficits may persist. Fatality rates vary from approximately 10% with EEE to as high as 70% with WEE.

Epidemiology and Control.   Most of these infections are zoonoses that are accidentally transmitted to man. The viruses survive by alternate cycles of replication in hematophagous arthropods and various vertebrate hosts. Normally when they are transmitted to a person by the bite of an insect, man is a dead-end host, i.e., the infection is generally not transmitted directly or by insect vectors from man to man. Several togaviral infections (yellow fever, dengue, and Chikungunya fever) are endemic to human or primate populations in tropical areas, however, and alternate

their infectious cycles between man and mosquito. The arthropod, usually a mosquito but sometimes a tick, becomes infected when it bites a viremic vertebrate. The virus replicates within the vector during what is referred to as the extrinsic incubation period. Upon subsequent feeding by the infected arthropod, virus is transmitted to a new vertebrate host via the arthropod's saliva. The virus then replicates in the vertebrate during the intrinsic incubation period prior to a viremia and potential transmission back to a biting arthropod. As an example, Figure 44.1 graphically presents the transmission cycle of WEE virus infections.

The distribution of arthropod-borne viral infections depends on the geographic range of the arthropod vector and the availability of a vertebrate host population. Three alphaviruses—EEE, WEE, and Venezuelan equine encephalitis (VEE) viruses—and two flaviviruses—St. Louis encephalitis virus and Powassan virus—are indigenous to the United States. EEE, WEE, and St. Louis encephalitis viruses cause zoonotic infections in birds, and VEE and Powassan viruses cause zoonotic infection in rodents. These viruses cause sporadic outbreaks in man and horses (EEE, WEE, VEE). Several members of the family Bunyaviridae are indigenous to the United States and cause undifferentiated fevers or encephalitis.

Control of arthropod-borne viral infections is actually dependent on controlling the arthropod vectors. Efforts to eliminate breeding sites for mosquitoes in

Table 44.2: Classification and Description of Arthropod-Borne Viruses and Clinically Related Viruses of Humans*

Family	Genus (Group)	Subgroup Complex	Viral Species	Vector	Clinical Disease(s) in Man	Geographic Distribution
Togaviridae†	*Alphavirus*	I	Eastern equine encephalitis (EEE)	Mosquito	Encephalitis	Eastern U.S., Canada, Brazil, Cuba, Panama, Philippines, Dominican Republic, Trinidad
		II	Venezuelan equine encephalitis (VEE)	Mosquito	Encephalitis	Brazil, Colombia, Ecuador, Trinidad, Venezuela, Mexico, Florida, Texas
		III	Western equine encephalitis (WEE)	Mosquito	Encephalitis	Western U.S., Canada, Mexico, Argentina, Brazil, British Guiana
			Sindbis	Mosquito	Subclinical or arthritis, rash	Egypt, India, South Africa, Australia, Sweden, Finland, Soviet Union
			(4 others) Semliki Forest	Mosquito	Fever or none	East Africa, West Africa
		IV	Chikungunya	Mosquito	Headache, fever, rash, joint and muscle pain	East Africa, South Africa, Southeast Asia
			Mayaro	Mosquito	Headache, fever, joint and muscle pain	Bolivia, Brazil, Colombia, Trinidad
		V–VII	Getah (each subgroup contains a single virus)	Mosquito	Subclinical or none known	
Flaviviridae	*Flavivirus*	I	St. Louis encephalitis	Mosquito	Encephalitis	U.S., Trinidad, Panama
			Japanese B encephalitis	Mosquito	Encephalitis	Japan, Guam, East Asian mainland, Malaya, India, Australia, New Guinea
			Murray Valley encephalitis	Mosquito	Encephalitis	Brazil, Guatemala, Trinidad, Honduras
			Ilheus	Mosquito	Encephalitis	
			West Nile	Mosquito	Headache, fever, myalgia, rash, lymphadenopathy	Egypt, Israel, India, Uganda, South Africa
			(8 other viruses)	Mosquito		
		II	Dengue (4 types)	Mosquito	Headache, fever, myalgia, prostration, rash (sometimes hemorrhagic)	Pacific Islands, South and Southeast Asia, Northern Australia, New Guinea, Greece, Caribbean islands, Nigeria, Central and South America, Republic of China
		III	Yellow fever	Mosquito	Fever, prostration, hepatitis, nephritis	Central and South America, Africa, Trinidad
		IV	Tick-borne group (Russian	Tick	Encephalitis, meningoencephalitis, hemorrhagic fever	Russian spring-summer encephalitis: U.S.S.R.,

Family	Genus	Group	Viruses	Disease	Transmission	Geographic distribution
		(...spring-summer encephalitis group)	15 viruses	Encephalitis	Mosquito	Canada, U.S.; others: Japan, Siberia, Central Europe, Finland, India, Malaya, Great Britain (louping ill)
		V–VII	(11 viruses)		Unrecognized	
			Rio Bravo (bat salivary gland) (16 others)		Unrecognized	California, Texas
Bunyaviridae	Bunyavirus (Bunyamwera supergroup)	C group	Marituba and 10 others	Headache, fever	Mosquito	Brazil (Belem), Panama, Trinidad, Florida
		Bunyamwera group	Bunyamwera and 17 others	Headache, fever, myalgia, fever only, or none	Mosquito	Uganda, South Africa, India, Malaya, Colombia, Brazil, Trinidad, West Africa, Finland, U.S.
		California group	California encephalitis and 10 others	Encephalitis	Mosquito	U.S, Trinidad, Brazil, Canada, Czechoslovakia, Mozambique
		10 other subgroups (3 ungrouped members of genus)	46 viruses			
	Phlebovirus fever group	Phlebotomus	37 viruses	Sandfly fever, headache, fever, myalgia	Phlebotomus	Italy, Egypt
	Nairovirus	Crimean–Congo hemorrhagic fever group (4 others)	19 viruses	Fever, headache, GI and renal symptoms, hemorrhages	Tick	Africa, Europe, Asia
	Uukuvirus	Uukuniemi group	Uukuniemi, 7 others; 8 unassigned viruses		Mosquito / Tick	Finland
Arenaviridae	*Arenavirus*	Tacaribe	Tacaribe, Junin, Tamiami, Machupo, Pichinde, and 3 others; Lymphocytic choriomeningitis; Lassa virus	Headache, fever, myalgia, hemorrhagic signs		South and Central America
Ungrouped			Silverwater	None known	Tick	Canada
			Rift Valley fever	Headache, fever, myalgia, joint pains, hemorrhagic signs, rash	Mosquito	Africa
			Crimean hemorrhagic fever	Headache, fever, myalgia, hemorrhagic signs	Tick	Southern U.S.S.R.
Others			36 others	None known	Mosquito	
			48 viruses (14 groups of 2–8 viruses)	None known in most cases	Mosquito	

*Reproduced with permission from R. Dulbecco and H. S. Ginsberg: *Virology*, Ed. 2. J. B. Lippincott Co., Philadelphia, 1988.
†Rubivirus (rubella, or German measles, virus), also a togavirus, is discussed in Chapter 45.

and around residential areas have significantly reduced the incidence of arthropod-borne human disease.

Natural Lassa virus infection apparently is limited to western Africa, although cases have occurred in other parts of the world due to nosocomial or laboratory transmission. No arthropod vector has yet been associated with infection, and attempts to isolate the virus from arthropods have been unsuccessful. The rodent *Mastomys natalensis* is the natural host of Lassa virus. Transmission in humans is apparently person-to-person via aerosols or direct contact with the body fluids of infected patients.

Many of the arboviruses can be transmitted by aerosols or via contact with specimens from infected patients. Precautions must be taken by personnel treating infected patients and by research or diagnostic laboratory workers who deal with these viruses or patient specimens. Class IV containment measures are required in laboratories handling arenaviruses or patient specimens of individuals possibly infected with these viruses.

An attenuated, live virus vaccine is available in the United States for immunization against yellow fever. It is recommended/required for persons traveling or living in areas of the world where yellow fever is endemic, currently parts of Africa and South America. Booster doses are required at intervals of 10 years. Effective vaccines against other arboviruses have not yet been developed in the United States.

Diagnosis and Treatment.   Either hemagglutination inhibition or complement fixation tests are most commonly used for serodiagnosis. In addition, neutralization tests, radioimmunoassay, EIA, and immunofluorescence tests are sometimes available. Dengue must be differentiated from murine typhus, yellow fever, Rocky Mountain spotted fever, leptospirosis, typhoid fever, and other insect-borne viral infections such as Colorado tick fever, caused by an *Orbivirus* (Reoviridae family). Yellow fever must be distinguished from dengue, influenza, hepatitis, malaria, typhoid fever, and leptospirosis. Differential diagnosis of arboviral encephalitides include both viral and bacterial CNS infections.

Treatment is primarily supportive rather than specific and involves careful monitoring of patient status and appropriate medical management upon presentation of symptoms. Immune serum globulin has shown some benefit in the management of arenavirus infections.

ADDITIONAL READING

Centers for Disease Control. 1988. Management of Patients with Suspected Viral Hemorrhagic Fever. MMWR, **37,** S-3.

Ginsberg, H. S. 1988. Togaviruses, Flaviviruses, Bunyaviruses, and Arenaviruses. In *Virology,* Ed. 2, p. 277, R. Dulbecco and H. S. Ginsberg. J. B. Lippincott Co., Philadelphia.

Halstead, S. B. 1990. Arboviruses. In *Laboratory Diagnosis of Viral Infections,* p. 147, edited by E. H. Lennette. Marcel Dekker, New York.

Johnson, K. M. 1985. Lymphocytic choriomeningitis virus, Lassa virus, and Other Arenaviruses. In *Principles and Practice of Infectious Diseases,* Ed. 3, p. 1329, edited by G. L. Mandell, R. G. Douglas, Jr., and J. E. Bennett. Churchill Livingstone, New York.

White, D. O., and Fenner, F. J. 1986. Arenaviruses, Bunyaviruses, Rhabdoviruses, and Filoviruses. In *Medical Virology,* Ed. 3, p. 547. Academic Press, New York.

45

Rubella: A Non-Arthropod-Borne Togavirus Infection

Virginia A. Merchant and Gretchen B. Caughman

Rubella, often referred to as German or 3-day measles, is a mild, even trivial, exanthematous disease in children and young adults that was first differentiated from other exanthems in the early 1800s. Later a viral etiology was suspected, but not until 1941 was the full impact of rubella's disease potential understood when it was realized that infections during pregnancy often resulted in devastating teratogenic effects in the developing fetus or fetal death.

Viral Properties

Rubella virus is classified as the single member of the *Rubivirus* genus of the family Togaviridae on the basis of its physical and chemical similarities to other togaviruses. However, it is not an arbovirus, has no animal reservoir, infects only humans, and is not related immunologically to other togaviruses. Structurally like the alphatogaviruses, rubella virus is an en-

veloped virus, 60 nm in diameter, with projecting peplomers. Beneath the envelope, an icosahedral capsid surrounds one molecule of single-stranded RNA. This RNA genome is positive-sense and has a molecular weight of about 3.8×10^6 daltons, significantly smaller than other togaviruses. Rubella virus replication occurs essentially as described for the alphatogaviruses (see Chap. 44).

Rubella Infection

Pathogenesis and Clinical Manifestations. Rubella is transmitted via inhalation of respiratory droplets. During the 12- to 23-day incubation period, the virus replicates first in the upper respiratory tract mucosa and the cervical lymph nodes; it infects leukocytes and is transported in the blood to other parts of the reticuloendothelial system. Following development of the second viremia, the characteristic rash or more, but it is rarely long-term. Thrombocytopenia and encephalitis are rare complications of rubella.

In intrauterine infection, the virus is transmitted across the placenta from the infected mother's bloodstream. The extent of teratogenicity depends on the age at which the fetus is infected. Frequently a persistent and chronic viral infection is established, and fetal growth is retarded by mitotic arrest or various degrees of chromosome damage. Tissue necrosis results, and hypoxia is created due to fetal vasculitis. This usually leads to spontaneous abortion or to an infant that is born as a rubella carrier, with varying degrees of congenital defects. Congenital rubella is a very serious infection and commonly results in fetal death or the development of severe defects. Some of these are listed in Table 45.1. Since the extent of the

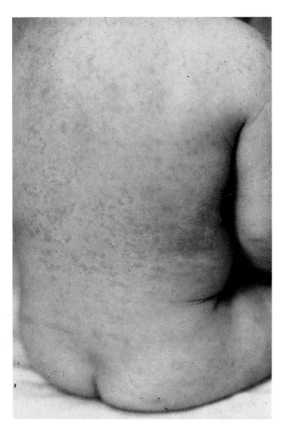

Figure 45.1: Maculopapular rash of rubella. (Centers for Disease Control ST69-3123.)

develops that is considered to be partly a hypersensitivity reaction, but also an infection of integumentary tissue.

A prodrome of malaise, fever, and anorexia lasting several days may occur in adults. Children do not usually experience prodromal symptoms. The major symptoms of rubella are lymphadenopathy and a discrete maculopapular rash (Fig. 45.1). Mild coryza and conjunctivitis may be seen in conjunction with the rash. The lymphadenopathy generally involves the posterior auricular, posterior cervical, and suboccipital lymph nodes. The rash, if present, lasts 3 to 5 days; it begins at the hairline and progresses down the body to involve the trunk and extremities within a 24-hour period. An enanthem of small petechial lesions is sometimes seen on the soft palate. These lesions are referred to as Forscheimer spots, but they are not pathognomonic of rubella.

Postnatal complications with rubella infection are rare. The most common is the development of arthritis or arthralgia in adults, particularly women, who are infected. This arthritis occurs in approximately one third of adult women and may last up to a month

Table 45.1: Manifestations of Congenital Rubella*

General	*Skin*
Intrauterine growth retardation	Purpuric or petechial rash
Postnatal growth retardation	Chronic rubelliform rash
Failure to thrive	
	Blood
Eye	Thrombocytopenia
Cataracts	Anemia
Retinopathy	Leukopenia
Microphthalmia	
Glaucoma	*Bones*
	Osteopathy
	Radiolucencies
Heart	
Patent ductus arteriosus	*Lungs*
Pulmonary arterial hypoplasia	Interstitial pneumonitis
Coarctation of the aorta	
	Genitourinary System
Ear	Undescended testicles
Sensorineural deafness	Polycystic kidney
	Hypospadias
Central Nervous System	
Encephalitis	*Gastrointestinal System*
Meningitis	Hepatitis
Microcephaly	Intestinal atresia
Psychomotor retardation	Chronic diarrhea
Speech and learning disabilities	
Behavior disorders	*Endocrine System*
Late-onset encephalopathy	Diabetes mellitus (early onset)
	Thyroiditis
Oral	
High arched palate	
Hypoplastic mandible	
Delayed tooth eruption	
Hypoplastic or aplastic enamel	

*Adapted with permission of the publisher from L. R. Stanberry and L. A. Glasgow: Viral Infections of the Fetus and Newborn. In *Virology,* edited by D. A. Stringfellow. The Upjohn Co., Kalamazoo, Mich., 1983.

effect on the fetus is generally related to fetal age, the greatest risk is during the first trimester of pregnancy, but congenital defects may occur from fetal infections during the fourth or even the fifth month. As a consequence of the severity of rubella in the fetus, therapeutic abortion is generally recommended to women infected during early pregnancy.

Epidemiology. Rubella is a moderately contagious disease, and, prior to the introduction of live attenuated rubella vaccine in 1969, 80% to 90% of adults had natural immunity to infection. Rubella outbreaks occurred during the late winter and spring in 5- to 9-year cycles and most commonly infected children between the ages of 5 and 9 years. More recently, with the decrease in susceptible children, outbreaks are being reported in adolescents and young adults who have not been immunized. There is only one serotype of rubella virus, so that multiple infections with different viruses do not occur. Reinfections in seropositive individuals, if they occur, are asymptomatic.

Rubella has a long incubation period, ranging from 12 to 23 days, with an average of 18 days. The virus is shed in respiratory secretions from 10 days before the eruption of the rash until 15 days after its appearance. Subclinical infection is common and is also accompanied by virus shedding. The prolonged period of contagion and the high incidence of subclinical infection increase the potential for transmission to nonimmune (seronegative) pregnant women.

Diagnosis. Rubella is easily confused with other exanthems, such as scarlet fever, mild measles, toxoplasmosis, roseola, erythema infectiosum, and certain enteroviral rashes. Definitive diagnosis can be made by serology, although it is rarely necessary except in cases where the possibility of fetal infection arises. The standard reference method for rubella serology, the hemagglutination inhibition test, remains the most widely used method for rubella diagnosis and immunity screening. A variety of other commercial kits are available, including ones that use enzyme-linked immunosorbent assays. Immunity testing, i.e., for determination of past rubella infection, can be rapidly performed using commercially available passive hemagglutination test kits. Virus isolation from throat swabs or from other body fluids or secretions is possible but has limited applicability for routine diagnosis.

Prevention and Treatment. Since symptoms are usually mild, no treatment is generally indicated. When needed, antipyretics or analgesics may be used for treatment of symptoms. Immune globulin is not recommended for exposed seronegative pregnant women since it could suppress symptoms of infection. Therapeutic abortions are frequently recommended for women infected early in pregnancy to avoid the development of congenital rubella.

Rubella vaccine is recommended for all children and young adults who are seronegative. Since there is a theoretical, although small, risk of congenital defects due to vaccine virus, pregnant women or those who anticipate pregnancy within 3 months should not be immunized. The live attenuated virus vaccine is usually administered to children at 15 months of age as a component of the measles–mumps–rubella (MMR) vaccine.

ADDITIONAL READING

Gershon, A. A. 1990. Rubella Virus (German Measles). In *Principles and Practice of Infectious Diseases,* Ed. 3, p. 1242, edited by G. L. Mandell, R. G. Douglas, Jr., and J. E. Bennett. Churchill Livingstone, New York.

Hermann, K. L. 1985. Rubella. In *Laboratory Diagnosis of Viral Infections,* p. 481, edited by E. H. Lennette. Marcel Dekker, New York.

White, D. O., and Fenner, F. J. 1986. Togaviruses and Flaviviruses. *Medical Virology,* Ed. 3, p. 479. Academic Press, New York.

46

Reoviruses, Caliciviruses, Astroviruses, and Norwalk Virus

Gretchen B. Caughman and Virginia A. Merchant

Reoviridae

The word *reovirus* is derived from *r*espiratory *e*nteric *o*rphan because the first viruses of this family were isolated from the respiratory and enteric tracts of humans and animals, but appeared to be orphans since they were not associated with clinical disease. However, as other reoviruses were discovered, the orphan status no longer held since some of the member viruses do cause severe disease. The family Reoviridae consists of six genera, three of which contain members that infect man. Viruses of the *Orthoreovirus* genus apparently cause asymptomatic or very mild infection in man, since the majority of adults possess antibodies to these viruses, but no disease has been associated with natural infection. All members of the *Orbivirus* genus are arboviruses, but only a few, including the Colorado tick fever virus, are known to infect man. By far the most significant genus of the Reoviridae with regard to human pathogens is *Rotavirus*. The rotaviruses are the major etiological

agents of acute nonbacterial gastroenteritis in infants and young children.

Properties. The reoviruses are unusual among the animal viruses in several respects. They are nonenveloped viruses but have a double capsid structure, 70 to 80 nm in outer diameter (Fig. 46.1). Both inner and outer capsid have icosahedral symmetry and together enclose the segmented, double-stranded RNA genome. The number of RNA segments, each representing a different gene, varies from 10 to 12, depending on the specific reovirus. After receptor-mediated endocytosis of the virion into a host cell, replication proceeds in the cytoplasm in association with lysosomes whose proteolytic enzymes partially hydrolyze the outer capsid. Thus, only partial uncoating of the core occurs and the genomic segments are not released free into the cytoplasm. Initially, early mRNAs are synthesized from only some of the genomic segments by the viral RNA-dependent RNA transcriptase. This stage is followed by late gene expression in which all genomic segments are trans-

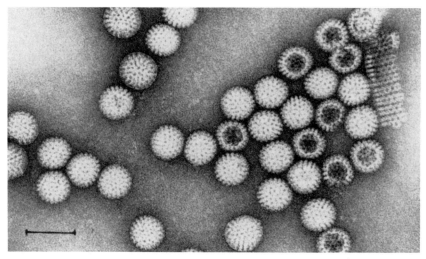

Figure 46.1: Negatively stained preparation of virions of human rotavirus. Bar = 100 nm. (Reproduced with permission from D. O. White and F. J. Fenner: *Medical Virology,* Ed. 3. Academic Press, Orlando, Fla., 1986.)

cribed and translated. Unlike the semiconservative replication of double-stranded DNA, replication of the reovirus double-stranded RNA genome occurs via a conservative mechanism such that neither strand of the parent RNA is present in any daughter RNA segment.

Orbivirus

Colorado tick fever is a self-limiting illness lasting 7 to 10 days following an incubation period of 3 to 6 days. It is characterized by biphasic fever, chills, headache, retroorbital pain, severe myalgia in the back and legs, lethargy, and prostration. The virus is endemic to small mammal populations in the western United States and is transmitted to man by the wood tick, *Dermacentor andersoni.*

Rotavirus

Pathogenesis and Clinical Manifestations. Rotaviruses have a distinct tropism for the differentiated enterocytes of the intestinal tract and replicate to very high titers in these cells. Large amounts of the virus are present in the fecal material of infected individuals and infection is spread by fecal–oral transmission, with fecal contamination of hands and food probably being a major route. Asymptomatic infection is the most common manifestation of infection in all age groups from neonates to adults. Infants and young children, however, frequently experience the sudden onset of vomiting and diarrhea following an incubation period of 1 to 3 days. Vomiting often precedes the onset of diarrhea. Diarrhea typically lasts 3 to 8 days and can lead to severe dehydration. The disease is normally self-limiting but can be fatal if lost

fluids and electrolytes are not replaced. Respiratory symptoms have sometimes been reported in association with rotaviral gastroenteritis.

Epidemiology. Symptomatic illness is most prevalent in children aged 6 to 24 months. Although neonates commonly excrete rotavirus, such infections are usually asymptomatic. Breast-fed infants are thought to derive some protection from antibodies present in colostrum. The majority of individuals beyond the age of 2 years show evidence of rotavirus infection in that they have acquired specific antibodies. Local intestinal antibodies (secretory IgA) appear to protect against reinfection; however, both symptomatic and subclinical reinfections do occur. In recent years, rotaviruses have been responsible for outbreaks of gastroenteritis in elderly patients, particularly in nursing homes, and an ongoing epidemic of adult diarrhea in China has been caused by a rotavirus strain that is quite different from those causing infantile diarrhea.

Illness is sporadic and occurs most often during the winter months in temperate regions. In developed countries, acute rotaviral infection is responsible for 30% to 50% of hospitalizations due to gastroenteritis of young children but is rarely fatal. In developing nations, however, rotaviral gastroenteritis is a very serious disease with a high mortality, resulting primarily from dehydration and electrolyte imbalance.

Diagnosis. Virus, which is present in large quantities in stool specimens, can be rapidly detected by antigen–antibody tests. The most commonly used procedures for diagnosis are probably EIA and the latex agglutination tests. However, the distinctive appearance of rotaviruses makes electron microscopy a satisfactory approach to diagnosis as well.

Prevention and Treatment. Since the virus is transmitted by the fecal–oral route, good personal hygiene is a first step in the prevention of outbreaks of infection. An attenuated vaccine is being developed for oral administration to infants or nursing mothers. Although a vaccine is unlikely to offer long-term protection against infection, it would reduce the incidence of clinical disease and particularly that of severe diarrhea requiring hospitalization.

Treatment is supportive and is directed at replacing lost fluids and electrolytes when necessary.

Caliciviridae

Members of the Caliciviridae are small (31 to 35 nm), icosahedral, nonenveloped, single-stranded RNA viruses characterized by their six-pointed starlike shape and cup-shaped indentations. Like rotaviruses, the caliciviruses primarily cause gastroenteritis in infants and young children. The clinical manifestations are similar to those of rotaviral gastroenteritis, including the severity, and the infections may be clinically indistinguishable. Asymptomatic infections are apparently common since most children throughout the world develop antibodies to calicivirus, although it is responsible for only a minority of hospitalized cases of viral gastroenteritis.

Astroviruses

Astroviruses are small, nonenveloped, icosahedral viruses whose taxonomic position has not yet been determined. They are responsible for approximately 5% of all cases of infantile gastroenteritis. They most frequently cause symptomatic disease in children from infancy to 5 to 7 years of age. The elderly are also susceptible to clinical disease since the Marin County agent, isolated from an outbreak of diarrhea in elderly convalescent patients and previously considered to be a Norwalk-like agent, has been determined to be an astrovirus. The symptoms of infection follow an incubation period of 24 to 36 hours and last from 12 hours to 3 to 4 days. Watery diarrhea or vomiting may occur. Illness is less severe than in rotaviral infection.

Norwalk Agent and Norwalk-like Viruses

The so-called Norwalk agent was identified first in an outbreak of gastroenteritis primarily among adults and older children in Norwalk, Ohio. It appears on electron microscopy of fecal specimens as a small round virus that is not cultivable by current laboratory methods. Several similar but serologically distinct agents have been isolated in other outbreaks and are designated as Norwalk-like viruses. Although these viruses generally are slightly smaller than typical *Calicivirus* members, they otherwise appear similar in overall morphology. Because of the similarities, they are usually grouped with the Caliciviridae; however, the Norwalk group remains officially unclassified.

Clinical Manifestations. The incubation period is usually 24 to 48 hours and is followed by the sudden onset of nausea and vomiting, thus the designation of "winter vomiting disease." Low-grade fever and mild diarrhea are common. Vomiting may occur without diarrhea, and vice versa. Abdominal pain or cramps, headache, and malaise may also occur. Symptoms generally resolve within 24 to 48 hours.

Epidemiology. Norwalk and Norwalk-like viruses are the major cause of outbreaks of viral gastroenteritis in older children and adults. The virus is transmitted fecal-orally and most often person-to-person; however, contaminated water supplies, raw oysters, cake frosting, and lettuce have been the sources for a number of outbreaks.

Antibodies do not protect against reinfection. Some individuals appear to be susceptible to repeated infections, and others apparently are resistant to infection. Certain individuals challenged with virus do not develop disease or antibodies. Others succumb to infection even in the presence of antibodies.

Diagnosis. Routine diagnosis is made on the basis of clinical presentation. Specific diagnosis is usually unnecessary since the symptoms are of short duration and self-limiting. The virus cannot be cultured at present, and diagnostic reagents for EIA are available only in certain research laboratories.

Prevention and Treatment. Prevention is primarily via good personal hygiene and the avoidance of contamination of water supplies with sewage. A vaccine is unlikely, given the poor protection afforded by the humoral immune response. Treatment is supportive, with replacement of fluids and electrolytes as necessary.

ADDITIONAL READING

Blacklow, N. R., and Cukor, G. 1981. Viral Gastroenteritis. N Engl J Med, **304**, 397.

Christensen, M. L. 1989. Human Viral Gastroenteritis. Clin Microbiol Rev, **2**, 51.

DuPont, H. L. 1984. Rotaviral Gastroenteritis: Some Recent Developments. J Infect Dis, **149**, 663.

Fairchild, P. G., and Blacklow, N. R. 1988. Viral Diarrhea. Infect Dis Clin North Am, **2**, 677.

Friedman, M. G., et al. 1988. Two Sequential Outbreaks of Rotavirus Gastroenteritis: Evidence for Symptomatic and Asymptomatic Reinfections. J Infect Dis, **158**, 814.

White, D. O., and Fenner, F. J. 1986. Picornaviruses and Caliciviruses. In *Medical Virology*, p. 451. Academic Press, New York.

White, D. O., and Fenner, F. J. 1986. Reoviruses. In *Medical Virology*, p. 575. Academic Press, New York.

47

Retroviruses

Virginia A. Merchant and Gretchen B. Caughman

Retroviruses were described first around the turn of the century as filterable agents capable of causing animal diseases such as equine infectious anemia as well as a variety of malignancies. Because of their association with cancer, this group of viruses was loosely referred to as RNA tumor viruses, although in fact many member viruses produce other disease syndromes and most retroviruses appear to be nonpathogenic. The term "retrovirus" was coined after the 1970 discovery that these viruses possess a novel enzyme, reverse transcriptase, which is capable of reversing the usual flow of genetic information by transcribing DNA from an RNA template. Although retroviruses had been characterized for many different animal species, including insects, fish and mammals, it was not until 1980 that the first human retrovirus, human T-cell lymphotropic virus type I (HTLV-I), was isolated.

The family Retroviridae has been divided into three subfamilies: spumavirinae, oncornavirinae, and lentivirinae. Five human retroviruses have now been described. HTLV-I, an oncornavirus, is etiologically linked to a distinct form of leukemia/lymphoma. The second human retrovirus, HTLV-II, also an oncornavirus, has not been clearly associated with any disease. Human immunodeficiency virus-1 (HIV-1) is the causative agent of acquired immunodeficiency syndrome (AIDS). The fourth human retrovirus, HIV-2, has been associated with an AIDS-like syndrome in patients of African origin. Both HIV-1 and HIV-2 are classified as lentiviruses. The fifth human virus, HTLV-V, was described recently in patients with a syndrome resembling mycosis fungoides, a cutaneous lymphoproliferative disease. The role of HTLV-V in the disease has not yet been defined conclusively. Although little is known about HTLV-V, it appears to be more closely related to HTLV-I.

Viral Properties

The typical retrovirion consists of an enveloped particle approximately 100 nm in diameter with a central core containing the single-stranded RNA genome associated with the reverse transcriptase (polymerase) enzyme. The envelope is a host membrane–derived structure studded with viral glycoproteins. The genome is diploid; that is, two identical RNA molecules linked together at their 5' ends are present in each virion. A cellular transfer RNA (tRNA) may also be present that acts as a primer in viral transcription.

After attachment to the host cell via a specific receptor and penetration, the virus is uncoated in the cytoplasm to release the RNA genome and reverse transcriptase. The reverse transcriptase first begins to synthesize negative-sense DNA (complementary to the virion RNA). Even before synthesis of the negative DNA strand is finished, synthesis of the positive DNA strand and concomitant degradation of the viral RNA occurs. These polymerase reactions are quite error prone, and this may contribute to the high degree of genetic drift seen in some viruses such as HIV-1. The double-stranded DNA molecules move to the nucleus, circularize, and integrate randomly into the host cell DNA as proviruses. Because of the manner in which the viral DNA is generated, sequences present only at either end of the RNA genome are transcribed to both ends of the DNA molecule so that it is several hundred nucleotides longer than the virion's RNA. The repeated sequences now appearing at both DNA termini are known as long terminal repeats (LTRs). The LTRs are essential for the integration of the viral DNA into the cellular DNA. Once integrated, the provirus may remain latent indefinitely, or gene expression, in the form of mRNA synthesis as well as progeny RNA genomes, may proceed. Because the proviral DNA integration is a permanent event, in some instances proviral sequences are transmitted in the germ line DNA from mother to offspring. These proviruses, termed endogenous retroviruses, often remain totally silent but some may be activated by various stimuli to produce virions. This vertical transmission of endogenous retroviruses is in contrast to the transmission mode of exogenous retroviruses, which are horizontally spread to contacts, as is typical of other infectious agents.

The retroviruses have several common genomic features. All have regions coding for group-specific core antigens (*gag*), the polymerase (*pol;* reverse transcriptase), and the envelope proteins (*env*). Some retroviruses (termed acutely transforming viruses) have additional genetic information in the form of an oncogene (*onc*); these viruses are capable of oncogenically transforming cells and inducing cancers. The *onc* genes often are viral counterparts to normal cellular genes which, when expressed inappropriately under viral control, may lead to malignant transformation. Because the *onc* gene sequences usually interrupt or replace viral genes, the acutely transforming viruses are defective and require a helper virus in

order to replicate. In addition to *gag, pol,* and *env* genes, the human retroviruses have a series of regulatory genes not previously observed in other animal retroviruses. Some of these genes produce proteins which act in *trans* to regulate the expression of other genes. These gene products orchestrate the complex events of the infection cycle and thereby modulate the pathogenesis of disease.

Human T-Cell Lymphotropic Virus Type I

HTLV-I is believed to be an etiologic agent for adult T-cell leukemia/lymphoma (ATL). The HTLV-I genome has been consistently found in ATL tumor cells, and virus has been isolated from patients with the disease. In addition, 80% to 100% of patients diagnosed with ATL have high titers of antibodies to the virus. Finally, there are clusters of individuals with high levels of HTLV-I antibodies in geographic areas where the disease is prevalent even though the virus is of low seroprevalence in these areas.

The major target for HTLV-I is the CD4-positive T-cell. The pathogenesis of infection is not yet clear, but the virus may cause disease by mechanisms similar to those of other leukemia viruses. Since no oncogenes have been detected in the HTLV-I genome, the virus may act by producing a trans-acting substance that induces prolonged proliferation of the infected T-cell. The leukemias are clonal in that the provirus is integrated at the same site in all the cells in an individual, but at different sites in different patients. This means that the leukemia results from the proliferation of a single infected cell. Since many T-cells are initially infected and harbor the provirus, there must be factors governing the eventual outgrowth of a single T-cell clone that are not yet understood.

ATL is primarily a disease of adults older than 40 years of age. The clinical course is usually an aggressive one with a mean survival time of approximately 6 months. Risk of developing disease is greatest in individuals born in areas where ATL is endemic, i.e., Japan and the Caribbean basin. Patients with ATL have also been seen from other areas, including sub-Saharan Africa, Latin America, Europe, the Middle East, and the southeastern United States. Although there are exceptions, the majority of patients have been either Japanese or black, from lower socioeconomic groups, and from warm climates.

HTLV-I also has been associated with tropical spastic paraparesis (TSP) in the Caribbean and with myelopathy in Japan. Evidence of HTLV-I as the causative agent of TSP, a slowly progressive neurological disorder affecting the pyramidal tracts and to some extent the sensory system, is less well established. An increased frequency of serum antibodies to HTLV-I has been found in cases versus controls, antibodies have been detected in the cerebrospinal fluid (CSF) of cases, and virus has recently been isolated from mononuclear cells in the serum and CSF of several cases. TSP is most often seen in areas where HTLV-I is endemic.

Recently, several studies of patients with multiple sclerosis (MS) have implicated HTLV-I as a possible etiological agent of this chronic, progressive neurological disorder, but the role of HTLV-I, if any, in this demyelinating disease remains to be seen. HTLV-I has not been associated with AIDS, and infection with HTLV-I does not imply infection with HIV.

A screening test for antibody to HTLV-I was licensed by the FDA in December 1988 and is recommended for screening of blood and cellular components donated for transfusion.

Human T-Cell Lymphotropic Virus Type II

HTLV-II is closely related to HTLV-I, and there is extensive serological cross-reactivity between the two viruses. The virus was isolated initially from two patients with hairy cell leukemias, but no serological evidence of infection has been found in other cases of hairy cell leukemia. No other information is available as yet on the seroepidemiology or the modes of transmission of this virus.

Human Immunodeficiency Virus

In 1981, the first reports were published of disease in individuals who were later designated as having acquired immunodeficiency syndrome (AIDS). A new disease, designated a syndrome because of its many presentations, had arisen to infect man. As the case definition evolved, it became evident that AIDS was a unique clinical entity. Patients with AIDS were found to be severely immunosuppressed, with a reversal of the normal T-helper cell to T-suppressor cell ratio (T4:T8), making them susceptible to a variety of opportunistic infections in which cell-mediated immunity was the major protective defense. These patients also developed neoplastic lesions, particularly Kaposi's sarcoma, a malignancy not usually seen in persons less than 60 years of age.

The epidemiological picture originally associated with the spread of AIDS suggested a viral etiology. In 1983–1984, a new virus, designated lymphadenopathy-associated virus (LAV) by French investigators and human T-cell lymphotropic virus-III (HTLV-III) or AIDS-associated retrovirus (ARV) by American researchers, was described and later determined to be the etiological agent of AIDS. The designation human immunodeficiency virus, or HIV, was made by an international committee.

Since its initial diagnosis, AIDS has become a pandemic. As of July 1989, 100,000 individuals in the United States had been diagnosed with AIDS, and more than 59,000 had died. Most other developed countries have similar numbers of cases and deaths per capita. In many African nations, however, AIDS has destroyed a significant portion of the population. It is estimated that as of mid-1989, 1 to 1.5 million persons have been infected with HIV in the United States.

Properties. Two HIV strains have been identified: HIV-1 and HIV-2. More is known about HIV-1, although HIV-2 is thought to be similar in many ways. The virions have bar-shaped nucleoid cores typical of the lentivirus subfamily. The envelope glycoprotein of HIV shows a marked propensity to undergo genetic drift, a feature that may have a serious impact on the potential use of purified envelope antigen as a vaccine. The lentiviruses also have larger genomes than the other retroviruses. In addition to the *gag, pol,* and *env* genes, the HIV genome contains six or possibly seven other small genes, some of which code for proteins that regulate gene expression. Unlike the situation for viruses in the other subfamilies, a large portion of lentiviral DNA transcribed during replication may remain unintegrated, although some molecules integrate as provirus and set up latent infection.

Pathogenesis and Clinical Manifestations. HIV infection is transmitted primarily by the transfer of blood or semen, although other body fluids can be potential hazards. HIV-1, like HTLV-I, infects helper T-cells displaying CD4 glycoproteins (T4 cells), but also other cells such as macrophages, dendritic cells, and nonneuronal brain cells that exhibit CD4 antigens. Infection can result in both productively infected cells and latently infected cells. Productive HIV-1 infection is cytocidal to the T-cells and macrophages, which produce large amounts of virus and die in just a few weeks. Subsequent activation of latently infected T4 cells by antigen results in productive infection and cell death. These cells transmit the virus to other susceptible cells, primarily by cell-to-cell contact. If enough T4 cells persist, individuals may remain asymptomatic carriers for very long periods of time. However, after a large proportion of the T4 cells and antigen-presenting macrophages have been depleted, immunosuppression ensues and the individual becomes susceptible to the constellation of opportunistic infections and malignancies that characterizes clinical AIDS.

Many aspects of the pathogenesis of HIV infection are not well understood. For instance, although the eventual consequence is a profound immunosuppression, some of the early manifestations of disease are not deficiencies but rather hyperactivities, such as hypergammaglobulinemia resulting from a reactive polyclonal activation of B-cells, and lymphoid hyperplasia. Also, autoimmune phenomena such as the occurrence of autoantibodies, development of glomerulonephritis, and inflammatory skin lesions are signs of hyperactivity and dysregulation of immune responses. Thus, AIDS might be regarded more properly as a syndrome not only of immune deficiency but also of dysregulation and dysfunction.

HIV infection may result in a wide range of clinical manifestations. The infection can be manifested as an acute primary infection or simply by seroconversion and the establishment of a latent infection in T4 lymphocytes. Given the recentness of AIDS as a recognized disease, it remains to be determined whether all infected individuals will eventually develop clinical manifestations or whether some individuals will simply seroconvert and remain asymptomatic indefinitely. Following the establishment of latency, overt disease may be manifested at some future time. The latent period varies from a few months to 10 or more years following primary infection before frank symptoms of immunodeficiency develop.

In some individuals, an acute infection, seen as a flu-like or mononucleosis-like episode, develops 5 days to 3 months after HIV exposure. This illness is characterized by malaise, fever, headache, pharyngitis, lymphadenopathy, myalgia, arthralgia, and a maculopapular rash. Other individuals may present with neurological manifestations, such as meningoencephalitis, myelopathy, peripheral neuropathy, radiculopathy, or Guillain–Barré syndrome. This acute illness has been associated with HIV seroconversion. The affected individual may apparently recover, entering a period of asymptomatic disease, or begin to manifest evidence of a suppressed immune system.

Prior to the development of full-blown AIDS as defined by the CDC, there are a series of syndromes that may be manifested either alone or as a progression of clinical manifestations now recognized as pre-AIDS conditions. Initially these conditions were lumped together as ARC, or the AIDS-related complex, but because of the broad spectrum of disease associated with this condition, several classification or staging systems have been developed to differentiate among these HIV-related illnesses. Pre-AIDS conditions include immune thrombocytopenic purpura, persistent generalized lymphadenopathy, oral and gastrointestinal manifestations, central nervous system (CNS) dysfunction, and the progressive wasting syndrome known as slim disease in central Africa. Certain of these conditions, i.e., CNS disease and the progressive wasting syndrome, ultimately lead to death, and patients may die without developing either AIDS-associated opportunistic infections or malignancies (now referred to by the CDC as indicator diseases).

The CDC defines AIDS as an illness characterized by one or more indicator diseases (Table 47.1) in conjunction with laboratory evidence of HIV infection or by certain indicator diseases diagnosed definitively, a T-helper/inducer (T4) lymphocyte count $<400/mm^3$, and no other cause of the immunodeficiency in the absence of laboratory evidence of HIV infection.

Pneumocystis carinii pneumonia, the first opportunistic infection to be associated with AIDS, occurs

---

Table 47.1: Indicator Diseases of AIDS in the Absence of Laboratory Evidence of HIV Infection as Defined by the CDC

1. Candidiasis of the esophagus, trachea, bronchi, or lungs
2. Cryptococcosis, extrapulmonary
3. Cryptosporidiosis with diarrhea persisting >1 month
4. Cytomegalovirus disease of an organ other than the liver, spleen, or lymph nodes in a patient >1 month of age
5. Herpes simplex virus infection causing a mucocutaneous ulcer that persists longer than 1 month; or bronchitis, pneumonitis, or esophagitis for any duration affecting a patient >1 month of age
6. Kaposi's sarcoma affecting a patient <60 years of age
7. Lymphoma of the brain (primary) affecting a patient <60 years of age
8. Lymphoid interstitial pneumonia and/or pulmonary lymphoid hyperplasia (LIP/PLH complex) affecting a child <13 years of age
9. *Mycobacterium avium/intracellulare* complex or *M. kansasii* disease, disseminated (at a site other than or in addition to lungs, skin, or cervical or hilar lymph nodes)
10. *Pneumocystis carinii* pneumonia
11. Progressive multifocal leukoencephalopathy
12. Toxoplasmosis of the brain affecting a patient >1 month of age

Table 47.2: Oral Lesions That Have Been Associated with HIV Infection

Fungal	*Bacterial*
Candidiasis	HIV-associated gingivitis
Pseudomembranous	HIV-associated periodontitis
Hyperplastic	Necrotizing stomatitis
Erythematous (atrophic)	*Mycobacterium avium/intracellulare*
Angular cheilitis	complex
Cryptococcosis	*Klebsiella* stomatitis
	Other gram-negative infections
Viral	
Herpes simplex infections	*Neoplastic*
Herpes zoster infections	Kaposi's sarcoma
Hairy leukoplakia	Non-Hodgkin's lymphoma
Molluscum contagiosum	Squamous cell carcinoma
Warts	

Other

Oral ulcerations
Idiopathic thrombocytopenic purpura
Xerostomia
Salivary gland enlargement

in approximately 85% of patients. Previously a rare sporadic disease, it is characterized by fever, non-productive cough, and shortness of breath. *P. carinii* pneumonia is the only one of the indicator diseases which if definitively diagnosed is in itself an indication of AIDS, even if laboratory studies for HIV infection are negative.

Kaposi's sarcoma is the most common neoplasm seen in AIDS patients. Its etiology has yet to be established, although the possibility of another virus as the causative agent has been frequently suggested. In AIDS patients, this malignancy can be quite aggressive, but it is rarely fatal except in cases of pulmonary invasion.

With the breakdown in the patient's immune system, most patients with AIDS experience multiple episodes of opportunistic infections. If treated, many patients will recover from these infections but later succumb to another infection or associated disease. The average patient survival following diagnosis of AIDS has been approximately 1 year, but this time is expected to increase with the use of chemotherapeutic agents.

Oral Manifestations. The first clinical signs of HIV infection and AIDS are often oral manifestations. Table 47.2 lists the oral lesions that have been associated with HIV infection.

Candidiasis is commonly seen in both pre-AIDS and full-blown disease and may take several forms, as indicated in Table 47.2. Oral candidiasis is now seen as a predictor of the development of overt disease. Oral infection may precede the development of pharyngeal or esophageal candidiasis.

A severe, rapidly progressive form of periodontal disease is often seen in HIV-infected patients. HIV-associated gingivitis (HIV-G) presents as a fiery red line on the free gingival margin but may also involve the attached gingiva and alveolar mucosa. HIV-G is often seen in clean mouths and does not respond to conventional periodontal therapy. HIV-associated periodontitis (HIV-P) shows extensive soft tissue necrosis, severe loss of periodontal attachment, and spontaneous bleeding (Fig. 47.1). Severe deep-seated pain is often the chief complaint of patients with HIV-P. This disease may progress from a mild gingivitis to advanced periodontal disease within a few months.

Oral hairy leukoplakia (HL) is a hyperplastic white

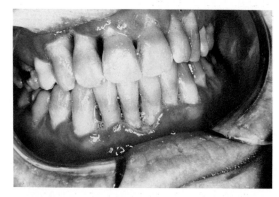

Figure 47.1: HIV-associated periodontitis. (Reproduced with permission from J. R. Winkler and P. A. Murray: Periodontal Disease. *Calif Dent Assoc J,* **15,** 22, 1987. Reprinted with permission from the *Journal of the California Dental Association.*)

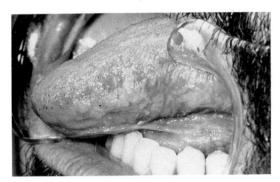

Figure 47.2: Hairy leukoplakia on the lateral border of the tongue. (Courtesy of Dr. D. Greenspan.)

lesion most commonly seen on the lateral borders of the tongue, but sometimes also on the buccal or labial mucosa (Fig. 47.2). The lesion may be smooth, corrugated, or markedly folded. HL is thought to be virally induced. The presence of Epstein–Barr virus (EBV) particles, EBV viral capsid antigen, and EBV DNA in its complete, fully replicating form in lesions of HL provides evidence for EBV as a potential etiological agent for HL. Originally described in male homosexuals infected with HIV, HL has now been reported from all groups of patients at risk for AIDS.

Oral warts, recurrent herpes simplex infections, and herpes zoster are all commonly seen in AIDS patients. In patients whose immune status is severely compromised, these infections are often extensive, severe, and prolonged. Oral ulcers resembling recurrent aphthous lesions are frequently seen in HIV patients and may be induced as a result of defects in the cell-mediated immune system.

The oral cavity is frequently the first site of appearance of the lesions of Kaposi's sarcoma. Oral Kaposi's sarcoma is most often seen on the hard palate, but the gingiva, soft palate, buccal mucosa, and tongue may also be involved. The lesions are red, blue, or purple and may be flat, raised, solitary, or multiple (Fig. 47.3).

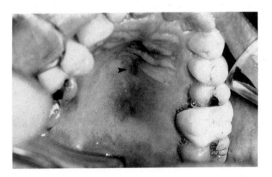

Figure 47.3: Kaposi's sarcoma on the hard palate. (Courtesy of Dr. D. Greenspan.)

Epidemiology. HIV infection has occurred throughout the world. HIV-1 was recognized first and has the widest distribution. HIV-2 was initially reported in West Africa in 1985 and was not isolated in the United States until December 1987. It is still most prevalent in West Africa, and all identified U.S. cases have been in West Africans residing in this country. The spectrum of disease and the modes of transmission of both viruses appear to be similar.

HIV has been isolated from blood, semen, vaginal secretions, saliva, tears, breast milk, urine, cerebrospinal fluid, and alveolar fluid. Infection is transmitted by sexual contact, by parenteral exposure to blood and blood products, and perinatally from mother to child. There is no evidence for transmission by casual contact or by other means such as fomites or vectors. Although HIV has been isolated from saliva, it is not frequently found and when present is in lower concentration than in blood or semen. A factor, at present unidentified, has been found in saliva that appears to inactivate HIV and may be responsible for the low concentration of virus detected as well as the fact that saliva apparently is not an effective mode of transmission.

AIDS was first recognized in homosexual men in New York and San Francisco. In the United States and other developed countries, the disease initially spread through the gay community. Because of the prolonged period of latency with no evidence of disease, transmission readily occurred from asymptomatic individuals to their sexual contacts. The virus was then transmitted into other communities via blood donations, the sharing of needles by intravenous drug users, and heterosexual contacts.

Groups at greatest risk for infection with HIV include male homosexuals, intravenous drug users, recipients of blood transfusions or blood products prior to 1985, sexual partners of the above groups, and children born to mothers belonging to any of the above groups. With the increased incidence of infection in the population and spread to contacts of many of these high-risk groups, the potential risk for HIV infection via a heterosexual contact has increased. Women who are infected with HIV can then transmit the infection to their infants during pregnancy, at parturition, or via breast-feeding.

Following HIV infection, antibodies develop and are usually detectable within 6 to 12 weeks of exposure. HIV infection, however, is persistent, and the individual may still be able to transmit virus. Detection of antibodies is indicative that infection with the virus has occurred; it does not imply viral clearance or loss of infectivity. Although seroconversion, i.e., the presence of detectable serum antibodies to HIV, usually occurs within several months of exposure, silent infections have been reported in which antibodies were not detectable for up to 36 months although viral proteins (antigens) were present.

Seroepidemiological surveys in the United States have been limited and have shown a very low level of seroprevalence in the general population (0.018% in voluntary blood donors, 0.14% in civilian applicants for military service) but much higher levels in groups of individuals at recognized risk, i.e., homosexual and bisexual men, IV drug users, and heterosexual partners of persons at risk. As of mid-1989, seroprevalence trends appeared to be relatively stable in most of these selected populations with the exception of IV drug users and their sexual partners. This suggests that the spread of HIV within the U.S. population has been slowed; however, the number of HIV-infected individuals will continue to increase, and the number of reported cases of AIDS will certainly increase as asymptomatically infected individuals develop frank AIDS. The numbers of infants and young children are also expected to increase as the result of more women being infected with HIV.

Diagnosis. The enzyme immunoassay (EIA) is most widely used for detection of antibody to HIV-1. If a serum sample is repeatedly reactive for HIV-1 antibody by EIA, the specimen should be retested via a more specific method. These include the Western blot test, antigen-capture tests, and the polymerase chain reaction. The Western blot test is the most commonly used.

The EIA tests for detection of HIV-1 currently used in the United States detect 42% to 92% of HIV-2 infections. Specific HIV-2 testing can be achieved using HIV-2 antigens in the tests. The only tests commercially available to date detect antibodies. Tests for the assay of HIV antigens are being developed and should allow earlier detection of infection, prior to seroconversion.

Diagnosis of AIDS is defined by the CDC and at least three staging systems for HIV infection have been developed. (See the discussion under Clinical Manifestations and the references listed at the end of the chapter for further information.) The diagnosis of opportunistic infections/indicator diseases associated with HIV infection and AIDS is dependent on specific diagnostic methodology associated with those infections/diseases.

Prevention and Treatment. The primary efforts of the U.S. Department of Health and Human Services in prevention of HIV infection have been directed at increasing public awareness through education. This endeavor initially met with strong resistance from many citizens since effective AIDS education required broader and more explicit discussions of sexual activities with young children as well as the dissemination of educational materials within the popular media. Public advertising warning against the sharing of needles and unprotected sex has now become commonplace in much of the country. Several large cities have set up needle exchange programs in efforts to control the spread of HIV among IV drug users.

Early efforts to prevent the spread of AIDS within the gay community led to the concept of safe sexual practices, i.e., the use of condoms and the avoidance of high-risk behaviors that might lead to exposure to blood, as well as limiting the numbers of sexual partners and thus decreasing the possibility of contact with an infected partner. The concept of safe sex has spread to the heterosexual population and had a major impact on sexual practices in the late 1980s.

To date, although the potential exposure to HIV in saliva and blood in the dental office has been substantial in certain areas, only two cases of seroconversion in dental professionals who were not members of high-risk groups have been seen. Therefore, the risk of HIV infection in dental practice is minimal and especially if recommended infection control practices are carefully followed. The concern of health care professionals over the potential transmission of HIV during patient care has been instrumental in the implementation of improved infection control protocols in both dentistry and medicine and was primarily responsible for the development of the concept of universal precautions (see Chap. 13). HIV seroconversion has occurred in health care workers as the result of needle-stick injuries, cuts, open-wound contamination, and mucous membrane exposures to the blood of HIV-infected patients; however, the seroprevalence rate in these exposed workers is extremely low (0.42%), indicating a low risk of seroconversion following exposure to the blood of HIV-infected individuals.

Several potential AIDS vaccines are under development, and clinical trials are under way. Progress in vaccine development has been impeded by our lack of understanding of protective immunity against HIV infection, the magnitude of genetic variation of the virus, and the lack of effective animal models. Preliminary results suggest, however, that an effective vaccine can probably be developed. Because of the high morbidity and mortality associated with HIV disease, the benefits of a vaccine providing protection against infection will outweigh some degree of risk.

Treatment of opportunistic infections in AIDS patients usually requires aggressive management in order to control the infection; refer to the chapters on these infectious diseases or the references regarding treatment modalities. Much effort has been directed at developing antiretroviral agents as well as therapeutic agents to restore the defective immune system. To date, the only drug that has proved effective in lengthening the survival of HIV-infected patients when used as monotherapy has been zidovudine (3'-azidothymidine; AZT). Zidovudine blocks HIV replication by inhibiting the virus-associated reverse transcriptase and was the first antiviral drug approved for AIDS therapy. Recent research results suggest that zidovudine can delay, if not prevent, the onset of full-blown AIDS when used prophylactically in asymptomatic HIV-infected individuals. As investigations continue, it is expected that either new agents will be proven effective or a combination of agents will be shown to be more efficacious than zidovudine alone. Combination trials of zidovudine with several other agents are in progress.

ADDITIONAL READING

AIDS Alert. A monthly update for health professionals. American Health Consultants Inc., 60 Peachtree Park Drive, NE, Atlanta, GA 30309-1397.

CDC AIDS Weekly. A weekly newsletter published privately for subscribers. P.O. Box 830409, Birmingham, AL 35283-0409.

Centers for Disease Control. 1986. Classification System for Human T-Lymphotropic Virus Type III/Lymphadenopathy Associated Virus Infection. MMWR, **35**, 334.

Centers for Disease Control. 1987. Revision of the CDC Surveillance Case Definition for Acquired Immunodeficiency Syndrome. MMWR, **36** (1S), 3S.

Friedland, G. H., and Klein, R. S. 1987. Transmission of the Human Immunodeficiency Virus. N Engl J Med, **317**, 1125.

Furman, P. A., and Barry, D. W. 1988. Spectrum of Antiviral Activity and Mechanism of Action of Zidovudine. Am J Med, **85**, Suppl 2A, 176.

Greenspan, D., Greenspan, J. S., Pindborg, J. J., and Schiodt, M. 1986. *AIDS and the Dental Team*. Munksgaard, Copenhagen.

Greenspan, J. S., and Greenspan, D. 1989. Oral Hairy Leukoplakia: Diagnosis and Management. Oral Surg Oral Med Oral Pathol, **67**, 396.

Hasse, A. T. 1986. Pathogenesis of Lentivirus Infections. Nature, **322**, 130.

Hirsch, M. S. 1988. Antiviral Drug Development for the Treatment of Human Immunodeficiency Virus Infection. Am J Med, **85**, Suppl 2A, 182.

Ho, D. D., Pomerantz, R. J., and Kaplan, J. C. 1987. Pathogenesis of Infection with Human Immunodeficiency Virus. N Engl J Med, **317**, 278.

Justice, A. C., Feinstein, A. R., and Wells, C. K. 1989. A New Prognostic Staging System for the Acquired Immunodeficiency Syndrome. N Engl J Med, **320**, 1388.

Koff, W. C., and Hoth, D. F. 1988. Development and Testing of AIDS Vaccines. Science, **241**, 426.

Levine, P. H., and Blattner, W. A. 1987. The Epidemiology of Diseases Associated with HTLV-I and HTLV-II. Infect Dis Clin North Am, **1**, 501.

Levy, J. A. 1986. The Multifaceted Retrovirus. Cancer Res **46**, 5457.

Marcus, R., et al. 1988. Surveillance of Health Care Workers Exposed to Blood from Patients Infected with the Human Immunodeficiency Virus. N Engl J Med, **319**, 1118.

Mims, C. A. 1988. Pathogenesis of Infection with the Human Immunodeficiency Virus: A Personal View. J Infection, **17**, 221.

Moellering, R. C., Jr. (Ed.) 1988. Medical Management of AIDS. Infect Dis Clin North Am, **2**, 285.

Redfield, R. R., Wright, D. C., and Tramont, E. C. 1986. The Walter Reed Staging Classification for HTLV-III/LAV Infection. N Engl J Med, **314**, 131.

Robertson, P. B., and Greenspan, J. S. (Eds.) 1988. *Perspectives on Oral Manifestations of AIDS: Diagnosis and Management of HIV-Associated Infections*. PSG Publishing Co., Littleton, Mass.

Weissman, I. 1988. Approaches to an Understanding of Pathogenetic Mechanisms in AIDS. Rev Infect Dis, **10**, 385.

48

Viral Hepatitis: Hepatitis A, Hepatitis B, Non-A, Non-B Hepatitis, and Delta Hepatitis

Virginia A. Merchant and Gretchen B. Caughman

Viral hepatitis in humans may be caused by several unrelated viruses. They are considered together in this chapter because of their similar, although not identical, clinical presentations and the need to accurately differentiate among them as to the etiological agent of any particular viral hepatitis case. All of the hepatitis viruses are difficult to cultivate and study by conventional means; a great deal has been learned recently about some of them, but about others we know almost nothing. Table 48.1 compares the characteristics of the hepatitis viruses as we currently recognize them.

Although outbreaks of epidemic jaundice have been noted since ancient times, only around the middle of this century was it realized that a number of different agents could cause hepatitis with jaundice. The term *infectious hepatitis* came to be used for one form of hepatitis that has a short incubation period

and is caused by the ingestion of contaminated food or water. Another form of disease follows injection of blood or blood products and has a long incubation period; this type came to be called *serum hepatitis*. The two diseases now are known as hepatitis A and hepatitis B, respectively, and can be differentiated by laboratory detection of specific antigens or antibodies. In the process of developing and using the specific assays, it became apparent that many hepatitis cases, particularly those following blood transfusions, were not due to hepatitis A virus or hepatitis B virus. Thus, by exclusion, these were termed non-A, non-B (NANB) hepatitis. Very little is known about the etiological agent(s) of NANB hepatitis, although recent studies indicate that at least two different viruses may be responsible. In the late 1970s, a previously unrecognized antigen was detected in the livers of some hepatitis B patients. This antigen was found to belong

Table 48.1: Characteristics and Clinical Manifestations of the Hepatitis Viruses

Property	HAV	HBV	NANB		HDV
Family	Picornaviridae	Hepadnaviridae	Togavirus-like?	?	Unclassified
Biological characteristics	Nonenveloped ssRNA	Enveloped; partially dsDNA, circular	ssRNA	?	ssRNA; HBsAg coat
Transmission	Fecal–oral	Blood, saliva, semen, other secretions?, mother to infant	Blood, probably sexual	Fecal–oral	Blood; requires HBV co-infection or HBsAg carrier state
Virus in feces	Late incubation period; Active phase	May be present	Unknown	Probably?	Unknown
Virus in blood	Late incubation period; Early acute phase	Late incubation period; Active phase may persist in carrier	Probably like HBV	?	Late incubation period; Early acute phase
Incubation period	1½–6 weeks (usually 30 days)	4–28 weeks (usually 60–180 days)	2–26 weeks (usually 35–70 days)	1½–6 weeks (usually 40 days)	Similar to HBV
Incidence of subclinical infection, i.e., nonicteric disease	Common, especially in children	Common	?	Apparently common in children	Apparently common
Type of onset	Usually abrupt	Usually insidious	Usually insidious	Abrupt?	Insidious?
Clinical symptoms	Fever, fatigue, myalgias, malaise, anorexia, nausea	Malaise, anorexia, nausea, headache, moderate fever	Mild symptoms similar to HBV	Similar to other viral hepatitis, but pruritus common	Similar to HBV
Duration of serum transaminase elevation	1–3 weeks	1–>6 months	1–2 years in up to 50% of pts; longer with persistent infection	?	2–>3 months
Fulminant infection	Very rare	<1%	Yes	Yes, especially in pregnant women	Common
Persistent infection	No	Occurs in 5%–10% of older children and adults and 90% of infants	Common, 10%–60%	No	Persistent infection common in survivors
Markers of persistent infection	—	HBsAg, HBeAg	Not defined	—	Anti-HD IgM
Mortality	<0.1%	1%–2%, but higher in adults over 40 years	Similar to HBV	High in pregnant women	High, ca. 20%
Possible outcomes of persistent infection	None	Cirrhosis, HCC	Cirrhosis	None	Cirrhosis

to a separate agent, the delta virus. Delta virus is a distinct virus, but it appears to be able to infect only patients who have active hepatitis B infections. It should be kept in mind that a number of viruses discussed in other chapters, including yellow fever virus, lassa virus, Epstein–Barr virus, cytomegalovirus, herpes simplex virus, and adenoviruses, also can produce liver inflammation and jaundice, but the liver is generally a secondary target for these viruses rather than the primary target organ as it is for the hepatitis viruses.

Hepatitis A

Originally designated as infectious hepatitis, hepatitis A, caused by the hepatitis A virus, is actually only one of the forms of hepatitis caused by infectious agents.

Properties. Hepatitis A virus (HAV) is a particularly fastidious member of the *Enterovirus* genus of the family Picornaviridae (see Chap. 40). Morphologically, it is a typical picornavirus: the virion consists of a nonenveloped, icosahedral capsid, 27 nm in diameter, surrounding one molecule of single-stranded positive-sense RNA. The physical and chemical properties of HAV are typical of the *Enterovirus* genus and this has led to its formal classification as enterovirus type 72.

Pathogenesis and Clinical Manifestations. HAV enters the body via the enteric tract, and, although there is no cellular evidence of HAV antigen synthesis in the gastrointestinal (GI) tract, the presence of viral antigen and antibodies in feces indicates that some epithelial cells of the GI tract must be susceptible to infection. From the GI tract, HAV disseminates to its primary target organ, the liver, where it replicates in the hepatocytes. Initial culturing of HAV was made difficult by the fact that virus freshly isolated from clinical samples had a very long adaptation period, produced no cytopathic effects, and did not appear to shut down any cellular processes. HAV has now been adapted to a number of cell lines, but viral replication is still relatively slow.

HAV disease may vary from completely asymptomatic with only minimal biochemical evidence of hepatitis (i.e., an increase in serum transaminases) to symptomatic disease with jaundice. HAV infection is relatively mild and does not result in chronic disease or persistent infection. Fulminant hepatitis leading to hepatic failure is extremely rare.

Following an incubation period of 2 to 6 weeks (usually about 4 weeks), fever, fatigue, myalgias, malaise, anorexia, and nausea may develop. The onset of symptoms is usually abrupt. Patients may or may not develop clinical evidence of liver inflammation including upper abdominal discomfort, dark urine, icterus, hepatomegaly, and splenomegaly. Clinical illness usually lasts 2 to 3 weeks but may be more prolonged in adults.

Figure 48.1 shows the course of production of viral antigen and antibodies. Hepatitis A antigen (HAAg) is detectable prior to the onset of clinical symptoms at about 30 days. The elevation of liver enzymes basically coincides with clinical disease but may remain at an increased level for some weeks following resolution of symptoms. The severity of disease appears to coincide with the level of detectable HAAg in feces and blood.

Epidemiology. HAV infection occurs worldwide with sporadic outbreaks occurring in developed countries such as the United States. In less developed regions of the world where sanitation is poor, HAV infection is common in children, and the majority (>90%) of individuals have been infected prior to adulthood. In developed countries such as the United States, only around 20% of adults have antibodies to HAV. Outbreaks in developed countries usually follow exposure to sewage-contaminated drinking water or uncooked or undercooked shellfish. Ingestion of contaminated water or food may lead to outbreaks in populations that are not normally exposed to sewage-contaminated water. Secondary fecal–oral transmission may occur, particularly among family members or in day-care centers for young children. Although there is a transient viremia following HAV infection, percutaneous or parenteral transmission is rare.

HAV infection is usually milder and of shorter duration in children than in adults. In fact, most infections in children are subclinical and anicteric. Overall, only about 10% of infections are clinically apparent. There is a single serotype of HAV, and long-lasting, protective immunity develops following infection.

Diagnosis. Acute HAV infection can be confirmed by demonstration of anti-HAAg IgM in serum. The presence of anti-HAAg IgG in the absence of anti-HAAg IgM is evidence of past infection or of passively acquired antibodies. Serodiagnosis by EIA (enzyme-linked immunosorbent assays) or RIA (radioimmunoassays) has replaced complement fixation assays and other tests previously employed.

Prevention and Treatment. Preexposure or postexposure prophylaxis with immune globulin is an effective method of preventing icteric disease but does not change the incidence of infection. Efforts to develop a vaccine to prevent HAV infection are promising, and either a live attenuated or component vaccine is anticipated within the next 10 years.

Treatment of hepatitis is nonspecific and consists of supportive measures, relief of symptoms, and avoidance of further liver damage. Bed rest is advised during the period of symptoms, and all but the most necessary medications should be avoided during the acute phase of disease.

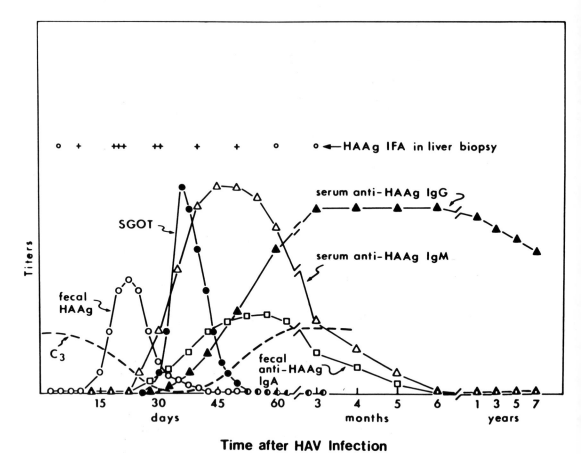

Figure 48.1: Course of hepatitis A infection. (Reproduced with permission from W. S. Robinson: Hepatitis A Virus. In *Principles and Practice of Infectious Diseases,* Ed. 3, edited by G. L. Mandell, R. G. Douglas, Jr., and J. E. Bennett. Churchill Livingstone, New York, 1990.)

Hepatitis B

Hepatitis B infection was originally known as serum hepatitis, but the term is no longer applicable, as we now recognize that all viral hepatides can be transmitted via exposure to blood (rare for hepatitis A). Although at the present time the highest incidence of hepatitis due to parenteral transmission is due to NANB hepatitis rather than to hepatitis B, the term serum hepatitis is still often identified with hepatitis B. Hepatitis B virus (HBV) is of major worldwide importance because chronic infection is one of the leading causes of death among adults, due to chronic liver disease and primary hepatocellular carcinoma (HCC).

Properties.   HBV belongs to a new virus family, Hepadnaviridae (*hepa* = hepatitis, *dna* = DNA genome). Several similar viruses of other animals, such as duck hepatitis virus and woodchuck hepatitis virus, also belong to this family. These viruses have been invaluable as research tools in animal model systems, since man is the only natural host of HBV and

it has yet to be cultivated in cell culture. HBV has several notable features, including a unique genome consisting of a circular DNA molecule that is partially single-stranded, a complex replication strategy that involves synthesis of an RNA intermediate and the activity of a viral-encoded reverse transcriptase (RNA-dependent DNA polymerase), and the production of very large amounts of one viral antigen, aggregates of which appear in infected serum as aberrant, noninfectious particles.

Three distinct particles are usually found in the serum of patients with clinical disease (Fig. 48.2). The Dane particle, the least frequent species, is the infectious virion. It is 42 nm in diameter and appears to be a complex sphere consisting of an electron-dense core surrounded by an envelope. The second type of particle is a 22-nm sphere, and the third type is comprised of filamentous forms, 22 nm in diameter and varying in length to more than 200 nm. The surfaces of these latter two particle types are similar to that of the Dane particle, and indeed they appear to be ag-

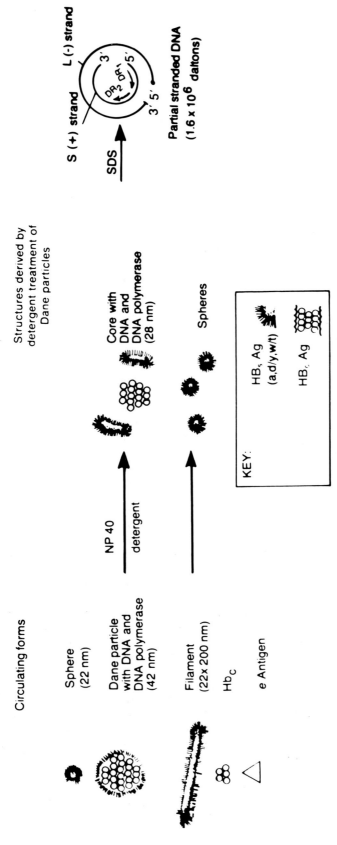

Figure 48.2: Schematic diagram of the circulating particles and antigens of HBV and the DNA structure. (Reproduced with permission from R. Dulbecco, and H. S. Ginsberg: *Virology*, Ed. 2, J. B. Lippincott Co., Philadelphia, 1988, as modified by permission of *The New England Journal of Medicine* from W. S. Robinson and L. I. Lutwick: *N Engl J Med*, **295**, 1232, 1976. Copyright by J. B. Lippincott.)

gregates of only one of the major viral proteins, the hepatitis B surface antigen (HBsAg). The 22-nm spheres and filaments are present in infected serum in extremely large amounts; concentrations of more than 10^{13} 22-nm particles per milliliter of serum have been reported. The concentration of Dane particles is usually at least a thousand-fold less.

In addition to HBsAg, the Dane particle contains another major antigen, the core antigen (HBcAg). HBcAg is found only in Dane particles, not in the other particle types. There are several HBsAg antigenic subtypes based on differences in its several antigenic determinants. The isolated polypeptides of HBsAg induce antibodies that offer protection from HBV infection and were therefore used as the component for the vaccine produced for immunization against HBV. (See Prevention and Treatment, below.) HBcAg is of a single antigenic type. Some patient sera also contain a third antigen, HBeAg, which is specific to HBV infection.

A unique model for HBV replication has been proposed based on information derived from the other hepadnavirus animal models and from identification of viral structures in the hepatocytes of patients with acute and chronic HBV. After uncoating of the virion, the viral DNA is conveyed to the cell nucleus where the virion-associated DNA polymerase completes the partially double-stranded molecule by filling in the single-stranded gap. Host cell DNA-dependent RNA polymerase then transcribes the minus strand DNA to complete RNA copies, as well as smaller capped mRNAs. These RNAs are transported to the cytoplasm where the core protein and the viral polymerase are translated from mRNA. Molecules of core protein encapsidate the complete RNA (pregenome RNA) as well as the viral polymerase enzyme, which has reverse transcriptase activity. The reverse transcriptase synthesizes DNA from the RNA pregenome template and all but a very small fragment of the RNA template is simultaneously degraded. The DNA synthesis reaction rarely goes to completion prior to egress of the viral particle, so that a single-stranded section of the genome remains to be filled at the onset of the next replication cycle.

Thus, like the retroviruses, the hepadnaviruses rely on a reverse transcriptase activity to replicate their genomes. However, the hepadnaviruses begin with DNA, go through an RNA intermediate, and end with DNA, whereas the retroviruses begin and end with RNA. Also, in most instances, the retroviruses' DNA intermediate must become integrated into the host cell's DNA in order to function; the hepadnaviruses have no such integration requirement. However, integration of HBV DNA does occur, particularly in association with hepatocellular carcinoma in patients with chronic HBV infection.

Destruction of HBV can be achieved by any method approved for sterilization. Additionally, it is assumed that any EPA-registered hospital tuberculocidal disinfectant when used appropriately will inactivate HBV. These include diluted hypochlorite solutions, glutaraldehydes, iodophors, and complex phenolics.

Pathogenesis and Clinical Manifestations. HBV is assumed to reach the liver via the bloodstream and to replicate predominantly or exclusively in hepatocytes. The lack of cell culture models for HBV makes our knowledge of cytopathic effects very sketchy. In experimental infections of chimpanzees, HBcAg appears in the nuclei of hepatocytes as early as 2 weeks after infection. It has been postulated that HBV is not highly cytopathic, but rather the infection induces cellular and humoral immune responses that severely damage or destroy the hepatocytes.

The majority of HBV infections are asymptomatic, self-limited, and completely resolve within 6 months of onset. Others can be symptomatic but self-limiting, can persist with or without evidence of clinical symptoms, or can be fulminant, often leading to hepatic failure and death. Chronic HBV infection can lead to the development of cirrhosis or hepatocellular carcinoma (HCC). Although HBV has not been proven unequivocably to be the etiological agent of HCC, the evidence strongly supports this conclusion.

In those patients who experience clinical manifestations, the incubation period from exposure to the appearance of symptoms ranges from 1 to 6 months. Acute hepatitis caused by HBV usually has a more insidious onset and a more prolonged course than that caused by HAV infection. Malaise and anorexia are usually the first symptoms to appear. Nausea, headache, and moderate fever are also commonly seen early in the course of disease. Symptomatic disease may be mild without jaundice, or more severe with associated icterus. Some patients experience fever, urticarial rash, and arthralgias in the preicteric phase, but icterus and dark urine are the most prominent features that develop. Icterus is most apparent in the sclera and on the ventral side of the tongue. Physical findings include right upper quadrant tenderness, mild to moderate hepatomegaly, and mild splenomegaly. The usual duration of symptoms ranges from approximately 2 weeks in children to 4 to 6 weeks in adults.

Increased levels of serum transaminases (either measured as serum glutamic-pyruvic transaminase [SGPT] and serum glutamic-oxalacetic transaminase [SGOT], or as alanine aminotransferase [ALT]) are almost invariably associated with hepatitis B infection, whether or not disease is apparent. The elevation in liver enzymes can usually be detected prior to the onset of symptoms and is frequently correlated with the extent of liver damage. SGPT levels usually exceed

SGOT levels. Serum bilirubin increases over a period of 10 to 14 days and then falls gradually over 2 to 4 weeks.

Although most cases of HBV infection are self-limiting, more severe disease is often seen. Some 5% to 10% of older children and adults infected with HBV will develop persistent or chronic disease. Of these patients, approximately 70% are silent carriers of HBV. These individuals have persistent infection, as evidenced by an HBs antigenemia. They may show evidence of elevated liver enzymes but otherwise appear healthy. The other 30% have chronic active hepatitis. These patients may or may not be jaundiced and often have progressive disease, which may lead to cirrhosis, hepatic failure, and death. In contrast to the rate of development of chronic disease in older individuals, 90% of infants infected perinatally develop chronic HBV infection.

On occasion, apparently mild cases of hepatitis B persist for 12 months or more. These may be difficult to distinguish from chronic hepatitis until the patient becomes HBsAg negative and the liver infection resolves. Relapses of hepatitis may also occur. These are usually associated with premature return to normal activity, consumption of alcohol, or treatment with corticosteroids and are seen as episodes of milder disease following apparent recovery from initial infection.

Fulminant hepatitis develops in a small percentage of patients (<1%) and is often fatal. Hepatic failure is accompanied by encephalopathy, culminating in coma and death. The incidence of fulminant hepatitis is increased when infection with delta hepatitis virus occurs concomitantly with HBV infection (see discussion under Delta Hepatitis).

Hepatocellular carcinoma (HCC) is a major cause of death in countries where HBV infection is endemic (see Epidemiology). It appears to follow persistent HBV infections of long duration. Viral DNA has been found in approximately 75% of tumors, and in many of these, the viral genomic material is integrated into the cellular DNA.

Serological Markers in Hepatitis B. Hepatitis B surface antigen (HBsAg), usually the first indication of active infection, may be detected in the blood as early as 1 week or as late as 12 weeks following exposure. This viral marker is detectable for 1 to 6 weeks in most patients with self-limited infections; however, it may persist up to 20 weeks. If clinical symptoms develop, they usually follow the appearance of HBsAg by approximately 4 weeks. In the majority of patients, HBsAg is no longer detectable after 20 weeks. In approximately 10%, antigenemia persists, indicating persistent infection, and the patient is classified as a hepatitis B carrier. Some patients with self-limited HBV infections never have detectable HBsAg in the blood.

Hepatitis B e antigen (HBeAg) may also be detected in serum and usually appears just after and disappears just before HBsAg. The level of HBeAg has been found to correlate with the level of infectious virus and thus can be related to the infectivity of a patient. Hepatitis B carriers who are also HBeAg positive are more infectious than HBsAg-positive individuals who are HBeAg negative. Unlike HBsAg and HBeAg, hepatitis B core antigen (HBcAg) is not free in serum, although it is found in circulating Dane particles.

Antibodies produced to hepatitis B antigens are important both in the diagnosis of infection and the prognosis of disease. Antibodies to HBsAg (anti-HBs) generally do not appear until the antigen disappears. Once HBsAg is no longer detectable, there is often a time interval, up to several months, during which neither free HBsAg nor anti-HBs is detected in serum samples. This period has been designated as the "window" or "core window" and may be important in evaluating recovery. Antibody to HBsAg typically persists for years and is associated with protection against reinfection. Since HBsAg is the viral component of hepatitis B vaccine, anti-HBs is produced following immunization and is the only HBV antibody that is evoked following vaccine administration.

Following natural infection, the immunocompetent individual also mounts an immune response to HBcAg and HBeAg. Antibodies to HBcAg are evoked early, usually within 3 to 5 weeks of appearance of HBsAg, and are the only antibodies detectable during acute clinical disease. This antibody is the only serological marker present in patients with recent HBV infection during the period of the "core window." Antibodies to HBeAg appear shortly after the antigen wanes and persist for 1 to 2 years. Since the presence of HBeAg in HBsAg carriers is an indication of viral replication and the potential for transmission, the presence of anti-HBe in an HBsAg carrier suggests a lessened risk of transmission.

Figures 48.3, 48.4, and 48.5 present schematics of the typical serological responses seen in self-limited HBV infections and in persistent HBV infection. Table 48.2 lists the serological markers associated with various stages of HBV infection.

Epidemiology. Hepatitis B has a worldwide distribution and is one of the leading causes of premature death in adults globally, due to the sequelae of chronic hepatitis: cirrhosis and HCC. At the close of the 1980s, over 200 million people worldwide had chronic HBV disease. The infection is endemic to Southeast Asia, China, tropical Africa, the Pacific Islands, the Amazon basin, and the Middle East, where there is a seropositivity rate of 70% to 95% with a carrier rate of 8% to 20%. Within North America, Western Europe, Australia, and temperate South

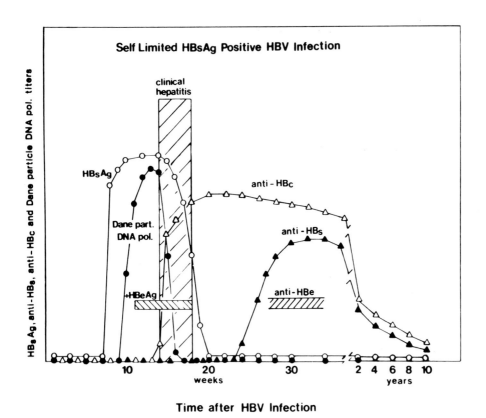

Figure 48.3: Schematic representation of viral markers in the blood throughout the course of self-limited HBsAb-positive primary HBV infection. (Reproduced with permission from W. S. Robinson: Hepatitis B Virus and the Delta Agent. In *Principles and Practice of Infectious Diseases,* Ed. 3, edited by G. L. Mandell, R. G. Douglas, Jr., and J. E. Bennett. Churchill Livingstone, New York, 1990.)

America, the prevalence of HBV infection is low in the general population, and the seropositivity rate is 4% to 6% with only 0.2% to 0.5% of the population being HBsAg carriers.

HBV is transmitted parenterally, sexually, from mother to infant, and by close personal contact via exchange of body secretions such as saliva. HBsAg has been found in blood and blood products, feces, urine, bile, sweat, tears, saliva, semen, breast milk, vaginal secretions, cerebrospinal fluid, synovial fluid, and cord blood.

In the areas of the world where HBV is endemic, transmission most frequently occurs from chronically infected mothers to their infants. Pregnant women who are both HBsAg positive and HBeAg positive have a 70% to 90% chance of transmitting the infection to their infant. Since 90% of infants infected perinatally develop chronic disease, they can then transmit the infection via secretions to other children with whom they come in contact. In areas of low endemicity such as the United States, transmission from mother to child is rare, and infection is more commonly spread by parenteral exposure or sexual contact. The risk of infection is directly related to the number of parenteral exposures or sexual contacts that an individual has. Those at greatest risk of infection are IV drug abusers, recipients of unscreened blood products, sexually active homosexual males, promiscuous heterosexuals, health care professionals exposed to blood or saliva, and the sexual contacts or children of these high-risk individuals. Another group at increased risk of HBV infection comprises institutionalized, developmentally disabled individuals, who are likely to be exposed to HBV-contaminated secretions.

The incidence of HBV infection in the United States has been estimated by the Centers for Disease Control (CDC) to be over 300,000 cases per year. Only about one quarter of these will have clinically confirmed disease, and approximately 10% would be expected to develop chronic infection with the potential for transmission to those at risk of infection.

The risk of hepatitis B in unimmunized, unpro-

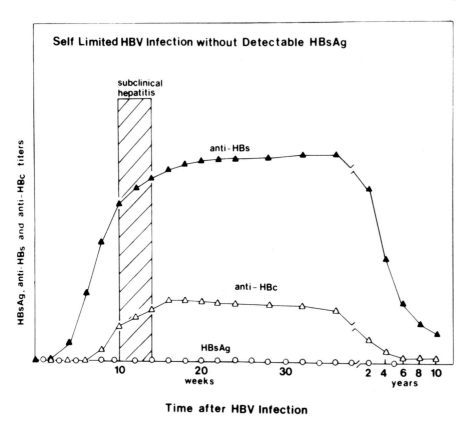

Figure 48.4: Schematic representation of the serological response throughout the course of HBsAg-negative primary HBV infection. (Reproduced with permission from W. S. Robinson: Hepatitis B Virus and the Delta Agent. In *Principles and Practice of Infectious Diseases,* Ed. 3, edited by G. L. Mandell, R. G. Douglas, Jr., and J. E. Bennett. Churchill Livingstone, New York, 1990.)

tected dental professionals is significant. A 1982 study to determine the prevalence of antibodies to HBV in a group of 963 dental professionals (dentists, hygienists, and other auxiliary personnel) revealed an overall prevalence of 16.2% for dentists, 16.9% for hygienists, 14.2% for laboratory technicians, 12.5% for assistants, and 8.9% for dental clerical workers. Oral and maxillofacial surgeons had the greatest incidence of markers, 24%, as might be expected since the prevalence of infection is directly related to the potential for blood exposure. In addition to the personal risk, a dentist infected in practice can transmit that infection to his or her spouse, children, and patients if precautions are not taken. Eleven outbreaks of hepatitis B have been traced to HBsAg-positive dentists. Dentists are not alone in transmitting infection to their patients; physicians have also been implicated as the source of hepatitis B outbreaks.

The incidence pattern of high-risk groups for hepatitis B in the United States changed during the 1980s, although the total number of cases remained about the same. A decreased incidence of hepatitis B was seen in sentinel populations of homosexual men and in health care workers from 1984 to 1987 while the incidence of infection increased by 80% in IV drug abusers and by 33% in heterosexuals. The decreased rate of infection in homosexual males was probably due to the decrease in high-risk sexual behaviors as part of AIDS prevention. The decreased rate of HBV infection seen in health care workers is probably the result of HBV vaccination and the increased precautions required for health care workers when there is potential for exposure to blood or other body fluids.

Diagnosis. When acute viral hepatitis is suspected, a diagnostic profile is usually requested and includes assay for anti-HAV IgM, HBsAg, and anti-HBc (Table 48.3). In patients who present with histories of unknown hepatitis, evaluation might include assay for anti-HAV IgG, anti-HBs, and HBsAg. If the individual is HBsAg positive, tests should be ordered for HBeAg and anti-HBe to determine the individual's probable infectivity.

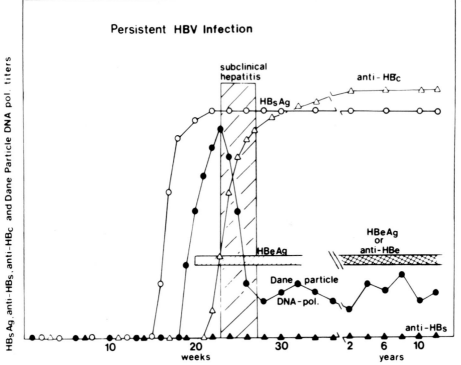

Figure 48.5: Schematic representation of viral markers in the blood throughout the course of HBV infection that becomes persistent. (Reproduced with permission from W. S. Robinson: Hepatitis B Virus and the Delta Agent. In *Principles and Practice of Infectious Diseases,* Ed. 3, edited by G. L. Mandell, R. G. Douglas, Jr., and J. E. Bennett. Churchill Livingstone, New York, 1990.)

Table 48.2: HBV Serological Markers in Different Stages of Infection and Convalescence*

| Stage of Infection | HBsAg | Anti-HBs | Anti-HBc | | HBeAg | Anti-HBe |
			IgG	IgM		
Late incubation period of hepatitis B	+	−	−	−	+/−	−
Acute hepatitis B	+	−	+	+	+	−
HBsAg-negative acute hepatitis B	−	−	+	+	−	−
Healthy HBsAg carrier	+	−	+ + +	+/−	−	−
Chronic hepatitis B	+	−	+ + +	+/−	+	−
HBV infection in recent past	−	+ +	+ +	+/−	−	+
HBV infection in distant past	−	+/−	+/−	−	−	−
Recent HBV vaccination	−	+ +	−	−	−	−

*Reproduced with permission from G. L. Mandell, et al.: *Principles and Practice of Infectious Diseases,* Ed. 3. Churchill Livingstone, New York, 1990.

Table 48.3: Interpretation of Results of Viral Hepatitis Diagnostic Profile

Anti-HAV IgM	HBsAg	Anti-HBc	Interpretation	Further Testing to Confirm
+	0	0	Acute HAV infection	None required
0	+	0	Acute HBV infection	Evaluate recovery*
0	+	+	Either acute or chronic HBV infection	anti-HBc IgM†
0	0	+	History of HBV infection, may be active	anti-HBs‡
0	0	0	Not HAV or HBV hepatitis	Rule out other causes§
+	+	+	Acute HAV infection in an HBsAg carrier	Determine infectivity‖

*Evaluate for seroconversion (anti-HBs). If HBsAg persists (HBsAg carrier), determine relative infectivity.

†If anti-HBc IgM is positive, acute HBV infection. See *asterisk* above. If anti-HBc IgM is negative, chronic HBV infection; see *parallels* below.

‡If anti-HBs is positive, recent or past history of HBV infection (indicates recovery). If patient is still symptomatic, evaluate for other causes of current illness. See *section mark*. If anti-HBs is negative, suggests recent HBV infection and currently in "window" phase. Reevaluate for seroconversion.

§If other infectious agents and environmental factors have been ruled out as causes of hepatitis, suggests probably NANB hepatitis.

‖If HBsAg carrier (chronic HBV infection) should determine relative infectivity by measuring HBeAg and anti-HBe. A positive HBeAg test indicates active viral replication and suggests that the individual is more likely to transmit infection than if HBeAg is negative and anti-HBe is positive.

Prevention and Treatment. Hepatitis B transmission can be effectively prevented by appropriate application of environmental control measures and immunization. Environmental control measures are the use of barriers and personal hygiene, particularly hand washing. Prior to the recommendations for universal precautions in the treatment of all dental patients (see Chap. 13, Sterilization and Disinfection), attempts were made to identify possible HBsAg-positive individuals by medical history and/or serological evaluation. These patients were then treated as infectious. With universal precautions, all dental patients are now treated as potentially infectious, making it unnecessary from an infection control standpoint to identify healthy HBsAg-positive individuals. Adherence to the recommendations for protection against occupational exposure to infectious agents as set forth by the Department of Health and Human Services and the CDC as well as various health care organizations is effective in preventing occupational exposure to hepatitis B virus as well as other hepatitis viruses. The use of barriers and personal hygiene also applies to individuals having household or other potential exposure to HBV.

Following extensive testing in more than 19,500 volunteers, many of whom were health care workers, Merck Sharp & Dohme began marketing its plasma-derived HB vaccine, Heptavax-B, in June 1982 (Table 48.4). This vaccine consists of purified, noninfectious HBsAg derived from the plasma of chronic carriers of HBV. Following purification of the HBsAg, three inactivation steps are undertaken consisting of treatments with pepsin at pH 2, 8 mol urea, and 1:4,000 formalin, treatments shown to inactivate HBV as well as other viral agents. The vaccine is administered as a three dose series. The vaccine is recommended for groups

Table 48.4: Immunization Against HBV

Preexposure:

Three intramuscular doses of HB vaccine, with second and third doses given 1 and 6 months, respectively, after the first.

(Three vaccines are currently available in the U.S.: Heptavax-B and Recombivax-HB, both marketed by Merck Sharp & Dohme, and Engerix-B by Smithkline Beckman.)

Postexposure (nonimmunized persons):

HBIG *and* initiation of HB vaccine series.

(Also applies to infants born to HBsAg-positive mothers.)

Table 48.5: Persons for Whom Hepatitis B Vaccine Is Recommended or Should Be Considered*

Preexposure:

Persons for whom vaccine is recommended:
  Health care workers having blood or needle-stick exposures
  Clients and staff of institutions for the developmentally disabled
  Hemodialysis patients
  Homosexually active men
  Users of illicit injectable drugs
  Individuals with clotting disorders who receive clotting factor concentrates
  Household and sexual contacts of HBV carriers
  Special high-risk populations

Persons for whom vaccine should be considered:
  Inmates of long-term correctional facilities
  Heterosexually active persons with multiple sexual partners
  International travelers to HBV endemic areas

Postexposure:
  Infants born to HBsAg-positive mothers
  Health care workers having needle-stick exposures to human blood

*Adapted with permission from Advisory Committee on Immunization Practices. Update on Hepatitis B Prevention. *MMWR,* **36,** 353, 1987.

considered to be at high risk for HBV infection (Table 48.5). In July 1986, a new, genetically engineered HB vaccine, the Recombivax-HB, was introduced, also marketed by Merck Sharp & Dohme. This vaccine is produced from HBsAg derived from *Saccharomyces cerevisiae* into which a plasmid containing the gene for HBsAg subtype *adw* has been inserted. The purified HBsAg protein is treated with formalin.

The only precautions in administering HB vaccines relate to the recombinant HB vaccine, which should not be used in individuals hypersensitive to yeast, in hemodialysis patients, or in other immunosuppressed persons. Since the vaccine contains only noninfectious particles, vaccination of a pregnant woman should not entail a risk to the woman or to the fetus. The Advisory Committee on Immunization Practices (ACIP) of the U.S. Department of Health and Human Services has stated that pregnancy should not be considered a contraindication for women in high-risk groups who are otherwise eligible to receive the vaccine.

The recombinant HB vaccine, which has been further improved since its introduction, and the plasma-derived HB vaccine are comparable in their immunogenicity. Following the three-dose series, over 95% of healthy adults develop protective antibody, anti-HBs. The vaccine should be given in the deltoid since immunogenicity is significantly lower when injections are given in the buttocks. The vaccine affords protection against hepatitis B and delta hepatitis in those who develop adequate antibody levels following vaccination.

Routine postvaccination serological testing to confirm immunity is not at present routinely recommended by the ACIP. Serological antibody testing is advisable, however, since a small but significant number of individuals (nonresponders) do not seroconvert following the three-dose series. Reasons for nonresponse in individuals vaccinated in the deltoid are not completely understood, although there appears to be a diminished vaccine effectiveness with increasing age. Initial testing should be done within 6 months of the third injection to differentiate vaccine responders from nonresponders since the results of testing after 6 months are more difficult to interpret. Revaccination results in adequate responsiveness in approximately one third of initial nonresponders. No recommendations for booster doses have yet been made by the ACIP for adults and children with normal immune status. Protection is considered to last for at least 5 years.

In 1988, the ACIP recommended routine screening of all pregnant women for HBsAg in an effort to prevent perinatal transmission of HBV and the immunization at birth of all infants born to HBsAg-positive mothers (see Table 48.4).

Prior to the licensure of the hepatitis B vaccine in 1982, only passive immunization against HBV was possible. Immune serum globulin contains very low levels of antibody to HBV, i.e., anti-HBs; therefore, it provides little protection against infection with HBV. Hepatitis immune serum globulin (HBIG), prepared from plasma preselected for high-titer anti-HBs, is about 75% effective in preventing infection following percutaneous or sexual exposure. Preexposure immunization by vaccination with HB vaccine is recommended for protection against hepatitis B in individuals at risk of exposure. If percutaneous or sexual exposure occurs without prior immunization, then HBIG should be administered. For exposed individuals at risk of repeat exposures, the HB vaccine series should be initiated simultaneously with the administration of HBIG. This recommendation also applies to infants born to HBsAg-positive mothers.

No therapeutic agent has shown a significant beneficial effect in the treatment of acute viral hepatitis. α-Interferon is effective in treating chronic hepatitis B and may lead to seroconversion for HBeAg in some patients and possible clearance of HBsAg. The efficacy of other antiviral agents has not been demonstrated. Corticosteroids have been used in severe disease, but results have been mixed.

Non-A, Non-B Hepatitis

Non-A, non-B hepatitis was first recognized in the mid-1970s. Although blood-donor screening for HBsAg had led to a significant reduction in posttransfusion hepatitis B, the incidence of hepatitis following transfusions remained high. Since hepatitis in these patients was not associated with any of the serological markers induced by either HAV or HBV, this form of hepatitis was designated non-A, non-B and was diagnosed by exclusion. Like hepatitis B, parenterally transmitted NANB hepatitis may result in chronic disease.

More recently, epidemiological evidence has implicated sewage contamination of common water sources as a cause of outbreaks of a form of NANB hepatitis in less developed countries of the world. The result is a mild disease except in pregnant women, in whom the mortality is very high. Unlike parenterally transmitted NANB hepatitis, no chronic disease has been associated with this enterically transmitted form, suggesting that there are at least two viruses responsible for NANB hepatitis.

Properties. Very little is known about the etiological agents of NANB hepatitis. At least two different viruses appear to be responsible. One of these has been transmitted to chimpanzees and appears to be a nonenveloped icosahedral virus about 27 nm in diameter. A second, blood-borne NANB agent which also is transmissible to chimpanzees appears to be a slightly larger, enveloped virus. This second virus may be identical to the agent characterized in a recent report from one research group which indicated that an enveloped, positive-stranded RNA togavirus-like agent is a major cause of NANB hepatitis. Little is known about the physical properties of these agents, although formalin has been shown to inactivate the infectivity of serum of patients having chronic NANB hepatitis.

Pathogenesis and Clinical Manifestations. The incubation period of NANB hepatitis appears to be intermediate between that of hepatitis A and hepatitis B, with most cases falling between 5 and 10 weeks, but a wide range has been noted and may be related to the fact that more than one agent causes the disease. Acute NANB hepatitis cannot be distinguished clinically from hepatitis A or hepatitis B. The acute infection tends to be mild, but fulminant cases occur. Chronic hepatitis is a frequent outcome of parenterally induced NANB hepatitis and, unlike the persistent HBV infection, is more often active. The risk for development of chronic NANB hepatitis appears to be inversely related to the severity of acute disease: patients are more likely to develop chronic NANB hepatitis if they are anicteric. Chronic disease leads to serious liver damage in some patients, but appears to resolve after several years, as evidenced by liver function tests, in others.

Epidemiology. Since there is no serological test for NANB hepatitis, information regarding the incidence of this infection within world populations is limited. Parenterally transmitted NANB hepatitis is responsible for 20% to 40% of acute viral hepatitis in the United States. NANB hepatitis has been associated most often with blood transfusions or the parenteral transfer of other blood products; however, only 8% to 11% of NANB hepatitis cases can be attributed to blood transfusion. Its greatest incidence is in IV drug users, who account for 23% to 42% of the cases. Unlike hepatitis B, this form of hepatitis is no more prevalent in male homosexuals than in the general population, although sexual transmission has been implicated in the disease. Late 1980s data from the CDC attributes 4% to 8% of NANB hepatitis cases to health care occupational exposure.

Apparently at least one form of NANB hepatitis is transmitted by the fecal–oral route, as evidenced by the outbreaks of NANB hepatitis associated with contaminated water sources in some undeveloped countries. This enterically transmitted disease has not been seen in the United States except as imported cases.

Diagnosis. Diagnosis is by exclusion. Other forms of viral hepatitis such as that caused by HAV, HBV, Epstein–Barr virus, or cytomegalovirus can be ruled out by serological testing. The differential diagnosis of this as well as any suspected viral hepatitis must also include other infectious agents (rickettsia, bacteria, protozoa, helminths), drug-induced or toxic hepatitis, biliary obstruction or primary biliary cirrhosis, Wilson's disease, α_1-antitrypsin deficiency, and neoplastic disease. If the virus recently implicated is the cause of parenterally transmitted NANB hepatitis, the serological assay developed for this agent will expedite diagnosis and establish it with certainty.

Prevention and Treatment. Avoiding parenteral exposure to blood when possible reduces the risk of NANB infection. By following the infection control guidelines for patient care recommended by the American Dental Association and the CDC, dental professionals can significantly reduce, if not eliminate, any risk they have of acquiring NANB hepatitis from a patient. Control measures for enterically transmitted NANB hepatitis are primarily in providing safe water supplies.

Until the virus(es) responsible for NANB hepatitis are conclusively identified, no specific assay for detection of virus will be possible. Two nonspecific screening tests for donor blood have shown promise in reducing the incidence of transfusion-induced disease. Several studies have shown that, by eliminating blood having elevated levels of serum amino acid aminotransferase (ALT) or testing positive for anti-HBc, the incidence of NANB hepatitis could be significantly reduced. Until specific antigen tests are available, however, the risk of NANB hepatitis following blood product transfusion cannot be eliminated.

No specific treatment is available, and the recommended management is basically the same as for other forms of infectious hepatitis.

Delta Hepatitis

First recognized in Italy in the 1970s, a new form of viral hepatitis often leading to fulminant disease was identified and attributed to a new viral form, the delta agent. Actually this virus is not as new as originally thought, since immune serum globulin collected in 1944 from U.S. soldiers was later shown to contain antibodies to delta virus (HDV), and cases appear to have occurred as far back as 1930 in South America.

Properties. HDV is a defective RNA virus that requires either HBV or another hepadnavirus (in other animal species) for complete expression and transmission in the host. The HDV particle is 35 to 38 nm in diameter, appears to be enveloped, and contains a small single-stranded RNA molecule that has no homology with HBV DNA. The outer coat is composed of HBsAg. This requirement for HBsAg apparently accounts for HDV's dependence on simultaneous active HBV infection since, as far as is known, it does not appear to require HBV at other steps in its replication. Thus, although replication of the HDV genome can occur in the absence of HBV, without the synthesis of HBsAg to provide the final coat, the delta hepatitis virus would not be infectious. HDV represents a new type of animal virus and has not been classified. Based on the present information, it seems to resemble most closely the satellite viruses of plants (virusoids).

Pathogenesis and Clinical Manifestations. HDV infection can occur simultaneously with HBV infection (co-infection) or as a superinfection in an individual who has chronic HBV infection, i.e., an HBsAg carrier. In co-infection the disease may be self-limited, as with the majority of HBV infections. The infection sometimes develops into fulminant hepatitis or a chronic infection with both HBV and HDV; however, the risk of developing severe disease with co-infection appears to be no greater than that with HBV infection alone. However, when superinfection occurs, fulminant infection or the development of severe, progressive, chronic active hepatitis is much more likely. The potential for HDV infection in carriers of HBsAg puts these individuals at increased risk of developing rapidly progressive disease. HBV carriers who survive HDV superinfection on occasion have a self-limited infection but more often develop chronic delta infection leading to progressive liver disease. Once HDV infection is established, HDV appears to compete with HBV, and a reduction in HBV antigens is seen.

Epidemiology. HDV infection is endemic in southern Italy, parts of South America, the Middle East, parts of Africa, Romania, and some parts of the Soviet Union. Most infections with HDV that have occurred in North America, Western Europe, and Australia have been in individuals at high risk for HBV infection: hemophilia, polytransfused, or hemodialysis patients, IV drug abusers, and promiscuous homosexual men. Any individual at risk of HBV infection, however, is susceptible to HDV co-infection, and carriers of HBsAg are at particular risk of disease. In the 1983–1984 outbreak of delta hepatitis in Worcester, Massachusetts, at least two health care professionals (a dentist and a physician) were infected. Nosocomial transmission has also been seen.

Diagnosis. Figures 48.6 and 48.7 show the typical course of virological and serological events during co-infection and superinfection. Detection of anti-HD, a nonneutralizing antibody present in serum during active delta infection, is valuable in diagnosing infection. This antibody may not be present or may be present only intermittently in a co-infection, and repeated testing may be necessary for accurate diagnosis. Serological testing for anti-HD IgM or HDAg once commercially available will be especially useful in diagnosis.

Prevention and Treatment. Prevention of HBV infection will prevent HDV infection; therefore, immunization against HBV also protects against HDV. Individuals who are HBsAg carriers or who have chronic HBV disease should be particularly careful to avoid superinfection with HDV. Environmental control measures recommended for hepatitis B protec-

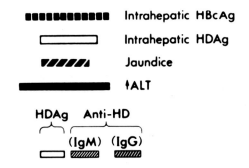

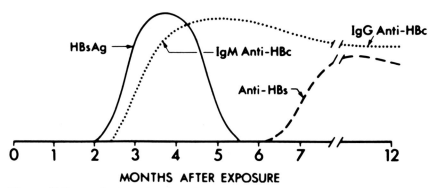

Figure 48.6: Typical course of virological and serological events during acute HDV and HBV co-infection. (Reproduced with permission from M. Chatzinoff and L. S. Friedman: *Infect Dis Clin North Am,* **1,** 535, 1987.)

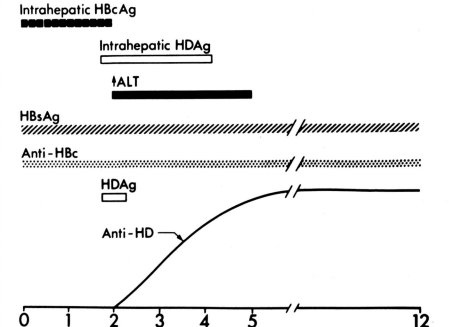

Figure 48.7: Typical course of virological and serological events during HDV superinfection of a chronic HBV carrier. (Reproduced with permission from M. Chatzinoff and L. S. Friedman: *Infect Dis Clin North Am,* **1,** 535, 1987.)

tion are appropriate for protection against HDV infection as well.

Treatment has been relatively unsuccessful. Corticosteroids and DNA viral inhibitors have been found to be ineffective. Although recombinant α_2-interferon has been shown to inhibit HDV replication, remission has not been sustained.

ADDITIONAL READING

Advisory Committee on Immunization Practices, U.S. Department of Health and Human Services. 1985. Recommendations for Protection Against Viral Hepatitis. MMWR, **34,** 313.

Advisory Committee on Immunization Practices, U.S. Department of Health and Human Services. 1987. Update on Hepatitis B Prevention. MMWR, **36,** 353.

Advisory Committee on Immunization Practices, U.S. Department of Health and Human Services. 1988. Prevention of Perinatal Transmission of Hepatitis B Virus: Prenatal Screening of All Pregnant Women for Hepatitis B Surface Antigen. MMWR, **37,** 341.

Chatzinoff, M., and Friedman, L. S. 1987. Delta Agent Hepatitis. Infect Dis Clin North Am, **1,** 529.

Choo, Q.-L., Kuo, G., Weiner, A. J., et al. 1989. Isolation of a cDNA Clone Derived from a Blood-Borne Non-A, Non-B Viral Hepatitis Genome. Science, **244,** 359.

Cottone, J. A. 1985. Hepatitis B Virus Infection in the Dental Profession. J Am Dent Assoc, **110,** 617.

Cottone, J. A. 1986. Delta Hepatitis: Another Concern for Dentistry. J Am Dent Assoc, **112,** 47.

Feinstone, S. M. 1990. Non-A, Non-B Hepatitis. In *Principles and Practice of Infectious Disease,* Ed. 3, p. 1407, edited by G. L. Mandell, R. G. Douglas, and J. E. Bennett. Churchill Livingstone, New York.

Hollinger, F. B. and Glombicki, A. P. 1990. Hepatitis A Virus. In *Principles and Practice of Infectious Disease,* Ed. 3, p. 1383, edited by G. L. Mandell, R. G. Douglas, and J. E. Bennett. Churchill Livingstone, New York.

Hollinger, F. B., and Melnick, J. L. 1985. Viral hepatitis. In *Laboratory Diagnosis of Viral Infections,* edited by E. H. Lennette. Marcel Dekker, New York.

Kane, M. A., and Lettau, L. A. 1985. Transmission of HBV from Dental Personnel to Patients. J Am Dent Assoc, **110,** 634.

Kuo, G., Choo, Q.-L., Alter, H. J., et al. 1989. An Assay for Circulating Antibodies to a Major Etiologic Virus of Human Non-A, Non-B Hepatitis. Science, **244,** 362.

Mullan, R. J., Baker, E. L., Bell, D. M., et al. 1989. Guidelines for Prevention of Transmission of Human Immunodeficiency Virus and Hepatitis B Virus to Health-Care and Public-Safety Workers. MMWR, **38** (S-6), 1.

Robinson, W. S. 1990. Hepatitis B Virus and Hepatitis Virus. In *Principles and Practice of Infectious Diseases,* Ed. 3, p. 1204, edited by G. L. Mandell, R. G. Douglas, Jr., and J. E. Bennett. Churchill Livingstone, New York.

Schiff, E. R., de Medina, M. D., Kline, S. N., et al. 1986. Veterans Administration Cooperative Study on Hepatitis and Dentistry. J Am Dent Assoc, **113,** 390.

Wanke, C. A., and Guerrant, R. L. 1987. Viral Hepatitis and Gastroenteritis Transmitted by Shellfish and Water. Infect Dis Clin North Am, **1,** 649.

West, D. J. 1984. The Risk of Hepatitis B Infection Among Health Professionals in the United States: A Review. Am J Med Sci, **287,** 26.

Part VIII

**Oral Microbiota
and Oral Disease**

49

The Oral Microbial Flora

Chris H. Miller

The human mouth supports one of the most complex microbial ecosystems of the body. The oral microbiota consists primarily of bacteria but may also include yeasts, protozoa, and occasionally viruses. Some of the characteristics of these microorganisms are described in this chapter; the ecological interactions and involvement in oral diseases are described in Chapters 50 to 53.

Even though considerable is known about the oral microbiota, our current information is not definitive. Some organisms found in the mouth have not yet been cultured in the laboratory. New organisms are being discovered and known organisms reclassified. The variability in the microbiota composition in different mouths and between different sites in the same mouth led to early confusion as to which microbes were actually members of the oral microbiota. The occurrence of transient organisms that exist in the mouth for only a short time tends to cloud the picture of the established members of the oral flora. Nevertheless, characterization of the oral microbiota and detailed studies of its members have provided invalu-

able information of aid in preventing and treating caries, periodontal diseases, soft tissue infections, and pulp and periapical infections.

General Nature of the Oral Microbiota Variability

Many of the problems associated with the culture and identification of oral bacteria were described in Chapter 2. Consideration must be given to the sampling site in the mouth, the method of sample collection, transport of the sample from the mouth to the laboratory, and the methods of sample dispersion, culturing, enumeration, and identification. The use of standardized techniques for collection, culturing, and identification of the oral microbiota has revealed a natural variability. This variability can be demonstrated by comparing the microbial composition of samples taken from similar sites in different mouths. Samples from the various areas, such as dental plaque, may show both qualitative and quantitative differences between indi-

Table 49.1: Incidence and Range of Viable Counts of 13 Bacterial Genera per Milligram of Oral Sample Isolated from Infants at Four Age Levels during the First Year of Life*

Genera	Mean Age in Days (No. of Subjects)							
	1.8 (51)		101 (44)		248 (29)		365 (29)	
	No. positive	Range	No. positive	Range	No. positive	Range	No. positive	Range
Aerobic incubation								
Total	42	0.8–1,600,000	44	11,000–1,900,000	29	12,000–2,400,000	29	15,000–690,000
Streptococcus salivarius	26	1.1–110,000	33	10–39,000	28	1.1–68,000	29	310–84,000
Staphylococcus	23	0.2–270	42	0.2–520	29	0.7–1,900	29	0.5–6,300
Neisseria	4	1.4–1,200	30	2–3,600	29	1.3–54,000	29	4–81,000
Nocardia	0	None	1	540	13	100–14,000	18	0.5–40,000
Lactobacillus	0	None	6	0.8–54	10	0.5–480	14	0.4–310
Corynebacterium	0	None	6	0.7–5	14	0.2–910	10	0.2–600
Candida	3	1.3–6	18	0.2–590	7	0.2–160	14	0.2–51
Coliforms	4	1–630,000	13	0.2–680	13	0.3–81,000	6	0.7–11
Anaerobic incubation								
Total	42	3–3,600,000	44	14,000–2,400,000	29	24,000–1,600,000	29	15,000–1,000,000
Streptococcus	38	2–1,100,000	44	2,200–860,000	29	17,000–1,300,000	29	7,000–690,000
Lactobacillus	9	1–14,000	16	1.4–150	16	0.2–30,000	15	0.2–7,700
Actinomyces	0	None	1	340	6	12–3,600	17	4.6–27,000
Veillonella	1	390	33	1.4–3,100	24	0.2–41,000	29	34–40,000
Fusobacterium	0	None	2	0.4–3	8	0.4–15,000	16	0.2–70,000
Bacteroides	0	None	2	5–100	3	49–580	13	22–2,700
Leptotrichia	0	None	3	0.2–9	15	0.2–5.9	12	0.1–80

*Reproduced with permission from C. McCarthy, M. L. Snyder, and R. B. Parker: The Indigenous Oral Flora of Man: I. The Newborn to the 1-Year-Old Infant. *Arch Oral Biol*, **10**, 61, 1965.

Table 49.2: Genera of Oral Bacteria*

Gram-Positive Genera	Gram-Negative Genera
Streptococcus	*Neisseria*
Micrococcus	*Moraxella*
Peptostreptococcus	*Veillonella*
Actinomyces	*Haemophilus*
Lactobacillus	*Actinobacillus*
Arachnia	*Capnocytophaga*
Propionibacterium	*Eikenella*
Bifidobacterium	*Campylobacter*
Eubacterium	*Selenomonas*
Rothia	*Centipeda*
Bacterionema	*Treponema*
	Bacteroides
	Fusobacterium
	Leptotrichia
	Wolinella

*Other genera appear occasionally but do not appear to be regular oral inhabitants. These include *Staphylococcus, Clostridium, Bacillus, Corynebacterium, Pseudomonas,* and various members of the Enterobacteriaceae.

viduals. Similarly, different sites in the oral cavity of one individual are colonized by a different microflora. Although each anatomical site may harbor most or all of the different types of organisms at some time, particular organisms tend to predominate in preferred ecological situations. For example, *Streptococcus mutans* resides primarily on the tooth surface, while *Streptococcus salivarius* resides primarily on the tongue and is washed off into the saliva, where it is found in high concentration. However, repeated sampling from the same site in a single individual on different occasions will often demonstrate a marked variation, both qualitative and quantitative, in the composition of the microflora.

The reasons for these variations in the oral microbiota, described more fully in Chapter 50, include differences in the ability of microorganisms to col-

onize different oral surfaces, differe[...] and physiological conditions of indiv[...] ent levels and frequencies of oral e[...] ent microorganisms. The qualitative a[...] variations in the oral microbiota are clearly demo[...] strated when the presence and levels of the same group of oral microorganisms are determined in the same people over a period of time (Table 49.1).

Microbial Types

Bacteria are by far the most predominant type of microorganisms present in the human mouth, with over 25 genera represented (Table 49.2). Some are regular members of the oral flora and are almost always present, others are recovered occasionally, yet others are transient or are recovered in very low numbers. Some people are oropharyngeal carriers of other types of microorganisms such as yeasts, protozoa, or certain viruses. Some of the characteristics of these oral microorganisms are described in the following sections.

Gram-Positive Cocci

Streptococci

Facultative streptococci are the most numerous single group in the oral cavity. In most surveys these organisms account for nearly half of the total viable counts in saliva and on the dorsum of the tongue and about a fourth of the viable counts in plaque and gingival sulcal samples (Fig. 49.1).

The most abundant of the oral streptococci are those referred to collectively as the viridans group. At different times these organisms have been classified by different criteria, and considerable confusion has surrounded their taxonomy and nomenclature. In ad-

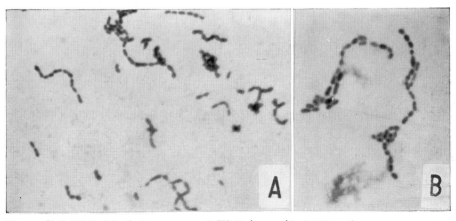

Figure 49.1: (**A**) Oral facultative streptococci. (**B**) Oral anaerobic streptococci.

on to α-hemolytic varieties, from which the name *viridans* is derived, some of the streptococci in this group may display either complete (β) hemolysis or be totally nonhemolytic. In any case, the character of hemolysis is not completely reliable and depends on the type of blood used and the culture conditions employed. Recent studies have clarified the taxonomy of the viridans streptococci and divided them into several distinct species on the basis of physiological and biochemical tests (Table 49.3). Some of these species can be further subdivided into serotypes, biotypes, or bacteriocin types.

The tests that have been employed for characterizing the streptococci include some commonly used biochemical tests, cell wall analysis, and serological methods. Some of the oral streptococci, including strains of *S. sanguis, S. salivarius,* and *S. mutans,* form distinctive colonies on media containing 5% (or more) sucrose. One such medium, mitis–salivarius agar, has been widely used for selective isolation of oral streptococci. In addition to sucrose, this medium contains trypan blue, crystal violet, and tellurite, which inhibit the growth of most organisms other than streptococci. Several other selective media have also been developed for isolation of oral streptococci.

Streptococcus mutans.   The mutans streptococci consist of oral streptococci that ferment mannitol and sorbitol, produce extracellular glucans from sucrose, and usually are cariogenic in animals (Table 49.4).

In 1924 Clarke isolated such bacteria from human carious teeth, and because their more oval than spherical shape suggested they were mutant streptococci, he called them *Streptococcus mutans.* Clarke attempted to associate these bacteria with human tooth decay, but since others could not corroborate this effort, interest in these bacteria declined. In the 1960s the recently developed technology of gnotobiotic animal research stimulated studies on the microbiology of caries. Streptococci from human carious lesions were shown to cause caries in animals under certain conditions. Taxonomic studies on these streptococci coupled with literature reviews resulted in the rediscovery of *S. mutans.* Further studies revealed serological and genetic differences among isolates of *S. mutans,* and this has resulted in proposing different specific epithets for members within the group that reflect the original mammalian source of isolation (see Table 49.4).

S. mutans contains strains of three different serotypes, c, e, and f, based on the carbohydrate composition of cell wall polysaccharides. The *c* serotype accounts for at least 70% of the human isolates. Most remaining human isolates possess d, g, or h carbohydrate antigens and represent the group *S. sobrinus.* *S. cricetus* (serotype a), *S. rattus* (serotype b), and *S.*

ferus (serotype c) are isolated from hamsters, rats, and wild rats, respectively; in addition, the first two have been recovered from humans. *S. macacae* is the most recently proposed addition to the *mutans* streptococci as a serotype c isolate from monkeys.

Selective isolation of the *mutans* streptococci from oral samples was greatly facilitated by the development of mitis–salivarius–bacitracin (MSB) agar, which contains mitis–salivarius agar supplemented with 20% sucrose and 0.5 mg of bacitracin per mL. This medium is selective for *S. mutans, S. sobrinus,* and *S. rattus* but will not permit growth of the bacitracin-sensitive species *S. cricetus* and *S. ferus*. Since this medium can be overselective, media containing 5.0% glucose, 5.0% sucrose, tellurite, and bacitracin (GSTB medium) or tryptone, yeast extract, cysteine, sucrose, and bacitracin (TYCSB medium) have recently been developed.

Mutans streptococci (in humans these are mainly *S. mutans* and to a lesser extent *S. sobrinus*) are the primary etiological agents in the formation of dental caries. *S. mutans, S. sobrinus, S. cricetus,* and *S. rattus* are cariogenic in animal models, and considerable clinical and epidemiological evidence in humans supports the key role played by *S. mutans* in caries initiation. The carcinogenic potential of this organism is primarily expressed in its acidogenic ability to ferment sugars to lactic acid and its aciduric ability to survive at the relatively low pH ("critical pH") required for demineralization of the tooth. *S. mutans* can also attach to the pellicle-coated enamel surface and produce extracellular dextran and mutan (glucans synthesized from sucrose). These properties aid the organism in attaching to and accumulating on tooth surfaces in plaque, particularly during high dietary sucrose intake. The actual number of *S. mutans* that may be found in plaque is variable and may be quite low, particularly in persons with a relatively low sucrose intake. In the presence of high dietary sucrose levels, *S. mutans* may constitute 50% or more of all organisms present.

Streptococcus sanguis.   *S. sanguis* was first isolated from the blood of a patient with subacute bacterial endocarditis in 1946. Later this bacterium was found to be a prominent member of the dental plaque microbiota, and an important relationship has since been established between a bacteremia-derived endocarditis and trauma in the mouth. *S. sanguis* is commonly isolated from plaque but also is frequently present on oral soft tissues and in saliva. It can usually be distinguished from other oral streptococci by its inability to ferment mannitol or sorbitol and its ability to produce ammonia and carbon dioxide from arginine. Most isolates produce extracellular glucans from sucrose, but of the water-soluble dextran type. Cells of *S. sanguis* can bind the more water-insoluble

Table 49.3: Some Characteristics for Identifying Oral Streptococci

	S. faecalis	S. sanguis	S. mitis/mitior	"S. mutans Group"	S. milleri	S. salivarius
Acid production from:						
Mannitol	+	–	–	+	–	–
Sorbitol	+	–	–	+	–	–
Glycerol	+	–	–	–	–	–
Production of:						
Acetoin from glucose	V	–	–*	+	+	V
Hydrogen peroxide	–	+	+	–*	+	–
Ammonia from arginine	+	+	V	–†	+	–
Extracellular polysaccharide from sucrose	–	Glucan	V	Glucan	–	Fructan
Hydrolysis of aesculin	+	+	–	+*	+	V
Growth in 6.5% NaCl	+	–	–	–*	–	–

Note: + denotes usually positive, – denotes usually negative, V denotes variable reactions.
*Some strains positive.
†Serotype b strains (S. rattus) positive.

Table 49.4: Differential Characteristics of the mutans Streptococci*

	Cariogenic		G + C DNA Content (mol%)	Serotype(s)	Cell Wall Carbohydrates	Acid Production From:			Resistance to Bacitracin	Arginine Hydrolysis	Predominant Glucan†
Species	Animals	Humans				Raffinose	Starch	Inulin			
S. mutans	+	+	36–38	c, e, f	Glucose, rhamnose	+	–	+	+	–	D > M
S. sobrinus	+	?	44–46	d, g, h	Glucose, galactose, rhamnose	–	–	–	+	–	M > D
S. cricetus	+	–	42–44	a	Glucose, galactose, rhamnose	+	–	+	–	–	M > D
S. rattus	+	–	41–43	b	Galactose, rhamnose	+	–	+	+	+	D > M
S. ferus	–	–	43–45	c	?	–	+	+	–	–	
S. macacae	?	?	35–36	c	Glucose, rhamnose	+	–	–	–	–	

*Reproduced with permission from W. J. Loesche: Role of Streptococcus mutans in human dental decay. Microbiol Rev 50, 356, 1986.
†D = dextran-type, water-soluble glucan; M = mutan-type, water-insoluble glucan.

sucrose-derived glucans (e.g., mutan) synthesized by *S. mutans*. These latter glucans may be more important than the water-soluble dextrans in attachment of streptococci to tooth surfaces. *S. sanguis* cells can attach to pellicle-coated enamel, and this species is thought to be one of the very early recolonizers of the cleaned tooth surface during initiation of plaque formation. Typical isolates from human plaque are commonly distinguished on sucrose-containing agar as having a firm attachment to the agar and a hard or rubbery consistency.

Although *S. sanguis* is commonly found in plaque and produces acids from sugar fermentation, it is not considered a highly cariogenic organism. This is primarily based on its low cariogenicity in animal models and lack of human clinical and epidemiological evidence indicating clear relationships to caries. This may be due to the fact that *S. sanguis* is not as aciduric as *S. mutans* or lactobacilli, both of which are important in dental caries.

Streptococcus salivarius. *S. salivarius* is one of the most regularly occurring organisms in the human mouth. It can be detected in the very young and very elderly. Its primary habitat in the mouth is the surface of the tongue, and it is frequently the predominant bacterium in saliva.

Typical isolates from the mouth produce mucoid "gumdrop" colonies on mitis–salivarius agar as a result of producing extracellular levan from the sucrose in the medium. Although *S. salivarius* is acidogenic and on occasion has been shown to produce dental caries as a monocontaminant in gnotobiotic rats, it is not considered an important cause of dental caries. *S. salivarius* is not commonly isolated from plaque on the tooth surface except as a contaminant from saliva. It does not have very efficient mechanisms that permit its accumulation in plaque, and if an oral organism does not colonize or accumulate on the tooth surface it can play only an indirect role, if any, in the cause of caries.

Streptococcus mitis (mitior). The species *S. mitis* or *S. mitior* is commonly used as a catch-all name for oral streptococci that cannot be identified as *S. mutans*, *S. salivarius*, *S. sanguis*, *S. milleri*, *S. faecalis*, or an anaerobic streptococcus. Other names used for this organism or group of organisms are *S. sanguis* biotype II, "nutritionally varient streptococci" (NVS), and, most recently, *S. oralis*. As shown in Table 49.3, most of the characteristics for differentiation of the streptococci are negative for *S. mitis (mitior)*, with no distinct characteristics to aid in its identification.

S. mitis (mitior) is present on the buccal mucosa and in plaque and frequently is detected in saliva. It is acidogenic and some strains produce extracellular polysaccharides. Nevertheless, it is not thought to be of significance in the etiology of dental caries.

Streptococcus milleri. *S. milleri* was first described in 1956 as an isolate from carious lesions. It was named after W. D. Miller, now known as the father of oral microbiology. The nomenclature for this organism or group of organisms known as the *S. anginosus–milleri* group remains controversial. The description of *S. milleri* includes organisms referred to as *S. anginosus*, *Streptococcus* MG, *Streptococcus constellatus*, *Streptococcus intermedius,* and small β-hemolytic streptococci of Lancefield groups F and G. Isolates identified as *S. milleri* have been detected in highest number in the gingival crevice and in plaque, and in low number on the tongue, buccal mucosa, and in saliva. It has been isolated from dental abscesses and from infections at other body sites.

Other Streptococci. The pyogenic species such as *Streptococcus pyogenes* (Lancefield group A) are not commonly found in the oral cavity and rarely cause local oral infections. When such streptococci are isolated from the mouth they probably derive from the oronasopharynx and should not be regarded as part of the resident flora. Enterococci (Lancefield group D) may be present in the human oral cavity of up to 75% of people, although usually in low number. These organisms are scarce on the tongue and average less than 10% of the streptococci from the gingival crevice. Enterococci are distinguished by their ability to grow under conditions that are inhibitory to most other streptococci (see Table 49.3) and by the presence of the Lancefield group D antigen. *Streptococcus faecalis* has been encountered more frequently than other enterococcal species. *Streptococcus bovis,* an extracellular dextran producer that also belongs to Lancefield group D, has not been reported as part of the normal oral flora. This streptococcus inhabits the human gut, is an occasional source of infective endocarditis, and is one of the species associated with bovine mastitis.

Streptococcus pneumoniae may not be considered part of the normal oral flora but is present in the oronasopharyngeal secretions of some people. About 33% of children and 10% of adults are asymptomatic carriers of *S. pneumoniae,* which is the primary cause of lobar pneumonia and middle ear infections.

Anaerobic Cocci

Obligately anaerobic gram-positive cocci of the genus *Peptostreptococcus* (family Peptococcaceae) have been estimated to average from 4% to 13% of the viable count in different sites in the oral cavity. They have been isolated from infected tooth pulp and dental abscesses. Considerable confusion surrounds the classification of this apparently heterogeneous genus. Several species previously regarded as peptostreptococci have subsequently proved to be facultatively anaerobic or carbon dioxide dependent and have been transferred to other genera and species, while others are only poorly characterized and described. The five species designations are *P. anaerobius, P. magnus, P. prevotii, P. asaccharolyticus,* and *P. tetradius.* The latter three were previously classified in the genus *Peptococcus.* One useful method for differentiating obligately anaerobic cocci from facultative cocci is to demonstrate their sensitivity to the antibiotic metronidazole by using a simple disk sensitivity test. Streptococci are invariably resistant to this agent.

Peptostreptococci are spherical to ovoid, 0.7 to 1.9 μm in diameter, and may occur in pairs, tetrads, clumps, or short or long chains. They are nonmotile, do not form spores, and are rarely hemolytic. The organisms are anaerobic and are generally quite sensitive to penicillins.

Besides being present in the mouth, various peptostreptococci are members of the gastrointestinal and vaginal floras and are important in pleuropulmonary disease, brain abscesses, and obstetrical and gynecological infections.

Staphylococci and Micrococci

Nearly every mouth harbors facultative, catalase-positive, gram-positive cocci that ferment glucose and nitrate and are accordingly identified as staphylococci or micrococci. Available data indicate that they primarily colonize the dorsum of the tongue. Staphylococci are not common in dental plaque and, when found, usually account for only a small proportion of the viable count. Such isolates, when found, are usually coagulase negative.

The tongue appears to provide the main ecological niche for one oral organism, *Micrococcus mucilagenosus* (formerly called *Staphylococcus salivarius*). This large coccus produces considerable amounts of an extracellular polysaccharide slime.

A number of reports agree that staphylococci counts range from 0 to around 50,000 per mL of saliva, with a mean of 5,000 mL. About half of subjects examined using single salivary samples yield some *S. aureus.* When swabbings of nose, throat, and mouth are cultured simultaneously, the total *S. aureus* carrier rate increases to about 80%. Although the number of salivary carriers equals the number of nasal carriers, the anterior nares are judged to harbor much larger quantities of *S. aureus.*

S. aureus may cause sinusitis, pneumonia, abscesses, and skin infections. However, exchange of *S. aureus* between dentists and patients does not seem to be a special public health problem. In 19 trials, transfer of *S. aureus* from a carrier dentist to a noncarrier patient could not be demonstrated during oral prophylaxis lasting half an hour. Likewise, the carrier rate of *S. aureus* by dental students did not increase during the clinical years of training.

Gram-Negative Cocci

Veillonellae

Gram-negative, obligately anaerobic cocci of the genus *Veillonella* are among the most numerous oral bacteria. These organisms account for 5% to 10% of the cultivable flora of saliva and on tongue surfaces. Estimates for their proportions in dental plaque vary from 0.1% to 28%, these differences possibly reflecting variation in sampling and laboratory methods.

The veillonellae are parasitic in the mouth and in the respiratory and intestinal tracts of humans and various animals. Recent taxonomic studies that considered DNA–DNA homology, in addition to other criteria, indicated that *V. alcalescens* and *V. parvula* are identical and should be combined under the latter name, which has priority. Other species that have been redefined as a result of these investigations are *V. dispar, V. atypica, V. rodentium, V. rattii, V. criceti,* and *V. carviae.* Several of these species have only been isolated from animals (guinea pigs, rats, rabbits, and hamsters), but *V. parvula, V. dispar,* and *V. atypica* have all been recovered from human sources.

Veillonella are nonmotile, nonsporulating cocci that average 0.3 to 0.5 μm in diameter. In culture they occur as spherical masses of diplococci or as short chains. Growth is good from 30 to 37°C at pH 6.5 to 8.0; cells do not survive at 60°C for 30 minutes. Veillonellae cannot ferment carbohydrates because they lack glucokinase and fructokinase, but evidently they have the other enzymes of a glycolytic system. Accordingly, they require for growth certain intermediate metabolites such as lactate, pyruvate, malate, fumarate, or oxalacetate. Carbon dioxide is indispensable for growth. Lactate is utilized with production of propionate, acetate, carbon dioxide, and hydrogen. Hydrogen sulfide is produced if the medium is supplemented with such substrates as cystine, glutathione, or thiosulfate. Gelatin is not liquefied. The veillonellae contain serologically specific lipopolysaccharide endotoxins that induce pyrogenicity and the Shwartzman reaction in rabbits.

Neisseriae and Moraxellae

Microorganisms designated as *Neisseria* have been found at several sites in the oral cavity, including the lips, tongue, cheek, plaque, and saliva. However, the mean proportions reported have generally been less than 1% to 2% of the cultivable flora, and the organisms do not appear to have any particular affinity for specific surfaces or sites within the mouth. As with many other groups of oral bacteria, the taxonomy of the family Neisseriaceae is far from fully understood. Two species of *Neisseria* were previously considered to be the predominant ones in the oral cavity, *Neisseria sicca* and *Neisseria catarrhalis*. The latter has more recently been transferred to the genus *Moraxella* subgenus *Branhamella* and is now designated *Moraxella (Branhamella) catarrhalis,* since it has been shown on the basis of biochemical, physiological, and genetic data to differ significantly from members of the genus *Neisseria*. The two genera may be distinguished by demonstrating the presence or absence of the enzyme glucose-6-phosphate dehydrogenase (absent in *M. (B.) catarrhalis*). Although oral *Neisseria* strains may be divided into broad groups according to their ability to produce polysaccharide and to ferment carbohydrates, it remains difficult at present to assign unknown isolates to named species with any confidence.

Gram-Positive Rod-Shaped Bacteria

The oral cavity supports the growth of large numbers of a surprisingly wide variety of gram-positive rods, including aerobic and facultatively and obligately anaerobic species. Although some, such as the lactobacilli, usually appear as rod-shaped cells, many are pleomorphic, assuming a range of microscopic forms from coccobacillary to filamentous. Some of the rods are club-shaped, and many show evidence of branching. Because of the morphological appearance of such organisms, they are often grouped together for descriptive purposes and referred to simply as diphtheroids or coryneforms. This broad morphological group of bacteria includes both facultative and anaerobic representatives. Facultative diphtheroids have been estimated to constitute 13% of the viable count from the dorsum of the tongue, 15% from the gingival sulcus, and 24% from plaque; obligately anaerobic strains average 8%, 20%, and 18% in the respective sites.

Identification of this group of oral bacteria to the genus and species level can be difficult on occasion, but their classification has been greatly facilitated in recent years by the application of chemotaxonomic techniques. Most of the strains initially isolated as diphtheroids appear not to be true *Corynebacterium* species; many turn out to be *Actinomyces,* including the catalase-positive species *Actinomyces viscosus,* which may account for many of the unidentified strains reported in earlier studies. Other genera that are found are *Arachnia, Propionibacterium, Bifidobacterium, Eubacterium, Rothia,* and *Bacterionema.*

Some of the distinguishing features of the various genera of pleomorphic gram-positive rods are summarized in Table 49.5.

Spore-forming genera, such as *Clostridium* and *Bacillus,* do not seem to be part of the normal oral flora, according to most investigators. However, there are a few published reports of the isolation of such organisms from particular populations.

Lactobacilli

Lactobacilli are a characteristic group of oral bacteria, although numerically a minor fraction. Their numbers vary according to circumstances to be discussed later in relation to dental caries. Some lactobacilli are likely present in all human oral cavities soon after birth, although probably not in significant proportions. The salivary *Lactobacillus* count in adults ranges from nearly 0 to about 100,000/mL or more, with a mean of about 70,000/mL—only a small fraction of a percent of the mean total viable count. Lactobacilli are widely distributed, also being found in the intestinal tracts of both infants and adults and in the vagina after puberty; in addition, they are found in milk and milk products (including pasteurized milk), compressed yeast, sour beer, soil, manure, feces of invertebrates, fishes, mammals, sewage, and many fermenting plant and animal products.

Lactobacilli are gram-positive, nonmotile (except for rare strains), nonsporulating, sometimes pleomorphic rods that divide in one plane only without branching. They tend to become gram negative in older cultures. A few species produce orange, rust, or brick-red pigment. In general they have very complex nutritional requirements for carbohydrates, fatty acids, inorganic ions, vitamins, nucleic acid precursors, peptides, and amino acids. In fact, many species are so specific in their amino acid requirements that they can be used for amino acid determination. Most oral lactobacilli grow best in or require a reducing medium containing a surface tension–reducing agent, adequately supplied with carbohydrate, and at a wide temperature range (15 to 45°C). They are aciduric with an optimal pH of usually 5.5 to 5.8. Isolation and enumeration of oral lactobacilli are greatly facilitated by selective agar media, which suppress the growth of practically all other oral microorganisms, owing to a high content of acetate and other salts, a surface tension depressant, and an acid pH (5.4), while providing adequate nourishment for lactobacilli. Most lactobacilli are not proteolytic. Carbohydrate fermentation by lactobacilli is variable with the species, although they are generally quite active. Differences in the action of oral lactobacilli on glucose divide them into homofermentative species, which produce principally lactic acid (above 65%), and heterofermentative

Table 49.5: Some Distinguishing Chemical Characteristics of Oral Pleomorphic Gram-Positive Rods*

| | Cell Wall Components | | | | | | | Acid End Products from Glucose | | | | | | DNA G+C Content (mol%) |
| | Dibasic Amino Acids | | | | Sugars | | Mycolic Acid | | | | | | | |
Genus	ORN	LYS	DL-DAP	LL-DAP	GAL	ARAB		A	P	B	C	L	S	
Actinomyces	+	+	–	–	V	–	–	+	–	–	–	+	+	60–63
Arachnia	–	–	V	V	+	–	–	+	+	–	–	–	±	63–65
Propionibacterium	–	–	–	+	+	–	–	+	+	–	–	–	–	57–60
Bifidobacterium	+	+	–	–	+	–	–	+	–	–	–	+	–	57–64
Eubacterium	–	–	+	–	V	–	NA	+	–	+	V	V	V	NA
Rothia	–	+	–	–	+	+	+	+	+	–	–	+	±	65–69
Bacterionema	–	–	+	–	+	+	+	+	+	–	–	±	–	55–57
Corynebacterium	–	–	+	–	+	+	+	+	+	–	–	±	–	57–60

Note: ORN = ornithine, LYS = lysine, DAP = diaminopimelic acid, GAL = galactose, ARAB = arabinose, A = acetic, P = propionic, B = butyric, C = caproic, L = lactic, S = succinic, + = usually positive, – = usually negative, ± = weakly positive, V = variable results reported, NA = data not available.

*Data from G. H. Bowden and J. M. Hardie, Oral Pleomorphic (coryneform) Gram-Positive Rods. In *Coryneform Bacteria*, p. 235, edited by D. J. Bousefield and A. G. Callely. Academic Press, New York, 1978.

Table 49.6: Some Characteristics Used to Classify Oral Lactobacilli

Lactobacillus Species	Optimum Temperature (°C)	DNA G+C Content (mol %)	Type of Lactic Acid	Fermentation				
				Lactose	Sucrose	Raffinose	Arabinose	Maltose
Homofermentative:								
L. acidophilus	35–38	36.7	DL	+	+	Some strains +	–	+
L. salivarius	35–40	34.7	Mainly L (+)	+	+	+	–	+
L. casei		46.4	Mainly L (+)	Some subsp. +	Some strains +	–	–	Some strains +
L. plantarum	30–35	45	DL	+	+	+	Some strains +	+
Heterofermentative:								
L. fermentum	41–42	53.4	DL	+	+	+	Some strains +	+
L. cellobiosus	30–35	53.1	DL	Weak	+	+	Some strains +	+
L. brevis	30	42.7–46.4	DL	Weak	Some strains +	Weak	+	+
L. buchneri	30	44.8	DL	Weak	Some strains +	Weak	+	+

species, which produce less lactic acid (less than 65%) and a number of other end products (principally acetic acid and ethanol), including gas (usually carbon dioxide).

The eighth edition of *Bergey's Manual of Determinative Bacteriology* recognized 27 homofermentative and heterofermentative species, grouped according to optimum temperature and metabolic patterns such as type of lactic acid produced and the differential fermentation of sugars (Table 49.6). Previous classifications were quite different from the present one. Indeed, from the time lactobacilli were first found in the oral cavity until relatively recently, there has been a tendency to assign all oral lactobacilli to the species *Lactobacillus acidophilus,* usually without supporting data. This is a most inaccurate practice, although it must be admitted that differentiation is often difficult.

Oral lactobacilli do not have efficient mechanisms for attachment and accumulation in plaque and when present constitute less than 1% of the total plaque flora. Nevertheless, lactobacilli are very important in pit and fissure caries and dentinal caries, likely as a result of their aciduric nature. Before the *"mutans* streptococci" era, many thought that lactobacilli were the cause of dental caries. Today they are believed to be important in the progression of carious lesions after the lesion has been initiated by the activities of other organisms, mainly *S. mutans* and *S. sobrinus.*

Actinomycetes

Actinomyces species are branched, filamentous rods commonly occurring in the mouths of humans and lower animals. They have been recovered from plaque, gingival crevice material, the oral soft tissues, and saliva. Oral species include *A. viscosus, A. naeslundii, A. israelii* and *A. odontolyticus.* The filamentous nature of the organisms in this genus convinced early pathologists that they were fungi. As a result, the name *Actinomyces* (meaning ray-fungus) has caused much confusion over the years. Members of this genus and of other genera in the family Actinomycetaceae are bacteria, not fungi. *Actinomyces* contains six species, five of which are found in the human mouth. *A. israelii* and *A. meyeri* are anaerobic and *A. viscosus, A. naelsundii,* and *A. odontolyticus* are facultative anaerobes. The *Actinomyces* genus can usually be differentiated from genera of other gram-positive rods without difficulty. Gas chromatographic analysis of acid end products from glucose fermentation is a key analysis in this regard (see Table 49.5). Additional biochemical and especially serological tests (immunofluorescence) are needed for accurate speciation within the genus.

Figure 49.2 shows the typical cellular morphology

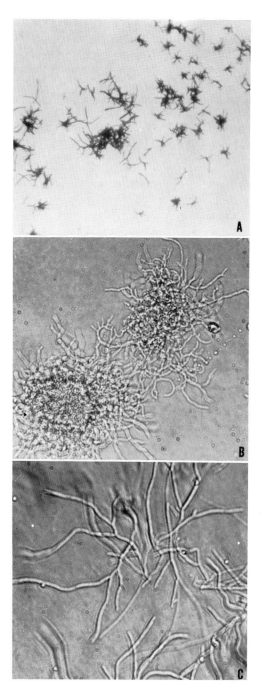

Figure 49.2: (**A**) Gram stain of *Actinomyces naeslundii* grown in thioglycolate medium. (**B**) Microcolony of *Actinomyces naeslundii* on 24-hour anaerobic brain–heart infusion agar culture. (**C**) Microcolony of *Actinomyces israelii* on 48-hour anaerobic brain–heart infusion agar culture. (Reproduced with permission from A. Howell, Jr., W. C. Murphy, E. Paul, and R. M. Stephan: Oral Strains of Actinomyces. *J Bacteriol,* **78,** 82, 1959.)

of *Actinomyces*. Microcolonies have a dense mass of diphtheroid cells and tangled filaments at their centers surrounded by a periphery of radiating, curved, and branched filaments. In liquid media, growth of *A. naeslundii* is frequently granular, particularly after the medium pH begins to drop. Although *A. naeslundii* is a facultative anaerobe, most strains will grow in air on agar media, but CO_2 enhances its growth. *A. naeslundii* colonizes the soft tissues of the human mouth at an early age. In adults, it is also found on the tooth surfaces in plaque. *A. naeslundii* strains isolated from plaque overlying human root surface caries have been repeatedly shown to induce root surface caries in rodent animal models. It has also been shown to induce alveolar bone destruction in laboratory rats. *A. viscosus* has been isolated from the oral cavity of hamsters, rats, and man. In liquid media, growth of this organism occurs with a viscous (although strain-variable) sediment. This produces a mucinous "string" when the media are swirled. *A viscosus* is a facultative anaerobe that grows better with CO_2. The organism synthesizes levan from sucrose and, in contrast to *A. naeslundii*, is catalase positive. *A. viscosus* (originally called *Odontomyces viscosus*) was originally isolated from hamsters and was shown to be responsible for causing periodontal destruction in these animals. Human strains also have been shown to induce periodontal destruction and root surface caries in laboratory rodents.

Both *A. naeslundii* and *A. viscosus* have surface fibrils or fimbriae that enhance their attachment to oral surfaces and to other bacterial cells. They are both prominent members of the plaque flora and are thought to play an important role in the colonization of crevicular and periodontal sites by gram-negative bacteria through direct cell binding.

Colonies of *A. odontolyticus* on blood agar may produce an area of greening around the colonies, resembling α-hemolytic streptococci. Some strains of *A. odontolyticus* may grow aerobically on blood agar. Colonies characteristically have a reddish brown center. Growth in liquid media is usually turbid and even, but sometimes may be flocculent. The normal habitat of this organism is the oral cavity of man. It may be isolated from deep dentinal caries, but its role in the caries process is undetermined.

A. israelii can be isolated from human plaque, tonsillar crypts, and calculus, but its role in plaque-associated disease is unknown. It is the most frequent cause of actinomycosis. Less frequent causes of this endogenous infectious disease are *Arachnia propionica* and *Actinomyces naeslundii* (see Chap. 24).

Even less is known about the oral ecology and disease potential of *A. meyeri*, which was earlier classified in the genus *Actinobacterium*. This species has been isolated from human plaque.

Rothiae

The genus *Rothia* is currently listed as a member of the family Actinomycetaceae. The organisms have a branching, filamentous morphology but appear in culture as coccoid, diphtheroid, or bacillary forms or a mixture of these. Largely because of these morphological features, rothiae were at one time considered to belong to *Norcardia*, but they are now recognized as a clearly distinct genus. *Rothia* is aerobic, although some strains may grow under anaerobic conditions. CO_2 is not stimulatory. Characteristic, usually white or cream-pigmented colonies are produced that often have a raised, rough appearance and may grow to several millimeters in diameter on aerobic blood agar plates.

At present, only one species is recognized, *R. dentocariosa*. However, several biotypes and serotypes have been described and it is likely that one or more new species designations will be proposed. Rothiae are commonly isolated from the normal human mouth, particularly from saliva, dental plaque, and calculus, and they have also been found in animals. No natural infections have been reported in man or animals, but abscess formation has been demonstrated experimentally in mice.

Bacterionemae

The genus *Bacterionema* was proposed to separate these branching filamentous organisms from the different *Leptotrichia*. There is a single species within the genus, *Bacterionema matruchotii*, which appears to be biochemically and serologically homogeneous. It is a gram-positive, non-acid-fast, nonmotile, usually facultative organism (some anaerobic strains have been described) with a characteristic cellular morphology. The cells are pleomorphic filaments 1 to 2 μm wide by 20 to 200 μm long, typically attached to a rectangular rod-shaped body 1.5 to 2.5 μm wide by 3 to 10 μm long. This combination of rod and filament gives rise to the so-called "whip handle" cells. Filamentous and rod forms also occur singly in microscopic preparations, and branching may be observed. *B. matruchotii* ferments carbohydrates to yield acid (predominantly acetic and propionic, with smaller amounts of lactic acid) and some CO_2. The optimal pH range is 6.5 to 7.5 and its optimal temperature is 37°C.

Bacterionema has been shown to be distinct from *Actinomyces*, *Norcardia*, and *Rothia*. Recent chemotaxonomic data, including cell wall composition, DNA-base ratios, and the presence of low molecular weight mycolic acid, indicate that *B. matruchotii* is closely related to *Corynebacterium* and should be reclassified with that genus.

Injection of these live organisms into mice produces nodules or abscesses. Similar lesions are produced following intraperitoneal or intravenous inoculation. *B. matruchotii* is found in the oral cavity of man and other primates, particularly in dental plaque and calculus.

Arachniae

The organisms now designated *Arachnia propionica* are anaerobic, gram-positive, pleomorphic bacteria that can resemble *Actinomyces israelii* both in colonial and microscopic appearance. They are catalase negative. This species was originally isolated from a case of lachrymal canaliculitis and has also been found in patients presenting with actinomycosis-like symptoms. Chemotaxonomic data indicate that this genus is distinct from *Actinomyces* and also from *Propionibacterium,* which it superficially resembles by virtue of producing propionic acid from glucose. Differences between strains of *Arachnia* indicate that there may be more than the one named species currently accepted. *Arachnia* has been isolated from dental plaque, carious dentin, and necrotic pulps, but the organism does not appear to be a numerically dominant member of the oral flora in most situations.

Bifidobacteria

These pleomorphic, anaerobic, gram-positive rods typically have bifid ends and have been classified at various times either with the Actinomycetaceae or the Lactobacillaceae. The characteristic ratio of fermentation products of the genus is three parts acetic to two parts lactic acid. Isolation of bifidobacteria from the mouth has been reported by several authors. The species found is *Bifidobacterium dentium,* previously known as *Actinomyces eriksonii.* Strains have been recovered from dental plaque and carious dentin, but their numbers appear to be relatively low. Their involvement in oral diseases is unknown.

Propionibacteria

This genus includes many of the organisms previously described as anaerobic coryneforms. They are anaerobic, gram-positive rods that produce a major peak of propionic acid when grown in glucose broth, and are catalase positive. Although primarily inhabitants of the skin, propionibacteria have been isolated from the mouth by a number of different workers and can therefore be regarded as part of the regular oral flora. Strains identified as *Propionibacterium acnes* have been isolated from dental plaque, carious dentin, and necrotic pulp and have also been detected microscopically in oral samples by immunofluorescence.

Corynebacteria

True animal corynebacteria have a typical cell wall composition, containing DL-DAP, galactose, and arabinose, possess a low molecular weight mycolic acid, and have a G + C ratio of 55% to 60%. With the exception of *B. matruchotii,* which may be a true *Corynebacterium,* the presence of corynebacteria in the mouth is uncertain. It is likely that many of the organisms described in the earlier literature as "diphtheroids" were not true corynebacteria, but a few isolates reported in more recent studies do appear to fit the description. Further research is required to clarify the uncertainty in this area.

Eubacteria

Anaerobic, nonsporulating, pleomorphic, gram-positive, rod-shaped or filamentous bacteria that cannot be allocated to any of the foregoing named genera may be classified in the genus *Eubacterium.* One useful trait for differentiation from other genera is the production of butyric acid from glucose fermentation (see Table 49.5). *E. suburreum* is commonly isolated from dental plaque, where it contributes to the mass of filamentous organisms present in mature supragingival deposits. Eubacteria have also reportedly been isolated from calculus, carious dentin, and necrotic pulps. Three additional species have been isolated from periodontal pockets in periodontitis patients: *E. timidum, E. brachy,* and *E. nodatum. E. timidum* cells are described as "small diphtheroids" that may produce trace amounts of acetate, formate, succinate, or lactate when grown in peptone–yeast extract broth. Unlike *Actinomyces* species, they do not ferment sugars. The cells of *E. brachy* are very short gram-positive rods arranged in chains, and those of *E. nodatum* are said to resemble *Actinomyces* morphologically. *E. nodatum* can be distinguished from *Actinomyces* species by its inability to ferment sugars and by the detection of butyric acid as a metabolic end product.

Gram-Negative Anaerobic Rod-Shaped Bacteria

Our knowledge of this important group of organisms has increased considerably in recent years, largely as a result of the application of more sophisticated anaerobic isolation techniques and identification methods. As a consequence of such improved isolation methods, many organisms have been found that cannot readily be identified by existing criteria and that may represent new taxa. The isolation of such previously undescribed organisms has stimulated a

Table 49.7: *Bacteroides* Detected in the Human Mouth*

Nonpigmented Species	Pigmented Species
B. oralis	*B. gingivalis*
B. buccae	*B. intermedius*
B. oris	*B. melaninogenicus*
B. zoogleoformans	*B. endodontalis*
B. forsythus	*B. loescheii*
B. gracilis	*B. denticola*
B. ureolyticus	
B. capillosus	
B. pneumosintes	
B. fragilis	

*B. pneumosintes and *B. fragilis* are not commonly found.

considerable amount of basic taxonomic work as research investigators attempt to characterize and classify the new isolates.

Anaerobic gram-negative rods generally belong to the family Bacteroidaceae. Oral representatives currently fall into one of five genera, *Bacteroides, Fusobacterium, Leptotrichia, Wolinella,* or *Selenomonas.*

Bacteroides

This genus comprises obligately anaerobic, gram-negative, sometimes pleomorphic rods with rounded ends and diameters greater than 0.3 μm. Most species produce acetic and succinic acid as end products of glucose metabolism, together with varying amounts of other acids. The eighth (1974) edition of *Bergey's Manual of Determinative Bacteriology* recognized 22 species which are primarily inhabitants of the intestinal tracts and mucous membranes of warm-blooded animals. This number was increased to 29 species by 1980 when the *Approved List of Bacterial Names* was published. The ninth (1984) edition of *Bergey's Manual of Systematic Bacteriology* lists 41 species of *Bacteroides.* To add to the taxonomic confusion, it seems that different investigators have given different names to the same "new species."

Bacteroides species that have been isolated from the human mouth are listed in Table 49.7. These can be broadly divided into black- (or brown-) pigmented and nonpigmented varieties. Members of the important group of *Bacteroides* associated with the intestinal tract, the *B. fragilis* group, which are frequently implicated in anaerobic infections, do not seem to occur as regular inhabitants of the oral cavity.

Pigmented *Bacteroides* Species. At one time all gram-negative anaerobic rods that yielded black or brown colonies on blood agar were referred to as *B. melaninogenicus.* Such strains were generally found to require hemin and menadione for growth;

pigmentation varied both in shade and speed of development. There was considerable interest in the potential pathogenic role of this "species" since it was often isolated from human infections and played an indispensable role in experimental mixed anaerobic infections in guinea pigs. Pigmented *Bacteroides* cells are frequently isolated from the mouth, particularly from the region of the gingival sulcus or periodontal pocket.

Subsequently it became clear that there were important biochemical differences between strains that produced black colonies. It was proposed that the species *B. melaninogenicus* be subdivided into several subspecies, namely *B. melaninogenicus* subsp. *intermedius, B. melaninogenicus* subsp. *asaccharolyticus, B. melaninogenicus* subsp. *melaninogenicus,* and *B. melaninogenicus* subsp. *levii.*

The *asaccharolyticus* subspecies was later found to be heterogeneous and has now been further split into two entities, each of which has been elevated to separate species status, namely *B. gingivalis* and *B. asaccharolyticus.* These species differ from one another in the electrophoretic mobility of their malate dehydrogenase (MDH) enzymes, lipid composition, and DNA base ratio (46.5% to 48.5% G + C and 51% to 52% G + C, respectively). *B. gingivalis* is the more common of the two in the mouth and is an important pathogen in human periodontal disease.

B. melaninogenicus subsp. *melaninogenicus* was divided into three new species, *B. melaninogenicus, B. loescheii,* and *B. denticola.* The latter is the accepted name for *B. socranskii.* These three species are detected in the human mouth and at periodontal disease sites. *B. melaninogenicus* subsp. *intermedius* was divided into two new species, *B. intermedius* (isolated from periodontal disease sites) and *B. corporis,* which is not normally found in the mouth.

B. endodontalis, one of the most recently described oral species, has been isolated from human dental abscesses and occasionally from plaque. Another variety of black-pigmented *Bacteroides* has been isolated from the mouths of monkeys and named *Bacteroides macacae. B. melaninogenicus* subsp. *levii* has been renamed *B. levii,* but this species is not normally found in the human mouth.

Nonpigmented *Bacteroides* Species. The taxonomic status of oral nonpigmented gram-negative rods is no less confusing and changeable than that of the pigmented species. *Bacteroides oralis* was described several years ago but there has been some difficulty in reaching international concensus on type and reference strains. However, the species is recognized and included in the *Approved List of Bacterial Names.* Several new species have been described by different authors since 1980, including *B. oris, B. buccae, B. buccalis,* and *B. gracilis.* The last mentioned in this list is one of several oral organisms that cause

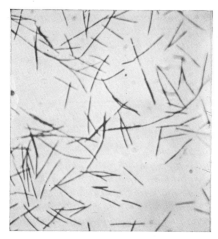

Figure 49.3: Oral fusiform organisms from the gingiva (×900). (Courtesy of Stig Schultz-Haudt.)

pitting or corrosion of the agar surface. Another corroding anaerobe is now called *Bacteroides ureolyticus;* this species was formerly designated *Bacteroides corrodens* and is quite distinct from the facultatively anaerobic, gram-negative rod *Eikenella corrodens.*

In view of the rapidly changing classification and nomenclature of the oral nonpigmented *Bacteroides* species, it is not possible at the moment to make much useful comment about their distribution in the mouth or their role in dental disease. However, *B. forsythus* and *B. gracilis* are present in subgingival plaque and the latter has been isolated from numerous infections at other body sites. *B. fragilis* has been occasionally detected in human oral samples and has been isolated from abscess-type infections at other body sites.

Fusobacteria

Members of the genus *Fusobacterium* are obligately anaerobic, gram-negative, nonsporulating rods (Fig. 49.3). Sixteen species of *Fusobacterium* that inhabit the natural cavities of the human body are currently recognized. Although several species have at one time or another been detected in the oral cavity, *F. nucleatum* is by far the most frequently isolated oral species. *F. nucleatum* produces small translucent colonies on horse blood agar. They are usually nonhemolytic and nonmotile. In the laboratory, fusobacteria are distinguished from other morphologically similar organisms by the production of major amounts of butyric acid from peptone or carbohydrate.

F. nucleatum has been isolated from infections of the upper respiratory tract, pleural cavity, and from the oral cavity. In fact, this bacterium is probably one of the most regularly occurring gram-negative an-

aerobic rods in the gingival crevice and subgingival plaque. Fusobacteria were first observed in ulcerative gingivitis in the 1880s and later they were associated with spirochetes in angina. Thus, the fusobacteria have long been associated with fusospirochetal disease, also called acute necrotizing ulcerative gingivitis or trenchmouth.

Leptotrichiae

The position of the genus *Leptotrichia* (a thin hair) has been ambiguous. Very early in the development of bacteriology, oral threadlike filamentous bacteria, differentiated almost entirely on the basis of their structure and oral habitat, were described by many and, after 1843, were generally classified in the genus *Leptothrix,* which originally referred to filamentous iron bacteria. In 1879, because of the obvious misnomer, Trevisan proposed the name *Leptotrichia buccalis* for these organisms, and in following years the status of the species was further confused by investigators placing any unbranched filamentous organisms, even sporulating bacilli, in it. Subsequently, *L. buccalis* was confused with *Bacillus fusiformis,* a synonym for *Fusobacterium nucleatum,* with *Fusobacterium plautivinterium nucleatum,* and even with *Bacterionema matruchotii.* Some authors have described *L. buccalis* as gram positive and related to the lactobacilli. However, early descriptions considered *Leptotrichia* to be gram negative and related to *Fusobacterium.* Also, the fine structure and lipopolysaccharides are characteristic of gram-negative organisms. *Leptotrichia* is now recognized as a valid genus with a single species, *L. buccalis.*

L. buccalis (Fig. 49.4) is an unbranching, nonmotile, nonsporulating, straight or slightly curved rod with a tendency for one or both ends to point. In young cultures it grows into short chains but in older cultures filaments of considerable length can be seen twisting around each other. Although cells in cultures less than 6 hours old are gram positive, by 24 hours they are gram negative but contain gram-positive granules. *L. buccalis* is anaerobic, but 5% carbon dioxide is essential for isolation and optimal growth. Carbohydrate fermentation follows a metabolic pattern similar to that of homofermentative lactobacilli.

Wolinella

Members of this genus are anaerobic, helical, curved or straight unbranched gram-negative rods that have a single polar flagellum. They neither require nor ferment carbohydrates, but growth is stimulated in fluid cultures by the presence of formate and fumarate. Hydrogen and formate can be used as energy sources, formate being oxidized to hydrogen and

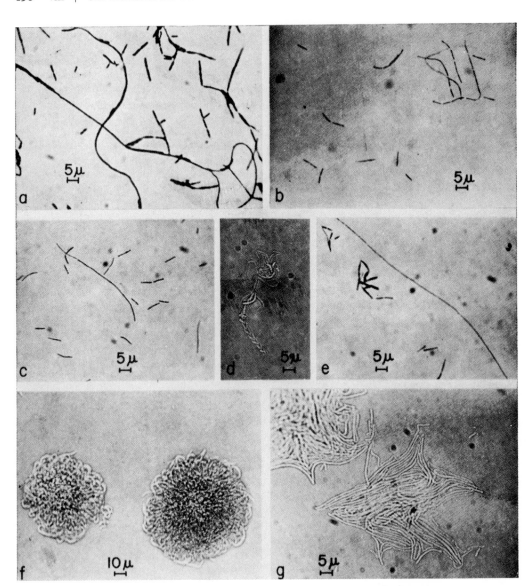

Figure 49.4: Cellular and colonial morphologies of *Leptotrichia buccalis,* originally described by Thiøtta, Hartmann, and Boe, 1939. (**A**) Gram stain of 12-hour thioglycolate broth culture with morphology ranging from short rods to long filaments, with branching evident. The cells are mostly gram positive but some are gram negative with gram-positive granules. (**B**) Gram stain of 48-hour anaerobic brain–heart infusion agar culture showing trichome formation and gram-negative cells. (**C**) Gram stain of 20-hour anaerobic brain–heart infusion agar culture showing gram-positive rods and short filaments. (**D**) Unstained microcolony on 12-hour anaerobic brain–heart infusion agar culture showing a braided filament. (**E**) Gram stain of a 20-hour anaerobic brain–heart infusion broth culture showing short gram-positive and gram-negative rods and one third of a filament. (**F**) Colony on a 48-hour, anaerobic brain–heart infusion agar culture. (**G**) Microcolony on a 16-hour anaerobic brain–heart infusion agar plate showing characteristic parallel arrangement of the cells. (Reproduced with permission from M. N. Gilmour, A. Howell, Jr., and B. G. Bibby: The Classification of Organisms Termed *Leptotrichia (Leptothrix) buccalis. Bacteriol Rev,* **25,** 131, 1961.)

carbon dioxide. The G + C ratio of the genus is 42 to 49 mol%. Colonies may be pale yellow to gray, transparent, convex, and agar pitting (corroding), or spreading and transparent with a matted appearance.

There are three species in the new genus: *W. succinogenes* (previously called *Vibrio succinogenes*), *W. recta,* and *W. curva.* Some strains of organisms previously classified as *Vibrio sputorum* have now been placed in the genus *Wolinella,* while other strains of *V. sputorum* have been reclassified as *Campylobacter sputorum.* All three species of *Wolinella* have been found in the human mouth but most of the information relates to *W. recta* and *W. succinogenes.* These two species differ from one another in cellular and ultrastructural morphology, antigenic structure, and susceptibility to dyes and antibiotics. They have also been shown to be distinct by DNA–DNA homology. *W. succinogenes* also requires succinate, or an immediate precursor, for growth.

W. recta has been detected in periodontal pockets of patients with periodontal disease, from necrotic root canals, and from periapical granulomas associated with nonvital teeth. It is found in higher proportions in periodontal sites of alveolar bone loss than in healthy sites. Also, it was one of the three predominant isolates from subgingival plaque in a study of periodontitis patients with non-insulin-dependent diabetes mellitus. The other two were *B. intermedius* and *B. gingivalis.*

Selenomonas

Cells in the gram-negative, anaerobic genus of *Selenomonas* are curved to helical rods. They may occur singly, in pairs, in short chains, and sometimes in clumps. Cells are motile, with active tumbling, and up to 16 flagella are arranged in a tuft near the center of the concave side of the cell (Fig. 49.5). Besides this unique flagellar arrangement, production of propionate as a major end product of glucose fermentation aids in differentiating *Selenomonas* from closely related genera. The species that has been detected in the human mouth is *Selenomonas sputigena* (originally known as *Spirillum sputigenum*). Although this species is found in the gingival crevice and has been isolated from subgingival material in periodontal pockets, the role (if any) that it plays in periodontal disease is unknown.

Centipeda

Centipeda periodontii is a newly described genus and species of bacteria that has been isolated from subgingival lesions of patients with chronic periodontitis and juvenile periodontitis, but not from healthy people or from healthy gingival sites in periodontitis

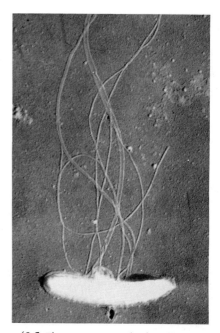

Figure 49.5: Electron micrograph of *Sprillum sputigenum* (*Selenomonas sputigena*), showing flagella originating on the concave side. (Reproduced with permission from J. B. MacDonald, E. M. Madlener, and S. S. Socransky: Observations on *Spirillum sputigenum* and Its Relationship to *Selenomonas* Species with Special Reference to Flagellation. *J Bacteriol,* **77,** 559, 1959.)

patients. It is a large, anaerobic, motile, rod-shaped, gram-negative bacterium with numerous flagella.

The role of *C. periodontii* in periodontal or other oral diseases has not been determined. However, some strains produce a soluble product that alters human lymphocyte function, which could have a local or systemic immunosuppressive effect.

Campylobacter

Although members of this genus are microaerophilic, they are considered here with the anaerobic gram-negative rods. *Campylobacter* organisms are gram-negative, slender, spirally curved rods that are microaerophilic and do not ferment carbohydrates. The cells may be as long as 8 μm and are motile with a corkscrew-like motion by means of a single polar flagellum. Two species have been detected in the gingival crevice and in subgingival material from humans: *C. sputorum* subsp. *sputorum,* and *C. concisus.* Microaerophilic growth occurs with *C. sputorum* subsp. *sputorum* in an atmosphere of 5% O_2, 10% CO_2, and 85% N_2. Anaerobic growth occurs in media containing fumarate. *C. concisus* grows microaerophilically with 5% O_2, 10% CO_2, and 10% to 85% H_2; the H_2 is required. Anaerobic growth occurs when both formate and fumarate are in the medium.

Table 49.8: Some Characteristics of Oral Facultative Gram-Negative Rods*

Characteristic	Eikenella corrodens	Actinobacillus actinomycetem-comitans	Capnocytophaga Species	Haemophilus Species
Oxidase	+	V	−	V
Catalase	−	+	−	− or V
Urease	−	−	−	− or V
Indole	−	−	−	−
Motility	−	−	V†	−
Acid from:				
Glucose	−	+	+	+
Mannitol	−	V	−	−
Lactose	−	−	V	V
Sucrose	−	−	+	+
Nitrate reduction	+	+	V	+
Pitting of agar	+	−	V	−
Major acid end products	A	A, S	A, S	A, S, L
Require V-factor	−	−	−	+ ‡
DNA G + C (mol%)	56	43	33–41	40–44

Note: A = acetic acid, S = succinic acid, L = lactic acid, V = variable reactions, + = most strains positive, − = most strains negative.
*Growth of all species is enhanced by 5% to 10% CO_2 in atmosphere.
†Capnocytophaga species display "gliding" motility.
‡*Haemophilus aphrophilus* does not require V-factor, unlike *H. segnis, H. paraphrophilus,* and *H. parainfluenzae.*

Both species are catalase negative, unlike other human *Campylobacter* isolates.

The importance of these two oral species in disease is not yet known. Other human species do have pathogenic potential in the intestinal tract. *C. jejuni* and *C. coli* can cause gastroenteritis, and *C. pylori* has recently been associated with and may be involved in the production of gastric and perhaps peptic ulcers.

Facultative Gram-Negative Rods

A number of facultatively anaerobic gram-negative rods occur in the oral cavity. Many of these are described as capnophilic because growth of colonies on solid media is enhanced by the addition of 5% to 10% CO_2 to the atmosphere. Bacteria of this group often were overlooked by most oral microbiologists until a few years ago, but recent studies on oral ecology and the flora associated with various types of periodontal disease have drawn attention to their presence and potential pathogenicity. The oral organisms included in this category are members of the genera *Haemophilus, Eikenella, Actinobacillus,* and *Capnocytophaga.* Some of the distinguishing features of these bacteria are listed in Table 49.8.

Haemophili

Haemophili are regularly present in dental plaque, saliva, and on soft tissue surfaces. They are gram-negative, facultatively anaerobic, rod-shaped or coccobacillary cells. The majority of haemophili isolated from the mouth, except *H. aphrophilus,* are V-factor (nicotinamide adenine dinucleotide, NAD) dependent but do not require X-factor (protoheme). Good growth is usually obtained on heated blood (chocolate) agar plates at 35 to 37°C, and most strains are enhanced by a moist atmosphere with the addition of 5% to 10% CO_2.

The species most commonly isolated from the mouth are *Haemophilus parainfluenzae, Haemophilus paraphrophilus* and *Haemophilus segnis. Haemophilus aphrophilus* is also found occasionally in dental plaque. *H. parainfluenzae* is the most common oral isolate and usually accounts for the majority of haemophili present in both saliva and mature plaque. This species has been implicated in cases of bacterial endocarditis but is not known to be associated with dental diseases. *H. segnis* is a recently described species in dental plaque. It forms smooth or granular, high convex, grayish white colonies up to 0.5 mm in diameter on chocolate agar and is nonhemolytic on blood-containing media. The cells are pleomorphic, nonmotile, and nonencapsulated, forming mainly irregular filaments with a few bacillary forms. Colonies of some strains of *H. parainfluenzae* are surrounded by zones of hemolysis on blood agar, and many resemble those of α-hemolytic streptococci. Some strains of *H. aphrophilus* and *H. paraphrophilus,* in contrast to *H. segnis,* can adhere to surfaces and undergo cell–cell aggregation in the absence of sucrose. However, their involvement in plaque formation in the mouth is unknown.

Encapsulated forms of *H. influenzae* are the most common cause of meningitis in children under age 4 and have been associated with epiglottitis. When present they usually inhabit the nasopharynx but may occur in the mouth. Nonencapsulated forms of *H. influenzae* are seldom pathogenic and are a common part of the normal nasopharyngeal flora.

Actinobacilli

Only one of five known species of the genus *Actinobacillus, Actinobacillus actinomycetemcomitans,* is found as an inhabitant of the mouth. Although it was originally described in 1912 it was renamed in 1936 because it had been frequently isolated from cases of actinomycosis in association with *Actinomyces israelii*. The species name is derived from *actinomyces* (ray fungus) and *comitans* (accompanying).

A. actinomycetemcomitans is a small, gram-negative, coccoid or coccobacillary organism that morphologically resembles *Haemophilus aphrophilus*. But unlike *H. aphrophilus,* it is catalase positive. Genetic analysis has shown *A. actinomycetemcomitans* to be more closely related to *Haemophilus* than to other species of *Actinobacillus*. Like other facultative gram-negative rods, growth on solid media, such as blood agar, is enhanced by an atmosphere with 5% to 10% CO_2. Distinguishing biochemical and physiological features are shown in Table 49.8.

The primary oral habitat of *A. actinomycetemcomitans* is supragingival and subgingival plaque, although it is capable of colonizing the buccal mucosa. It is usually present in high concentrations in subgingival material from patients with juvenile periodontitis and has been strongly implicated in the etiology of this form of periodontitis (see Chap. 52). This organism also has been isolated from patients with infective endocarditis.

Capnocytophagae

Organisms that require greater concentrations of CO_2 than are present in air are referred to as capnophilic. *Capnocytophaga* is the genus name that has been proposed for a group of fastidious, CO_2-requiring, gram-negative, fusiform rods isolated from the oral cavity. These organisms are characteristically described as gliding or surface translocating bacteria. Colonies tend to have a spreading, fringelike edge and may be gray-white, pink, or yellow in color. Some strains produce pitting of the agar surface. Three species have been described within the new genus: *Capnocytophaga ochracea, Capnocytophaga sputigena,* and *Capnocytophaga gingivalis.* These can be distinguished on the basis of lactose and galactose fermentation and nitrate reduction. Although the names are new, *C. ochracea* in fact corresponds to an organism previously known by various other titles (including *Fusiformis nucleatus* var. *orchraceus* and *Bacteroides ochraceus*). Isolates of *Capnocytophaga* are clearly differentiated from both *Fusobacterium* and *Bacteroides* on the basis of their ability to grow in air + CO_2, fermentation of carbohydrates, end products of glucose metabolism, and DNA base composition. Interest has been aroused in these organisms because of their association with juvenile periodontitis and possibly other forms of destructive periodontal disease.

Eikenella corrodens

Eikenella corrodens is a facultatively anaerobic organism that characteristically "corrodes" or causes "pitting" of the surface of agar media. Several other bacterial species also produce similar corroding colonies, and this property has caused some confusion in the past. In particular, *E. corrodens* has been confused with the obligately anaerobic organism *Bacteroides corrodens* (now designated *Bacteroides ureolyticus*), although it is known that they differ in several important respects, including DNA base ratio.

The cells of *E. corrodens* are small, non-spore-forming, nonencapsulated, nonmotile, microaerophilic, asaccharolytic, gram-negative coccobacilli. The organism grows on blood or chocolate agar and is enhanced by the presence of 3% to 10% CO_2. It is found in the mouth and upper respiratory tract as part of the normal commensal flora and has also been isolated from abscesses in various parts of the body, usually in mixed infections. Strains are usually sensitive to penicillin, ampicillin, chloramphenicol, and tetracycline but resistant to clindamycin and aminoglycosides. DNA homology studies indicate that strains designated *E. corrodens* constitute a genetically homogeneous species, although some antigenic and biotype differences have been demonstrated. This organism can be recovered from periodontal pockets in humans and has been shown to induce a particular type of periodontal disease in gnotobiotic rats. Its role in human disease is still being defined.

Enterics and Pseudomonads

The gram-negative, facultatively anaerobic enteric rods (Enterobacteriaceae) and the gram-negative aerobic rods of *Pseudomonas* are not considered prominent members of the normal oral flora. However, they have been detected in some people at various oral sites and have been occasionally associated with postextraction infections and mucosal and en-

Table 49.9: Characteristics of Oral *Treponema* Species

Species	Number of Axial Fibrils*	Length (μm)	Width (μm)	Ferments Sugars	Requires Serum	DNA G + C (mol%)
T. vincentii	4–6	5–16	0.2–0.25	Yes	Yes	44
T. denticola	2–3	6–15	0.15–0.20	Yes	Yes	37–38
T. socranskii	1	6–15	0.16–0.18	No	No	51
T. pectinovorum	2	7–15	0.28–0.30	Pectin†	No	39
T. macrodentium	1	5–16	0.10–0.25	No	Yes	39
T. scoliodontium	1	6–16	0.15–0.20	Yes	Yes	39–43
T. orale	2	6–16	0.10–0.25	Yes	Yes	37

*Number of axial fibrils inserted into each end of the bacterium.
†Ferments only pectin, polygalacturonic acid, glucuronic acid, and galacturonic acid.

dodontic lesions. Recently, a survey for these organisms in subgingival material from patients with refractory periodontitis revealed their presence in about 10% of the 500 patients examined. When enteric rods were found they constituted over 20% of the total flora. The most frequently detected enterics were *Enterobacter cloacae, Enterobacter agglomerans, Proteus mirabilis, Klebsiella pneumoniae,* and *Klebsiella oxytoca. Pseudomonas aeruginosa* was found in 10 of the 500 patients. Since most of these patients with refractory periodontitis had received antibiotic therapy, it is likely that the enterics and pseudomonads present in some of the patients responded to antibiotics selectively, resulting in opportunistic infections.

Spirochetes

Spirochetes are common inhabitants of the oral cavity, particularly of the gingival crevices and subgingival areas. In 1875 one of the first references was made to an oral spirochete, *Treponema buccale,* and in 1877 another oral spirochete was given the name *Treponema dentium* by Robert Koch. W. D. Miller made numerous microscopic observations of the oral spirochetes, referring to them collectively under the name *Spirochaeta dentium,* but was unable to culture any of them. Among the first references to a possible association between the oral spirochetes and diseases of the oral cavity or upper respiratory tract was that of Plaut in 1894, who observed such organisms in angina caused by a throat infection. Vincent in 1896 and 1898 also observed spirochetes and fusiform bacilli in "hospital gangrene" and in angina. Later Noguchi isolated and described six species, based on morphological characteristics and the motions of the organisms in fluid culture media. Noguchi's classification of the oral spirochetes gradually fell into disrepute because other workers could not substantiate his findings. Subsequently, so many new strains were described

that more than 40 names for oral spirochetes were recorded in an appendix to the family Treponemataceae in the 1957 edition of *Bergey's Manual.*

Today seven species of oral spirochetes are recognized, all belonging to the genus *Treponema.* Others exist in the human mouth and will be periodically added to the list as techniques are discovered to permit their isolation, followed by culture and characterization.

Oral spirochetes are easily detected through dark-field or phase-contrast microscopic observation of oral samples. Thus, they have been categorized according to size as small (less than 0.3 μm in diameter and up to 10 μm long), intermediate (about 0.2 to 0.5 μm in diameter and up to 15 μm long), and large (0.5 μm in width and up to 20 μm long). Ultrastructural components of these unique bacteria also are used to aid in their classification, and many of the spirochetes that can be isolated and cultured have been analyzed for some phenotypic and genotypic properties (Table 49.9).

Oral *Treponema* organisms are helical rod-shaped, anaerobic, gram-negative bacteria that have regular or irregular spirals. They are 5 to 16 mm long and 0.1 to 0.25 mm in diameter. The cells possess flagella-like structures called axial fibrils, axial filaments, or periplasmic flagella. These structures are inserted into the ends of the cells and lie adjacent to the length of the cells between the cytoplasmic membrane and the external surface of the outer envelope. They are actively motile, with a rapid jerky motion. All of the oral spirochetes listed in Table 49.9 have been cultivated, and all are considered to be small spirochetes except the intermediate-sized *T. vincentii.* Microscopic observation of subgingival material from periodontitis patients reveals the presence of small, intermediate, and large spirochetes. Thus, many of the oral spirochetes have never been cultivated or characterized, most likely because of a lack of specifically required nutrients in the isolating medium. Additional problems relate to lysis of delicate spirochetes by the methods used to disperse plaque samples prior to plating on agar media. Even if the appropriate nutrients are used and care is taken not to lyse the spirochetes during dispersion, special techniques are required to separate the spirochetes from all of the other bacteria in the oral samples. Isolating spirochetes during primary culture is difficult because of their tendency to spread over the surface of agar. However, isolation techniques that take advantage of this motility have been developed. One method involves placing the sample onto filters that are lying on the surface of an agar growth medium. The filter (pore size of 0.22 to 0.45 μm) retains most of the plaque bacteria but allows the thin motile spirochetes to penetrate to the underlying surface of the agar and grow. Another method involves placing the sample in recessed wells made in an agar growth medium. The motile organisms, including spirochetes, migrate from the well into the surrounding agar. The outermost edge of this "spirochetal" zone is removed and subcultured in broth. Purification is accomplished by subculturing dilutions of the broth cultures. Development and use of DNA probes (see Chap. 2) for the cultivable *Treponema* species will greatly facilitate the detection of these bacteria in oral sites.

There is overwhelming evidence that the proportion of spirochetes (percentage of total microscopic count) in subgingival plaque greatly increases in gingivitis and most forms of periodontitis when compared to the healthy gingival state. Percentages in nondiseased sites range from 0% to 4% and in adult periodontitis sites may be as high as 56% of the total microscopic count. This along with other information described in Chapter 52 (Periodontal Disease) at least suggests that spirochetes are important in such diseases. Penetration of periodontal tissues in ANUG by spirochetes was first demonstrated by Listegarten about 25 years ago, but at that time little work had been done on the characterization and identification of the pathogenic properties of these bacteria. Now that cultivable strains of *Treponema* are available, more and more information is being gathered on their pathogenic properties in relation to periodontal disease.

Mycoplasmas

Mycoplasma is a unique genus of bacteria that do not have a cell wall. The organisms range in size from 0.2 to 0.8 μm in diameter and their cytoplasmic membrane contains cholesterol.

The highly pleomorphic bacteria of the genus *Mycoplasma* are regular oral residents. *Mycoplasma* species have been isolated from throat swabs, dental

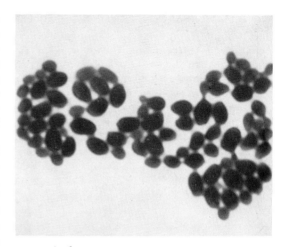

Figure 49.6: Oral yeast.

plaque and calculus, root canals, inflamed pulp, carious lesions, healthy and diseased gingival crevices, and periodontal pockets. These organisms are found more frequently in the gingival area than at other oral sites. Seven species have been isolated from the human oropharyngeal area: *M. pneumoniae, M. hominis, M. orale, M. salivarium, M. faucium,* and *M. lipophilum.* The predominant species is apparently *M. salivarium.* Although one report shows *M. salivarium* has been isolated in significantly higher percentages from people with periodontal disease (87%) as compared with a healthy control group (32%), strong evidence for a role in periodontal disease is currently lacking.

Fungi

Oral yeasts (Fig. 49.6) are by far the most common fungus detected in the human mouth. *Candida albicans* is the most frequently detected oral yeast. Its reported incidence in the mouth and throat of healthy people varies considerably, ranging from 10% to 80%. The range of counts in positive mouths is from 10 to 10,000; in 90% the count per milliliter is 1,000 or less. *Candida tropicalis, Candida stellatoidea, Candida pseudotropicalis, Cryptococcus* species, and several unidentified species of *Candida* have also been detected in lower concentrations in healthy mouths. *C. albicans* and other yeasts have been detected in high numbers in the subgingival flora or in the gingival tissues of acute periodontal abscesses, in advancing periodontitis, in HIV-infected patients, and in juvenile periodontitis and refractory periodontitis lesions.

As discussed in Chapter 33, *Candida* species are opportunistic pathogens that may cause harmful infections following suppression of the normal bacterial flora or of host defense mechanisms. Typical examples are oral candidiasis following long-term tetracy-cline therapy or immunosuppression resulting from HIV infection. A recent example of this opportunistic potential was described as a result of determining the level of yeasts in subgingival sites in patients with re-fractory periodontitis. These patients are not respon-sive to the mechanical treatment methods and are commonly given broad-spectrum antibiotics. They are also commonly nonresponsive to the antibiotic ther-apy. Of the 500 patients studied, 16.8% had *Candida* species at the disease sites. In those sites that were positive, *Candida* made up 21% to 39% of the cultiv-able flora. *C. albicans* was detected in about 83% of the yeast-infected sites. *C. parapsilosus, C. tropicalis,* and *C. lipolytica* were detected in 8%, 5% and 2%, respectively, of the yeast-infected sites. Gram-negative enteric rods and *Pseudomonas* were also detected in some of these patients.

Other fungi that have been isolated from the hu-man mouth are *Penicillium* species, *Scopulariopsis brevicularis, Geotrichum asteroides, Hormodendrum compactum, Aspergillus* species, and *Hemispora stel-lata,* but these fungi are not considered normal oral inhabitants.

Protozoa

Protozoa are not uncommon in the oral cavity, the most common being *Entamoeba gingivalis* and *Trichomonas tenax.* It was found that the oral cavities of 39% of 700 patients contained *E. gingivalis,* while 23% contained *T. tenax* and 17.7% contained both. Distribution was also related to the condition of the oral cavity. Of "clean and healthy" mouths, 26.4% con-tained *E. gingivalis,* 11.2% contained *T. tenax,* and 6.4% contained both. In early periodontal disease, 62.5% contained *E. gingivalis,* 48.2% contained *T. tenax,* and 39% contained both. In advanced pe-riodontal disease, 100% contained *E. gingivalis,* 80% contained *T. tenax,* and 80% contained both. *E. gingi-valis* and *T. tenax* were absent from the oral cavities of children 6 to 12 years of age but were present in increasing proportions with age. There was no rela-tionship between the number of carious lesions and the prevalence of the protozoa. Protozoal infestation was approximately equally prevalent in men and women.

Viruses

Most viruses that are detected in the mouth or in saliva are oral transients present only during active infec-tions or during asymptomatic carrier states. Herpes simplex virus infection occurs in a large proportion of the population, for approximately 70% to 90% of adults continuously maintain significant levels of ho-mologous circulating antibody. This fact and the re-current nature of vesicular lesions in or near the oral cavity indicate the persistence of the virus throughout life. Between the recurrent episodes (latency), the vi-rus persists in the trigeminal ganglia. Herpes simplex virus is excreted in saliva for as long as 2 months after complete recovery from the infection. It has been demonstrated in the saliva of slightly less than 3% of asymptomatic adults.

It is estimated that about 80% of the population is infected with cytomegalovirus. Most show no symp-toms. The virus has been detected in all body se-cretions, including saliva. Symptomatic infections re-sult in birth defects from congenital transmission, and opportunistic infections occur in immunocom-promised patients (renal and bone marrow transplant recipients and persons with HIV infection).

Symptomatic or asymptomatic, blood-borne viral diseases (e.g., hepatitis B and HIV infection) may re-sult in the virus being present in saliva. Other viruses such as varicella–zoster (chickenpox, shingles), Ep-stein–Barr (infectious mononucleosis), mumps, mea-sles, and influenza viruses and numerous respiratory viruses may be present in the oropharyngeal fluids on a transient basis.

ADDITIONAL READING

Ashamaony, L., Goodfellow, M., Minnikin, D. E., Bowden, G. H. W., and Hardie, J. M. 1977. Fatty and Mycolic Acid Composition of *Bacterionema matruchotii* and Related Organisms. J Gen Microbiol, **98,** 205.

Berg, J-O., and Nord, C-E. 1972. Isolation of Peptococci and Peptostreptococci in Developing Human Dental Plaque by Maintaining Continuous Anaerobiosis. Acta Odont Scand, **30,** 503.

Bowden, G. H., and Hardie, J. M. 1973. Commensal and Pathogenic *Actinomyces* Species in Man. In *Actinomy-cetales: Characteristics and Practical Importance,* p. 277, edited by G. Sykes and F. A. Skinner. Academic Press, New York.

Bowden, G. H., and Hardie, J. M. 1978. Oral Pleomorphic (coryneform) Gram-Positive Rods. In *Coryneform Bac-teria,* p. 235, edited by I. J. Bousefield and A. G. Callely. Academic Press, New York.

Bratthall, D. 1970. Demonstration of Five Serological Groups of Streptococcal Strains Resembling *Streptococcus mu-tans.* Odontol Rev, **21,** 143.

Brooks, G. F., O'Donoghue, J. M., Rissing, J. P., Soapes, K., and Smith, J. W. 1974. *Eikenella corrodens,* a Recently Recog-nized Pathogen. Medicine, **53,** 325.

Collins, P. A., Gerencser, M. A., and Slack, J. M. 1973. Enu-meration and Identification of Actinomycetaceae in Hu-man Dental Calculus Using the Fluorescent Antibody Technique. Arch Oral Biol, **18,** 145.

Coykendall, A. L. 1977. Proposal to Elevate the Subspecies of *Streptococcus mutans* to Species Status, Based on Their Molecular Composition. Int J Syst Bacteriol, **27,** 26.

Coykendall, A. L., and Munzenmaier, A. J. 1979. Deoxyribonucleic Acid Hybridization Among Strains of *Actinomyces viscosus* and *Actinomyces naeslundii*. Int J Syst Bacteriol, **29**, 234.

Coykendall, A. L., Kaczmarek, F. S., and Slots, J. 1980. Genetic Heterogeneity in *Bacteroides asaccharolyticus* (Holdeman and Moore, 1970), Finegold and Barnes, 1977 (Approved Lists, 1980) and Proposal of *Bacteroides gingivalis* sp. nov. and *Bacteroides macacae* (Slots and Genco) comb. nov. Int J Syst Bacteriol, **30**, 559.

Dent, V. E. 1982. Identification of Oral *Neisseria* Species of Animals. J Appl Bacteriol, **52**, 21.

Dzink, J. L., Gibbons, R. J., Childs, III, W. C., and Socransky, S. S. 1989. The Predominant Cultivable Microbiota of Crevicular Epithelial Cells. Oral Microbiol Immunol, **4**, 4, 1.

Dzink, J. L., Socransky, S. S., and Haffajee, A. D. 1988. The Predominant Cultivable Microbiota of Active and Inactive Lesions of Destructive Periodontal Diseases. J Clin Periodontol, **15**, 316.

Gillespie, J., Holt, S. C. 1987. Growth Studies of *Wolinella recta,* a Gram-negative Periodontopathogen. Oral Microbiol Immunol, **2**, 105.

Gold, O. G., Jordan, H. V., and Van Houte, J. 1975. The Prevalence of Enterococci in the Human Mouth and their Pathogenicity in Animal Models. Arch Oral Biol, **20**, 473.

Hamada, S., and Slade, J. D. 1980. Biology, Immunology, and Cariogenicity of *Streptococcus mutans*. Microbiol Rev, **44**, 331.

Hammond, B. F. 1967. Studies on Encapsulated Lactobacilli: III. Human Oral Strains. J Dent Res, **46**, 340.

Hardie, J. M., and Bowden, G. H. 1971. Carbohydrate Components of the Cell Walls of *Streptococcus mutans* and the Possible Value in Serological Grouping. Caries Res, **6**, 80.

Hardie, J. M., and Bowden, G. H. 1974. The Normal Microbial Flora of the Mouth. In *The Normal Microbial Flora of Man,* p. 47, edited by F. A. Skinner and J. G. Carr. Academic Press, London.

Hardie, J. M., and Bowden, G. H. 1976. Physiological Classification of Oral Viridans Streptococci. J Dent Res, **55**, A166.

Hardie, J. M., and Marsh, P. D. 1978. Streptococci and the Human Oral Flora. In *Streptococci,* p. 157, edited by F. A. Skinner and L. Quesnell. Academic Press, New York.

Holdeman, L. V., Cato, E. P., Burmeister, J. A., and Moore, W. E. C. 1980. Descriptions of *Eubacterium timidum* sp. nov., *Eubacterium brachy* sp. nov. and *Eubacterium nodatum* sp. nov., isolated from human periodontitis. Int J Syst Bacteriol, **30**, 163.

Holdeman, L. V., Cato, E. P., and Moore, W. E. C. (Eds.) 1977. *Anaerobe Laboratory Manual,* Ed. 4. Virginia Polytechnic Institute and State University Anaerobe Laboratory, Blacksburg.

Holdeman, L. V., Johnson, J. L., and Moore, W. E. C. 1981. Pigmenting *Bacteroides* in Periodontal Samples. J Dent Res, **60**, Special Issue A, 414.

Holdeman, L. V., Moore, W. E. C., Churn, P. J., and Johnson, J. L. 1982. *Bacteroides oris* and *Bacteroides buccae,* New Species from Human Periodontitis and Other Human Infections. Int J Syst Bacteriol, **32**, 125.

Jordan, H. V., and Hammond, B. F. 1972. Filamentous Bacteria Isolated from Human Root Surface Caries. Arch Oral Biol, **17**, 1333.

Kilian, M. 1976. A Taxonomic Study of the Genus *Haemophilus* with the Proposal of a New Species. J Gen Microbiol, **93**, 9.

Krieg, N. R., and Holt, J. G. (Eds.) 1984. *Bergey's Manual of Systematic Bacteriology,* Vol. 1. Williams & Wilkins, Baltimore.

Kumagai, K., Iwabuchi, T., Hinuma, Y., Yuri, K., and Ishida, N. 1971. Incidence, Species, and Significance of *Mycoplasma* Species in the Mouth. J Infect Dis, **123**, 16.

Lai, C., Listgarten, M. A., Shirakawa, M., Slots, J. 1987. *Bacteroides forsythus* in Adult Gingivitis and Periodontitis. Oral Microbiol Immunol, **2**, 152.

Leadbetter, E. R., Holt, S. C., and Socransky, S. S. 1979. *Capnocytophaga:* New Genus of Gram-Negative Gliding Bacteria. I. General Characteristics, Taxonomic Considerations and Significance. Arch Microbiol, **122**, 9.

Loesche, W. J. 1986. Role of *Streptococcus mutans* in Dental Decay. Microbiol Rev, **50**, 353.

Loesche, W. J., and Syed, S. A. 1973. The Predominant Cultivable Flora of Carious Plaque and Carious Dentine. Caries Res, **7**, 201.

Mayrand, D., and Holt, S. C. 1988. Biology of Asaccharolytic Black-Pigmented *Bacteroides* Species. Microbiol Rev, **52**, 134.

Mays, T. D., Holdeman, L. V., Moore, W. E. C., Rogosa, M., and Johnson, J. L. 1982. Taxonomy of the Genus *Veillonella* Prevot. Int J Syst Bacteriol, **32**, 28.

McCarthy, C., Snyder, M. L., and Parker, R. B. 1965. The Indigenous Oral Flora of Man: I. The Newborn to the 1-Year-Old Infant. Arch Oral Biol, **10**, 61.

Mejare, B., and Edwardsson, S. 1975. *Streptococcus milleri* (Guthof): An Indigenous Organism of the Human Oral Cavity. Arch Oral Biol, **20**, 757.

Perch, B. E., Kjems, E., and Ravn, T. 1974. Biochemical and Serological Properties of *Streptococcus mutans* from Various Human and Animal Sources. Acta Pathol Microbiol Scand, **82**, 357.

Progulske, A., Holt, S. C. 1987. Studies on the Growth of *Eikenella corrodens* Strain 23834. Oral Microbiol Immunol, **2**, 2.

Rasmussen, E. G., Gibbons, R. J., and Socransky, S. S. 1966. Taxonomic Study of 50 Gram-Positive Anaerobic Diphtheroids Isolated from the Oral Cavity. Arch Oral Biol, **11**, 573.

Schofield, G. M., and Schaal, K. P. 1981. A Numerical Taxonomic Study of Members of the Actinomycetaceae and Related Taxa. J Gen Microbiol, **127**, 237.

Shah, H. N., and Collins, M. D. 1981. *Bacteroides buccalis,* sp. nov., *Bacteroides denticola,* sp. nov., and *Bacteroides pentosaceus,* sp. nov., New Species of the Genus *Bacteroides* from the Oral Cavity. Zentralbl Bakteriol Mikrobiol Hyg, Part I. Orig. **C2**, 235.

Shah, H. N., and Collins, M. D. 1988. Proposal for Reclassification of *Bacteroides asaccharolyticus, Bacteroides gingivalis,* and *Bacteroides endodontalis* in a New Genus, *Porphyromonas*. Int J Syst Bacteriol, **38**, 128.

Sharpe, M. E. 1979. Identification of the Lactic Acid Bacteria. In *Identification Methods for Microbiologists,* Ed. 2, edited by F. A. Skinner and D. W. Lovelock. Academic Press, New York.

Shenker, B. J., Berthold, P., Dougherty, P., and Porter, K. K. 1987. Immunosuppressive Effects of *Centipeda periodontii:* Selective Cytotoxicity for Lymphocytes and Monocytes. Infect Immun, **55**, 2332.

Shklair, I. L., and Keene, H. J. 1974. A Biochemical Scheme for the Separation of the Five Varieties of *Streptococcus mutans*. Arch Oral Biol, **19**, 1079.

Skerman, V. D. B., McGowan, V., and Sneath, P. H. A. (Eds.) 1980. *Approved List of Bacterial Names*. Int J Syst Bacteriol, **30**, 225.

Slack, J. M., and Gerencser, M. A. 1975. *Actinomyces, Filamentous Bacteria. Biology and Pathogenicity*. Burgess Publishing Company, Minneapolis.

Slots, J., Rams, T. E., Listgarten, M. A. 1988. Yeasts, Enteric

Rods and Pseudomonads in the Subgingival Flora of Severe Adult Periodontitis. Oral Microbiol Immunol, **3,** 47.

Smibert, R. M. 1978. The genus *Campylobacter.* Annu Rev Microbiol, **32,** 673.

Smibert, R. M., and Burmeister, J. A. 1983. *Treponema pectinovorum* sp. nov. Isolated from Humans with Periodontitis. Int J Syst Bacteriol, **34,** 852.

Smibert, R. M., Johnson, J. L., and Ranney, R. R. 1984. *Treponema socranskii* nov., *Treponema socranskii* subsp. *buccale* subsp. nov., and *Treponema socranskii* subsp. *paredis* subsp. nov. Isolated from the Human Periodontia. Int J Syst Bacteriol, **34,** 457.

Socransky, S. S., Holt, S. C., Leadbetter, E. R., Tanner, A. C. R., Savitt, E., and Hammond, B. F. 1979. *Capnocytophaga:* A New Genus of Gram-Negative Gliding Bacteria. III. Physiological Characterization. Arch Microbiol, **122,** 29.

Socransky, S. S., and Manganiello, S. D. 1971. The Oral Microbiota of Man from Birth to Senility. J Periodontol, **42,** 485.

Tanner, A. C. R., Badger, S., Lai, C-H., Listgarten, M. A., Visconti, R. A., and Socransky, S. S. 1981. *Wolinella* gen. nov., *Wolinella succinogenes (Vibrio succinogenes* Wolin et al.) comb. nov., and Description of *Bacteroides gracilis* sp. nov., *Wolinella recta* sp. nov., *Campylobacter concisus* sp. nov. and *Eikenella corrodens* from Humans with Periodontal Disease. Int J Syst Bacteriol, **31,** 432.

Tanner, A. C. R., Dzink, J. L., Ebersole, J. L., and Socransky, S. S. 1987. *Wolinella recta, Campylobacter concisus, Bacteroides gracilis,* and *Eikenella corrodens* from Periodontal Lesions. J Periodont Res, **22,** 327.

Van Steenbergen, T. J. M., Vlaanderen, C. A., and De Graaff, J. 1981. Confirmation of *Bacteroides gingivalis* as a Species Distinct from *Bacteroides asaccharolyticus.* Int J Syst Bacteriol, **31,** 236.

Van Winkelhoff, A. J., Van Steenbergen, T. J. M., and De Graaff, J. 1988. The Role of Black-pigmented *Bacteroides* in Human Oral Infections. J Clin Periodontol, **15,** 145.

50

Microbial Ecology of the Oral Cavity

Chris H. Miller

The oral cavity supports one of the most concentrated and varied of microbial populations of any area of the body. Particularly high numbers of microorganisms are found on the dorsum of the tongue, around the gingival sulcus, and on the tooth surface. On tooth surfaces, the soft, noncalcified accumulations of bacteria and their products are referred to as dental plaque. Dental plaque is a bacterial mass tenaciously attached to the tooth surface. It is not merely an accumulation of food debris. Calcified dental plaque is called calculus (tartar).

The total microscopic count of saliva, which is derived mainly from the tongue, ranges from 43 million to 5.5 billion/mL, with an average of 750 million/mL. One can easily culture from 10 million to over 100 million live bacteria per 1 mL of saliva. The microbial concentration about the gingival sulcus and in plaque is approximately 200 billion cells per gram of sample. This is equivalent to the density of centrifugally packed cells from a broth culture or of a bacterial colony on agar medium.

A variety of physical and chemical environmental factors influence the survival and growth of microorganisms in the mouth. These include the availability of organic and inorganic nutrients, levels of oxygen and carbon dioxide, pH, the presence of antimicrobial substances, the anatomy of the oral structures, abrasive forces associated with oral surfaces, temperature, and the availability of water. These factors are associated with several microbial and host activities or conditions (Table 50.1), which reciprocally select for the types and levels of microbes that exist in the mouth. The results of these selective pressures are readily seen in the variability of the normal microbiota at different body sites (Table 50.2), including different sites in the mouth (Table 50.3).

Acquisition of an Oral Microbiota

The human is edentulous at birth and has a flora that is characteristic of this condition. When the primary teeth begin to erupt, there is a significant change in the environment that is reflected in changes in the

Table 50.1: Microbial and Host Factors That Affect the Oral Microbiota

Microbial	Host
Synthesis of antimicrobial agents	Flow and composition of oral fluids
Susceptibility to antimicrobial agents	Oral immune defenses
Nutritional requirements	Oral and systemic diseases
Metabolic capability	Diet
Adherence properties	Oral hygiene
	Oral anatomy

oral flora. When the primary dentition is complete, the conditions are relatively stable until the permanent teeth begin to erupt. During the period of mixed dentition, conditions vary as teeth are lost and new ones erupt, producing varied environmental conditions that can affect the oral flora. Once the permanent dentition is present, conditions become somewhat more stable.

In utero the fetus is normally free of bacteria. During birth, the infant is exposed to the normal flora of the mother's genital tract, including lactobacilli, corynebacteria, micrococci, coliforms, facultative streptococci, anaerobic cocci, yeasts, protozoa, and possibly viruses. Nevertheless, the oral cavity is usually sterile at birth. From about 8 hours after birth there is a rapid increase in the number of detectable organisms. However, the composition of the bacterial flora varies considerably for the first few days of life. Several species of lactobacilli, streptococci, staphylococci, pneumococci, enterococci, coliforms, sarcinae, and neisseriae can be detected, but with the exception of *Streptococcus salivarius,* most of these organisms are found sporadically and not in high numbers. Even though it is exposed to a wide range of organisms during the first few days, the mouth of a newborn

Table 50.2: Distribution of Indigenous Microorganisms in Man

Organism	Mouth	Oropharynx	Naso-pharynx	Intestine	Skin	Eye	External Genitalia	Vagina
α-Streptococcus	1	1	2	2	0	0	2	2
β-Streptococcus	tr	3	tr	2*	0	0	0	tr
γ-Streptococcus	2	2	tr	2	0	0	2	2
Anaerobic streptococcus	2	2	0	2	0	0	2	2
Pneumococcus	tr	3	tr	0	0	0	0	0
Staphylococcus epidermidis	2	tr	3	2	1	2	2	2
Staphylococcus aureus	2	2	3	2	0	0	0	tr
Other staphylococci	2	2	tr	2	tr	tr	tr	2
Corynebacterium†	1	2	2	2	1	1	2	2‡
Lactobacillus	2	0	0	2	0	0	0	1
Leptotrichia	2	0	0	0	0	0	0	0
Actinomyces	2	2	0	0	0	0	0	0
Bacteroides	2	tr	tr	1	0	0	tr	tr
Fusobacterium	2	tr	0	2	0	0	2	0
Spirochetes	2	tr	0	2	0	0	2	0
Anaerobic vibrios	2	tr	tr	0	0	0	0	tr
Neisseria meningitidis	0	3	3	0	0	0	0	0
Other neisseriae	2	1	1	0	0	0	tr	tr
Veillonella	1	2	2	0	0	0	0	2
Haemophilus	tr	3	3	0	0	0	0	0
Mycoplasmas	2	2	0	2	0	0	2	2
Coliform bacteria	tr	tr	tr	1	0	0	2	2
Proteus	0	0	0	2	0	0	tr	0
Pseudomonas	tr	0	0	tr	0	0	tr	0
Clostridium	0	0	0	2	0	0	0	0
Bacillus	0	0	0	0	0	0	0	0
Mycobacterium	0	0	0	tr	tr	0	3	0
Yeasts	2	2	0	2	2	0	2	2‡
Protozoa	2	tr	0	3	0	0	3	3

Note: 1 = generally present and constituting a principal fraction of the regional microbial flora; 2 = generally present but constituting a minor fraction of the regional microbial flora; 3 = carriers found frequently in whom the organisms may constitute a prominent fraction of the regional microbial flora; tr = often found, usually in small numbers, as a trace component or a transient; 0 = if found, may be assumed to be a transient.

   *Group D hemolytic enterococci.

   †A very small proportion of the populace acts as the reservoir of diphtheria, owing to the persistence of *C. diphtheriae* in the nasopharynx.

   ‡During the period of ovarian activity.

Table 50.3: Mean Percentages of Cultivable Organisms in the Adult Oral Cavity*

Organism	Gingival Crevice Area	Dental Plaque	Tongue	Saliva
Gram-positive facultative cocci	28.8	28.2	44.8	46.2
Streptococci	27.1	27.9	38.3	41.0
S. salivarius	ND	ND	8.2	4.6
Enterococci	7.2		ND	1.3
Staphylococci	1.7	0.3	6.5	4.0
Gram-positive anaerobic cocci	7.4	12.6	4.2	13.0
Gram-negative facultative cocci	0.4	0.4	3.4	1.2
Gram-negative anaerobic cocci	10.7	6.4	16.0	15.9
Gram-positive facultative rods	15.3	23.8	13.0	11.8
Gram-positive anaerobic rods	20.2	18.4	8.2	4.8
Gram-negative facultative rods	1.2	ND	3.2	2.3
Gram-negative anaerobic rods	16.1	10.4	8.2	4.8
Fusobacterium	1.9	4.1	0.7	0.3
B. melaninogenicus	4.7	ND	0.2	ND
V. sputorum	3.8	1.3	2.2	2.1
Other Bacteroides	5.6	4.8	5.1	2.4
Spirochetes	1.0	ND	ND	ND

Note: ND = not detected.
*Reproduced with permission from S. S. Socransky and S. D. Manganiello: The Oral Microbiota of Man from Birth to Senility. *J Periodontol,* **42,** 485, 1971.

infant is a selective habitat. Consequently, few of the bacteria common to adult mouths become established, and practically none of the species present in the general environment do so, except occasionally as transients. Organisms different from those harbored by immediate contacts may be acquired; for example, identical twins may harbor different strains of the same species. Some selectivity continues into adulthood.

At least by the end of the third month, all mouths support a recognizable resident microflora. Even at the end of 1 year, however, only streptococci, staphylococci, veillonellae, and neisseriae are generally found in all mouths. Actinomycetes, rothiae, lactobacilli, and fusobacteria can be isolated from about half of the mouths, while bacteroids, leptotrichiae, corynebacteria, and coliforms are present in less than half of the mouths. By 1 year, streptococci, although still numerically dominant, account for only about 70% of the viable count. The early period is dominated by facultative and aerobic species, to which are gradually added the various obligate anaerobes, but numerically the facultative types generally dominate at all ages.

A major change in the oral environment occurs at around age 6 months with the eruption of the first deciduous teeth. The appearance of hard enamel surfaces in the mouth apparently favors the establishment of *Streptococcus sanguis,* an organism not usually isolated prior to the eruption of the deciduous incisors (Fig. 50.1). Other organisms, including *Strep-*

tococcus mutans, preferentially colonize the tooth surface and become regular oral inhabitants from about the age of 1 year. In one Swedish study, lactobacilli were recovered only in low numbers from infants and those less than 2 years old and appeared to be mostly transients (Fig. 50.2). Throughout child-

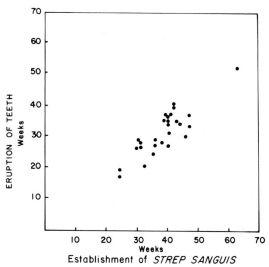

Figure 50.1: Relation between the eruption time of the teeth and the time when *Streptococcus sanguis* was established in the mouths of 27 infants. (Reproduced with permission from J. Carlsson, H. Grahnen, G. Jonsson, and S. Wilkner: Establishment of *Streptococcus sanguis* in the mouths of infants. *Arch Oral Biol,* **15,** 1143, 1970. Copyright 1970, Pergamon Press, Ltd.)

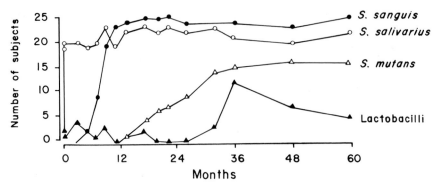

Figure 50.2: Presence of *S. salivarius, S. sanguis, S. mutans,* and lactobacilli in samples taken from the mouths of infants during a 5-year period. (Reproduced with permission from J. Carlsson, H. Grahnen, and G. Jonsson: Lactobacilli and streptococci in the mouths of children. *Caries Res, 9,* 333, 1975. S. Karger, Basel.)

hood the bacterial populations increase. Black-pigmented *Bacteroides* and spirochetes, which are strict anaerobes, are not present in the gingival crevice of all children. By adolescence, these *Bacteroides* species are present in virtually all individuals, and spirochetes also increase in incidence with age. The increase in these and other anaerobic organisms may be related to the concurrent increase in the prevalence of gingivitis that occurs during the same period.

The development of dental caries creates a new set of environmental conditions for microorganisms. The resulting cavities provide a protected and retentive niche, thus favoring organisms with little adhesive capability and which are poorly adapted for colonization of exposed tooth surfaces. The lesion also provides new substrates, a more acid pH, and decreased exposure to salivary antimicrobial factors. As indicated in Table 50.3, which lists the predominant genera and species found in various sites, the cultivable microbiota of different regions of the oral cavity of the adult is quite complex. Certain species have a predilection for particular sites, probably because some nutritional or physical requirement is met at that site. As the individual ages, some changes occur in the microflora, primarily associated with the loss of teeth. Spirochetes, lactobacilli, and some strains of streptococci are reduced. Oral disease will further alter the flora, the specific changes depending on which disease is present.

The extraction of all remaining teeth and the placement of complete dentures influences both the total numbers of the oral microorganisms and the prevalence of particular species (Fig. 50.3). Various studies have demonstrated that *Streptococcus mutans, Streptococcus sanguis,* yeasts, lactobacilli, and spirochetes are reduced in number or virtually eliminated during the edentulous period. The studies of Shklair and Mazzerella indicate that lactobacilli and

yeasts virtually disappear during the edentulous period and that *Streptococcus salivarius* increases. During the first 2 weeks after placement of the denture, streptococci remain at a high level, while lactobacilli and yeasts gradually return but remain at a low level. After 3 to 5 weeks the lactobacilli and yeasts increase and the streptococci decrease to preextraction levels. Throughout the entire period of this study, little fluctuation was observed in the number of staphylococci.

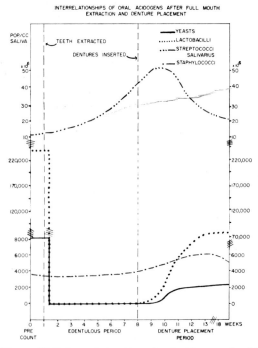

Figure 50.3: Interrelationships of oral acidogens after full mouth extraction and denture placement. (Reproduced with permission from I. L. Shklair and M. A. Mazzarella: Salivary Microbial Changes as a Result of Full Mouth Extraction. Dental Research Facility. U. S. Naval Training Center, Great Lakes, Ill. Project MR-005. 12-5004 NM 750127, 1960.)

A 1969 study on full denture wearers by Carlsson et al. showed that *S. sanguis, S. mutans,* and *S. salivarius* were present in samples of plaque from the dentures and in saliva from most subjects. When the dentures were left out of the mouth for 2 days, *S. sanguis* and *S. mutans* were no longer detected in saliva, whereas the prevalence of *S. salivarius* was unaffected. After the dentures had been worn again for 2 to 4 days, *S. sanguis* was again found in all subjects and *S. mutans* was found in five out of seven.

The organisms that colonize the mouth are in constant interaction with the host and with each other. These interactions are reflected in the terms *symbiosis* (mutually beneficial interactions), *antibiosis* (antagonistic to one), *probiosis* (beneficial to one), and *amphibiosis* (no harmful or beneficial interaction). The following sections will describe bacteria–host interactions and interbacterial interactions.

Bacteria–Host Interactions

Microbial Growth Factors from the Host

As is the case with any habitat, the composition of the oral microflora reflects its environment. The organisms that inhabit the mouth have several physicochemical and nutritional requirements and must be able to survive various physiological, mechanical, and defense activities of the host. The growth requirements of the microorganisms can be provided by the diet and tissues of the host, or by other microorganisms. Although saliva does not have continued access to all colonized sites in the mouth (e.g., deep pits and fissures, subgingival plaque), saliva is involved in regulating at least a portion of the oral microbiota. This fluid serves as the culture medium in which many of the oral microorganisms must live, grow, reproduce, and carry out their various functions. Growth and survival in saliva may even influence the establishment of bacteria in dental plaque and on epithelial surfaces. For example, *S. mutans* and *S. sanguis* must reach certain threshold levels in saliva before they are found with any degree of regularity on the tooth surface. Recolonization of cleaned tooth surfaces also occurs from organisms present in saliva or oral soft tissues.

"Whole saliva" is a complex mixture of the secretions of the parotid, submaxillary, and sublingual glands and of numerous lesser glands of the mucous membranes of the oral cavity; other substances that may be taken into the mouth from time to time and their degradation products; leukocytes, shed epithelial cells, and their products; gingival crevice fluid; and the oral microbiota and its metabolic products. Since the secretions of the various salivary glands are distinctive and subject to change by various reflex stimulations, the composition and amount of saliva secreted vary. Furthermore, the enzymatic activity of the oral microbiota must produce profound but extremely variable changes in the excreted saliva and its dissolved foods. On the average, saliva is composed of about 99.5% water and 0.5% solids, of which about half is inorganic (mostly chloride, bicarbonate, phosphate, sodium, calcium, potassium, trace elements, and dissolved carbon dioxide, oxygen, and nitrogen), and half is organic (proteins, cholesterol, hormone-like substances, free amino acids, urea, ammonia, vitamins, and antibacterial and antienzymatic factors). In addition, various foods and their breakdown products are transitorily present in saliva during and after their ingestion.

Mineral Content and Ionic Strength. The mineral content of saliva influences the microbiota through osmotic pressure, buffering capacity, E_h and pH; or the minerals act as essential metabolites or as activators or inhibitors of enzymes. Based on the mean inorganic content of saliva as reported in the literature, the calculated ionic strength of saliva is 0.046. The salivary proteins presumably contribute slightly but not enough to bring the ionic strength up to isotonicity. Although this is only about one-fourth to one-third that of tissue fluids or common bacterial culture media, the osmotic tolerance of bacteria is quite great, for many organisms can grow in either an extremely hypotonic or hypertonic environment.

The values for concentrations of inorganic constituents of saliva vary considerably. Only potassium and phosphate ions are more concentrated in saliva than in blood. Most attention has been given to salivary calcium and phosphate, because of their relationship to the teeth and to calculus formation. Their mean concentrations in saliva are respectively 5.8 mg/100 mL (range, 2.2 to 11.3 mg/100 mL) and 52.0 mg/100 mL (range, 19 to 220 mg/100 mL). The calcium is about 60% ionized, the remainder being mostly bound to protein. Saliva is probably saturated with calcium phosphate, which helps prevent the dissolution of the calcified tissues of the tooth. On the other hand, saturation leads to precipitation of calcium phosphate as dental calculus. Although it is true that an increase in alkalinity of saliva causes the precipitation of calcium phosphate, this seems to occur locally (i.e., calculus formation) rather than generally. The specific mechanisms causing the local precipitation of calcium phosphate have not been determined precisely. A number of investigators have suggested that it is due to the action of the oral microbiota, since calculus is mineralized plaque. However, calculus formation has been shown to occur in germ-free rats, but germ-free conditions do not exist in the human mouth.

The precise influence of inorganic ions on the oral

microbiota is difficult to evaluate because we lack adequate information about the inorganic ion requirements of bacteria. Most culture media contain at least available sodium, potassium, magnesium, manganese, calcium, iron, chloride, sulfate, phosphate, and carbonate. It is difficult to determine how essential each of these ions may be, for some, such as sodium chloride and sodium and potassium phosphate, are present in part to give the medium sufficient ionic strength and osmotic pressure and to provide a balanced ionic environment. Others have been shown definitely to be either essential or stimulatory to certain microbial species. Iron, for instance, is required particularly for microorganisms with a high cytochrome content, e.g., strongly aerobic bacteria such as *Pseudomonas aeruginosa*.

Most of the inorganic ions required for or stimulatory to bacteria function as activators or essential components of enzymes. If such ions were deficient in saliva, bacteria requiring them would be severely limited. Such ions, particularly trace ions, could be supplied in foodstuffs. Also, inorganic ions could indirectly influence the oral microbiota by activating salivary enzymes, which would help supply the necessary substrates for growth.

Buffer System. Salivary buffering capacity is directly related to the secretion rate, for more buffer is available per unit of time in rapid secretors than in slow secretors. The buffering capacity of saliva is mainly related to its bicarbonate system, which contributes about 64% to 85% of the total capacity. Microorganisms, mucoids, and proteins contribute little buffering capacity between pH 4.0 and 7.0. Most of the buffering capacity of salivary sediment is due to adsorbed bicarbonate. The buffering capacity of dental plaque is not due to bicarbonate but probably to bacterial products. It is generally agreed that the excretion of carbon dioxide and hence the buffering capacity of the saliva is increased fourfold to fivefold by stimulation of the glands and that it returns to its previous level within about one-half hour after cessation of stimulation. Hence, the buffering capacity of saliva is maximal at meals and is minimal between meals. As a corollary, the abrasive action of mastication may reduce the total microbial flora during the period of greatest buffering, after which the flora increases to a maximum in the interval between meals, when buffering capacity is minimal. On the other hand, local acid production, as in dental plaque or in carious lesions, would be greatest when buffering capacity is maximal.

The pH of the saliva is thought to have an important influence in the regulation of the oral microbial flora. The pH of freshly collected saliva varies between 5.7 and 7.0, with the mean near 6.7, which is satisfactory for the growth of a wide variety of microorganisms. It may vary by as much as 1 unit in normal circum-

stances of chewing, fatigue, change in breathing rate, and general metabolic influences. Such changes, if prolonged, would affect the oral microbial flora, since most bacteria grow only within a restricted pH range. If the saliva became too alkaline, acidophilic organisms would be unable to grow; if too acid, such proteolytic bacteria as staphylococci, streptococci, and *Bacillus* species could not maintain themselves. However, no relationship has been established between the pH of saliva and the incidence of caries, which would reflect changes in the microbial flora. The actual pH is determined by the ratio between the concentrations of bicarbonate ion and dissolved carbon dioxide, whereas the buffer capacity at a given pH depends on their total amounts. Ultimately, both depend on the carbon dioxide–secreting capacity of the salivary glands. Thus, an increase in carbon dioxide would lower the pH and at the same time increase the buffer capacity. Since carbon dioxide is essential for the growth of all bacteria and stimulates some species more than others, an increase in the buffer capacity of the saliva may favor the growth of certain oral microorganisms both indirectly, by increasing the content of carbon dioxide, and directly, by stabilizing the pH at a favorable value. Of course, the effective buffer capacity of saliva is enhanced by its rate of flow, whereby the buffer is continually renewed. Consequently, in areas of stagnation the production of acids or alkalis by bacterial action soon exceeds the effective buffer capacity of saliva and favors the establishment of bacteria that grow best in an acid or alkaline environment, as the case may be. Thus, despite its own considerable additional buffer capacity, dental plaque rapidly becomes quite acid in response to the ingestion of sugars and tends to favor aciduric microorganisms. Conversely, the gingival crevice is definitely alkaline and is characterized by proteolysis and putrefaction.

Oxidation–Reduction Potential. Another indirect effect of pH is through the oxidation–reduction potential (E_h), which becomes more positive (oxidative) as the pH decreases and vice versa, although the relationship appears not to hold as rigidly in saliva as in simple systems.

Although the E_h of saliva has been shown to vary over a considerable range, there was no significant variation in the E_h of the saliva of individuals tested under identical conditions. The E_h did not vary greatly during the day, although the pH did. Determination of the E_h for stimulated saliva in open vessels showed that the mean E_h for 50 caries-resistant persons was $+309 \pm 4.7$ mV, and for 50 caries-active persons it was $+237 \pm 9.9$ mV, the difference between the two groups being statistically significant. The saliva samples from the caries-resistant persons were oxygen saturated, whence the strongly oxidative E_h, which could not be raised by passing pure oxygen through the saliva. Nevertheless, the high oxidative potential of all salivas favors aerobic microorganisms. A typical aerobic culture broth has an E_h of $+300$ mV, and cultures of bacteria that produce hydrogen peroxide may go as high as $+429$ mV. Facultative and obligate anaerobes require a negative E_h. For instance, cultures of oral lactobacilli have an E_h of -130 to -240 mV, while clostridial cultures have an E_h of -300 to -400 mV.

How do so many anaerobes grow in saliva? Saliva does, of course, possess reducing substances and tends to drift fairly rapidly toward a negative E_h. More important, it is unlikely that free-flowing saliva is the primary habitat of the oral anaerobes, for these organisms are scarce in the edentulous mouth. Dental plaque has E_h levels as low as -200 mV and the gingival crevice area has E_h levels over the range of $+100$ to -300 mV.

Gases. The principal gases in saliva are carbon dioxide, oxygen, and nitrogen. The carbon dioxide content of saliva ranges from about 13 to 85 mL/100 mL, depending largely on the degree of stimulation of the salivary glands. About half of the carbon dioxide in stimulated saliva is in the form of bicarbonate at pH 6.9. The remaining portion is extremely labile. Being present in saliva in greater concentration than in air, it tends to escape, with concomitant changes in salivary pH, E_h, and buffering capacity. Not only does carbon dioxide influence the oral microbiota by regulating the physical environment (cell permeability, pH, E_h, buffering capacity), but it is also an essential metabolite for many microorganisms.

The oxygen content of saliva from caries-inactive (or caries-resistant) and caries-active persons differs, averaging respectively about 1.35 and 0.51 mL/100 mL. The high oxygen content of the saliva of caries-inactive persons may be associated with a predominantly aerobic oral microbiota, for oxygen uptake by the microbiota of unstimulated saliva of caries-resistant persons is greater than that of the saliva of caries-susceptible persons. The predominantly aerobic flora of caries-resistant persons may also influence the oral microbiota by rapid oxidation of the acids formed by the anaerobic degradation of carbohydrates by the anaerobic components of the flora.

The nitrogen content of saliva, ranging from 0.48 to 2.78 mL/100 mL, has not been shown to relate to caries activity or to any component of the oral microbial flora.

Organic Content. As it is secreted, saliva contains many organic constitutents. Some are derived from or similar to those of plasma, others are distinctive secretions of the glands. In addition, a multitude of organic substances are introduced into saliva via the diet, the metabolism of the oral microbiota, and

products released from dead host and microbial cells. Some of these substances are transitory but others remain in the oral environment for sufficient time to influence the oral microbiota. Some, such as amino acids and proteins, carbohydrates, vitamins, purines, and pyrimidines, serve as nutrients for the oral microbiota, limiting or promoting various bacterial species, depending on their availability and on the degree of nutritional dependence of the bacteria. Enzymes such as lysozyme may limit bacterial growth. Other enzymes in saliva (Table 50.4) promote bacterial growth by breaking down complex salivary or dietary substances into components that are suitable nutrients. Salivary organic constituents may also affect the oral microbiota by their influence on the physical environment (viscosity, ionic strength, osmotic pressure, attachment sites).

Proteins. Nonenzyme proteins make up the major portion of the organic constituents of saliva. The principal salivary protein-containing material is mucin, about two thirds of which is protein and one third polysaccharide. Mucin is derived principally but not exclusively from sublingual and submaxillary glands. Mucin imparts viscosity to saliva primarily through its bound polysaccharide. It is not known whether mucin serves as a nutrient for the oral microbiota under the conditions that exist in the oral cavity, for mucin preparations in general are poor culture media for bacteria. However, mucin breaks down considerably if saliva stands for any length of time, and its components then are available for bacterial nutrition. Involvement of salivary glycoproteins in the attachment of bacteria to oral surfaces is discussed later.

Carbohydrates. Although salivary glycoproteins may supply minute amounts of carbohydrates to microorganisms, it is thought that most carbohydrates available to oral bacteria come as refined sugars (sucrose, glucose, fructose) in the host's diet. Lactose also is available from milk and maltose and subsequently glucose is available through the hydrolysis of dietary starch by salivary and to a lesser extent microbial amylases and maltases. A relatively large amount of salivary amylase is present in the mouth. However, the rapid passage of most foods through the mouth and the solvent action of saliva may preclude the digestion of starch as a very significant source of nutrient for the oral microbiota, except (importantly) when starchy food is retained about the teeth. Dietary refined sugars are probably more significant because of their proved relationship to caries activity (see Chap. 51). One example to be cited here is that the presence of sucrose in the diet enhances the amount of plaque formed on the teeth and the proportion of *S. mutans* in the plaque.

Amino Acids. Amino acids have been found essential for all oral bacteria whose nutritional require-

Table 50.4: Oral Enzymes*

Enzymes	Source		
	Saliva	Bacteria	Leukocytes
Carbohydrases			
Amylase	+	+	
Maltase		+	+
Invertase		+	
Dextran hydrolase		+	
Fructan hydrolase		+	
β-Glucuronidase	+	+	+
β-D-Galactosidase		+	+
Lysozyme	+		+
Hyaluronidase		+	+
Neuraminidase		+	
Esterases			
Acid/alkaline phosphatases	+	+	+
Hexosediphosphatase		+	
Aliesterase	+	+	+
Lipase	+	+	+
Acetylcholinesterase	+		+
Chondrosulfatase		+	
Arylsulfatase		+	+
Transferring enzymes			
Glucosyltransferase		+	
Fructosyltransferase		+	
Catalase		+	
Peroxidase	+		+
Phenyloxidase		+	
Hexokinase		+	+
Proteolytic enzymes			
Proteases		+	+
Peptidases		+	+
Urease		+	
Other enzymes			
Carbonic anhydrase	+		
Pyrophosphatase		+	
Aldolase	+	+	+

*Adapted with permission from H. H. Chauncey: Salivary enzymes. *J Am Dent Assoc,* **63,** 360, 1961.

ments have been even partly defined. For example, most strains of *Streptococcus sobrinus* require about seven different amino acids. Aspartic and glumatic acids, threonine, serine, glycine, alanine, phenylalanine, leucine, and isoleucine are regularly present in whole saliva, but there is considerable variation in proline, cystine, valine, methionine, tyrosine, tryptophan, histidine, lysine, and arginine. The free amino acids in whole saliva range from 3.44 to 4.78 mg/100 mL. Amino acids may provide a source of substrate for salivary microorganisms in the absence of dietary substrates. In addition to free amino acids in saliva, peptides and proteins also may act as a potential source of amino acids.

Urea and Ammonia. Ammonia is the simplest salivary nitrogen source available to the oral microbiota, although apparently few organisms use it significantly. Urea appears to be derived by the salivary glands by filtration from blood, but ammonia is not secreted by the salivary glands in significant amounts. Rather, ammonia is considered to be derived from urea or by deamination of amino acids by bacterial enzymes. Staphylococci produce considerable urease, while many of the common oral gram-negative bacteria produce deaminases. These enzymes are not present in the glandular secretion, for ammonia is not produced in saliva that has been filtered to remove the bacteria.

Vitamins. Vitamins of the B group are essential for the growth of many members of the oral microbiota, particularly streptococci and lactobacilli. Hence, the vitamin B content of saliva could either enhance or limit microbial growth as well as determine the nature of the oral microbiota. Little or no vitamin A is normally present in saliva. The ascorbic acid (vitamin C) content of saliva averages less than that of whole blood, urine, or gastric juice. There is no correlation between the vitamin C contents of saliva and other body fluids. The concentrations of B vitamins present in whole saliva, as reported by various investigators, show considerable variation. One study found pantothenate in whole saliva only after it was incubated, suggesting that microbial activity is a source of vitamins in saliva. Oral yeasts, particularly *Candida albicans*, are a potent source of vitamins essential to oral lactic acid bacteria, particularly lactobacilli. Many other common oral bacteria are sources of B vitamins. Nevertheless, the actual amounts of these vitamins in saliva are barely adequate, particularly for lactic acid bacteria.

As demonstrated in a study of 18 strains of oral streptococci, vitamin requirements do not appear to be related to cariogenicity, nor do they account for the preferential colonization of various sites in the oral cavity. However, they may affect the overall ecological picture of the oral flora.

Colonization of Oral Surfaces

To be a part of the indigenous microbiota, organisms must first be retained in the oral cavity and then must be able to multiply at the site where retained. If not retained, they will be cleared from the mouth as a result of salivary flow and swallowing mechanisms. If they cannot multiply, their numbers will rapidly become diluted and obscure. Bacteria may be retained by adhesion to oral structures, by attachment to other organisms, or by mechanical retention. Several different mechanisms are involved in microbial adhesion, and different bacteria have different affinities for particular types of surfaces.

Thus, bacterial adherence is very important to oral microbial ecology, for it determines the specific habitats of various species within the mouth. *Streptococcus salivarius* has a high affinity for the dorsum of the tongue, where it is found in abundance naturally, but it has relatively poor ability to adhere to the tooth surface. In contrast, strains of *Streptococcus sanguis* have been shown to attach strongly to the coronal surfaces of the teeth and in moderate degree to oral epithelial surfaces.

Host polymers interact with the surfaces of oral bacteria to facilitate bacterial adherence. For example, salivary glycoproteins adsorb into the tooth surface to form a pellicle which then serves as the initial surface for bacterial adherence and accumulation. *S. mitis, S. sanguis, S. mutans, A. naeslundi,* and *A. viscosus* all have the ability to adhere to saliva-coated surfaces. Salivary glycoproteins also may become incorporated into plaque by binding to bacteria, and as the bacteria proliferate, more salivary constitutents attach, building up the mass of material. The binding of bacterial cells and salivary components contributes to the cohesive nature of the plaque. One mechanism associated with this type of adherence involves the interaction of lectin-like protein molecules on the bacterial cell surface (called adhesins) with the carbohydrate components of salivary or pellicle glycoproteins.

Adherence and bacterial accumulation in the mouth also involve interbacterial relationships that are described below. Nonadherent organisms, or those with low affinity for various oral structures, may be retained mechanically, as in the pits and fissures of teeth, in the gingival crevice, in the periodontal pocket, or in carious lesions. For example, lactobacilli appear to have a low affinity for the tooth surface compared to other bacteria, such as *S. sanguis*. The observed association between lactobacilli and carious lesions is due to mechanical retention within the altered tooth structure coupled with selective growth as a result of the aciduric nature of these bacteria.

Infection vs. Disease

Dental caries, periodontal diseases, and pulp and periapical infections are endogenous diseases caused by bacteria that are members of the oral microbiota. Our mouths are continuously infected, but, unless given the opportunity to do so, resident bacteria do not cause damage. However, disturbance in the microbial ecology of the mouth (resulting from a defect or change in the host defenses, from bacterial accumulation above some threshold level, from selective multiplication of certain species, or from bacterial entrance into normally sterile tissues) can result in damage to the host referred to as an infectious disease. Chapters 7 and 51 through 53 describe specific interactions between oral bacteria and the host that lead to oral disease states.

Beneficial Aspects of the Oral Microbiota

Very little definitive information is available on the beneficial aspects of the oral microbiota in respect to their partially supplying certain nutrients needed by the host, aiding in food digestion, and protecting against invading and endogenous pathogens. Nevertheless, it is important to be aware of theoretical aspects in this area. Although we may swallow a few grams of bacteria daily, it is obvious that this cannot supply all of our dietary needs. However, oral bacteria like some intestinal strains do produce vitamins and cofactors needed by humans (e.g., vitamin K, biotin, riboflavin).

Microbial enzymes released into saliva (e.g., amylase, proteases, lipases) may aid in food digestion, although any such contribution would be minor in relation to the overall digestive process. Members of the oral microbiota may provide some degree of protection against invading pathogenic microorganisms. For example, it may be difficult for some bacteria to establish themselves in the mouth in the presence of the already existing oral flora. This could relate to competition for binding sites or sensitivity to antimicrobial substances produced by the oral strains. In the laboratory, *S. mitior* has been shown to inhibit the growth of some strains of *Corynebacterium diphtheriae, Streptococcus pyogenes, Staphylococcus aureus, Streptococcus pneumoniae,* and *Escherichia coli.* Also, proliferation of oral *Candida albicans* to a level that becomes harmful (oral candidiasis) in some instances has been related to the decrease in oral bacteria that occurs with broad-spectrum antibacterial therapy. Some strains of *Streptococcus salivarius* produce a substance called enocin that is bacteriostatic to group A streptococci. Enocin apparently interferes with the utilization of pantothenate. Lastly, some strains of *S. mitior* and *S. sanguis* produce cross-reacting antibodies that can react with some strains of *S. pneumoniae,* the leading cause of bacterial pneumonia. If these antibodies are produced in the body as a result of involvement of the oral bacteria in bacteremias, then such antibodies may provide some small degree of protection against invading *S. pneumoniae.* The oral microbiota also may aid in the maturation of the immune system of the host. Indirect supporting evidence for this function is that animals born and raised in a germ-free environment have poorly developed lymphoid tissues and low levels of serum immunoglobulins.

Antimicrobial Factors from the Host

Details of host defense mechanisms active in the mouth are found in the chapters on immunology and periodontal disease. The information presented here summarizes the oral antimicrobial activities that may influence oral microbial ecology.

Self-cleansing Mechanisms.   The flow of saliva and the movements of the tongue and musculature of cheeks promote natural self-cleansing of the dentition. This tends to reduce the rate of supragingival plaque formation on smooth tooth surfaces. Plaque accumulation occurs at a faster rate on the non-self-cleansing surfaces such as in pits and fissures, interproximally, in the gingival crevice, and in coronal defects. The suppression of salivary flow may also result in the more rapid accumulation of the oral microbiota, owing to reduced rinsing and oral clearing action and to reduced exposure to antimicrobial factors in saliva. This suppression can also affect the composition of the oral flora by reducing buffering action and the supply of essential nutrients.

Antimicrobial Chemicals.   Whole saliva inhibits the growth of such organisms as some lactobacilli and streptococci. Although little evidence is

available to describe what salivary agents may indeed be active in the mouth, several antimicrobial substances have been characterized. It should be noted that these substances are not totally effective or the oral microbiota would not exist.

Lysozyme is present in most body secretions, including saliva. This enzyme lyses susceptible bacteria by degrading the polysaccharide component of cell wall peptidoglycan. The lysozyme content of saliva is about the same as that of blood but much less than that of other areas of the body where bacteria are not abundant; it is about 1/300 that of tears and about 1/45 that of nasal mucus.

Lactoferrin is an iron-binding protein in saliva that may scavenge iron from saliva, preventing uptake by oral bacteria. Organisms undergoing respiration involving cytochromes require iron. Some immunoglobulins have been shown to bind lactoferrin, and this would bring the iron-scavenging protein directly to the surface of antibody-coated bacteria, which could impair nutrition.

Saliva also contains lactoperoxidase, which converts salivary thiocyanate (SCN^-) to hypothiocyanite ion ($OSCN^-$) in the presence of hydrogen peroxide (H_2O_2) generated at the surface of catalase-negative bacteria. The $OSCN^-$ can then enter the bacterial cell and oxidize compounds such as proteins containing sulfhydryl groups ($-SH$). This changes the conformation of proteins, causing them to lose enzyme activity, which can stop metabolism. Thus, the salivary peroxidase system has the potential to inhibit glycolytic enzymes of streptococci. Unfortunately, this system is mainly bacteriostatic rather than bactericidal. A peroxidase system is also active in lysosomal vacuoles of phagocytes.

Secretory IgA (sIgA) is the predominant immunoglobulin in saliva, and other immunoglobulins (IgG, IgM) may enter the mouth through gingival crevice fluid. Although sIgA is not generally considered to be bactericidal, it is thought to play an important role in reducing bacterial colonization of oral surfaces. sIgA can bind to and agglutinate bacteria, thus masking cell-surface receptors important in binding to oral surfaces. Stimulation of specific sIgA has been shown to reduce colonization of oral surfaces by the homologous strain of *S. mutans.* This function of sIgA could serve, in part, to control the balance of the indigenous flora, as well as to exert a protective function by limiting exogenous pathogens. Whereas pathogens might enter the oral cavity, adhere to various structures, and multiply, their advantage would be only temporary. Once sIgA increases to a sufficient level, the bacteria would be aggregated and their colonization impaired, permitting them to be washed away and eliminated.

Chapter 52 (Periodontal Disease) provides further

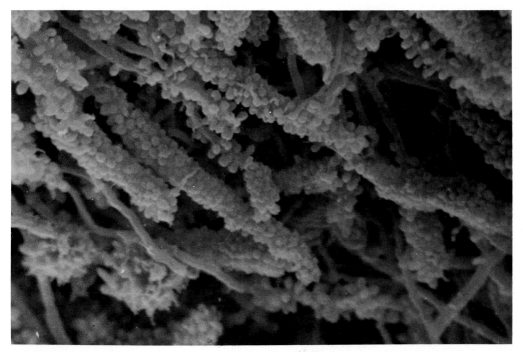

Figure 50.4: "Corn-on-the-cob" formations in plaque, with coccoid forms coating filamentous organisms. (Photograph courtesy of Dr. Sheila Jones, University College, London. Adapted with permission from S. A. Jones: Special Relationship Between Spherical and Filamentous Microorganisms in Mature Human Dental Plaque. *Arch Oral Biol,* **17,** 613, 1972.)

information on the role of antibodies in gingival crevice fluid and inflamed gingival tissues against subgingival bacteria.

Interbacterial Interactions

Plaque Formation

Interbacterial interactions play a very important role in the cohesive nature of plaque and are one of several mechanisms involved in the initiation of plaque formation. One example of microbial coaggregation is vividly illustrated in Figure 50.4. Another example of interspecies coaggregation involves gram-negative bacteria such as *Bacteroides gingivalis,* which has only a very limited ability to attach to clean oral surfaces. This and other gram-negative species such as *Fusobacterium, Capnocytophaga, Eikenella,* and *Veillonella* can attach to gram-positive *Actinomyces* species (or in some cases *Streptococcus* species) that may already by retained at a site through other mechanisms of adherence. This "piggyback" mechanism of adherence is thought to play an important role in colonization of subgingival sites by periodontopathic gram-negative bacteria that have little ability to initiate plaque formation on their own. Mechanisms of inter-

species coaggregation may involve interaction of surface fibrils present on many oral species. A lectin-like interaction has been shown to be involved in the specific coaggregation of *A. viscosus* with *S. sanguis,* two organisms that predominate in the early recolonization of cleaned tooth surfaces.

Oral bacteria produce a variety of extracellular products that may participate in adherence to oral surfaces or to bacterial cells of the same or different species. The best-known mechanism of this type involves the extracellular glucans (dextran and mutan) synthesized from sucrose by most strains of *mutans* streptococci. In general, these streptococci possess enzymatic and nonenzymatic glucan-binding sites on their cell surface that allow the cells to bind to extracellular glucans, linking them to other glucan-coated bacterial or oral surfaces. The glucosyltransferases (GTF) that synthesize the glucans from sucrose may be bound to the cell surface (the enzymatic glucan-binding site mentioned above) or may be released into the extracellular environment to adsorb to the tooth surface or bacterial surfaces. The adsorbed GTF may then produce a mutan (α-1,3 glucan) that serves as a binding site for cells with glucan surface receptors. Thus, the glucan-synthesizing system of the mutans streptococci appears to be involved in both coaggregation and direct binding to tooth surfaces.

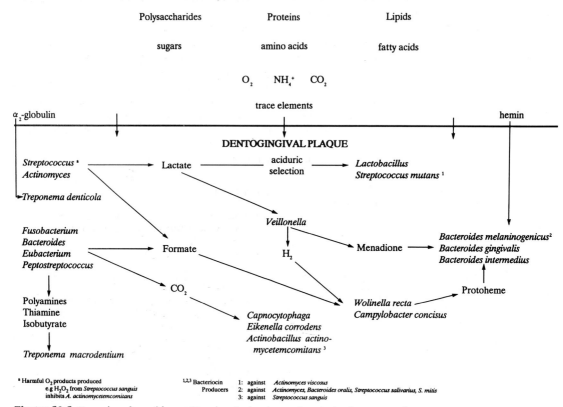

GINGIVAL CREVICE FLUID - DIET - SALIVA

Figure 50.5: Examples of possible nutritional and other interactions in the dentogingival area. (Adapted with permission from J. Carlsson: Microbiology of Plaque Associated Periodontal Disease. In *Textbook of Clinical Periodontology,* edited by J. Lindhe. Munksgaard, Copenhagen, 1984.)

Nutritional Interactions

Bacteria survive at specific sites, or ecological niches, in the mouth where they are retained, supplied with required nutrients, survive antimicrobial activities, and thrive at the oxidation–reduction potentials present. The survival and growth of each member of a niche influences the other microbes present by constantly changing the environment. The possible number of interactions actually occurring within a given oral ecosystem are numerous and are likely never to be completely defined. Nevertheless, knowing specific nutritional requirement and chemical sensitivities of individual species and knowing what species are commonly detected at specific oral sites permits postulations of interactions that might influence the ecology of an oral site (Fig. 50.5).

Some spirochetes, and *Bacteroides melaninogenicus, Bacteroides gingivalis,* and *Capnocytophaga,* have specific nutritional requirements that are best met by exposure to gingival crevice fluids. The black-pigmented bacteroides require hemin and are at least stimulated by vitamin K and some human hormones. *Treponema macrodentium* requires spermine or

other polyamines, and other spirochetes require α_2-globulin, which is present only in human serum or fluids of serum origin. These spirochetes and other gram-negative bacteria preferentially colonize the gingival crevice and subgingival plaque, where required nutrients are supplied in crevicular fluid or during gingival bleeding. Other possible interactions involve production of lactic acid from carbohydrates by plaque streptococci and *Actinomyces.* Lactic acid is utilized for growth by the asaccharolytic *Veillonella.* As the lactic acid is utilized, the low plaque pH increases. This permits nonaciduric streptococci such as *S. sanguis* and *S. mitior* to resume metabolism and growth. The *Veillonella* produces vitamin K (menidione) required by black-pigmented bacteroides, and H_2 utilized by *Wolinella.* Formate produced by many bacteria is required by *Wolinella* and *Campylobacter. Fusobacterium, Bacteroides, Peptostreptococcus, Eubacterium,* and many other bacteria produce CO_2 required by capnophilic species of *Capnocytophaga, Eikenella,* and *Actinobacillus.* Fusobacteria and eubacteria can produce isobutyrate, thiamine, and putrescine needed to support growth of

Treponema. Nutrients supplied by the host, such as hemin and α_2-globulin, stimulate growth of certain *Bacteroides* species and spirochetes, respectively. Production of acid end products tends to select for aciduric lactobacilli and mutans streptococci, and the use of available oxygen in the respiratory metabolism of anaerobes or facultative anaerobes would favor growth of obligate anaerobes. Antibiosis interactions also seem plausible and might involve inhibition of nonaciduric bacteria resulting from acid production by acidogens. Also, formation of reduced metabolites would lower the E_h, favoring anaerobes but inhibiting others. Production of bacteriocins, superoxide radicals, hydrogen peroxide, and other antimicrobial substances would selectively inhibit certain species.

Interactions between microbial species have been primarily investigated in the laboratory or in animal models. For example, coculturing of *W. recta* and *B. melaninogenicus* shows that the former stimulates growth of the latter by producing a protoheme (compound related to hemin). Such activity by *W. recta* in subgingival plaque might replace serum (gingival crevice fluid) as a source of hemin required for growth of *Bacteroides.* This laboratory coculturing technique also demonstrates growth stimulation of *W. recta* by the formate produced by *B. melaninogenicus.* Experimental mixed anaerobic infections in animals involving *B. gingivalis* show that interbacterial cooperation is very important in that most infectious mixtures contain one strain that aids the growth of *B. gingivalis.* Such growth factors have been identified as naphthoquinone (a compound related to vitamin K) and succinate, which can be used by at least some *Bacteroides* species in place of hemin.

Very little information is available that describes microbial interactions known to occur in the human mouth. *Streptococcus sanguis* II, *Streptococcus uberis,* and *Actinomyces viscosus* have been shown to inhibit the growth of *A. actinomycetemcomitans* in vitro. The mechanism of inhibition by *S. sanguis* II involves formation of hydrogen peroxide, and this negative association between *S. sanguis* II and *A. actinomycetemcomitans* has been demonstrated to occur in human subgingival plaque. Recent work by S. Socransky and co-workers also suggests other possible microbial interactions based on a determination of the odds ratio of a subgingival site being infected by one of several suspected periodontal pathogens in the presence of one or more of 22 other species. In general, species of streptococci, *Actinomyces* species, and *Propionibacterium acnes* showed a negative association with the suspected pathogens (*B. gingivalis, B. forsythus, P. micros, W. recta, B. melaninogenicus, B. intermedius,* or *A. actinomycetemcomitans*). Gram-negative species tended to show more positive associations with these suspected pathogens.

Additional work in the area of oral microbial ecology will be important in determining potentially "beneficial" species that may be antagonistic to caries or periodontal pathogens, or at least compatible with the host. One might even envision approaches to control oral disease by manipulation of the normal oral flora to a composition that favors health. This might involve specific enhancement of certain species or the use of antimicrobial agents with a more defined spectrum of activity. Other approaches might include local destruction or sequestering of special nutrients required by known pathogens.

ADDITIONAL READING

Berkowitz, R. J., Jordan, H. V., and White, G. 1975. The Early Establishment of *Streptococcus mutans* in the Mouths of Infants. Arch Oral Biol, **20,** 171.

Bowden, G. H. W., Ellwood, D. C., and Hamilton, I. R. 1979. Microbial Ecology of the Oral Cavity. In *Advances in Microbial Ecology,* vol. 3, M. Alexander, ed. Plenum Press, New York.

Carlsson, J. 1984. Microbiology of Plaque Associated with Periodontal Disease. In *Textbook of Clinical Periodontology,* pp. 125–153, J. Lindhe, ed. Munksgaard.

Carlsson, J., Grahnen, H., Jonsson, G., and Wikner, S. 1970. Establishment of *Streptococcus sanguis* in the Mouth of Infants. Arch Oral Biol, **15,** 1143.

Carlsson, J., Grahnen, H., and Jonsson, G. 1975. Lactobacilli and Streptococci in the Mouth of Children. Caries Res, **9,** 333.

Carlsson, J., Soderholm, G., and Almfelt, I. 1969. Prevalence of *Streptococcus sanguis* and *Streptococcus mutans* in the Mouth of Persons Wearing Full Dentures. Arch Oral Biol, **14,** 243.

Cisar, J. O. 1982. Coaggregation Reactions Between Oral Bacteria. In *Host-Parasite Interactions in Periodontal Disease,* pp. 121–131, R. J. Genco and S. E. Mergenhagen, eds. American Society of Microbiology, Washington, D.C.

Cowman, R. A., Perrella, M. M., and Fitzgerald, R. J. 1974. Influence of Incubation Atmosphere on Growth and Amino Acid Requirements of *Streptococcus mutans.* Appl Microbiol, **27,** 86.

Eskow, R. N., and Loesch, W. J. 1971. Oxygen Tensions in the Human Oral Cavity. Arch Oral Biol, **16,** 1127.

Gibbons, R. J., and Van Houte, J. 1975. Bacterial Adherence in Oral Microbial Ecology. Annu Rev Microbiol, **29,** 19.

Grenier, D., and Mayrand, D. 1986. Nutritional Relationships between Oral Bacteria. Infect Immun, **53,** 616.

Hammond, B. F., Lillard, S. E., and Stevens, R. N. 1987. A Bacteriocin of *Actinobacillus actinomycetemcomitans.* Infect Immun, **55,** 686.

Hillman, J. D., and Socransky, S. S. 1982. Bacterial Interference in the Oral Ecology of *Actinobacillus actinomycetemcomitans* and Its Relationship to Human Periodontosis. Arch Oral Biol, **27,** 75.

Holmberg, K., and Hallander, H. O. 1972. Interference Between Gram-Positive Microorganisms in Dental Plaque. J Dent Res, **51,** 588.

Kleinberg, I., Ellison, S. A., and Mandel, I. D. (Eds.) 1979. *Saliva and Dental Caries.* Information Retrieval, Inc., New York.

Mayrand, D. 1985. Virulence Promotion by Mixed Bacterial Infections. In *Bayer-Symposium VIII: The Pathogenesis of Bacterial Infections,* pp. 281–291. Springer-Verlag, Berlin.

Morehart, R. E., and Fitzgerald, R. J. 1976. Nutritional Determinants of the Ecology of the Oral Flora. Dent Clin North Am, **20,** 473.

Parker, R. B. 1970. Paired Culture Interaction of the Oral Microbiota. J Dent Res, **49,** 804.

Rogers, A. H. 1973. The Vitamin Requirements of Some Oral Streptococci. Arch Oral Biol, **18,** 227.

Rogers, A. H., Van Der Hoeven, J. S., and Mikx, F. N. M. 1978. Inhibition of *Actinomyces viscosus* by Bacteriocin-Producing Strains of *Streptococcus mutans* in the Dental Plaque of Gnotobiotic Rats. Arch Oral Biol, **23,** 477.

Rosebury, T. 1962. *Microorganisms Indigenous to Man.* McGraw-Hill, New York.

Sirisinha, S., and Charupatana, C. 1971. Antibodies to Indigenous Bacteria in Human Serum, Secretions, and Urine. Can J Microbiol, **17,** 1471.

Socransky, S. S., Haffajee, A. D., Dzink, J. L., and Hillman, J. D. 1988. Associations between Microbial Species in Subgingival Plaque Samples. Oral Microbiol Immunol, **3,** 1.

Socransky, S. S., Loesche, W. J., Hubersak, C., Macdonald, J. B. 1964. Dependency of *Treponema macrodentium* on Other Oral Organisms for Isobutyrate, Polyamines and a Controlled Oxidation-Reduction Potential. J Bacteriol, **88,** 200.

Van Winkelhoff, A. J., Van Steenbergen, T. J. M., and Degraaff, J. 1988. The Role of Black-Pigmented *Bacteroides* in Human Oral Infections. J Clin Periodontol, **15,** 145.

Williams, R. C., and Gibbons, R. J. 1975. Inhibition of Streptococcal Attachment to Receptors on Human Buccal Epithelial Cells by Antigenically Similar Salivary Glycoproteins. Infect Immun, **11,** 711.

51

Dental Caries

Charles F. Schachtele

Definition and Magnitude of the Problem

In dentistry, the term *caries* (Latin: decay; rottenness; dry rot) refers to a disease in which the calcified tissues of the teeth are modified and eventually dissolved. Because of the frequent occurrence of this destructive process, dental caries ranks as one of the more significant diseases affecting humans. Although some surveys in the past decade have indicated a significant reduction in the prevalence of caries in several countries, including the United States, this disease remains a major public health problem which is costly, can cause considerable discomfort, and can have a significant effect on personality and overall health.

Dental scientists have made great progress toward understanding the etiology of caries formation in humans. Starting with the basic premise that carious lesions result from localized demineralization of the tooth by organic acids produced by bacteria which ferment dietary carbohydrate, knowledge has evolved to identification of the etiological agents. The major interactions during disease development involve the teeth, as part of the entire oral cavity; the oral bacterial flora, as part of the total human indigenous microbiota; and the diet, as an essential, intermittent source of cariogenic, cariostatic, and anticariogenic components. By determining the exact details of these interactions, dental researchers are continuously supplying new leads for disease control or prevention.

It is important that dental caries is considered an endogenous bacterial disease. In an exogenous microbial disease, by contrast, the pathogen is relatively foreign to the host and creates an infection on colonization of a susceptible site. Caries involves potentially pathogenic bacteria that are indigenous to the oral cavity of humans. The disease results from conditions in which the resistance of the host is lowered or the cariogenic challenge from the diet increases and specific bacterial strains proliferate to high levels and express detrimental traits. The challenge to dental scientists is to understand how and why this transition

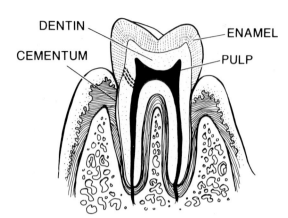

DENTIN

CEMENTUM

ENAMEL

PULP

Figure 51.1: Schematic drawing illustrating the four tissues of a human tooth. *Dashed lines* indicate the relative location of representative dentinal tubules.

from a friendly symbiotic state to a harmful relationship takes place at specific times and at unique locations in the human dentition.

The Carious Process

Tooth Structure and Chemistry

The mature erupted human tooth is made up of four distinct tissues: pulp, dentin, cementum, and enamel (Fig. 51.1). Each of these tissues has been analyzed by biochemists and its ultrastructure carefully determined. Although much of our understanding of the details of carious lesion development has resulted from studies on the outermost tissue, the enamel, the other three tissues play important roles as lesions progress from the early or incipient stage to actual cavitation. Indeed, as disease progresses through the enamel toward the pulp, the microenvironment of the lesion changes. This is reflected in the complex microbial etiology of caries where various types of bacteria may be involved in the different phases of tooth destruction.

Pulp. Pulp makes up the core of the tooth and has been described as a special type of connective tissue. It is like most other soft tissues which, on average, contain 25% organic material and 75% water. The basic structural entities of the dental pulp are connective tissue cells, fibers, and ground substance. The cells are predominantly fibroblasts, but undifferentiated mesenchymal cells, macrophages, lymphocytes, plasma cells, and eosinophilic granulocytes are occasionally observed. In inflamed pulps mast cells can be found. The fibers in the pulp increase in number with age and are mainly collagenous in nature. The ground substance of the pulp includes various molecules, including complex carbohydrates, glycoproteins, and acid mucopolysaccharides. The carbohydrate com-

plexes are predominant during tooth development and decrease in quantity during aging.

The presence of this wide range of materials that provide growth substrates and water under conditions when the pulp is exposed to the oral environment, whether through caries or traumatic exposure, sets up a situation in which serious bacterial infections can occur. Since the pulp contains arteries, veins, lymphatic vessels, and nerves, all entering through an apical foramen, infections of this tissue can spread to the rest of the body.

Dentin. Encasing and physically protecting the pulp is a calcified collagenous tissue called dentin. On a wet weight basis this tissue contains approximately 70% inorganic material, 18% organic material, and 12% water. The water phase is labile and its in situ concentration is not known. The basic structural entities of dentin are the odontoblast, the odontoblast process, the dentinal tubule, the periodontoblastic space, the peritubular dentin, and the intertubular dentin. The odontoblasts are specialized cells whose long cytoplasmic extensions, the odontoblast processes, are located within the dentinal tubules and extend through the entire width of the dentin. The diameter and volume of the dentinal tubules vary according to location in the dentin and age of the tooth. In young teeth the diameter of the tubules may be 4 to 5 μm. Close to the pulp the lumina of the tubules may make up 80% of the total volume of the dentin. In the peripheral dentin they may make up only about 4% of the volume. On average there are about 35,000 tubules per square millimeter of dentin. With regard to caries, the tubules are large and nutritive enough to be invaded by bacteria and to serve as a pathway for lesion progression. Although bacteria do not normally penetrate dentin, owing to the presence of a fine layer of "microcrystalline debris," if acid has modified the surface, bacterial invasion can occur. Acid etching of dentin could occur either from the carious process or during restorative procedures.

The periodontoblastic space intervenes between the wall of the dentinal tubule and the odontoblast process. This region contains tissue fluid and some organic components such as collagen fibers. This is an important area because tissue changes in dentin occur in this location. The peritubular and intertubular dentin are mineralized, with the latter containing abundant quantities of collagen. Dentin collagen normally is tightly complexed to the mineral phase and is not accessible to stains or proteolytic enzymes. Dentin is a vital tissue in that its odontoblasts exchange solutes through their extensions into the tubules. In addition, the odontoblasts can lay down a layer of secondary dentin, relatively lacking in tubules, in response to irritation resulting from caries, operative procedures, erosion, or attrition.

The inorganic portion of dentin consists mainly of hydroxyapatite crystals. The crystals are similar in size to those found in cementum and bone but are significantly smaller than those found in enamel. Of the total dry weight, dentin contains 26% calcium and 13% phosphorus. Since dentin forms the structural bulk of the tooth and has a unique chemical and structural composition, caries of the dentin is a very critical phase in destruction of the tooth.

Cementum. Radicular dentin is covered by a 20- to 200-μm-thick layer of calcified tissue, called cementum, which is laid down in incremental zones of high and low mineral content by cementoblasts derived from the periodontal ligament. Cementum is the least mineralized of the three dental hard tissues, being slightly less calcified than dentin. On a wet weight basis the mineral content of cementum is approximately 65%, the organic content is 23%, and the remaining 12% is water.

Like dentin and bone, the organic material of cementum is largely highly cross-linked insoluble collagen. Cementum anchors the periodontal ligament fibers to the tooth. From midroot to the cemento-enamel junction, cementum is acellular; increasingly toward the apex, the cementoblasts become embedded in the developing mineral phase and are then referred to as cementocytes. Cementum is continuously deposited throughout life and can triple in thickness from 10 to 70 years of age.

Enamel. Coronal dentin is covered by the hardest and most highly calcified tissue in the body. More than 95% of enamel is inorganic material, essentially all in the crystalline state. Mature enamel is acellular and contains less than 1% organic material. Only about 3% of this tissue is water. Enamel is not the inert system that one would predict from its chemical composition. In fact, within the oral cavity, tooth enamel is an active chemical system, participating in ion-exchange reactions with saliva and demineralization–remineralization processes. These reactions influence the rate of caries development. To appreciate the formation of carious lesions we must understand the structural and chemical nature of this unique tissue.

The largest structural components of enamel are the rods or prisms. These entities are approximately 4 to 6 μm in diameter and can be up to 3 mm long. In most cases the rods extend perpendicularly from the enamel–dentin junction to the tooth surface. In cross-section the rods have a characteristic keyhole shape. The dense packing of the rods gives enamel most of its physical properties, such as hardness, that we normally associate with the teeth. Closer inspection reveals that the rods are composed of millions of small elongated crystallites arranged in a characteristic pattern. The crystallites are approximately 1,000 angstroms in length and thus are 5 to 10 times larger than those in bone. The large size of the crystallites is an important factor in maintaining the structural integrity of enamel and markedly influences the ability of teeth to resist attacks from bacterial or dietary acids.

The enamel crystallites are made up of thousands of stacked subunits called unit cells. These cells are about 10 angstroms across and are made up of highly ordered arrangements of atoms including oxygen, hydrogen, calcium, and phosphorus. X-ray diffraction analysis of enamel reveals patterns that are characteristic of apatite structures. Apatite represents a general class of minerals characterized by similar stoichiometry and crystal structure. Chemically, apatites have compositions that are variants of the formula D_5T_3M, where D is a divalent cation, T is a trivalent tetrahedral compound anion, and M is a monovalent anion. The unit of cell apatite crystals contains two of the formula units and thus has the formula $D_{10}T_6M_2$. The mineral components of enamel are often described as impure forms of hydroxyapatite, $Ca_{10}(PO_4)_6(OH)_2$. The basic formula of hydroxyapatite allows many partial substitutions to occur without changing the crystal lattice. To some extent calcium may be replaced by strontium, barium, lead, and radium; phosphate may be partially replaced by carbonate, arsenate, and vanadate; and hydroxyl may be replaced by fluoride and chloride. A broad range of ions can be incorporated secondarily. Since hydroxyapatite behaves as a highly active ion-exchange medium, after eruption the outer layer of enamel acquires a number of ions, depending mainly on dietary intake.

With regard to caries, it is important that variations in enamel composition extend over broader ranges than from unit cell to unit cell. The chemical composition of enamel varies considerably from person to person, from tooth to tooth, and from site to site within a given section of enamel. In addition to the influence of ions present in the oral cavity at any given time, the enamel composition is also determined by the presence and concentration of various ions at different stages of tooth development. Concentrations of several of the components vary according to the distance from the tooth surface. For example, the concentration of fluoride is normally higher in samples of enamel close to the tooth surface and decreases toward the enamel–dentin junction. On the other hand, the concentration of carbonate is lower at the tooth surface and increases toward the enamel–dentin junction. Some ions such as strontium appear to be uniformly distributed through the enamel. It is clear that dental enamel is not a simple substance but contains a large variety of minor components that can be distributed in various patterns within the mineral. The solubility of the enamel is influenced by the presence of the minor components: carbonate, magnesium, sodium, and citrate can increase acidic dissolution, while fluoride decreases it.

Hydroxyapatite can exist in equilibrium with an aqueous phase at neutrality where its solubility is such that the product of calcium and phosphate ion activities in the solution is equivalent to about 100 mg/L of the ions. The daily oral passage of more than 1L of saliva might be expected to leach out tooth mineral. Significant leaching does not occur because saliva is normally supersaturated with respect to calcium and phosphate. Only when the pH of the environment markedly drops will the supersaturation of saliva be overcome and loss of mineral from the enamel commence. This level of acidity, estimated by in vitro studies to be pH 5.2, has been termed the critical pH for initiation of caries, but it is an operational concept and not subject to exact calculation. The exact pH at which tooth minerals begins to be lost in situ is an important issue that will be discussed later in the context of evaluating the cariogenic potential of foods.

Caries Mechanism

Chemical analyses have demonstrated that the main process occurring during caries development is demineralization, followed by replacement of the dissolved mineral with loosely bound water. For simplicity, one can discuss the mechanism of caries formation as acid dissolution of enamel. In enamel, acidic demineralization also suffices to destroy the protein phase. Enamel protein goes into solution concomitantly with sufficient loss of mineral. In dentin, demineralization leaves the collagenous matrix intact. This residue is either digested by proteases from bacteria or converted to a leather-like material.

To the unaided eye, caries first becomes discernible as a white spot. Such incipient caries reflects opacity caused by demineralized subsurface enamel. Early white spot lesions are not easily distinguishable from areas of developmental hypocalcification. However, long before this stage the initiation of coronal caries is delineated by microscopic changes.

Demineralization does not proceed uniformly within enamel but selectively along regular pathways. The earliest structural changes include roughening of exposed ends of enamel rods, resulting in grainlike defects and spreading to the inter-rod area. Individual crystallites become smaller, widening the spaces between them. These spaces tend to fill with organic matter (acquired pellicle), which might actually slow the carious process. Surface indentations appear in the acquired pellicle and underlying enamel surface, conforming to the shape and location of plaque bacteria. Even as demineralization proceeds, a relatively intact surface zone averaging 30 μm deep remains over an increasingly radiolucent area. Demineralizing

acids apparently diffuse through an outer, less readily soluble layer of involved enamel at one or more undefined microscopic points of entry. Whatever the points of entry, demineralization radiates primarily laterally along the striae of Retzius beneath the intact surface zone, gradually creating a roughly cone-shaped lesion with its base parallel to the surface. Examination by polarized light reveals a translucent zone at the advancing edge of the lesion, indicating the presence of about 1% of spaces only large enough to admit molecules the size of water or smaller. Toward the surface is a dark, almost opaque, positively birefringent zone, calculated to contain 2% to 4% of larger spaces. The body or central zone of the lesion is negatively birefringent and contains from 5% to 25% of still larger spaces. The surface layer is still highly mineralized and radiopaque. Density measurements indicate an average volume loss of 1% mineral in the translucent zone, 6% in the dark zone, 24% in the body of the lesion, and 10% in the surface layer. The net effect is thinning, shortening and eventual disappearance of crystallites, creating microcavities, mainly along the striae of Retzius, and enlargement of the interstices between rods. Deeper planes of enamel are attacked via the interstices between rods. Demineralization of rod cores proceeds from their peripheries inward. This whole process may extend as deep as a millimeter and even involve the dentin superficially, while the enamel surface remains grossly intact. Finally, however, this surface zone either demineralizes or collapses from loss of supporting structure. The classic cavity has now developed, and bacterial invasion becomes evident.

The rate of caries development varies greatly. The median rate for occlusal surfaces (mostly fissure caries) is from 20 to 24 months in enamel, with a range of less than 3 months to more than 48; the median time to mild dentinal involvement is 36 months. The median time from initial detection in enamel to dentinal involvement is about 4 years, but some lesions do not progress for several years or longer. White spot lesions that developed within 1½ years of eruption on free smooth surfaces have been followed to determine their fate. A small proportion soon progressed to cavitation, but most remained unchanged for up to 8 years, and a small proportion even reverted to "normalcy." These data indicate that remineralization of enamel by saliva is a real and clinically important phenomenon. Indeed, the rate of lesion development at a particular site depends on the frequency and strength of attack by bacterial acids and the remineralizing potential of plaque and saliva at that site.

In dentin the carious process is characterized by primary bacterial invasion of the tubules; gram-positive cocci predominate but gram-positive bacilli and filaments are not infrequent. Demineralization proceeds in advance of bacterial growth. The lesion expands most rapidly laterally via cross-connections between tubules but also continues to penetrate inward toward the pulp on a relatively broad front. Further destruction of enamel mostly results from the lateral spread of the destructive process in dentin, which undermines the enamel. After demineralization, the collagenous dentinal matrix is usually degraded by bacterial proteases. Alternatively, in slow or arrested caries the dentin matrix remains as a tough leatherlike mass.

Unless halted by sclerosis (occlusion of tubules by mineralization), formation of reparative dentin, or reparative dentistry, bacterial invasion of the tubules eventually penetrates to the pulp, which becomes infected, inflamed, and ultimately undergoes necrosis. Subsequent infection, inflammation, and necrosis of the periapical tissue lead to formation of a periapical abscess, which may expand into cancellous bone and eventually establish fistulas to a body cavity or to the outside.

Caries in cementum (root surface caries) is characterized by an overlying bacterial mat containing an abundance of filamentous forms. Underneath this mat there is a roughening and softening on a rather broad scale, and brownish discoloration. The lesion may encircle the tooth cervically without spreading apically, and adjacent enamel is often undermined. Demineralization far in advance of the bacteria is not common in cemental caries.

Chemistry of Caries

Acidity. The paramount chemical fact about the carious lesion is that its prevailing acidity is sufficient to account for demineralization. Numerous publications attest to the general acidity of caries in both enamel and dentin, determined both colorimetrically with pH indicators and electrometrically with antimony and glass electrodes. The range observed at different depths of clinically different types of cavities is exemplified by the data in Table 51.1. Acidity is greatest in cavities with small openings and deeper layers. In some cavities judged clinically to be inactive, the pH at the base of the cavity was between 3.5 and 4.8. A neutral or even slightly alkaline reaction in a minority of cavity layers presumably indicates temporary neutralization or a quiescent period. Neutralization has only a temporary effect, suggesting either continual production of acid or a reservoir of acid in the deeper layers. Cavity acidity can persist for a long time without additional external substrate. The mean pH of an area of a carious lesion need not remain below the critical point for demineralization. The necessary acid

condition need prevail only transiently in the hydration shell of the hydroxyapatite.

Associated Chemical Changes. Even superficial demineralization not only exposes the respective organic phases of enamel and dentin to chemical change but also strikingly increases the reactivity of the mineral phase. These changes imply that the close complexing between organic and inorganic phases in the sound tooth reduces the chemical reactivity of both and impedes their solubilization. They imply also the possibility of remineralization by uptake of calcium and phosphate from saliva or redeposition of calcium phosphate. Another possibility is increased resistance to progress of the lesion by increased uptake of fluoride. Fluoride also accelerates remineralization of enamel. Arrested lesions in dentin contain a fluoride-rich surface zone.

Caries removes calcium and phosphate from enamel and dentin in essentially the same proportion as they occur in the sound tissues. Magnesium and carbonate are lost preferentially, indicating that they are held by only weak bonds. Fluoride is not leached from enamel caries in situ by acid buffers. Thus, fluoride increases fivefold in carious enamel and tenfold in carious dentin.

The fate of the organic phase of enamel during caries is incompletely understood. Dentin undergoes proteolysis or turns yellow to brown, and undergoes marked change in composition: an average 25% reduction in the content of arginine, hydroxyproline, and proline, doubling of phenylalanine, and tripling of tyrosine. These changes result in a collagenase-resistant fraction that is deficient in arginine but contains 14% carbohydrate. Sound dentin matrix is nearly carbohydrate free. The resistant fraction results from reactions between demineralized matrix and such sugars as glucose and glucosamine, or intermediary products of their fermentation.

Chemically Induced Enamel Caries. Since acids are the cause of dental caries, it should be possible to form a carious lesion simply by immersing a tooth in an acid solution. Actually, it was reported in 1926 that 8 weeks of exposure of teeth in vitro to a flow of carbon dioxide–free water etched the enamel surface, producing discernible opaque white spots. However, in subsequent studies in which teeth were exposed to acid solutions, the changes resembled erosive dissolution of the enamel and not dental caries. Since the mid-1950s, however, investigators have reproduced the successive zones typical of enamel caries by acid demineralization in the pH range 3.4 to 5.5. Enamel was untouched by acidity as low as pH 3.5 if the buffer was initially saturated with calcium phosphate. White spot enamel caries occurs regularly in an organic acid buffer (usually lactate or acetate) in the pH range 3 to 6 (most often 4.5), with strict avoidance

Table 51.1: Mean pH of Carious Cavities at Different Depths*†

Cavity Type‡	No. of Cavities	Surface			Cavity Layers Intermediate			Bottom		
		pH	S.D.	Range	pH	S.D.	Range	pH	S.D.	Range
I	31	4.9	0.75	3.5–6.6	4.2	0.51	3.2–5.7	3.9	0.40	3.2–4.9
II	42	5.8	0.74	4.0–7.7	4.9	0.74	3.3–7.2	4.5	0.77	3.3–6.8
III	16	6.3	0.63	5.2–7.3	—§	—	—	5.4	1.22	3.5–7.3

*Adapted with permission from T. R. Dirksen, M. F. Little, and B. G. Bibby: The pH of Carious Cavities: II. The pH at Different Depths of Isolated Cavities. *Arch Oral Biol*, **8**, 91, 1963.

†Isolated from saliva by rubber dam and excavated progressively; pH determined in situ by antimony microelectrode. Hours after eating, 1–15; median, 2.

‡Type I, small clinical opening, thick layer of decay; type II, large clinical opening, thick layer of decay; type III, large clinical opening, thin layer of decay, designated as "inactive" or "arrested."

§Thickness of decay insufficient for adequate measurements on intermediate layers.

of agitation and inclusion of a colloid. Unless agitation is avoided, simple surface diffusion results. The added colloid simulates the role played in vivo by the acquired pellicle and overlying plaque.

The nature of the resistant surface layer of enamel is incompletely understood. The outer few micrometers of normal enamel are indeed harder and less soluble than the subjacent tissue. If this outer layer is polished off and the enamel then subjected to an in vitro caries test, a radiodense surface zone results nonetheless. There is a transient initial demineralization at the very surface, with regeneration of a seemingly sound surface. Calcium phosphate redeposits from a saturated solution, diffusing outward from the subsurface demineralized area. In natural caries both an inherently more resistant surface layer and redeposition of calcium phosphate are involved.

The entire sequence of events seen in dentinal caries cannot be reproduced by the action of acids alone. The collagenous matrix is resistant to the degree of acidity that prevails in dentinal caries. Changes in the organic phase must be attributed to bacterial invasion. However, the organic phase of dentin must be demineralized to be susceptible to degradative reactions. The abundant organic matter released from dentin and the invading bacteria may sequester calcium in soluble complexes and may be an important ancillary factor in dentinal caries.

Dynamics. Kinetic analyses of physical models of dental caries show that the rate of solution of calcium and phosphate is diffusion controlled. It increases with increasing concentrations of hydrogen ion and undissociated acid and, using different acids, with decreasing dissociation constants of the acids and of their anionic complex with calcium. Carious demineralization commences then after initial diffusion of undissociated acid (mainly lactic) through the resistant surface layer into subsurface enamel. The ambient concentration of hydrogen ions would be small relative to that of undissociated acid and they would be a minor component of the inward diffusion. Within the hydroxyapatite hydration shell, the acid would dissociate and convert hydroxyapatite into relatively soluble $CaHPO_4 \cdot 2H_2O$, $Ca(H_2PO_4)_2 \cdot H_2O$, and calcium lactate, plus their several cognate ionic species and complexes. The controlling solid surface phase on the enamel crystallite becomes $CaHPO_4 \cdot 2H_2O$. These solutes must diffuse outward to the oral environment, a process that is opposed by the concentrations of calcium and phosphate in plaque and by the neutralizing action of the salivary bicarbonate system. Controlling diffusion in caries is the permeability of the plaque matrix (calcium, phosphate, bicarbonate, bacterial nutrients, particularly sugars, and bacterial metabolic products, particularly acids). Also involved are the permeabilities of the acquired pellicle, relatively intact surface layer, partially demineralized subsurface zones, sound portions of enamel, and ultimately of dentin.

Whether the outcome in enamel is demineralization, steady state, or remineralization depends on the relative concentrations of the products from a complex series of competing chemical reactions. Demineralization would be most active at the interface between sound enamel and organic acid and would tend toward an equilibrium value in intermediate zones. Remineralization would be most likely near the surface. The key variable is the external concentration of organic acid. The rates of the individual reactions are not critical determinants of the overall outcome, which is controlled by much slower diffusion processes. Mathematical formulations have been derived that describe reasonably well the dissolution rate of enamel during the formation of white spot caries in the experimental models. An important requirement is a correction factor for complex formation between calcium ion and the anion of the demineralizing acid.

Etiology of Caries

Dental caries has a multifactorial etiology. To the well-known triad of host, microbial, and substrate factors should be added a time factor, since this parameter emphasizes the need for a prolonged simultaneous interaction of the various contributors to the disease (Fig. 51.2).

Bacteria and Caries

One of the most rapidly progressing areas of microbiology is the study of the indigenous oral flora of man. The stimulus for interest in oral microbiology came from a series of discoveries showing that dental caries was a transmissible disease dependent on bacteria with unique properties. The discovery and analysis of a group of bacteria often simply called *Streptococcus mutans* has led to an understanding of bacteria that have essentially every feature one could desire in microorganisms designed to cause carious lesions. *S. mutans* lives only on the teeth. It can utilize sucrose in very clever ways to foster its colonization while using virtually every sugar in the diet for acid production. It resists attempts at removal by most oral hygiene procedures and can be selected for among other plaque bacteria, owing to its ability to tolerate the presence of acids. Once a carious lesion is initiated, other bacteria such as the acidogenic lactobacilli can take over, and this ensures that the destructive process progresses rapidly. *S. mutans* has to be given credit for attracting many basic scientists into dental research and for stimulating oral microbiology research.

A

B

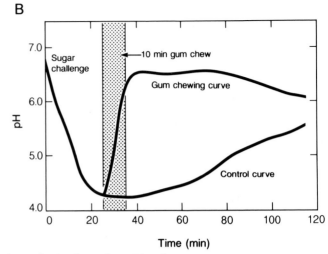

Figure 51.2: **(A)** Interaction of factors known to be involved in the etiology of dental caries. **(B)** Stephan curve illustrating the plaque pH response observed following interaction of bacteria on the surface of the teeth with dietary fermentable carbohydrate. Immediately after the sugar challenge the pH drops as acid is produced and then slowly rises toward neutrality with time. The chewing of gum causes the pH to rise rapidly due to the supplying of buffers through the stimulation of the flow of saliva.

Bacterial plaques develop on the tooth surface, and under normal conditions the end products of their metabolism are not harmful. However, under the right conditions plaque can develop enhanced cariogenic potential. This is reflected in higher levels of acidogenic bacteria, such as *S. mutans,* and possibly changes in the physical nature of the plaque that alter the diffusion of harmful acids away from the teeth and the penetration of protective buffers from saliva.

Carbohydrate and Caries

Although dental plaque can form when no food is ingested, food components can play a major role in converting plaque from an innocuous to a cariogenic substance. Carbohydrates are the substrates that cause the production of harmful acids and changes in the plaque microflora. It is not the absolute quantity of carbohydrate that is critical for disease development but the frequency with which it is presented to the dentition during ingestion. The low-plaque pH produced from carbohydrate fermentation will kill acid-sensitive bacteria and select for strains that are acid tolerant. As discussed later, the bacteria involved in caries are aciduric and can survive at low pH. In addition, it will be shown that many fermentable dietary carbohydrates can contribute to caries formation.

Acid Dissolution

This phenomenon was discussed in detail when the carious process was analyzed. However, the actual cause of caries is best visualized if the plaque bacteria are supplied in situ with fermentable carbohydrate and the pH of the plaque is monitored for a period of time. The data obtained allow the drawing of what has been termed a Stephan curve (see Fig. 51.2). Prior to carbohydrate ingestion the pH value is normally only slightly acidic or alkaline. Immediately after exposure to carbohydrate the plaque pH rapidly drops 2 or more pH units, indicating an increase in hydrogen ion concentration of almost 1,000-fold. With time the pH slowly rises, owing primarily to the diffusion of salivary buffers into the plaque. Theoretically, plaque pH curves could be equated with the acidic challenge to the teeth and the strength of the attack could be calculated from some feature of the curve. The length of time that the curve remains low may be critically related to the challenge to the tooth surface.

Dental Plaque and Caries

The oral environment and the nonmineralized coverings of the teeth play an essential role in the initiation and continuation of caries. As a tooth erupts into the oral environment, its coronal surface is covered by an inner acellular structure called the primary enamel cuticle. Covering it is a cellular structure, the reduced enamel epithelium. As the tooth erupts, the epithelium of the oral mucosa may also fuse with the reduced enamel epithelium. After the tooth erupts, its coronal surfaces may acquire a number of distinctive deposits that are categorized as acquired pellicle, dental plaque, dental calculus, food debris, or materia alba. Some of these structures play an important role in maintaining the integrity of the coronal enamel surface, others are involved in both dental caries and periodontal disease.

The roles of the primary enamel cuticle and of the reduced enamel epithelium in dental caries have not been clearly defined. Once the tooth has erupted they are rapidly lost from the enamel surfaces that are subject to abrasion during mastication. Due to their origin they cannot reform. The organic matrices of the enamel surface are quite resistant to enzymes and acids and bases, but they are permeable to organic acids and to microbial products formed in dental plaque. The primary enamel cuticle is involved in the attachment of the other dental integuments and deposits on the coronal surfaces. However, the one-time contribution of the primary enamel cuticle and reduced enamel epithelium to the formation of additional nonmineralized coatings of the teeth probably makes their role in caries formation inconsequential.

The Acquired Pellicle

External to the primary enamel cuticle and reduced epithelium, exposed coronal enamel is normally covered by an acquired pellicle that is generally described as acellular, structureless, bacteria free, and of salivary origin. This pellicle forms as the tooth erupts, and when fully matured after several weeks it is either colorless, light brown, or gray. It can be removed by vigorous brushing with an abrasive dentrifice, but when the enamel is reexposed to saliva it rapidly reforms as an almost invisible film. At maturity, when it is about 8 μm thick, it is sufficiently pigmented to be visible, and it is insoluble in acids. The acquired pellicle has been divided into surface, subsurface, colorless, and pigmented types. The subsurface type occurs when the enamel surface is partially decalcified, especially in interproximal areas, or when it is abraded. Colorless or pigmented pellicles have no particular significance except that they seem to represent young and older pellicles, respectively. The pellicle is primarily derived from salivary mucins, and it contains carbohydrates, neutral polysaccharides complexed with protein, and some lipid; it is not collagenous and it is not keratinous. It is quite resistant to hydrolysis, is stable at room or body temperature, and is relatively insoluble. Even when freed from the enamel surface, it is very resistant to proteolytic enzymes.

Initially, the acquired pellicle is essentially free of bacteria. However, although oral microorganisms are not directly involved in pellicle formation, at maturity it often contains muramic acid, indicative of bacterial cell walls. It is very difficult to obtain naturally formed pellicle free of bacterial contamination. In vitro studies, where "experimental" pellicles have been created by suspending enamel in different glandular salivas, have shown that there are present in both submandibular and parotid salivas similar glycoproteins that are selectively deposited onto etched enamel as an initial pellicle.

Acquired pellicle is a diffusion barrier to acids present in some foods and beverages, if it is not exposed to them for a long time, and to a certain extent to acids formed by the glycolytic metabolism of oral bacteria; hence, it serves as a deterrent to the initiation of dental caries. It may also impregnate minor defects in enamel and prevent cariogenic bacteria from entering and colonizing. If the subsurface pellicle can be mineralized, minor damage to the enamel surface may be repaired. Pellicle may also function as a lubricating medium between opposing enamel surfaces. A controversial function of pellicle is its role in the utilization of fluoride as an anticaries agent. Normally, prior to topically applying fluoride the dentist recommends a thorough prophylaxis with abrasives. Since the outer layer of enamel is known to contain the highest levels of fluoride it is possible that thorough cleaning with an abrasive is not the ideal preparation for the application of fluoride. Brushing and flossing prior to treatment may be adequate and preferred. Others have suggested that the pellicle can block ionic interactions of fluoride with the enamel and should be removed. There is also the possibility that the pellicle acts as a reservoir for fluoride and causes enhanced interactions with the enamel over an extended interval of time. More work on the role of pellicle in interactions with the enamel of various agents would be beneficial.

Plaque Formation

Dental plaques are dense, nonmineralized bacterial masses that are so firmly attached to the tooth surface that they are not removed by the flow of saliva or a gentle stream of water. After tooth cleaning, plaque develops on the acquired pellicle as distinct bacterial aggregates that form colonies and eventually grow and coalesce to form a continuous layer of bacteria. The mass of the plaque grows until it is limited by the abrasive forces exerted by the surrounding oral tissues. A unique feature of such plaques is their heterogeneity. The microbial composition of plaque varies not only between individuals but between different teeth in the same mouth and, more critically, between different sites on an individual tooth surface. This point will be emphasized when the oral ecology of the cariogenic bacterium *S. mutans* is discussed. It is reasonable to state that the microbial content of a dental plaque is unique to its site at any given time.

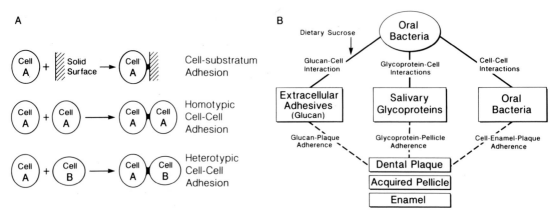

Figure 51.3: (**A**) Basic interactions involved in the formation of bacterial plaque on teeth. (**B**) Some of the factors involved in the interactions that occur during dental plaque formation.

The consequences of this microbial heterogeneity are great. Differences in biochemical activity exist throughout plaque, as reflected in the localized production of bacterial end products. With regard to dental caries, the pattern of disease in the dentition indicates that the production and accumulation of acid at localized sites is essential for lesion development. An interesting and not thoroughly understood process essential to caries formation is the transition from a plaque with minimal cariogenic potential to a cariogenic plaque.

After initial formation, plaque matures through a series of phases involving growth of the original microorganisms, continued attachment of additional bacteria to the tooth and the early colonizers, changes in the flora, and accumulation of extracellular substances.

Various investigators have studied the development of plaque during its initial stages. Young developing plaque consists mostly of gram-positive and gram-negative cocci and short rods and some filaments in an amorphous or finely granular matrix. Some dental scientists have divided plaque development into an initial phase, about 8 hours long, during which initial colonization occurs; a phase of rapid growth, lasting for an additional 16 hours, when the numbers of organisms increase rapidly; and a third phase, in which the numbers of bacteria remain constant but remodeling occurs. In this study *Streptococcus sanguis,* which was consistently present, made up 15% to 35% of the plaque isolates during the initial phase. *Streptococcus mitis* was present in some of the early samples but later disappeared, while *Streptococcus salivarius* was present only transiently. *Veillonella alcalescens* and peptostreptococci were irregularly present in early samples but were more frequently isolated after 1 day. Several unidentified gram-positive cocci were also found in the early samples. Organisms considered to

be corynebacteria were present during the first few hours, then disappeared. *Actinomyces viscosus* was present in proportions ranging from 15% to 50% through the initial phase.

Generally, cocci increase rapidly within developing plaque and in a few days make up 80% to 90% of the resident flora. *S. sanguis can* reach between 60% and 70% of the cultivated bacteria during the second phase. The proportion of *Actinomyces* decreases during this stage, most likely due to an increase in the number of other bacteria which grew more rapidly. By the end of the second phase other actinomycetes can be detected and their numbers increase, reaching proportions of 10% to almost 30% of the total flora. After a week or so cocci are reduced to about 50% of the plaque flora, having been replaced by bacteria such as fusobacteria, nocardiae, neisseriae, vibrios, and spirochetes. In older plaque, the total number of bacteria remains about the same, but again there are changes in relative proportions. The percentages of streptococci decrease but they remain prominent, along with actinomycetes and veillonellae. Some plaques consist mostly of filamentous bacteria at the end of 2 weeks.

In summary, these types of studies illustrate that plaque is a complex, dynamic system that can undergo relatively rapid changes. The nature of these changes is regulated by the site where the plaque is forming and by the local environment at the time of plaque formation.

Adhesive Interactions.   As illustrated in Figure 51.3, three basic cell interactions must be involved in plaque formation. The bacteria in saliva must interact with the tooth surface, cells of the same type can attach to each other (homotypic adherence), and different types of cells can attach to each other (heterotypic adherence). The first interaction in plaque formation involves the selective sorption of bacteria from saliva onto pellicle-coated enamel. This type of adherence is governed in part by the concentration of each bacterium in saliva. This determines the relative frequency with which a bacterium comes in contact with the tooth surface. Another factor involves the affinity of each bacterium to binding sites on the pellicle. The greater the affinity, the greater its chances for becoming irreversibly bound. Adherence to pellicle can be divided into two stages. The initial interaction is reversible and the bacterium can return to saliva. Some of the bacteria that interact with the pellicle become irreversibly bound (stage 2) through one of several mechanisms. Adherence and the homotypic and heterotypic cell–cell interactions are all influenced by extracellular products produced by the bacteria, specific factors present in saliva, and specific binding sites on the surfaces of the various bacteria.

Extracellular Polymers. The most intensely studied example of the role of extracellular material in plaque formation involves the production of glucan from sucrose by *S. mutans*. The relationship between this phenomenon and the cariogenic potential of this bacterium will be discussed in detail later in this chapter.

Extracellular glucan production from sucrose is not limited to *S. mutans* since other oral streptococci produce these types of polymers. However, the chemical bonds in the glucans and the degree of branching in the glucans formed by these other bacteria are different from those produced by *S. mutans* enzymes, and the glucan is clearly not essential for their colonization of the tooth surface. For example, *S. sanguis* is one of the primary colonizers of human teeth, and although this bacterium can produce glucan from sucrose, the presence of this disaccharide in the diet is neither required for *S. sanguis* colonization nor does it stimulate accumulation of this organism on the tooth surface. *S. sanguis* does not have glucan-specific binding sites on its cell surface, as does *S. mutans,* and this may be a partial explanation for these observations.

It has recently been demonstrated that additional plaque bacteria such as some of the *Actinomyces* can bind glucan and aggregate. The function of this interaction in human plaque formation is not known. As yet there is no evidence that the level of these bacteria in plaque is markedly increased with increases in dietary sucrose.

Certain oral bacteria produce extracellular products that enhance their ability to participate in plaque formation. Strains of *A. viscosus* produce a polymer that is not a glucan; this material allows them to form in vitro plaquelike masses on solid surfaces. It is worth emphasizing that heterogeneous dental plaques can form on the teeth of subjects who receive their diet by nonoral means. Thus, most plaque bacteria have mechanisms to become a part of plaque that are unrelated to the presence of factors in the diet. As we will see, some bacteria, such as *S. mutans,* have mechanisms that allow them to take advantage of substrates in the diet to become dominant members of the plaque flora at specific sites.

Salivary Constituents. Various components in human saliva are critically involved in plaque formation. The chemical composition of the saliva components that form the acquired pellicle governs the capacity of bacteria to be primary colonizers of a cleaned tooth surface. It has been demonstrated that strains of *S. sanguis, S. mutans, S. mitior,* and several *Actinomyces* aggregate when mixed with whole human saliva. Saliva glycoproteins and calcium ions appear to be involved in aggregate formation. There are separate agglutinins for the different streptococci, and the interactions appear to be chemically specific. In one study a high molecular weight mucin glycoprotein agglutinated both *S. sanguis* and *S. mutans.* When the sialic acid residues were removed from the agglutinin, the polymer no longer caused the agglutination of *S. sanguis* but was still capable of agglutinating *S. mutans.* Other investigators have reported that oral bacteria can selectively bind lysozyme and blood group reactive mucins from saliva. The latter material appears to be present in some samples of acquired pellicle.

The specificity of the interaction between oral bacteria and saliva components which may be a part of the acquired pellicle can be demonstrated utilizing hydroxyapatite that has been treated with saliva to form a layer of pellicle-like material. By studying the adherence of bacteria to saliva-coated hydroxyapatite it has been demonstrated that lactose and *N*-actylgalactosamine inhibit the attachment of *Leptotrichia buccalis,* that hexosamines and other amines can block adherence of *S. mutans,* and that various simple sugars are capable of blocking attachment of *Actinomyces naeslundii.* Thus, it appears that some of the components from saliva which adhere to the enamel tooth surface provide unique sites where specific oral bacteria can adhere. An analogy which supports this mechanism of plaque formation involves the "lectin-receptor" type of interaction where specific proteins selectively bind to carbohydrate receptors. These types of interactions would partially explain the bacterial specificity of early plaque formation. It is important that the binding of salivary components to bacteria could also prevent adherence to teeth or plaque by masking of binding sites and/or enhancing their removal from the oral cavity via swallowing.

Cell-to-Cell Attachment. Under certain conditions plaque bacteria can be shown to undergo heterotypic interactions in the absence of exogenous

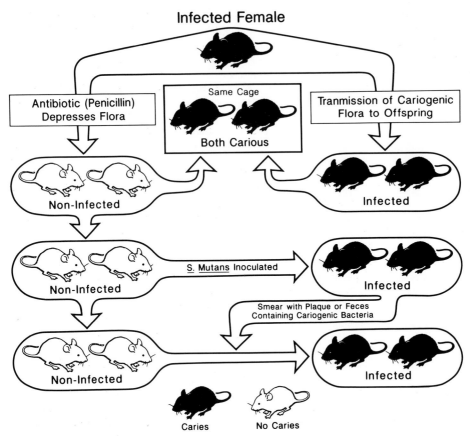

Figure 51.4: Diagram of caries formation due to passage of bacteria from rat dams to their pups, elimination of the disease by treatment of animals with antibiotics, and the occurrence of caries following various types of inoculations. The infection was reintroduced by contact with infected animals, inoculation with isolated strains of "caries-inducing" streptococci, and transfer of bacterial plaque or feces.

factors. For example, strains of *A. viscosus* will aggregate with certain strains of *S. sanguis, Neisseria, Leptotrichia, Veillonella,* and *Nocardia* when cell suspensions are mixed together. Interactions of this type may be directly visualized by microscopic examination of plaque, although it is difficult to exclude participation of salivary components under these conditions. It is difficult to estimate the contribution of direct cell-to-cell interactions to in situ plaque formation.

Microbiology of Dental Caries

Evidence for Bacterial Etiology

Despite the known involvement of microorganisms in many diseases of animals and humans, it was not until the 1880s that W. D. Miller performed experiments which placed dental caries in the category of a bacterially dependent problem. In one experiment

Miller exposed extracted human teeth to salivary bacteria and carbohydrate and demonstrated demineralization of tooth enamel. Miller postulated that bacteria were the etiological agents of dental caries and that their acidic and proteolytic products caused destruction of the mineral and organic components of the teeth, respectively. This chemicoparasitic theory of caries formation eventually gained substantial support through a wide range of investigations.

In the 1950s a series of studies in rodents demonstrated that the development of caries was absolutely dependent on the presence of bacteria. Rats raised under bacteria-free conditions did not develop caries when supplied with a carbohydrate-containing diet capable of producing the disease in animals with a normal bacterial flora. When the germ-free animals were orally infected with selected bacteria they developed carious lesions.

In 1960 Keyes performed a series of experiments that established dental caries as an infectious disease (Fig. 51.4). The offspring of caries-active animal dams did not develop caries if the mothers were treated with antibiotics during pregnancy and lactation. Caries-inactive animals failed to develop extensive lesions unless they were caged with animals exhibiting rampant decay or were supplied with fecal material from carious animals and consequently became orally infected due to coprophagious habits. Caries was shown to involve transmission of antibiotic-sensitive bacteria.

Specific Bacteria and Caries

During his investigations Miller isolated several types of plaque bacteria capable of producing large amounts of acid. Consequently, he concluded that no single species was responsible for dental caries but that the process resulted from any microorganism that could produce acid and degrade protein. Considerable subsequent investigation has involved searches to determine the type and number of bacteria that contribute to caries formation in humans. Plaques from both carious lesions and sound tooth surfaces are best described as microbiologically variable and complex. However, significant differences in bacterial composition from such plaques have been demonstrated.

Based on the work of early investigators, several principles were formulated as a guide to scientists attempting to study the microbial etiology of human caries:

1. The causative organism should be the most acidogenic species that could be found in the oral cavity and in carious lesions.
2. The causative agent should be able to endure the acidity that it produces in the carious lesion.
3. The causative microorganism must be isolated from all stages of the carious lesion and grown in pure culture.
4. The pure culture of the microorganisms must be able to produce caries when inoculated into the oral cavity or directly onto the tooth, and no other organism should be able to do so.
5. The causative microorganism should be absent from the surfaces of teeth that do not undergo carious decalcification and from the saliva of "caries-free" individuals.
6. Other microorganisms that produce sufficient acid to decalcify enamel and dentin must not be present in any stage of the carious process. If they are present, it must be proved that they cannot produce a carious lesion.

These rather stringent principles had a reasonable basis at the time of their development. However, it is now clear that dental caries should probably be divided into a number of unique diseases or disease states defined by the site of microbial attack, the time at which the attack is occurring, and the nature of the dietary substrate being provided. By clearly defining the clinical parameters associated with the disease, a clearer picture of the microbial etiology of caries can be developed.

Lactobacilli. These bacteria were thought to play an important role in caries etiology when it was first found that early carious plaque contained elevated levels of lactobacilli, compared with plaque from noncarious surfaces. By exploiting the ability of lactobacilli to grow on acidified culture media it was possible to detect low numbers of these bacteria in oral samplings containing mixtures of bacteria. Consequently, lactobacilli were isolated from saliva, plaque, and carious lesions, and it was possible to correlate high lactobacillus numbers in saliva with caries activity in groups of subjects. For example, in a group of caries-free children the mean number of lactobacilli per 1 mL of saliva was in the hundreds, while in caries-active children the mean number per 1 mL was in the range of 100,000.

Further evidence for the role of lactobacilli in caries came from investigations showing that a rise in salivary lactobacilli preceded the formation of cavities by 3 to 6 months. Increases or decreases in the level of fermentable carbohydrate in the diet were also shown to cause corresponding changes in the level of salivary lactobacilli. Studies by Jay in 1947 that demonstrated that the level of oral lactobacilli could be reduced by restricting the intake of dietary carbohydrate represented one of the first conclusive associations of a quantitative change in the level of an oral bacterium with a shift in diet. Interestingly, Jay also demonstrated that elimination of carious lesions in humans by placement of restorations caused a precipitous reduction in the level of salivary lactobacilli. In a study of 39 patients the mean number of lactobacilli was 138,000/1 mL prior to restorative work. One week after completion of the operative procedures the mean number of lactobacilli was 1,600/1 mL.

The early observations on changes in *Lactobacillus* levels in the oral cavity led many dental scientists to consider these bacteria as the specific microbial etiological factor in human caries. For example, Snyder and co-workers designed a simple laboratory test for the assessment of caries activity by monitoring salivary *Lactobacillus* populations. The method is based on the rate of acid production in a glucose medium by oral acidogenic microorganisms that will grow at a pH from 4.7 to 5.0 (principally lactobacilli). From 0.1 to 0.2 mL of saliva is mixed thoroughly with 10 mL of melted medium in a test tube. During incubation at 37°C the production of acid is detected by an indicator, bromcresol green, which changes from blue-green (pH 4.7 to 5.0) to green (pH 4.2 to 4.6) to yellow (pH 4.0 or lower). Yellow indicates a positive test after incubation for 72 hours. Unfortunately, when attempts were made to use such tests for predicting future caries activity in a given individual, the correlation was not sufficient to allow these tests to be fully accepted. It is worth pointing out that *Lactobacillus* counts remained higher after restoration of the lesions. It might be advisable to have the dentist look for undetected lesions or restorations with poor marginal adaptation. An additional situation in which bacterial counts might be useful is in monitoring a patient's dietary habits and ability to restrict the level of dietary carbohydrate. Such techniques have been used successfully in certain populations in Sweden.

For a number of reasons, the lactobacilli failed to qualify as an exclusive etiological agent in human caries formation. Lactobacilli are found in saliva in proportions far exceeding those in dental plaque because they also colonize the dorsum of the tongue, vestibular mucosa, and hard palate. The affinity of lactobacilli for tooth surfaces is low; they represent less than 0.01% of the cultivable flora of plaque on intact tooth surfaces. Although high levels of lactobacilli tend to exist after caries has developed, caries can frequently be initiated in children in the absence of detectable lactobacilli. Loesche and Syed reported that lactobacilli made up 0% to 11% (average, 4%) of the flora in six samples of plaque from approximal lesions, indicating that lactobacilli in some, but not all, cases increased after decay had started. In corresponding samples of plaque from carious dentin, the lactobacilli made up 0% to 85% (average, 21%) of the flora. These types of data have supported the conclusion that the lactobacilli are secondary invaders in some carious lesions where they may contribute to the progression of decay due to their acidogenic and aciduric properties. The level of these bacteria in saliva may reflect spillover from lesions that contain high concentrations of lactobacilli.

Attempts to produce caries in experimental animals by inoculation with lactobacilli have shown that when these bacteria have been established in rodents, they produce caries less regularly and less extensively than several other microbial species. In the rat model, caries development is normally associated with the molar fissures where this bacterium is most easily established.

Streptococci. From the time that Miller found streptococci in the oral cavity and associated them with caries formation, these bacteria have received considerable attention from dental scientists. Initially, oral streptococci were implicated in caries due to their abundance in the mouth, their presence in deep dentinal carious lesions, and their consistent association with pulpitis, accompanying dentinal caries where the pulp had not been exposed. Understanding of the role of streptococci in dental caries has been greatly advanced by studies with animal model systems, in vitro laboratory studies, and investigations with human subjects including analysis of plaque from various sites on the tooth surface.

Fitzgerald and Keyes in 1960 isolated certain streptococci from carious lesions in hamsters. When these bacteria were inoculated into the mouths of caries-inactive albino hamsters, rampant decay developed. Subsequent testing of other bacteria, including lactobacilli and acidogenic streptococci, indicated that caries formation in the hamsters was specifically related to the presence of strains of bacteria with characteristics similar to the isolates used in the initial studies. It is now known that the bacteria responsible for producing extensive smooth enamel decay in the hamster model belonged to a group of bacteria designated *S. mutans*. The hamster model is clearly a good system to evaluate the ability of a bacterium to colonize smooth tooth surfaces and initiate carious lesions. However, failure to cause caries in this model may partially reflect the fact that some strains of acidogenic oral bacteria are simply unable to colonize the hamster tooth surface under the conditions used, and it is possible that changes in the diet or time and mode of infection might provide different results. Formation of adequate quantities of plaque is surely a prerequisite for significant lesion development.

When germ-free and conventional rats were used to evaluate the cariogenic potential of various oral bacteria, the relationship was not nearly as specific as with hamsters. As presented in Table 51.2, a large number of bacteria proved capable of causing caries in germ-free rats. Although the microbial specificity for attack on the smooth surfaces was retained, fissure lesions could be initiated by a greater variety of streptococci and by other bacterial types. In contrast to the hamster, the molar teeth of rats contain occlusal fissures similar in relative size to those of human molars. These stagnant areas foster accumulation of bacteria that are incapable of colonizing smooth non-retentive tooth surfaces. A wide range of acidogenic streptococci can consequently produce lesions in the occlusal fissures of rat teeth. It is worth noting that in all of these studies the animals were provided with a caries-promoting diet containing high concentrations of sucrose.

Several oral streptococci have been shown to produce root surface lesions in germ-free rats. Strains of *S. mutans* appear to be the more versatile bacteria since they cause caries on buccal and lingual smooth surfaces, in pits and fissures, and on root surfaces in the rat model.

In vitro studies with the oral streptococci have

Table 51.2: Bacteria Capable of Producing Carious Lesions at Different Sites in the Dentition of Germ-free Rats

Bacterium	Site		
	Smooth Surfaces	Occlusal Fissures	Root Surfaces
Lactobacillus acidophilus	−	+	−
Lactobacillus casei	−	+	−
Streptococcus mutans	+	+	+
Streptococcus sanguis	−	+	−
Streptococcus salivarius	+	+	+
Streptococcus mitior	−	+	−
Streptococcus milleri	+	+	−
Streptococcus faecalis	−	+	−
Actinomyces viscosus	−	+	+
Actinomyces naeslundii	−	+	+
Actinomyces israelii	−	+	+
Rothia sp.	−	−	+

demonstrated many features that support their role as cariogenic agents:

1. They have a relatively rapid generation time, and dense liquid cultures can be obtained in less than 12 hours following subculturing. Although the rate of growth of streptococci in the oral cavity is surely not this rapid, when these bacteria are compared with other oral bacteria, there is no doubt that they have the capacity to grow faster when provided with the appropriate environment.

2. They produce large quantities of acid during growth, and the terminal pH in broth cultures is normally close to 4.0. Although the rate and extent of acid production depend on the growth conditions, the high acidogenicity of the oral streptococci has been repeatedly observed.

3. The various oral streptococci do not appear to be as aciduric as the lactobacilli. Most oral streptococci do not grow well at pH 5.5 and die within 48 hours at pH 4.2. However, these in vitro observations may not be applicable to the oral cavity, since these bacteria can clearly form large quantities of plaque on teeth under conditions where fermentable carbohydrate is being supplied in high concentrations. The buffering capacity of saliva, plaque, and enamel is apparently adequate to protect the streptococci from their acidic end products. A possible explanation for variations in the capacity of various strains of *S. mutans* to produce caries in model systems may reflect differences in acid tolerance.

4. The streptococci can utilize a wide range of fermentable carbohydrates, including all the predominant simple sugars found in the human diet. Selected strains can ferment mannitol and sorbitol.

5. They can store carbohydrate intracellularly for prolonged utilization as an energy or carbon source with the subsequent production of acid.

6. They can produce extracellular polysaccharides from sucrose. These polymers can function as storage polysaccharides and facilitate colonization of the streptococci on tooth surfaces.

7. They can be manipulated to form plaque on various surfaces under conditions simulating the in vivo situations which they normally encounter.

Each of these properties of the oral streptococci will be discussed in more detail when we analyze *S. mutans* as a cariogenic bacterium.

Studies on the ecology of oral streptococci have strengthened the argument for their relationship to dental caries formation. Plaques from human teeth can contain up to 10^{11} streptococci per gram of wet weight. Collectively, the various oral streptococci can make up 30% to 60% of the total bacterial populations which live at various sites in the human oral cavity. If the distribution of these bacteria in the mouth is examined (Table 51.3), it is clear that the various strains have a predilection for particular sites within the oral cavity. The localization of *S. mutans* on the tooth surface indicates that this particular bacterium has a rather limited but critically important ecological niche.

For practical, methodological, and ethical reasons, evidence for the role of streptococci in human dental caries formation cannot be directly obtained. Consequently, epidemiological approaches have been used to correlate the presence of streptococci in samples of plaque and saliva with caries activity, to correlate the presence of streptococci in plaque from carious lesions with results with plaque from adjacent tooth surfaces, and to establish longitudinal studies where

Table 51.3: Distribution of Oral Streptococci at Various Sites in the Human Oral Cavity*

Streptococcus	Site			
	Plaque	Tongue	Saliva	Gingival Crevice
S. mutans	0–50	0–1	0–1	0–30
S. sanguis	40–60	10–20	10–30	10–20
S. salivarius	0–1	40–60	40–60	0–1
S. mitior	20–40	10–30	30–50	10–20
S. milleri	3–25	0–1	0–1	14–56

*All values are reported as a percentage of the total cultivable facultative streptococci.

periodic sampling at caries-prone sites is used to develop an association between the presence of streptococci, or other bacteria, and the development of disease. Briefly, it appears that the streptococci capable of causing caries in rats are also associated with human caries.

In conclusion, the oral streptococci represent a predominant group of bacteria in the human oral cavity. Selected species can cause caries at distinct sites in the dentition of rodents. These bacteria have a number of biochemical properties that can be directly related to their cariogenic potential. The oral streptococci are likely candidates for primary involvement in dental caries formation in humans.

Other Cariogenic Bacteria. As indicated in Table 51.2, caries formation in the rat is not restricted to the lactobacilli and streptococci. Animals infected with *A. viscosus* and *A. naeslundii* exhibit large plaque accumulations along the gingival margin rather than on the occlusal surfaces, as is observed with streptococci. Under the appropriate conditions the accumulation of such plaque leads to breakdown of the periodontal tissues. Although these bacteria are not as acidogenic as the lactobacilli and streptococci, they do produce enough acid to cause slight damage to enamel and much greater disruption to the less mineralized cementum. The *Actinomyces* species and other gram-positive rods may be involved in the initiation of lesions on root surfaces of human teeth. In plaques over root surface lesions in humans *S. mutans* may be absent or may make up to 30% of the total flora. In the latter case *S. sanguis* can make up approximately 48% of the total flora. In both cases *A. viscosus* was the dominant microorganism. It may be relevant that *A. viscosus* has proved to be significantly more resistant to fluoride than other oral bacteria such as *S. mutans*. Whether this lack of sensitivity to fluoride by the *Actinomyces* is important for treatment plans involving root surface lesions is not known at this time.

The complexity of caries formation in humans is emphasized when the microbial content of deep dentinal lesions is analyzed. In this unique environment the incidence of streptococci is often very low and lactobacilli are dominant. However, other bacteria frequently isolated from such sites include members of the following genera: *Actinomyces, Arachnia, Bacillus, Bifidobacterium, Eubacterium, Propionibacterium,* and *Rothia.* Whether these bacteria contribute positively or negatively to lesion progression is not known.

There is precedence for the concept that certain bacterial strains could be antagonistic to caries production. Members of the genus *Veillonella* are obligate anaerobes and are found in significant numbers in dental plaque and saliva from humans. Members of this genera are asaccharolytic due to lesions in their glycolytic pathway but can readily metabolize a variety of short chain acids, including lactic acid. Lactate is converted to propionate, acetate, CO_2, and H_2. Consequently, within plaque these bacteria have the capacity to utilize lactic acid and convert it to less harmful products. The production of weaker acids from lactate could cause a reduction in caries formation. Although a study in humans has not been performed where the level of caries has been compared to levels of *Veillonella,* there is clear evidence from animal studies that such an investigation might provide important data. If germ-free rats are provided with a high sucrose diet and infected with both *S. mutans* and *V. alcalescens,* less caries is formed than in animals that are infected with *S. mutans* alone.

Streptococcus mutans and Dental Caries

The great progress made in oral microbiology research in the past decade has been tied to a series of discoveries on a unique group of bacteria. The story that has evolved relating the formation of dental caries to these bacteria involves the uncovering of a fascinating relationship between a specific host tissue, the presence of sucrose and other fermentable carbohydrates in the diet, and a group of bacteria called *S. mutans*. There is little doubt that *S. mutans* is intimately involved in caries formation in humans, and detailed evidence will be presented to support this conclusion. However, it is important that our discussion of *S. mutans* be placed in proper perspective. The oral cavity, and specifically dental plaque, contains a complex mixture of bacteria in an environment that is almost continuously changing. Oral biologists have documented many fluctuations that occur in the mouth as a consequence of almost every human activity. The complexity of the environment and the microbial community on the tooth surface combined with the impossibility for repeating in humans the infectivity studies done in germ-free rats makes it unlikely that one bacterium could ever be implicated as the sole etiological agent in human caries formation. Indeed, when caries is regarded as a process involving lesion initiation and lesion extension, and when the microbial composition at the various sites at which caries occurs is analyzed, it begins to appear that the disease results from a concerted effort by specific bacteria that can be positively or negatively effected by their microbial neighbors.

It is reasonable to focus on *S. mutans* as a model to study the possibility of reducing or eliminating a specific bacterium from the oral cavity. Using the *S. mutans* model, dental scientists are assessing the possibility of controlling a member of man's indigenous oral flora. The results of this work could open the door to the control of other odontopathic bacteria and possibly lead to reductions in the incidence of caries in humans. An interesting question that dental scientists are close to answering is what effect will the elimination of *S. mutans* from the human oral cavity have on the development of dental caries? To evaluate current attempts to answer this question, we must understand the uniqueness of *S. mutans* as a cariogenic bacterium.

Historical Perspective

S. mutans is a bacterium whose rise to prominence required time and insight. In the early 1920s Clark attempted to evaluate the etiology of caries by analyzing the microbial content of plaque from human carious lesions. A streptococcal bacterium was consistently isolated from the samples, and its pleomorphic nature (ranging from cocci to rods, depending on the culture conditions) caused it to be named *Streptococcus mutans*. After this initial report there were sporadic publications on bacteria with similar characteristics, but not until nearly four decades later were intense investigations of *S. mutans* initiated. The impetus for this work came from investigations performed at the National Institute of Dental Research in the 1960s. In an expansion of the pioneering studies of Orland and his co-workers, who had conclusively demonstrated that microorganisms were required for the initiation of dental caries in rats, Keyes and Fitzgerald showed that in rats, caries is an infectious and transmissible disease, and that specific streptococci from carious lesions in animals could induce extensive decay in hamsters. Streptococci with characteristics very similar to those of the animal-infective strains were subsequently isolated from human mouths and shown to be capable of causing caries when implanted in rodents. More recently it was demonstrated that the cariogenic potential of *S. mutans* from caries-active and caries-resistant adults is similar when tested in the hamster model system.

The bacteria used in many of the early studies were designated as *S. mutans* due to their expression of traits which we now use to identify these microorganisms. In general, *S. mutans* is recognized by its ability to 1) produce a distinctive colonial morphology when grown under standardized conditions on a sucrose-containing selective medium called mitis–salivarius agar; 2) synthesize extracellular polysaccharide from sucrose; 3) undergo cell–cell aggregation when mixed with sucrose or the polymer of glucose called dextran; 4) grow in the presence of the antibiotics sulfadimetine and bacitracin; and 5) ferment mannitol and/or sorbitol. The extent of the expression of these traits may vary from isolate to isolate.

Streptococcus mutans and Human Caries

The only feasible approaches to studying the association between a specific oral bacterium and caries formation in humans are epidemiological. Unfortunately, causation in the epidemiological sense cannot provide unequivocal answers in defining the microbial etiology of dental caries. However, such investigations have greatly increased our understanding of the role of bacteria in caries formation in humans.

Based on the results from the rodent model systems, where *S. mutans* was shown to have great cariogenic potential, a large number of investigations have focused on relating this bacterium to disease. Initial studies revealed that *S. mutans* normally makes up 5% to 10% of the total bacteria present in pooled plaque samples obtained from caries-active subjects. In contrast, *S. mutans* represents less than 1% of the flora in pooled plaque from caries-inactive individuals. Unfortunately, pooled plaque samples do not actually reflect the concentrations of *S. mutans* on specific sites of the teeth. Data from pooled samples represent a significant underestimation of the levels of *S. mutans,* owing to the dilution of the samples with plaque from sites in the dentition that do not harbor high concentrations of the bacterium. *S. mutans* is found mainly at retentive sites such as carious lesions, occlusal surface pits and fissures, and approximal areas.

When disease-prone or diseased sites are analyzed, the association between *S. mutans* and caries becomes stronger. For example, plaque samples taken from a defined interproximal surface in 164 young adults revealed that *S. mutans* was present in 72% of the cases where radiographs subsequently revealed lesions (83 total lesions). A strong positive correlation was observed between early detectable lesions and *S. mutans*. In another large study where the areas of sampling included retentive sites, a significant association between percentage levels of *S. mutans* and caries was found in plaques taken from a single occlusive fissure and pooled plaques from representative occlusal and approximal molar surfaces. Saliva samples, however, were equivocal in demonstrating a relationship between *S. mutans* and decay.

In spite of the observation by many investigators that *S. mutans* can be associated with human decay in cross-sectional, association-type studies, such investigations fail to indicate whether these bacteria are present as the cause or the result of dental decay. Some of the problems in these types of studies have been circumvented; others remain. Dental caries is a chronic disease where it may take months for the destruction to progress to a clinically detectable level. It is also very difficult to diagnose the incipient carious lesion. The complex nature of the oral flora poses technical problems that are often difficult to avoid. Plaque samples should be analyzed immediately after collection since the levels of *S. mutans* and other viable bacteria can decrease during storage. *S. mutans* is usually reported as a percentage of the total streptococcal flora which grows on mitis–salivarius agar. This and other selective media may cause underestimation of the *S. mutans* counts. In addition, the results give a false impression of *S. mutans* relative to the total plaque flora. Finally, plaque sampling is a problem in that retentive areas are difficult if not impossible to examine, and the ability of *S. mutans* to exist as dense polysaccharide-coated microcolonies close to the enamel may make their collection and dispersion for quantitation difficult.

Longitudinal studies can be proposed as a means for demonstrating whether an increase in caries development coincides with an increase in *S. mutans* counts. There are several inherent difficulties in performing such studies. They are expensive and labor intensive, since a large number of subjects are needed to provide for patient loss and to increase the likelihood that a selected tooth surface will become carious during the time of the study. Other factors that could complicate such studies involve changes in dietary habits, exposure to fluoride, utilization of medications, oral hygiene habits, composition and flow rate of saliva, microbial interactions within plaque, and the immunological state of the subjects. All of these factors influence caries formation in man. The design of a longitudinal caries study in humans will probably always be less than ideal.

A large longitudinal study in England yielded some interesting findings. As a part of a much larger sample, 19 subjects were followed for 2 years, with bilateral plaque samples taken at 6-month intervals from the distal surface of the upper first premolars. Radiographs were used to document caries development, and extensive microbiological analyses were performed on each of 224 plaque samples. During the 2-year interval, caries developed at 20% of the target sites. In general, the microbial composition of plaque samples from caries-free sites and from carious sites before and after radiographic detection of lesions was similar. In 2 of 15 sites *S. mutans* became numerically dominant before detection of a lesion. Pooled data from the sites that developed decay indicated a rise in the isolation frequency and mean numbers of *S. mutans* after detection of caries. Of interest, in 2 of 15 cases, *S. mutans* was not isolated from sites that developed caries. From this study it was concluded that no single species of bacteria was uniquely associated with the onset of dental caries. It is worth noting that an abrasive strip was used to obtain the plaque samples, and it is possible that the level of cariogenic bacteria was diluted by the presence of supragingival plaque from gingival margins.

In a longitudinal study of the role of *S. mutans* in human fissure decay in which great care was taken to define disease and sites, the proportions of *S. mutans* in carious fissures were significantly higher than the proportions from caries-free fissures. More direct evidence for involvement of *S. mutans* has been obtained using a fissure sampling technique where the fissure is removed with a bur in a high-speed handpiece under conditions in which the entire microbial content of the fissure could be retained for analysis. In samples from 48 carious teeth, the only bacterium found in every case was *S. mutans*. Other bacteria present in some of the samples included *S. sanguis, A. viscosus,* and lactobacilli. These studies indicate that *S. mutans* is significantly involved in occlusal fissure decay. This is important, since decay in these sites normally occurs prior to caries development on smooth surfaces and represents the most prevalent form of tooth decay in children.

Ecology of *Streptococcus mutans*

To appreciate attempts to eradicate *S. mutans* from the oral cavity, the ecology of this bacterium must be considered. In the broadest sense, *S. mutans* exists in worldwide distribution. More specifically, the only natural habitat of *S. mutans* appears to be the mouth of humans and some animals. This bacterium requires a nondesquamating surface for colonization of the mouth and consequently is found primarily in plaque on the surfaces of teeth. *S. mutans* does not colonize the mouth of predentate infants but appears shortly after teeth have erupted. It disappears from the human mouth after the loss of teeth. The bacterium will remain or reappear if dentures are placed, either immediately or at a later date. The explanation for these phenomena is that although the teeth are *S. mutans'* primary ecological niche, this bacterium does not have a high affinity for the tooth surface. For example, it takes only about 1×10^3 *S. sanguis* cells in saliva to cause adherence of this bacterium to the tooth surface, whereas approximately 5×10^4 cells of *S. mutans* are required before adherence to the teeth is noticeable. Since *S. mutans* appears unable to colonize the mucosal surfaces of the oral cavity, the reservoir for this microorganism is limited to the sites on the teeth that have been previously colonized. Removal of these sites can cause dramatic decreases in *S. mutans* levels in the mouth. Perhaps as a consequence of this need for a stable surface in the mouth for colonization, *S. mutans* has developed mechanisms that allow it to become very firmly attached to the tooth surface. As will be discussed later, the mechanisms for fixation involve a complex interaction between *S. mutans* and dietary sucrose.

Our current knowledge concerning acquisition of *S. mutans* by children indicates that maternal transfer is a likely possibility. Parental or sibling reservoirs of *S. mutans* are a potential source of bacterial infection for infants whose erupting teeth are being colonized for the first time. Using growth inhibitory bacteriocins to identify specific types of *S. mutans,* investigators can sometimes identify the person providing the initial effective oral inoculum. This person is most likely to be someone who has close contact with the infant at the time of tooth arrival in the oral cavity. In adult subjects the situation appears to be much more complicated. It is difficult to experimentally establish characterized strains of *S. mutans* in the mouths of individuals with a well-established oral flora. Rinsing the mouth with cultures of *S. mutans* usually does not lead to implantation, and the bacterium is quickly cleared from the oral cavity. Interestingly, one of the most effective ways to implant strains of *S. mutans* on human adult teeth is to place a drop of a culture of this bacterium onto a piece of dental floss and to work the floss at an approximal site. The procedure may need to be repeated on consecutive days. Intense localization of high densities of *S. mutans* at specific sites appears to overcome some of the suppressors of colonization. The floss implantation technique has significant implications for the proper use of this material during an individual's oral hygiene procedures.

It is known that the factors that can regulate the interoral spreading of *S. mutans* include the frequency and time of exposure to the bacterium, the dose received during each exposure; the nature and quantity of antibacterial substances present in saliva at the time of exposure, the flow rate of saliva, the nature of the indigenous flora at the sites of initial tooth contact, and other factors related to the specific adherence mechanisms of *S. mutans.*

A key concept related to *S. mutans* infections and caries involves the results: this bacterium colonizes teeth in a very localized manner, and the sites that harbor high concentrations of *S. mutans* are the sites that most readily become diseased. In humans, *S. mutans* is isolated with greatest frequency from occlusal surface pits and fissures, approximal areas, and close to the gingival margin. It is well documented that fissure decay is the most prevalent form of human dental caries and that the smooth surfaces of teeth are attacked less readily. A role for *S. mutans* in smooth surface decay has recently been supported with data obtained by taking small plaque samples from directly over and adjacent to incipient white spot lesions on buccal tooth surfaces in children. The proportions of *S. mutans* in samples from carious areas were significantly higher than those from the adjacent sound surface areas. In the samples from the lesions, lactobacilli were not detected. This supports a role for lactobacilli as secondary invaders of carious lesions where the retentiveness and acidic environment are enhanced.

Another issue of concern related to the ecology of *S. mutans* is the intraoral spreading of this bacterium. In a normal infectious disease the invading pathogen spreads from an infected site until endogenous or exogenous forces suppress the infection. In the dental floss implantation study discussed previously, the established *S. mutans* strains were rarely subsequently isolated from plaque obtained from teeth on the other side of the mouth. Confirmation of the limited intraoral movement of *S. mutans* has been obtained by the placement of *S. mutans* "seeded" artificial fissures into the mouth of human volunteers. In these studies streptomycin-resistant strains of *S. mutans* spread relatively slowly to the adjacent teeth and even more slowly to teeth in the opposing arch or on the other side of the mouth. The intraoral establishment and spread of the implanted *S. mutans* were favored under conditions of high salivary concentrations of endogenous strains of *S. mutans* and high caries experience. There are clearly strong inhibitors that prevent *S. mutans* from spreading in a manner analogous to the more rapidly disseminating bacterial infections.

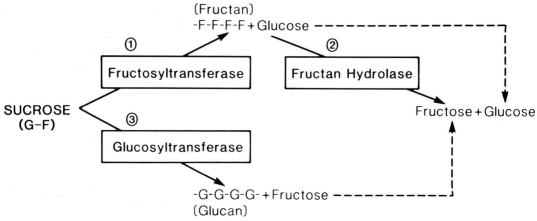

Figure 51.5: Extracellular sucrose metabolism by *Streptococcus mutans.* The disaccharide is cleaved, releasing the hexoses glucose and fructose and forming the polysaccharides fructan (*Step 1*) and glucan (*Step 3*). The fructan can be degraded to free fructose (*Step 2*), which is available for cell metabolism. Formation of glucan enhances *S. mutans'* ability to colonize human teeth.

Elucidation of these factors would provide interesting information relative to ongoing attempts to prevent caries by suppressing *S. mutans* infections.

The limited intraoral movement of *S. mutans* has direct implications for clinical dentistry when we consider the possible effects of various techniques routinely used by the practitioner. The most striking finding is the recent demonstration that by probing with a dental explorer, one can transfer *S. mutans* from a fissure on one side of the mouth to a fissure on the other side and, most important, establish the bacterium at the new site. The high frequency with which this transfer was achieved emphasizes that alteration of the microbial content of caries-prone sites on human teeth with a dental explorer is surely worthy of additional study.

S. mutans and Sucrose

One of the more unique features of *S. mutans* is the ability to utilize dietary sucrose to enhance colonization of the oral cavity. In the rodent models, sucrose significantly enhanced *S. mutans*–induced caries formation. In studies in humans the level of *S. mutans* in the oral cavity can be raised or lowered by increasing or decreasing, respectively, the quantity of dietary sucrose.

S. mutans has the ability to metabolize the disaccharide sucrose by several pathways. Two extracellular sucrose-dependent polysaccharide-forming enzymes are constitutively produced and excreted from the cell by *S. mutans* (Fig. 51.5). By taking advantage of the energy in the bond between the glucosyl and fructosyl moieties of sucrose, the *S. mutans* enzymes produce extracellular polysaccharides containing either fructose or glucose.

The fructans produced by *S. mutans* predominantly consist of fructose moieties attached together through β(2→1)-fructofuranoside linkages. The quantity of fructan synthesized by the *S. mutans* fructosyltransferase varies from strain to strain, depending on the cultural conditions. Although there are no reports that *S. mutans* produces a fructan hydrolase, many bacteria in plaque do produce such enzymes. The fructans may thus be classified as extracellular storage polysaccharides that may benefit the survival of *S. mutans* in the presence of other bacteria that cause the release of fructose for metabolism.

The production of extracellular glucans by *S. mutans* is considered to be the critical reaction in the oral accumulation and cariogenicity of this bacterium. The reaction involves the conversion of sucrose to polyglucans with the release of free fructose (Fig. 51.6). Dextransucrase or glucosyltransferase (GTF) is the enzyme responsible for glucan production. The importance of this enzyme is emphasized by the fact that mutants of *S. mutans* that produce elevated or reduced levels of the enzyme initiate correspondingly higher or lower levels of caries when tested in rodent model systems. The goal of several current approaches to reducing caries formation in humans involves attempts to inhibit GTF activity in the mouth with antibodies, enzyme-active site inhibitors, or enzymes capable of altering glucan synthesis by destruction of polymer as it is synthesized.

Great effort has been directed toward purifying the *S. mutans* GTF and understanding the mechanism of glucan formation. Several points can be made:

1. GTF is produced in several forms by *S. mutans,* and the various enzyme activities appear to work together to produce complex water-soluble and water-insoluble glucan products.

2. Although many laboratories have attempted to purify the various GTF enzymes, only recently have pure forms become available. This has been achieved with molecular biology techniques where the genes coding for the enzymes have been cloned and the gene products isolated. Detailed chemical and immunological analysis will eventually provide important new information about these enzymes. In addition, the different GTF genes from various strains of S. *mutans* are being sequenced so that detailed comparisons can be made.

3. The activity of GTF can be stimulated by various entities, including dextran [an α(1→6)-linked glucan], phospholipids, and various surface active agents such as detergents.

4. When glucan is formed by GTF, the products contain varying proportions of α(1→6) and α(1→3) linkages. The ratio of the linkages can vary greatly, depending on the enzyme source and reaction conditions. The α(1→3) linkages are critically important in that as their proportion increases, the glucan becomes less soluble in water. This water-insolubility may give unique properties to colonies of S. *mutans* on the tooth surface. Indeed, glucan-coated colonies of S. *mutans* adjacent to the tooth enamel surface may limit access to the site of buffering or antibacterial entities from saliva and block diffusion of acid away from the teeth. In addition, aggregated compact colonies of S. *mutans* might be less susceptible to disruption and removal for analysis. This could affect the efficiency of certain oral hygiene procedures and complicate attempts to perform longitudinal caries studies. Greater

problems can be envisioned when S. *mutans* colonize retentive areas with limited accessibility.

5. Glucan production may be affected by the presence of enzymes that can degrade or modify the polysaccharide as it is being synthesized. S. *mutans* produces a dextranase activity that is capable of breaking the α(1→6) bonds in glucan. Interestingly, the enzyme is endohydrolytic, which means that it fragments the glucans into pieces. The fragments may modify glucan synthesis in several ways, resulting in changes in the final polysaccharide product. In order for the fragments to be metabolized to fermentable glucose units they must be degraded by additional enzymes. The presence of significant numbers of dextranase-producing bacteria in human dental plaque has been demonstrated, so that under certain conditions the extracellular glucans may function as an energy source. It is significant that the glucan remaining after such interactions would be highly enriched for α(1→3) linkages.

Sugar Metabolism by *Streptococcus mutans*

The extracellular metabolism of sucrose by S. *mutans* involves utilization of only a small portion of the substrate that may be available to the bacterium. Most of the sucrose is directly transported into the S. *mutans* cell by a membrane-associated phosphoenolpyruvate (PEP)-dependent phosphotransferase system. The sucrose is phosphorylated by the PEP during

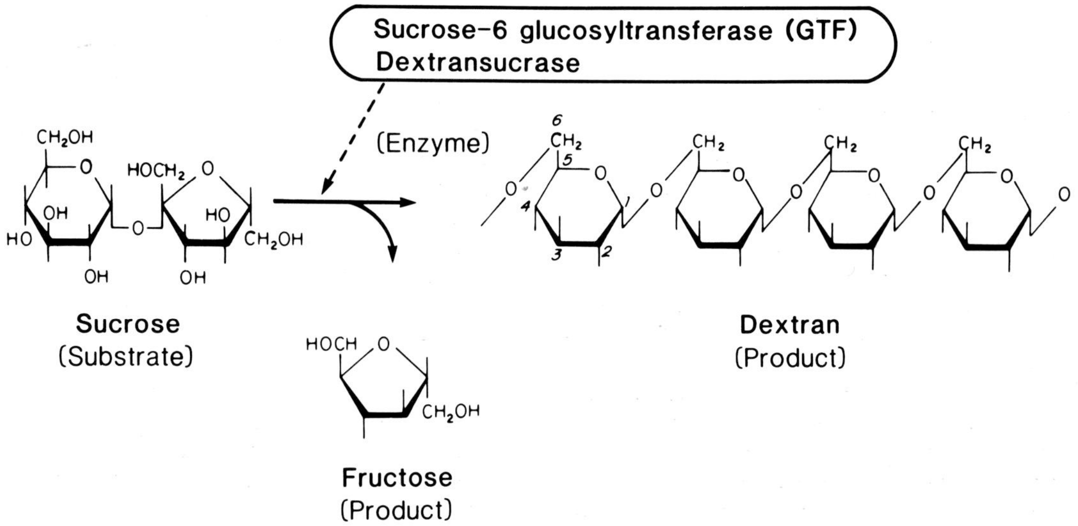

Figure 51.6: Schematic drawing of the conversion of the glucosyl moiety of sucrose to dextran by the enzyme glucosyltransferase (*GTF,* dextransucrase). This enzyme is essential for the production of extracellular glucans by *Streptococcus mutans* and is the prime candidate antigen for immunization against S. *mutans*–dependent dental caries.

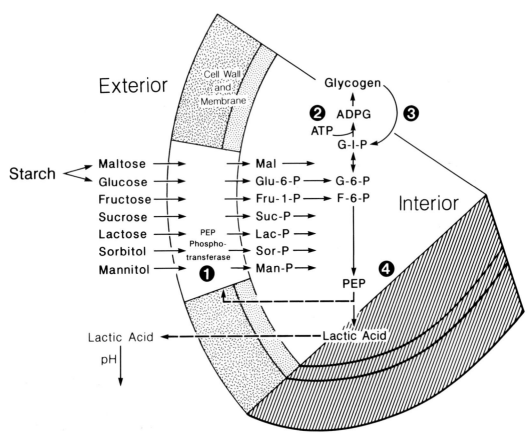

Figure 51.7: Schematic drawing of fermentable carbohydrate metabolism by *Streptococcus mutans*. Carbohydrates are transported into the cell by a PEP-dependent phosphotransferase system (*Step 1*) and can be stored in the form of glycogen (*Pathway 2*) which can be subsequently degraded (*Step 3*). Carbohydrates can also be metabolized to lactic acid (*Pathway 4*). Enolase is an enzyme in the glycolytic pathway which can be inhibited with fluoride. When this enzyme is inhibited, carbohydrate transport is reduced, due to a lack of PEP.

transport and when inside the cell the molecule is cleaved by an enzyme called invertase (Fig. 51.7). The products of this reaction can be incorporated into the glycolytic metabolic pathway. In addition to sucrose *S. mutans* can readily ferment essentially all of the simple sugars found in the "normal" human diet (see Fig. 51.7). The polyols sorbitol and mannitol can be utilized by certain strains of *S. mutans*.

After entering the cell, sugar molecules can go in either of two directions. Under conditions of sugar excess *S. mutans* is capable of storing glucose as an intracellular glycogen-like polysaccharide that can be metabolized when necessary for growth and maintenance. The ability to store glucose in this manner may be important for *S. mutans* survival and may also be related to its cariogenic potential. Plaques associated with high caries activity have been shown to contain significantly higher proportions of glycogen-storing bacteria than plaques from sound enamel surfaces. Electron microscopic analyses of plaque overlying

carious lesions have revealed large numbers of bacteria containing glycogen-like granules.

The other direction that sugars can take after entering the cell involves fermentation. *S. mutans* has been historically designated as a homofermentative lactic acid bacterium. However, under certain environmental conditions *S. mutans* may produce end products other than lactic acid. Both in vitro and in vivo studies have demonstrated that *S. mutans* can produce significant amounts of formate, acetate, and ethanol. Glucose limitation caused these products to be formed in in vitro studies. When excess glucose or sucrose is made available to *S. mutans,* this bacterium is also capable of producing mannitol.

S. mutans can utilize sucrose at a significantly faster rate than other oral bacteria such as *S. sanguis, S. mitis,* and *A. viscosus.* In a study in which the pH of colonies of *S. mutans, S. sanguis,* and *S. mitis* was determined, it was demonstrated that under carefully controlled conditions, *S. mutans* produced greater

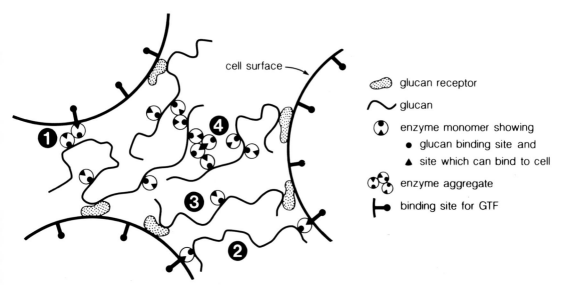

cell surface

glucan receptor

glucan

enzyme monomer showing
• glucan binding site and
▲ site which can bind to cell

enzyme aggregate

binding site for GTF

Figure 51.8: Schematic representation of the association of GTF and glucan with the *Streptococcus mutans* and their participation in cellular aggregation. *1,* Binding of GTF to cell surface receptor; *2,* cell-to-cell attachment via glucan–enzyme interactions; *3,* cell-to-cell attachment via glucan–glucan receptor interactions; and *4,* enzyme aggregate involvement in glucan-mediated cell aggregation.

quantities of acid which could be measured in the agar directly below the bacterial colonies. Support for the high metabolic potential of S. *mutans* was obtained in a study where the utilization of sucrose to form various products was monitored in small plaque samples from carious lesions and samples from sound tooth surfaces. The plaque from the lesions metabolized significantly more sucrose and produced higher levels of metabolic end products. Since S. *mutans* was, on average, the numerically dominant species in the samples taken from the lesions, these results support the concept that this bacterium is metabolically dominant in plaque associated with carious lesions.

Adherence of *Streptococcus mutans*

When washed-cell suspensions of S. *mutans* are supplied with sucrose, the cells become firmly attached to the walls of their container. This phenomenon involves the conversion of sucrose to glucan by GTF enzyme present on the bacterial cell surface. From these observations the term "adherent glucans" evolved. Unfortunately, glucans with $\alpha(1{\rightarrow}6)$ and $\alpha(1{\rightarrow}3)$ linkages are not adherent by themselves and have little affinity for solid surfaces. The charge needed to achieve firm adherence to a surface by S. *mutans* must be supplied by some other bacterial molecule, with glucan acting as a carrier and matrix former. Many cellular products could be involved in the in vitro adherence; lipoteichoic acids and phospholipids are possible contributers.

In addition, when washed cells of S. *mutans* are

provided with dextran they undergo a clumping reaction. This dramatic demonstration of bacterial–polymer interaction is best explained by the presence of dextran-binding sites on the bacterial cell surface. Proteins capable of binding dextrans have been isolated from S. *mutans.* Several models have been proposed to explain the interactions between S. *mutans,* GTF, sucrose, and glucans (Fig. 51.8).

The relationship of the sucrose-dependent adherence reactions and dextran-induced cell clumping to in vivo adherence is not fully understood. Since dental plaque can accumulate on teeth in the absence of sucrose, it is clear that the disaccharide is not involved in plaque formation by many plaque bacteria. Since S. *mutans* can grow on a variety of carbohydrate sources, the ability of sucrose to enhance accumulation of this bacterium on teeth appears to be due to the stimulation of cell–cell interactions. The studies in which glucan synthesis enhanced colonization of the teeth of rodents and the in vitro adherence and aggregation data have led to the conclusion that glucan formation is necessary for the initial attachment of S. *mutans* to the teeth. Evidence from a number of studies indicates that this conclusion is probably not valid and that sucrose is not required for the initial attachment of S. *mutans* to the tooth surface. It appears that attachment to pellicle-coated enamel involves a glycoprotein in the pellicle and a polysaccharide on the bacterial surface. However, the presence of the components could be reversed, with the protein residing on the bacterial surface. It has been proposed that lectins are involved in the initial attachment of S. *mu-*

Table 51.4: Characteristics of the Various Types of *Streptococcus mutans*

Serotype	Biotype	Antigenic Determinants	Guanine and Cytosine Content of DNA (%)	Distinguishing Biochemical Characteristics	Proposed Species Name
c, e, f	I	Glc-α(1,4)-Glc Glc-α(1,6)-Glc Glc-β(1,4)-Glc Glc-β(1,6)-Glc	36–38	—	*S. mutans*
b	II	α-Gal	41–43	Ammonia from arginine, grows at 45°C	*S. rattus*
a	III	Glc-β(1,6)-Glc	42–44	Bacitracin sensitive	*S. cricetus*
d, g	IV	Gal-β(1,6)-Glc	44–46	Fails to ferment raffinose, produces H_2O_2	*S. sobrinas*
c	—	Glc-α(1,4)-Glc	43–45	Fails to ferment raffinose, bacitracin sensitive	*S. ferus*
e	V	Glc-β(1,6)-Glc Glc-β(1,4)-Glc	—	—	—

Note: Glc = glucose; gal = galactose.

tans to the tooth surface. Such carbohydrate-binding proteins make reasonable candidates for some of the interactions that occur during plaque formation. Little is known about the adherence of *S. mutans* to preformed layers of dental plaque, although such interactions are likely involved in colonization by this bacterium.

Classification of *Streptococcus mutans*

The characterization of *S. mutans* isolates has become relatively sophisticated (Table 51.4). This group of bacteria has a number of important phenotypic characteristics in common, but the members show significant heterogeneity when studied serologically, genetically, and biochemically. Various serotypes of *S. mutans* have been identified (a through g), and the specific antigen that allows the typing has been purified and characterized chemically. A biochemical scheme has been developed for separating strains of *S. mutans* into biotypes (I through V). Although the biotyping cannot be completely correlated with the serotypes, the system has proved useful. Based on analysis of the deoxyribonucleic acid (DNA) is has been proposed that the subspecies of *S. mutans* be given species names which would include *S. mutans*, *S. rattus*, *S. cricetus*, *S. sobrinus*, and *S. ferus* (see Table 51.4). Although further work on these bacteria will be necessary before the taxonomy of *S. mutans*–like strains can be thoroughly established, it is very clear that there are differences in these bacteria with regard to their cariogenic potential. For example, strains of *S. ferus* form plaques on the teeth of rats, but the plaques do not cover the surfaces of the teeth to the extent observed with other strains. Minimal caries de-

veloped in the *S. ferus*–infected animals under conditions where other strains were highly cariogenic. This failure to initiate decay was attributed to a lack of copius plaque formation and production of less acid.

Immunological Aspects of *Streptococcus mutans*

Serotyping of *S. mutans* allowed investigations on distribution in plaques from 14 different human populations. The c serotype is found most frequently—in 80% of total isolates, irrespective of the age of the subject, place of residence, site of plaque sampling, or the isolation and serotyping procedures used. Serotypes d, e, f and g have been detected in human plaques, but a and b types are very rare. The dominance of the c serotype has been confirmed with the biochemical biotyping method. At this time it is not known why c strains dominate in human plaques. They are clearly well suited to survive in the human oral cavity.

Antibodies raised against whole *S. mutans* or isolated fractions of this bacterium have provided important information. Sites involved in various cellular activities can be blocked, and this has allowed clarification of some of the reactions involved in in vitro sucrose-dependent adherence of *S. mutans*. For example, antibody specific for the a-d site of the serotype a, *S. mutans* inhibits binding of GTF to the cell surface and subsequent sucrose-induced adherence. In addition, cross-reactions between the GTF from the various *S. mutans* groups have been observed. These types of studies have supported the possibility that immunization against *S. mutans* might cause a reduction in the ability to colonize the oral cavity.

Genetics of *Streptococcus mutans*

The genetic analysis of *S. mutans* is in its infancy. However, advances in streptococcal genetic systems are being made very rapidly, and many current findings may be applicable to *S. mutans*. Although a variety of mutants of *S. mutans* have been isolated and partially characterized, the technology to determine the type or degree of mutation is not yet available. The variants have been used in attempts to define certain "virulence factors" for *S. mutans* and have been helpful in understanding the production and role of extracellular glucans. Development of a system where *S. mutans* DNA could be analyzed in detail and a genetic map created would greatly facilitate work in this area. Until such a system is available, studies with mutated strains of *S. mutans* must be evaluated with considerable caution. Recent reports have indicated that DNA can be transferred into *S. mutans* by transformation, and this will eventually allow advanced genetic studies. A few strains of *S. mutans* contain extrachromosomal elements known as plasmids. No function for these pieces of DNA has been determined, although in many other bacterial systems they are known to contribute to a wide range of cell properties, including fermentation of sugars, the production of toxins, bacteriocins, and antigens, and antibiotic resistance.

Caries Prevention and Control

The formation of dental caries in humans may be prevented by the systematic application of measures currently available to the dental profession. Reductions in caries development can result from utilization of fluoride and occlusal surface sealants in a manner that optimizes their effectiveness, through application of appropriate oral hygiene procedures, and through dietary changes, particularly in the ingestion of foodstuffs containing fermentable carbohydrate. Unfortunately, these control measures require either changes in individual habits, development of adequate dexterity and skills, or strong motivation. Few individuals prescribe their lives in a manner that supports these measures, especially for control of a chronic problem that is not life-threatening. In addition, the disease primarily affects children and young adults, who are usually not concerned with oral hygiene. In light of these problems, dental scientists have attempted to develop means for caries prevention that require minimal effort and cooperation by the public.

The current approaches to preventing caries formation in humans are all based on attempts to disrupt the etiological factors responsible for the disease. In every case the attempts to prevent and control caries have a significant effect on the oral microbial flora.

Protecting the Teeth

A major approach to caries prevention entails protecting the teeth from the acid attacks that occur due to metabolism of carbohydrate by the plaque flora. This approach has proved to be the most effective.

Fluoride. The cariostatic effects of the fluoride ion have been thoroughly documented. Water fluoridation, salt fluoridation, and fluoride-containing tablets, dentifrices, mouthrinses, and gels have all been shown to be capable of preventing caries in populations or selected subjects. It is now believed that there are three primary means by which fluoride exerts its cariostatic effect. First, by the conversion of hydroxyapatite to fluoroapatite the solubility of enamel apatite is changed and it becomes more resistant to acid attack. Second, the fluoride ion fosters remineralization of enamel with deposition of a mixture of fluoride-containing salts. Third, fluoride can decrease acid production by plaque bacteria.

The hydroxyl groups in hydroxyapatite are arranged in columns that are surrounded by channels formed by triangles of calcium ions. Fluoride ions become incorporated into this structure by substituting for hydroxyl groups. X-ray diffraction studies of fluorapatite show that the fluoride ions, in contrast to the original hydroxyl groups, are situated in the planes of the calcium triangles equidistant from the three calcium ions. Fluoride substitution can exert several significant effects on the chemical and physical properties of hydroxyapatite. The smaller fluoride ion is able to form interactions with the calcium ions which are stronger than the interactions of the hydroxyl ions with the calcium. The calcium ions are actually pulled in closer to the fluoride. In addition, the substituting fluoride ions can establish hydrogen bonding interactions with neighboring hydroxyl groups. Consequently, the enamel structure is more stable and is less soluble in acid. Trace quantities of fluoride can have profound effects on enamel solubility, and in the normal oral environment fluoroapatite is relatively insoluble. Optimum utilization of fluoride clearly can make the tooth enamel more resistant to attack by bacterial acids.

One of the most important effects of fluoride relative to caries involves the enhancement of remineralization of the enamel surface. The shifting of the demineralization–remineralization balance toward the latter process would retard the progression of incipient carious lesions. The exact mechanism of fluoride enhancement of remineralization is not fully known, but it appears that fluoride salts can accumulate in the microspaces in subsurface carious lesions. This mechanism of fluoride action emphasizes the importance of achieving optimum concentrations of the ion in the oral cavity when the teeth are undergoing acid attack and when they are being repaired through remineralization.

Good information supports the antimicrobial effects of fluoride. The principal mechanism of fluoride action on oral bacteria involves inhibition of acid production. In the streptococci, fluoride inhibits the enzyme enolase (see Fig. 51.7), which converts 2-phosphoglycerate to PEP in the glycolytic pathway. Production of lactic acid is thus prevented. In addition, by decreasing the availability of PEP in the cell, the transport of sugars into the bacterium is also suppressed. As illustrated in Figure 51.7, PEP is involved in the transport of many of the sugars utilized by *S. mutans*. Due to the blockage of glucose-6-phosphate formation, the storage of glucose in the form of intracellular glycogen-like polysaccharides is also inhibited.

Fluoride may have a selective effect on certain members of the oral flora. For example, daily applications of acidulated phosphate fluoride reduced *S. mutans* levels in plaque from the occlusal surfaces of human teeth. The effect was site specific in that there was little effect on *S. mutans* at approximal sites. The level of *S. sanguis* was unaffected at both of the sampling sites. In a study with rats consuming high levels of fluoride in their drinking water, the levels of *S. sanguis* and *A. viscosus* actually increased in the presence of the ion. It may be important that certain strains of the latter organism are resistant to the higher levels of fluoride, while *S. sanguis* is fluoride sensitive. No attempt was made to look for fluoride-resistant strains of *S. sanguis,* although such bacteria have been induced by prolonged growth in the presence of increasing concentrations of the ion. The issue of the development of fluoride-resistant oral bacteria has not been carefully addressed by oral microbiologists, although many in vitro studies have demonstrated the phenomenon.

A very dramatic effect of fluoride on oral bacteria is observed during the treatment of patients with radiation-induced xerostomia. In this situation a marked change in the oral flora occurs concomitantly with a decrease in saliva flow. *S. mutans* shows a rapid increase in numbers which parallels the onset of rampant caries. Daily utilization of a 1% sodium fluoride gel as a topical treatment can significantly reduce the rate of increase of *S. mutans* while preventing lesion development. Since the fluoride regimen only delays the increases in *S. mutans* the fluoride must have additional effects in inhibiting caries formation. The ion proved capable of blocking caries development in the presence of a highly cariogenic flora.

The presence of fluoride in drinking water or supplementation with fluoride from birth has little effect on the presence of *S. mutans* in human dental plaque. It has been proposed that fluoride may affect plaque formation by interfering with the binding of plaque components to the enamel surface and by altering the production of extracellular polysaccharides by oral streptococci. Further studies will be necessary to confirm that such effects can actually occur and consequently affect the formation of dental caries.

Three new approaches to delivering fluoride more effectively to the human oral cavity are being developed. The technology takes advantage of recent advances in controlled drug release, where there is a need to ensure that an agent gets to the correct site at a concentration and for a period of time that will allow it to exert its maximal effect. An agent can be delivered in vivo at a constant or slowly declining rate if it is encased in a protective polymeric sheath that allows release by either diffusion or erosion. Sodium fluoride has been incorporated into capsules that when chewed or sucked in the mouth release 10% to 15% of the encased ion. When the capsule is swallowed, the remaining fluoride is released in the gastrointestinal tract over a 2-day period. The net effect is that fluoride is immediately available for local oral interactions and then for a prolonged interval through elevated levels in blood and saliva. A related approach involves attempts to develop an oral aerosol delivery system that would cause fluoride-containing microcapsules to adhere directly to the teeth. It is envisioned that the adherent capsules would enhance fluoride uptake by plaque and enamel over a prolonged interval. Probably the most advanced utilization of time-release technology is in the development of fluoride-containing "sandwiches." A very small trilaminate device consisting of an inner core of a fluoride-containing copolymer surrounded by a copolymer membrane can be made and attached to or near the teeth. Fluoride is slowly released from the biocompatible device at a constant predetermined linear rate for at least 6 months. Attempts to stimulate remineralization by utilization of "artificial saliva" containing fluoride and appropriate minerals have been successful in some clinical trials. This approach appears to be promising in light of what is known about the repair capability of enamel due to interactions with saliva.

Sealants.   Fluoride is most effective in reducing caries on the smooth surfaces of teeth, i.e. the approximal, buccal, and lingual surfaces. Fluoride used at the concentration normally available is much less effective in reducing caries development on occlusal surfaces. Unfortunately, occlusal caries accounts for approximately 40% of all carious surfaces in 6- and

7-year-old children. This probably reflects the normally inaccessible pits and fissures which are found on these surfaces and which can collect oral debris and bacteria. Consequently, efforts have been made to develop materials that can seal and protect these surfaces. Excellent materials that firmly adhere to the enamel surfaces of teeth and block caries formation have become available. Although the sealing of occlusal tooth surfaces is undertaken as part of some preventative dentistry programs, these materials are underused by the dental profession. In a study in which human carious lesions were covered with sealant for 5 years, few bacteria survived under the material, and they were not capable of continuing destruction of the teeth. In addition, sealants remove one of the primary sites in the mouth that can harbor high concentrations of S. mutans. One could predict that sealing decreases the overall cariogenic challenge to the teeth by reducing the level of infection.

Combating Cariogenic Bacteria

Focus on *Streptococcus mutans*. We have emphasized that dental caries in humans is associated with S. mutans. Great progress in caries control could be made by specifically reducing or blocking infections of tooth surfaces by this bacterium. Success would greatly clarify the microbial specificity of human caries and possibly open the door to disease eradication.

By accepting S. mutans as a target we are endorsing the "specific plaque hypothesis." Most dental scientists believe that only certain plaques cause harmful infections due to the presence of elevated levels of certain indigenous plaque bacteria. Perturbations of the homeostatic state in the oral cavity have been shown to result in this exact type of detrimental change in the oral flora. Changes in the level and frequency of fermentable carbohydrate intake into the oral cavity, alterations in saliva flow with the use of drugs capable of causing minor xerostomic effects, and the frequent use of topical fluorides all represent changes in the oral environment that have an effect on the oral flora. The first two situations can result in increases in the levels of S. mutans in plaque; the third situation can cause a decline in S. mutans. These changes cause an alteration in the cariogenic challenge to the teeth.

Attempts to selectively remove S. mutans from the complex plaque flora have met with varying success. As our understanding of the virulence factors of S. mutans grows, more approaches become available for testing. There are many effective tools and techniques available to the researcher that have not moved into the daily practice of dentistry. It is hoped that, as with fluoride and sealants, many of the caries-preventing techniques based on antimicrobial effects will become available to the practitioner. In several instances clinical trials are being performed; in other cases a significant amount of basic research is still needed.

Antimicrobial Agents

General Considerations. There are several advantages to treating dental caries as an infectious disease with a distinct microbial etiology. By focusing on specific microbial targets one can avoid the problems involved in causing gross changes in the oral flora. Superinfections by exogenous pathogens or marked increases in indigenous oral bacteria with latent pathogenic potential are less likely to occur if most of the indigenous flora remains intact. An obvious example of the problems that can occur when the indigenous flora is modified is the increase in yeasts or fungi when certain antibiotics are used to treat oral bacterial infections.

The formation of dental plaque on teeth is a natural process that reflects the presence of a dense oral flora that does not normally cause disease. In fact there is evidence that the indigenous oral flora can contribute to our nutrition, induce the production of potentially protective antibodies, and influence the development of various organs and tissues. We are just beginning to appreciate the developmental and immunological consequences of the several grams of oral bacteria that humans swallow each day. The generation time of bacteria on the tooth surface has been estimated to be 8 to 12 hours. Great fluctuations in generation times are probably caused by changes in the quantity and quality of saliva, the periodic supplying of fermentable substrates, and the microbial content of the plaque in each microenvironment. Timing of the utilization of antimicrobial agents may be critical to their effectiveness, and this will be governed by the properties of the agent and its mode of utilization.

The testing of potential anticaries agents is complex and, based on the nature of the drug, consideration must be given to the type of subjects who will be used, how long the study will continue, the means for delivery of the agent, the quantity of agent to be used, the frequency of utilization, and how the effectiveness of the agent will be assessed. Each of these considerations can be determined through in vitro studies and animal models prior to human application. Selection of a drug for testing must take into account effects not only on the target bacteria but on the host as well. The ideal agent would have the following properties: it would be safe for intraoral use in humans; it would promote rapid and effective killing to avoid selection of strains resistant to the agent; it would be capable of penetrating into caries-prone sites; it would not be needed for the treatment of life-threatening diseases; it would not affect the intestinal flora; it could be effectively distributed and utilized without loss of activity; and it would have reasonable organoleptic properties to foster patient compliance.

The mode of application of an agent can be either topical or systemic; the former is the more reasonable. Agents have been tested using mouthrinses, dentifrices, gels, varnishes, and, as discussed previously with fluoride, slow release delivery systems. The selection in this area is governed by the properties of the agent, including its mechanism of action.

Antibiotics. Initial studies with antibiotics and dental caries were encouraging due to findings from animals supplied with antibiotics in their food and water and epidemiological evidence from patients receiving penicillin each day for rheumatic fever or chronic respiratory diseases. In both instances reductions in caries development were observed. Frustration was encountered when broad-spectrum antibiotics were used, owing to the creation of imbalances in the oral and intestinal flora with the overgrowth of resistant microorganisms and the development of allergic and anaphylactic reactions. An appreciation of the specific microbial etiology of caries has stimulated attempts to find antibiotics with a limited antimicrobial spectrum and properties amenable for use in the oral cavity.

The cariostatic effects of a large number of antibiotics have been studied including penicillin, kanamycin, vancomycin, Aureomycin, bacitracin, chloromycetin, streptomycin, Terramycin, panthenol, tyrothricin, actinobolin, subtilin, and spiramycin. Important observations have been made with several of the drugs. Penicillin can kill gram-positive streptococci by inhibition of cell wall synthesis. When placed in the drinking water of rats the drug almost completely blocks caries formation. However, when penicillin-containing dentifrices were tested in children, few positive data were obtained, probably owing to ineffective delivery at suboptimal concentrations. Although the effectiveness of penicillin in preventing caries in humans was demonstrated in the retrospective studies mentioned previously, there is little justification for long-term systemic administration of this important drug for dental caries prevention. Short-term use under defined conditions might be justified in cases of severe rampant caries where for some reason other preventive methods cannot be effectively utilized.

Vancomycin is another inhibitor of bacterial cell wall synthesis effective against gram-positive bacteria. Since this drug is not absorbed into the body, it has been tested as a topical anticaries agent. In a series of clinical studies the drug suppressed levels of S. mutans on occlusal surfaces but had little effect on S. mutans on approximal surfaces. After daily application for prolonged intervals, a 20% reduction in caries could be achieved. Since it was most effective in retentive areas such as the occlusal pits and fissures, it is possible that the antibiotic did not effectively inhibit bacteria on surfaces where the drug could not be retained for a prolonged interval. The drug may need to be retained at a site for a long time, owing to the slow growth rates of the bacteria in plaque. It is also possible that the drug did not get to the approximal surfaces at adequate concentrations because of the mode of delivery. In a study in which subjects used a solution of vancomycin three times a day for 5 days, the proportion of gram-negative bacteria significantly increased. Because of the suspected role of such bacteria in human periodontal disease, vancomycin may be considered unsuitable for further investigations on caries.

The use of kanamycin as an anticaries agent has provided insight into the functioning of drugs relative to bacterial specificity and the specific plaque hypothesis. Patients with significant active decay used a 5% kanamycin or placebo gel in an applicator tray twice a day for 1 week prior to placement of all necessary dental restorations. Treatment was continued for 1 additional week. Surprisingly, within 10 months after treatment the number of new carious lesions in the kanamycin group was greater than in the control group. However, during the subsequent 2 years the kanamycin patients developed few new lesions while the control patients continued to develop lesions to a level that exceeded that in the kanamycin patients. After the entire study was completed, the kanamycin patients had a net caries reduction of 45% when compared with the placebo group. Based on these findings, Loesche formulated the "white spot hypothesis." Briefly, the incipient white spot lesion is considered a reservoir for cariogenic bacteria. When the tooth is treated with an antimicrobial agent there is a nonspecific reduction in the entire flora. If the agent fails to penetrate the white spot lesion, either due to the agent's structure or blockage by embedded bacterial cells, the cariogenic bacteria may rapidly grow and become dominant in the nascent plaques. This would accelerate decay. The reason for the long-term reduction in caries at sites where no lesions were present would be due to a reduction in the overall level of cariogenic bacteria in the mouth due to the agent. As discussed previously, establishment of a cariogenic plaque at the sites would require considerable time.

In an interesting test of the white spot hypothesis, relatively high concentrations of fluoride were used in an attempt to eradicate the bacteria in incipient lesions. The penetrability of fluoride present in gels was shown to provide the desired effect via a reduction in caries in comparison to controls and application of the agent in a less effective vehicle, a mouth rinse. The consequences of these important studies are great since they confirm previous ideas and emphasize that treatment of caries by antimicrobial agents must be carried out under conditions which guarantee the complete destruction of the cariogenic bacterial flora. A challenge to investigators in this area is to develop agents that will penetrate and kill cariogenic bacteria in the depths of occlusal surface pits and fissures. If for some reason sealants cannot be used on these surfaces, such an agent would be extremely useful.

Topical Antiseptics

Chlorhexidine. Repeated clinical trials have shown that this cationic detergent is an effective antiplaque agent. The structure of this compound includes hydrophobic and hydrophilic groups with a net positive charge at neutral pH. Consequently it can effectively kill a wide range of bacteria. Its antiplaque properties can be related to its retention in the mouth for long intervals due to extensive binding to various surfaces. An effective mouth rinse is now available by prescription in the United States.

Chlorhexidine is capable of reducing *S. mutans* populations when applied topically, although it has not been extensively employed as an anticaries agent. Under the proper conditions the compound would be expected to be markedly inhibitory to caries development. Negative aspects of chlorhexidine include its bitter taste, staining of enamel and the tongue, and development of resistant microorganisms. However, the concept that antimicrobial agents with unique structures could be retained in the oral cavity for prolonged intervals is important and might be useful in the development of new agents.

Iodine. The use of iodine as an anticaries agent has recently been proposed as a way to take advantage of the specific plaque hypothesis and the limited capacity for interoral and intraoral transfer of *S. mutans*. Iodine has been used in medicine and dentistry for many years as an antiseptic, and thus there is precedence and approval for its use in the oral cavity. Low toxicity and the ability to kill bacteria on contact are attractive features. Several studies in humans have shown that iodine in the form of I_2-KI solutions can reduce *S. mutans* levels on smooth surfaces for prolonged intervals. Lack of iodine penetration of occlusal pits and fissures or rapid recolonization of these sites caused a less prolonged reduction of *S. mutans* at these sites. It is possible that this halogen will join fluoride as an effective means for reducing dental caries in humans.

Enzyme Preparations. A large number of enzymes believed to be capable of disrupting plaque have been tested. Because of the emphasis on the role of glucan in *S. mutans* colonization, attempts to disrupt plaque with polysaccharide-destroying enzymes have been undertaken in animals and human subjects. A dextranase preparation capable of hydrolyzing $\alpha(1{\rightarrow}6)$-linked glucans was tested as a mouth rinse in several groups of subjects, with equivocal results. In retrospect, these studies were premature; it is now known that the glucans in plaque have a high proportion of $\alpha(1{\rightarrow}3)$ linkages and consequently are water insoluble as well as resistant to $\alpha(1{\rightarrow}6)$-specific hydrolases. Subsequently it has been shown that there are dextranase-producing bacteria in plaque and endogenous levels of the enzyme may actually be higher than those used in the mouth rinse studies. Enzymes capable of hydrolyzing $\alpha(1{\rightarrow}3)$-linked glucans have been used in several studies, with some promising results.

A unique combination of enzymes has recently been tested with a dentifrice as the vehicle. Amyloglucosidase and glucose oxidase are proposed to activate a naturally occurring antibacterial system that involves lactoperoxidase-catalyzed oxidation of thiocyanate with hydrogen peroxide, resulting in the formation of hypothiocyanite. The latter compound oxidizes thiol groups and interferes with bacterial sugar metabolism. Tests in rats have failed to support some of the conclusions drawn from the human trials.

Problems with the use of enzymes as an antiplaque or anticaries agents include retaining the enzymes at the needed site for an adequate interval and getting the enzymes to penetrate to areas of the dentition that are difficult to reach by conventional hygiene techniques. Sensitization of the host to the protein enzymes must also be considered.

Immunization against Caries

An approach to caries prevention that has received ongoing publicity is the development of an anticaries vaccine. A reason for optimism is our increased understanding of the microbial etiology of human caries and man's secretory immunological system. Since enhanced colonization of teeth by *S. mutans* involves production of glucans from dietary sucrose, it is possible that inhibition by antibodies of the enzyme involved in glucan synthesis could prevent *S. mutans*–induced caries. Indeed, the *S. mutans* dextransucrase is a primary candidate for the antigen to be used in a caries vaccine (see Fig. 51.6). When crude preparations of the enzyme are injected in the salivary gland region of rats and hamsters, a local protective secretory immune response is induced. Scientists are using genetic engineering to isolate and manipulate the *S. mutans* DNA, which codes for the production of GTF and other antigens. Large quantities of pure antigen are now available and will greatly accelerate attempts to determine if a caries vaccine can be developed.

Caries immunization studies with rodents and primates have clearly suggested a role for secretory immunoglobulin A (sIgA) antibodies in protection against caries. The secretory immune system's role in regulating the human oral flora is being studied with increasing intensity. Briefly, the external secretions of the body, including saliva, contain sIgA as their predominant immunoglobulin. These fluids bathe the mucous membrane surfaces of the body and their immunoglobulins are involved in first-line defenses such as the trapping of microorganisms at mucous surfaces, coating of bacteria and inhibition of their adherence, viral and toxin neutralization, lysis of bacteria, and opsonization. With regard to caries, local injection followed by direct instillation of S. mutans antigen into the parotid duct of monkeys induced the production of sIgA, which reduced the levels of S. mutans on the animal's teeth.

Recent excitement in caries immunization stems from the observation that oral or intragastric administration of antigens results in the appearance of sIgA antibodies in saliva and other external secretions. It has been proposed that antibody-producing lymphoid cells originate and are stimulated in the gut-associated lymphoid tissue. These cells can migrate through the lymphatics via the mesenteric lymph nodes and home to secretory tissues located in various parts of the body. When they are in the environment of these tissues the lymphocytes differentiate into mature IgA-secreting plasma cells with antibody specificity directed to the ingested antigen. Local synthesis of antibody would result in enhanced levels in the corresponding secretion.

Our advancing knowledge of secretory immunity stimulated a pioneering study by investigators at the University of Alabama in Birmingham. Four adult volunteers ingested gelatin capsules filled with 100 mg of formalin-killed S. mutans cells for 14 consecutive days. Antibodies to the strain of S. mutans used in the capsules could be detected in samples in saliva and tears within 1 week of immunization. A second cycle of antigen ingestion in capsules produced a more rapid and pronounced increase in antibody levels. The immunoglobulins were shown to be sIgA and were not present in the subjects' serum. The data are consistent with the concept that the ingested antigen stimulated precursor IgA cells in the gut-associated lymphoid tissue and that homing of cells to the salivary glands resulted in the localized production of specific antibodies. This approach to immunization eliminates some of the many problems previously encountered during attempts to immunize against caries by injections in the region of the salivary glands. An interesting point to be made here is that

due to the swallowing of oral bacteria each day, it is likely that we are being continuously immunized against our indigenous oral flora. Indeed, when saliva from patients is analyzed, antibody against various serotypes of S. mutans can be detected. Due to the low titers obtained in the S. mutans ingestion study it appears that a means to elevate the concentration of sIgA with a designated specificity is an essential next step in this work. A potential problem in this area involves studies that have demonstrated antigenic drift among bacteria residing in the oral cavity. This may reflect the selective pressure applied by the continuous production of secretory antibodies.

Another facet of caries immunization involves the passive transfer or direct supply to the oral cavity of antibodies specific for S. mutans. Rat dams immunized by various methods to S. mutans have high levels of antibody to this bacterium in colostrum, milk, and serum. When offspring suckling these dams were challenged with S. mutans, fewer carious lesions developed in the pups. Passive transfer and immunity could be important to man, since caries primarily affects children at a time when they may be consuming large quantities of milk. It is possible that bovine milk supplemented with antibody or milk from cows immunized with the appropriate cariogenic bacteria could be used as part of a caries prevention program. What is exciting about this approach to suppression of S. mutans infections is that breakthroughs in the area of monoclonal antibody production will make available large quantities of human antibodies specific for S. mutans. The supplying of such molecules to the human oral cavity at appropriate times could markedly suppress S. mutans infections and possibly eliminate this bacterium as a member of the human oral flora. Sequestering of other oral bacteria with cariogenic potential might also be accomplished.

Modification of Cariogenic Bacteria

Evidence has been presented in several systems that certain bacterial infections may be controlled by allowing colonization of the host with nonvirulent variants of bacteria with disease-producing potential. Mutants of S. mutans have been isolated that lack the enzyme lactate dehydrogenase. These isolates produce less acid from glucose than wild-type strains but can still colonize the oral cavity to high levels. Replacement therapy would involve supplying the mutants to the mouths of subjects either prior to colonization of the teeth by cariogenic strains of S. mutans or after reduction in the levels of S. mutans by various methods (i.e., iodine application). It is possible that the mutant strains could occupy the sites normally colonized by S. mutans. The mutants would be expected to reduce the capacity of superinfecting acid-

---

Table 51.5: Factors Capable of Influencing the Cariogenic Potential of a Food at the Time of Ingestion

---

Host factors

Buffering capacity of saliva
Calcium and phosphate concentration of saliva
Flow rate and viscosity of saliva
Presence and age of plaque at caries-prone sites
Composition of the plaque matrix
Anatomy of the dentition
Microstructure of the enamel
Fluoride content of enamel and plaque
Pattern of mastication, sucking, rinsing, swallowing
Breathing by mouth
Frequency of food ingestion

Microbial factors

Concentration of acidogenic bacteria at specific sites on teeth
Acidogenic potential of bacteria on mucosal surfaces and in saliva
Concentration of acid-utilizing bacteria in plaque

Substrate factors

Total fermentable carbohydrate
Concentration of mono-, di-, oligo-, and polysaccharides
Concentration and types of proteins and fats
Physical form, including factors that affect oral retention
Presence of fluoride, calcium, phosphate, and trace elements
Total buffering capacity
Presence and quantity of sialagogues, metabolic inhibitors, flavors, and organic phosphates
Acidity of the food
Sequences of ingestion relative to other foods

---

producing strains of *S. mutans* to become established in the oral cavity, and consequently there would be a reduction in the cariogenic challenge to the teeth.

An additional and related approach entails the creation of unique oral bacteria by genetic engineering techniques. Recombinant DNA methods could be used to selectively remove from or add to oral bacteria specific characteristics that would alter the microorganisms' cariogenic or anticariogenic properties. Progress in molecular biology and our increasing knowledge of oral bacteria may lead to new approaches to caries prevention.

Diet Modification

The role of foods in caries development has led to attempts to prevent the disease either by reducing the availability of fermentable carbohydrate or by supplying agents that could minimize the consequences of bacterial acids produced at the time of food ingestion. Such attempts need to include the nutritional status of the oral bacterial flora and the individual as well as the interactions that occur when potential substrates for acid production are ingested (Table 51.5).

Compared to other microbial niches in nature, the oral cavity is rich in growth substrates. This environment supports a complex and fastidious mixture of bacteria with substrates from the host, other oral bacteria, and the diet. The localized entry into the mouth of various host fluids has a significant influence on the composition and metabolic activity of bacteria at different locations in the oral cavity. Saliva and gingival crevicular fluid contain many potential bacterial substrates, and in vitro growth in these fluids can be demonstrated. The contribution of the host is supported by data showing that a complex bacterial flora exists, and that plaque accumulates on the teeth of human subjects who receive all of their food by stomach tube. The plaque that accumulates under such conditions has diminished acid-producing potential. This emphasizes that exogenous fermentable carbohydrate is involved in development of an acidogenic plaque flora. This probably occurs through the acid killing selection process discussed previously. Although certain diets can conceivably affect the oral flora by altering the normally homeostatic oral environment, little information is available on the effect of various types of diets and the consequent changes in the mouth on the flora.

Role of Fermentable Carbohydrate. Research with animals and epidemiological analyses have strongly implicated fermentable carbohydrate, in particular simple sugars, in human dental caries formation. It has been concluded that decay in humans is associated with both the frequency of ingestion of readily fermentable carbohydrate and the duration of time the substrate is retained in the mouth. Alterations in the ingested levels of carbohydrate can dramatically influence the oral concentrations of certain types of bacteria. Specifically, we know that the *S. mutans* concentrations in the mouth can be markedly elevated by increasing the quantity of sucrose and that replacement of this disaccharide with other carbohydrates causes a decrease in the numbers of *S. mutans* on the teeth. Similar results have been observed with the lactobacilli where the total fermentable carbohydrate in the diet can cause population changes at retentive sites in the dentition. These observations on the response of acidogenic bacteria to dietary carbohydrate may be the key to much of the controversy concerning the role of dietary components in caries etiology. Studies comparing the cariogenic potential of fermentable carbohydrates have not always considered the effect of changing microbial populations on disease development.

Few clinical trials designed to determine the cariogenicity of different sugars in humans have been performed. One of the most significant studies was reported from Turku, Finland. One group of subjects was supplied with a diet containing a "normal" level of sucrose. Another group received a diet that consisted of similar food products made with fructose in place of the sucrose. A third group consumed a similar diet with the minimally fermentable polyol xylitol in place of the sucrose. This study provided unequivocal support for the role of fermentable sugar in human caries formation. After 2 years on the various diets, the group consuming sucrose had a mean increment in the number of decayed, missing, and filled tooth surfaces (DMFS) of 7.2. The DMFS index of the group consuming the fructose diet was 3.8, while in the xylitol group it was 0.0.

Sucrose Replacement.   It has been proposed that caries could be prevented by replacing sucrose with a less cariogenic substrate. This would be difficult for a number of reasons. Briefly, sucrose has many properties that have caused it to be used in many foodstuffs. In addition to cost considerations, sucrose increases the sweetness, osmotic pressure, viscosity, boiling point, and moisture retention of foods. Sucrose also enhances flavor and appearance by improving clarity, luster, and gloss. Finally, the disaccharide provides calories, affects the solubility of other ingredients, imparts plasticity, provides bulk and body, and assists emulsification and color development. These properties make attempts to substitute other agents extremely difficult. In addition, it would be necessary to consider such things as the absorp-

tion, metabolism, and safety of the compound, practical problems in using the substitute in various foodstuffs, and the legal and regulatory aspects of its utilization.

Sorbitol is a sugar alcohol that meets many of the criteria for a sugar substitute. Although there are technical limitations to its use in some foodstuffs, sorbitol has been generally accepted in chewing gums, and a significant portion of chewing gum is of the sugarless type. Some producers have labeled their sorbitol gums as not promoting tooth decay. In animal model studies where sorbitol and sucrose are compared, the latter is clearly more cariogenic. Supplying sorbitol to dental plaque either in vivo or in vitro causes a minimal pH drop due to limited production of acid. There are few bacteria in the oral cavity capable of utilizing sorbitol for growth. However, as illustrated in Figure 51.7, *S. mutans* has the capacity to transport sorbitol and metabolize it for energy and possibly to produce acid. Competition between oral bacteria for substrates makes it possible that polyols give *S. mutans* a selective advantage over other bacteria. Since individuals ingesting sorbitol are probably also obtaining sucrose in their diet, *S. mutans* colonization might be enhanced under these conditions. Although the enzymes to metabolize sorbitol may be repressed in *S. mutans* within plaque, the metabolic capabilities of this bacterium when it is in the mouth are not known. *S. mutans* may make the enzymes to metabolize sorbitol under conditions where more readily fermentable carbohydrates are not available. Although end products other than acid may be produced from sorbitol, the supplying of this substrate between meals might be aiding a bacterium with documented cariogenic potential.

Aspartame is a methyl ester of a dipeptide consisting of the amino acids aspartate and phenylalanine. The compound is 150 to 200 times sweeter than sucrose and has been approved by the Food and Drug Administration for utilization in a wide range of foods. Aspartame would be expected to be noncariogenic and the experimental data indicate that this is true. In addition, the dipeptide has been shown to reduce sucrose-dependent in vitro plaque formation by *S. mutans* and decrease the production of lactic acid from glucose by the bacteria in whole human saliva. The compound may eventually be shown to be slightly anticariogenic.

Decreasing Sucrose in the Diet.   A reduction in the consumption of refined and other processed sugars, including foods high in sugars such as soft drinks, cereal and bakery products and confections, is a common recommendation from nutrition experts. However, with regard to dental caries, it is difficult to project changes in the level disease. Dose-response studies in rats have shown that very low

Table 51.6: Selected List of Acidogenic Foods as Determined by Interproximal Plaque pH Telemetry

Apples, dried	Corn starch	Oatmeal, cooked
Apples, fresh	Crackers, rye	Oats, rolled
Apple drink	Crackers, soda	Oranges
Apple cider	Crackers, wheat	Orange juice
Apricots, dried	Cupcakes, frosted	Pasta
Bananas	Dates	Peaches
Beans, baked	Doughnuts, jelly	Peanut butter
Beans, green, canned	Doughnuts, plain	Pears, fresh
Bread, white	Fruit bars	Pears, dried
Bread, whole wheat	French fries	Peas, canned
Bread, high fiber	Gelatin, sweetened	Potato, amylose
Cake, chocolate	Graham crackers	Potato, boiled
Caramel	Granola cereal	Potato chips
Carrots, cooked	Granola bar	Raisins
Cereals, nonpresweet.	Grapes	Rice, instant, cooked
Cereals, presweetened	Grape juice	Soft drinks, sugarless
Chocolate, milk	Gumdrops	Sponge cake, filled
Cola, beverage	Milk, whole	Tomato, fresh
Cookies, cream-filled	Milk, 2%	Wheat flakes
Cookies, sugar	Milk, chocolate	Yogurt, fruit
Cookies, vanilla, sugar	Nut, fruit mix	Yogurt, plain

levels of sucrose (1%) can support significant *S. mutans*–induced caries. The frequency of ingestion and the form of the carbohydrate are the most critical parameters regarding caries enhancement through food consumption.

Controversy exists concerning the relative cariogenicity of different carbohydrates. In general, monosaccharides and disaccharides are more cariogenic than starch, and sucrose is considered the most cariogenic sugar. However, there are conflicting data on this subject, and some animal studies indicate there is little difference in the cariogenicity of sucrose, glucose, and fructose. It should be emphasized that monitoring which surfaces of the teeth are being attacked in such studies and the type of bacterial flora present on the teeth before, during, and at the termination of the experiment is very important. The level of *S. mutans* in the animals or humans under study is important since high levels of this bacterium have been associated with elevated decay on the smooth surfaces of teeth. As illustrated in Figure 51.7, *S. mutans* can readily transport the predominant sugars found in the typical human diet. Thus, considerable caution should be used when attempting to evaluate studies in which multiple types of fermentable carbohydrate are available. Another problem would be in diet shifting studies. A subject with high or moderate levels of *S. mutans* might develop significant caries after changing to a diet free of sucrose if the new diet contained quantities of a carbohydrate that this bacterium could readily ferment. There are no simple answers when discussing the relative cariogenicity of various fermentable carbohydrates.

Cariogenicity of Foods

Recent research has provided important information with regard to the role of specific foods in human dental caries formation. Several key findings bear emphasis.

Only a few foods do not contribute to human plaque acid production. Dental scientists have used various types of pH microelectrodes in human volunteers to demonstrate that most commonly ingested foods contain sufficient carbohydrate to cause the production of plaque acids. All of the foods in Table 51.6 cause the pH at interproximal sites in the dentition to fall to close to pH 4. These findings reflect the presence of some fermentable carbohydrate in most foods and the capacity of plaque to rapidly metabolize low concentrations of a wide range of dietary carbohydrates. The range of highly acidogenic products emphasizes the amazing breadth of the cariogenic challenge presented by the human diet.

Table 51.7 lists foods that are hypoacidogenic, nonacidogenic, or minimally acidogenic when tested by interproximal plaque pH telemetry. This limited range of "safe for the teeth" products illustrates the problems involved in attempting to make dietary recommendations for oral health.

Few natural foods or food components have cariostatic or anticariogenic properties. Scientists have repeatedly tested foods and food components for anticaries effects, with limited success. The practical use of entities with reported anticaries activities such as cheese, cocoa, dicalcium phosphate, fatty acids, lipids, seed hulls, sodium trimetaphosphate, sorghum, and

Table 51.7: Food Products That are Hypoacidogenic, Nonacidogenic or Minimally Acidogenic as Determined by Interproximal Plaque pH Telemetry

Almonds	Edam cheese	Pecans
Beef jerky	Flounder fish	Pepperoni
Beef steak	Gouda cheese	Popcorn (plain)
Bologna	Green pepper	Port du salut cheese
Brie cheese	Gummi bears	Red snapper fish
Broccoli	Ham	Sugarless candy
Carrots, raw	Hazelnuts	Sugarless gum
Cauliflower	Monterey jack cheese	Swiss cheese
Celery	Mozzarella cheese	Tilsit cheese
Cheddar cheese (aged)	Muenster cheese	Trout fish
Cucumber	Peanuts, plain	Walleye fish

tea for disease prevention in humans has not been demonstrated. There are many problems with using specific foods or food components for decreasing caries formation, including the probable need for frequent ingestion of relatively high concentrations. However, it is important that a large number of animal and human studies have supported the cariostatic properties of relatively low concentrations of the naturally occurring nonacidogenic sweetener xylitol.

The attack on the human teeth from plaque acids may be far greater than previously envisioned. Plaque pH studies using biotelemetry (Fig. 51.9) have clearly demonstrated that up to 1,000-fold increases in plaque acid concentrations, from approximately pH 7 to pH 4,

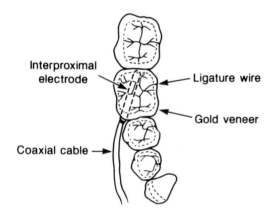

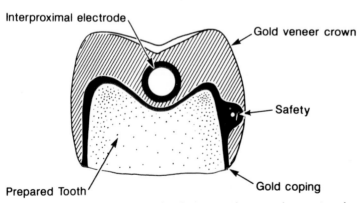

Figure 51.9: Schematic drawing of a telemetric appliance used to monitor plaque pH. Plaque is allowed to accumulate on the electrode and the production of acid can be monitored continuously following the ingestion of fermentable carbohydrate.

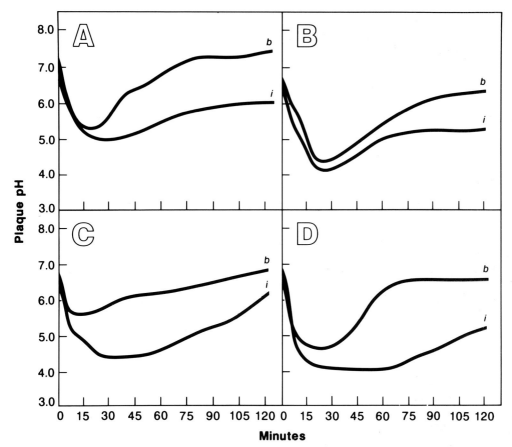

Figure 51.10: Recordings of plaque pH changes in four human subjects following rinsing with a sucrose solution. Data were obtained from plaque-coated microelectrodes positioned at buccal and interproximal sites. In each case the upper curve represents the buccal (*b*) electrode and the lower curve the interproximal (*i*) electrode. The caries-prone interproximal site retains greater quantities of acid for a longer period of time. (Reproduced with permission from M. E. Jensen, C. F. Schachtele, and P. J. Polansky: *Foods, Nutrition and Dental Health,* Vol. 3. Pathotox Publishers, Inc., Park Forest South, Ill.)

can occur at caries-prone sites between the teeth, and that the resulting low pH can be maintained at these sites for 2 or more hours. This prolonged interval at low pH provides an ideal environment for extensive enamel demineralization (Fig. 51.10).

Stimulation of the flow of saliva can aid in clearance of food particles from the mouth and can have a dramatic effect on the level of plaque acids. Human saliva has a high buffering capacity, due to the presence of carbonic acid-bicarbonate, phosphate, proteins, ammonia and urea. Saliva flow can be physically stimulated by the mechanics of chewing or chemically by the presence of sialogogues, such as citric acid, in a food. Consequently, when the pH at interdental sites has decreased due to the ingestion of carbohydrate-containing food, the pH can be dramatically elevated toward neutrality by chewing paraffin wax or gum (see Fig. 51.2).

Stimulation of saliva flow brings into the mouth various components capable of enhancing the repair of enamel damaged by plaque acids. Saliva contains high concentrations of calcium and phosphorus, essential for remineralization. Preliminary studies in laboratory rats and human volunteers have demonstrated remineralization due to the ingestion of nonacidogenic products. It is possible that enhanced remineralization of damaged tooth enamel may occur due to enhanced availability of elevated levels of the appropriate ions during and after ingestion of nonacidogenic snacks.

Nonacidogenic Snack Foods

Because of limited knowledge of the exact nutritional needs of humans and the apparent relationships between diet and many chronic and sometimes fatal diseases, it is difficult to justify making dramatic dietary recommendations based on a non-life-threatening problem such as dental caries. However, the cariogenic challenge to the human dentition can be significantly reduced by providing the consumer with a wide range of snack foods that do not contribute to plaque acid production. The ingestion between meals of nonacidogenic snack foods will 1) not result in the production of harmful plaque acids, 2) cause the stimulation of saliva flow, which will enhance the removal of food particles and plaque acids through washing and buffering actions, and 3) enhance remineralization of damaged enamel by providing more saliva with minerals necessary for this natural repair process.

Through a series of pioneering studies, Hans Mühlemann in Zurich, Switzerland, demonstrated that foods could be divided into two classes: Minimally acidogenic or hypoacidogenic products, of which there were few, and acidogenic products which represented the majority of foods tested. Based on these observations, Mühleman directed his attention toward the development of snacks that would not harm the teeth. He developed a unique wire biotelemetry system in which oral appliances containing small glass pH electrodes were carried in the mouth of human volunteers. The ion-sensitive tip of the electrodes resided in the interdental space found between teeth. After placement in the mouth the electrodes become covered with dental plaque. The hydronium ion concentration in vivo under an undisturbed layer of interdental plaque could thus be continuously monitored following food ingestion. This work led the Swiss Health Authorities to issue regulations that foods or drugs could be advertised as *zahnschönend* (i.e., kind or friendly to teeth) if the pH of interdental plaque did not fall below 5.7 within 30 minutes after ingestion due to the glycolytic activity of the plaque.

Of great importance was the dramatic increase in sales of products that were labeled "tooth friendly." In Switzerland the sales of sugar-free products (sweets, chewing gum, and chocolate) grew from 1400 tons in 1981 to 3100 tons in 1989, representing 16.1% of the total market. Of such products sold in 1989, approximately 89% carried a logo designating that the product was safe for the teeth.

Nonacidogenic snack foods should aid in eliminating the promotion of food cariogenicity ranking where unfair comparisons are often made between acidogenic products. Although the cariogenic potential of a variety of foods can be determined in laboratory rats and by plaque pH studies, it remains impossible to control individual eating habits involving the mixing of foods, the manner of ingestion, and above all the frequency with which the foods or food mixtures are consumed by individual subjects. It is diffi-

cult to envision a ranking system for acidogenic food products that cause a reduction in caries through diet modification.

ADDITIONAL READING

Bibby, B. G., and Shern, R. J. (Eds.) 1978. Proceedings: Methods of Caries Prediction, Special Supplement. Microbiology Abstracts, Information Retrieval Inc., Washington, D.C.

Bowden, G. H. W., Ellwood, D. C., and Hamilton, I. R. 1979. Microbial Ecology of the Oral Cavity. In *Advances in Microbial Ecology*, Vol. 3, p. 135. Plenum Press, New York.

Bowen, W. H., Genco, R. J., and O'Brien, T. C. 1976. Immunologic Aspects of Dental Caries, Special Supplement. Immunology Abstracts, Information Retrieval Inc., Washington, D.C.

Dawes, C. 1968. The Nature of Dental Plaque, Films, and Calcareous Deposits. Ann NY Acad Sci, **153**, 102.

Ellen, R. P. 1976. Microbiological Assays for Dental Caries and Periodontal Disease Susceptibility. Oral Sci Rev, **8**, 3.

Gibbons, R. J., and Van Houte, J. 1973. On the Formation of Dental Plaques. J Periodontol, **44**, 347.

Gibbons, R. J., and Van Houte, J. 1975. Bacterial Adherence in Oral Microbial Ecology. Annu Rev Microbiol, **29**, 19.

Gibbons, R. J., and Van Houte, J. 1975. Dental Caries. Annu Rev Med, **26**, 121.

Hamada, S., and Slade, H. D. 1980. Biology, Immunology, and Cariogenicity of *Streptococcus mutans*. Microbiol Rev, **44**, 331.

Hefferren, J. J., and Koehler, H. M. 1981. *Foods, Nutrition and Dental Health*, Vol. 1. Pathotox Publishers, Inc., Park Forest South, Ill.

Kleinberg, I. (Ed.) 1979. Proceedings: Saliva and Dental Caries, Special Supplement. Microbiology Abstracts, Information Retrieval Inc., Washington, D.C.

Lazzari, E. P. 1976. *Dental Biochemistry*. Lea & Febiger, Philadelphia.

Leach, S. A. (Ed.) 1980. Proceedings: Dental Plaque and Surface Interactions in the Oral Cavity. Information Retrieval Ltd., London.

Lehner, T. 1977. *The Borderland between Caries and Periodontal Disease*. Academic Press, London.

Listgarten, M. A. 1976. Structure of Surface Coatings on Teeth: A Review. J Periodontol, **47**, 139.

Loesche, W. J. 1975. Chemotherapy of Dental Plaque Infections. Oral Sci Rev, **9**, 65.

McGhee, J. R., Mestecky, J., and Babb, J. L. (Eds.) 1977. *Secretory Immunity and Infection*. Plenum Press, New York.

McGhee, J. R., and Michalek, S. M. 1981. Immunobiology of Dental Caries: Microbial Aspects and Local Immunity. Annu Rev Microbiol, **35**, 595.

McHugh, W. D. (Ed.) 1970. *Dental Plaque*. E. & S. Livingstone Ltd., London.

Menaker, L. (Ed.) 1980. *The Biologic Basis of Dental Caries*. Harper & Row, Hagerstown, Md.

Mergenhagen, S. E., and Scherp, H. W. (Eds.) 1973. Comparative Immunology of the Oral Cavity. DHEW Publication No. (NIH) 73-438. U.S. Government Printing Office, Washington, D.C.

Mjor, I. A., and Pindborg, J. J. (Eds.) 1973. *Histology of the Human Tooth*. Munksgaard, Copenhagen.

Navia, J. M. 1977. *Animal Models in Dental Research*. University of Alabama Press, Birmingham, Ala.

Newbrun, E. (Ed.) 1975. *Fluorides and Dental Caries*. Charles C Thomas, Springfield, Ill.

Newbrun, E. 1978. *Cariology*. Williams & Wilkins, Baltimore.

Newman, H. N. 1980. *Dental Plaque: The Ecology of the Flora on Human Teeth*. Charles C Thomas, Springfield, Ill.

Roit, I. M., and Lehner, T. 1980. *Immunology of Oral Diseases*. Blackwell Scientific Publications, London.

Rolla, G., Sonju, T., and Embery, G. (Eds.) 1981. Tooth Surface Interactions and Preventive Dentistry. Information Retrieval Ltd., London.

Shaw, J. H., and Roussos, G. G. (Eds.) 1978. Sweeteners and Dental Caries. Information Retrieval Inc., Washington, D.C.

Shaw, J. H., Sweeney, E. A., Cappucino, C. C., and Meller, S. M. 1978. *Textbook of Oral Biology*. W. G. Saunders, Philadelphia.

Silverstone, L. M., Johnson, N. W., Hardie, J. M., and Williams, R. A. D. 1981. *Dental Caries: Aetiology, Pathology and Prevention*. Macmillan, London.

Stiles, H. M., Loesche, W. J., and O'Brien, T. C. (Eds.) 1976. Proceedings: Microbial Aspects of Dental Caries, Special Supplement, Microbiology Abstracts, Vols. I, II, III. Information Retrieval, Washington, D.C.

Tanzer, J. M. (Ed.) 1981. Animal Models in Cariology. Information Retrieval Inc., Washington, D.C.

Tomasi, T. B. 1976. *The Immune System of Secretions*. Prentice-Hall, Englewood Cliffs, N.J.

52

Periodontal Disease

Mark R. Patters

Diseases of the periodontium are among the most common afflictions of mankind. Bone resorption consistent with periodontitis has been observed in the fossil remains of Neanderthal man, and detailed descriptions of periodontal disease appeared in Chinese and Egyptian writings more than 4000 years ago. Epidemiological surveys conducted during this century suggest that essentially all of the world's populations have experienced some form of periodontal disease. This chapter examines factors involved in the etiology and progression of inflammatory periodontal disease in man.

Four structures collectively termed the periodontium invest the teeth and support them in functional relationship to each other. These structures are 1) the alveolar bone, which is formed around the root of the developing tooth; 2) the cementum, a calcified matrix laid down on the root of the tooth by differentiated cells of the periodontal ligament (or membrane); 3) the periodontal ligament proper, which has transverse collagen fibers anchoring the tooth by embedment in alveolar bone and cementum; and 4) the gin-

giva, which in health is tightly adapted to the neck of the tooth.

The periodontium is subject to a variety of pathoses, collectively but loosely termed periodontal disease. The unmodified term periodontal disease usually means a chronic, slowly progressive, and destructive inflammatory process affecting one or more of the four components of the periodontium—literally, chronic periodontitis. The term *gingivitis* is used for readily reversible inflammation involving marginal gingiva and *periodontitis* for inflammation extending deeper into the periodontium.

The principal features of inflammatory periodontal disease are 1) occurrence most frequently in otherwise healthy persons; 2) accumulation of bacterial plaque at the gingival margin, which may mineralize to form calculus; 3) chronic inflammation of the gingiva and periodontal ligament, with degeneration of connective tissue ground substance and collagen fibers; 4) apical migration of epithelium with formation of periodontal pockets in which additional bacteria accumulate, often accompanied by purulent exudate; and 5) resorption of alveolar bone and destruction of the periodontal collagen fiber insertion into cementum and consequent mobility and eventual exfoliation of the teeth. Fundamentally, periodontal disease is a pathosis of connective tissue.

Research has defined many of the microbial and host factors involved in periodontal disease. The early phases may involve the action of cytotoxic substances and histolytic enzymes from plaque bacteria on cells and the intercellular substance of gingival junctional epithelium. Later, destruction of periodontal tissues and alveolar bone may result from an excessive and continued host inflammatory response that is sustained by chemotactic and toxic bacterial products and by hypersensitivity.

Periodontal disease is a major global public health problem. Nearly all adults have gingival inflammation or periodontitis. After age 35 years, this syndrome causes two to three times as many extractions as dental caries.

Epidemiology of Chronic Inflammatory Periodontal Disease

Surveys conducted in the past 40 years indicate that most adults in North America have some periodontal disease. About half of those who still retain some teeth at age 50 have extensive periodontal tissue destruction. As a consequence of caries before age 35 years and of periodontal disease thereafter, between 20 and 30 million adults in the United States have lost all of their teeth; the eventual total loss from each disease is about the same. However, recent studies suggest that these figures are decreasing as awareness of periodontal disease increases in the population.

Periodontal and Oral Hygiene Indices

Critical quantitative data on a scale sufficient to substantiate the relative importance of various etiological factors have become available only recently as adequate indices have been developed. Operational necessity has limited a large fraction of periodontal studies to scoring the reversible inflammatory involvement of the gingiva. In the PMA (papillary, marginal, attached) gingival index, the P and M components score increasing involvement about each tooth on a scale of 5, culminating in atrophy, loss of papillae, and recession of marginal gingiva below the cementoenamel junction; the A component allows scoring of periodontitis with pocket formation.

Many recent studies have used the gingival index (GI), which scores the mesial, distal, buccal, and lingual gingival areas around each tooth from 0 (no inflammation) to 3 (severe inflammation, ulceration, spontaneous bleeding).

The periodontal index (PI), which enables quantitative assessment of the more advanced stages of tissue destruction, has been widely used to assess the periodontal status of populations. In determining the PI, each tooth is scored as follows: 0, health; 1, mild gingivitis in a discrete region; 2, marginal gingivitis circumscribing the tooth without pocket formation; 6, gingivitis with pocket formation; and 8, advanced periodontal destruction with loss of masticatory function. The PI for a given mouth is the sum of the scores of individual teeth divided by the number of teeth examined.

An alternative periodontal disease index (PDI) depends on assessment of gingivitis and attachment loss as measured from the bottom of the gingival sulcus to the cementoenamel junction. The recommended clinical examination also provides data for indices of occlusal and incisal attrition, tooth mobility, lack of contact, plaque, and calculus.

Oral hygiene indices of unmineralized bacteria plus calculus have been described. For the oral hygiene index—the simplified oral hygiene index (OHI-S), the condition of each of six tooth surfaces is scored according to the fraction of exposed tooth surface covered by loose soft debris (plaque) and calculus, respectively; 0, none; 1, up to one third; 2, between one and two thirds; 3, more than two thirds, or a continuous heavy band of subgingival calculus around the cervical portion of the tooth. Ordinarily the buccal surfaces of the upper first molars, the lingual surfaces of the lower first molars, and the labial surfaces of the upper right and lower left central incisors are scored. The mean debris index score (DI-S) plus the mean calculus index score (CI-S) gives the OHI-S, the maximum possible score.

The plaque index measures the thickness of plaque at the gingival margin on the buccal, lingual, mesial, and distal aspects of each tooth. The scores used are 0, none; 1, plaque that is not visible to the eye but that can be seen on an instrument when scraped along the gingival margin of the tooth surface; 2, plaque that can be seen with the unaided eye; and 3, gross accumulation of plaque. In conjunction with the gingival index, the plaque index has been used extensively in research to yield the current knowledge of the relationship of plaque accumulation to gingival inflammation.

Other plaque indices have been developed that measure the surface area of tooth covered with plaque after staining the teeth with a dye that reveals plaque. These indices usually do not correlate well with gingival inflammation because they measure plaque distant from the area of the gingival margin, which has little effect on inflammation.

Epidemiological Findings

Gingivitis is negligible during the first 5 years of life. However, by age 7 it affects at least two thirds of suburban children. Prevalence remains at about this level through the third decade. The PMA score rises with increasing age but does not correlate with the prevalence of caries. Gingivitis increases rapidly to a peak at the onset of puberty, presumably due to hormonal factors, and decreases somewhat to reach a plateau from age 16 to age 25 years, when a very slow, long-term rise begins.

Periodontal disease has often been considered to be antagonistic to dental caries in the sense that the oral environment associated with periodontal disease is not conducive to the development of caries, and vice versa. Epidemiological analysis does not support this concept.

Surveys measuring the prevalence and severity of periodontal disease without exception indicate a correlation of increasing oral uncleanliness and age with increasing prevalence and severity of periodontal disease. When the group data are equalized for oral hygiene and age by statistical analysis, no correlation has yet been established between periodontal index and geography, water fluoride levels, race, ABO blood group, sex, molar attrition, total serum protein, hemoglobin, socioeconomic factors, or nutritional status with respect to vitamin A, ascorbic acid, thiamine, riboflavin, or nicotinamide.

The rising prevalence of periodontal disease with age and the correlated onset of periodontitis are illustrated in Figure 52.1, from a study by Barros and Witkop. In that study, signs of periodontal disease were

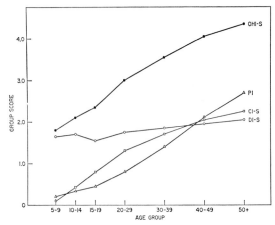

Figure 52.2: Correlation of periodontal index (*PI*), debris index (*DI-S*), calculus index (*CI-S*), oral hygiene index (*OHI-S* = DI-S + CI-S), and age group. Combined data for civilians in Ecuador (1959) and Montana (1961). (Reproduced with permission from J. C. Greene: Oral Hygiene and Periodontal Disease. *Am J Public Health,* **53,** 913, 1963. Copyright by the American Journal of Public Health, Inc.)

common in childhood, and the percentage of persons with obvious disease reached 60% in the 20- to 24-year-old age group, but only 9% of these had pockets. In the next 5-year period, the diseased population increased only to 68%, but the proportion of those with pockets rose sharply to 23%. This increase continued steadily thereafter, reaching 68% after age 45 years. Evidence of periodontal destruction generally does not appear until the third decade of life.

Figure 52.2 illustrates the correlation of periodontal index, debris index, calculus index, and age group. The group periodontal index and the group oral hygiene index increase roughly in parallel with increasing age. When the two components of the oral hygiene index are considered separately, the debris index reaches a high level early in life and increases only slightly with time. The cumulative rise in the oral hygiene index is caused mostly by a steady rise in the calculus index with age. Progressive accumulation of calculus is recognized repeatedly as a close correlate of increasing severity of periodontitis.

In a given oral hygiene score group, the severity of periodontal disease increases progressively with age, especially after 25 years (Fig. 52.3). Evidently throughout the teen years one can have an extraordinarily dirty mouth (OHI-S score of 4.1 or greater) with an average risk of developing nothing worse than gingivitis (PI score of about 1.0 or less).

Periodontitis is uncommon before 25 years but becomes increasingly more prevalent thereafter. If one maintains only moderately good oral hygiene (OHI-S of 2.1 to 3.0), eventually one is likely to develop severe periodontitis. If one maintains good oral hygiene

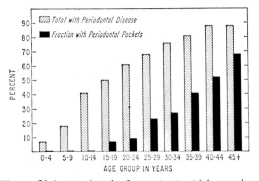

Figure 52.1: Periodontal inflammation is widely prevalent early in life but pocket formation remains infrequent until the third decade. *Hatched bars:* percent distribution by age group of persons with manifest periodontal disease, periodontal index score greater than zero. *Solid bars:* percent of those periodontally diseased who had developed periodontal pockets. Data for 1877 subjects. (Reproduced with permission from L. Barros and C. J. Witkop, Jr.: Oral and Genetic Study of Chileans, 1960: III. Periodontal Disease and Nutritional Factors. *Arch Oral Biol,* **8,** 195, 1963.)

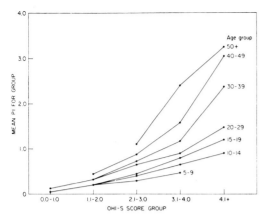

Figure 52.3: In a given oral hygiene index score (*OHI-S*) group, the severity of periodontitis increases with age. Combined data for civilians in Ecuador (1959) and Montana (1961). (Reproduced with permission from J. C. Greene: Oral Hygiene and Periodontal Disease. *Am J Public Health,* **53,** 913, 1963. Copyright by the American Journal of Public Health, Inc.)

(OHI-S of 2.0 or below) from age 5 to age 50 years, one has a good chance of avoiding periodontitis.

Structure and Physiology of the Periodontium

The anatomical relationships of the periodontium are diagrammed in Figure 52.4. The term *sulcus* applies to the proportionately long (1.5 to 2.5 mm) area of contact between the junctional epithelium and the enamel; the term *periodontal pocket* designates the clinically patent gingival pouch that develops under pathological conditions.

Mucous membrane entirely lines the oral cavity except for the erupted teeth. The *gingiva* is that part of the mucosa that is attached to the teeth and

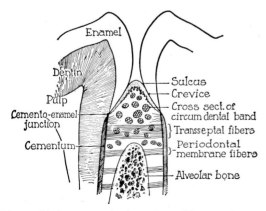

Figure 52.4: Anatomical relationships of the periodontium.

alveolar bone. It consists of keratinized surface epithelium overlying dense connective tissue. A well-differentiated submucosa cannot be recognized in the gingiva. *Oral epithelium* extends from the alveolar mucosa over the tip of the marginal gingiva into the sulcus, where the superficial cells become less keratinized. Apically, sulcular epithelium merges with so-called *junctional epithelium,* which interposes between gingival connective tissue and tooth surface from the bottom of the sulcus, where it is 15 to 30 cells thick. Throughout this area the junctional epithelium normally adheres to the enamel of the fully erupted tooth as far as the cementoenamel junction. The attachment between epithelium and tooth is maintained by hemidesmosomes and has been termed the *epithelial attachment.* In humans, monkeys, and dogs, junctional epithelium does not keratinize.

The marginal gingiva surrounding one tooth joins the marginal gingiva of an adjacent tooth to form interdental papillae. The papillae seen at the oral and vestibular aspects do not necessarily extend across the interproximal space. Particularly between recently erupted teeth, the interproximal gingiva falls to form a *col* between the two peaks. The sulcus may be correspondingly shallow in the col area. With newly erupted teeth in apposition, the col is covered by reduced enamel epithelium, a not very dynamic vestigial tissue, which ordinarily is gradually undergrown and replaced by stratified squamous epithelium from the adjacent papillae.

The lamina propria underlies and supports the gingival epithelium, with which it forms an undulating margin (epithelial ridges). The lamina propria is typical dense connective tissue. In this tissue many of the collagenous bundles are disordered but others are embedded at one end in the cementum (dentogingival fibers) or alveolar bone (alveologingival fibers), thereby anchoring the attached gingiva. Other functional groups are the circumdental fibers, which form interlacing bands around the tooth, and the transseptal fibers, which run interproximally between adjacent teeth and are embedded in cementum at the ends.

Connective tissues consist largely of collagens, a family of fibrous proteins produced by fibroblasts and characterized by several unique chemical and physical properties. As extruded from fibroblasts, the collagen molecule (*tropocollagen*) comprises three polypeptide chains, each of about 1,000 amino acids and a molecular weight of 120,000 daltons, held together by hydrogen bonds in a triple helix about 300 nm long and 1.4 nm in diameter. Under physiological conditions of salinity, pH, and temperature, collagen molecules aggregate spontaneously in an overlapping manner with their axes parallel to form submicroscopic collagen fibrils, held together by labile noncovalent bonds. Extracellularly, specific amino groups on lysine and hydroxylysine residues are oxidized enzymatically to aldehyde groups, which react nonenzymatically to form covalent intermolecular cross-links either by aldol condensation of two aldehyde groups or by Schiff base formation between an aldehyde group and a residual amino group on lysine or hydroxylysine. Thus, fibrils are united into the collagen fibers of tissue. Cross-links via glycosaminoglycans may also be involved. Such mature collagens are variably insoluble in aqueous media and, unless denatured, resist proteases other than specific collagenases. Mature collagens tend to be metabolically inert but vary widely; tendon collagen turns over minimally, whereas periodontal ligament collagen is quite dynamic.

The ground substance of connective tissue consists of a colloid-rich, water-poor, viscid gel matrix, enclosing submicroscopic vacuoles (0.05 to 0.2 μm) with protein-rich walls and containing chiefly water. The gel phase consists primarily of complexes of proteins and the acid mucopolysaccharides hyaluronic acid, chondroitin, chondroitin sulfates (A, B, C), and keratosulfate. Glycoproteins, plasma proteins, and other soluble components of plasma are also present.

The acid mucopolysaccharides are products of fibroblasts and perhaps mast cells, with molecular weights of many millions. Hyaluronic acid and chondroitin sulfates have been demonstrated in human gingiva. Also present is sialic acid. So-called neutral heteropolysaccharides have been found in ground substance glycoprotein.

The ground substance is the medium through which water, salts, gases, nutrients, metabolic products, and internal secretions are exchanged selectively between blood and parenchymal cells. It functions as a selectively permeable barrier, controlling the distribution of solutes in part by Donnan equilibrium. Because of its net excess of acidic groups, the ground substance acts also like a cation-exchange resin. Its permeability is readily altered by a variety of physiological and pathological factors that alter its degree of polymerization. Ground substance is subject to disaggregation by mucopolysaccharases (hyaluronidase, chondroitinase, chondrosulfatase) and proteases. The production of such enzymes by oral bacteria and their possible pathogenic role in periodontal disease is discussed later in this chapter.

Alveolar bone, which serves as the rigid support of the periodontium, closely resembles ordinary bone. The principal fiber bundles of the periodontal ligament continue as Sharpey's fibers into the adjacent alveolar bone, giving rise to the term *bundle bone*. The outer portion of alveolar bone consists of periosteum covering cortical plates. The cortical plate invaginates into the interstitial bone, forming the sockets in which the teeth are held by the principal fibers of the periodontal ligament.

By its nature, alveolar bone is regularly subjected to asymmetrical forces and therefore the bone must be highly adaptable. Normally, alveolar bone is constantly in a state of remodeling. The failure of formation to match resorption of alveolar bone is one of the most serious and least understood features of chronic periodontitis.

The periodontal ligament consists of a sheet of connective tissue between the root of the tooth and the alveolar bone, from 0.15 to 0.38 mm in width and continuous with the gingival lamina propria. Its principal collagenous fibers attach tooth to bone. Failure of these fibers to re-embed in newly formed cementum is an important feature of periodontal disease.

Cementum is the specialized calcified connective tissue that covers the anatomical root of the tooth to a depth of 0.02 to 0.2 mm and attaches it to the principal fibers of the periodontal membrane. Cementoblasts induce disordered collagen fibrils, ground substance, and hydroxyapatite crystals to be laid down on the dentin of the root. Cementum apposition continues throughout life by gradual mineralization of the periodontal ligament. Cementum closely resembles bone in chemical composition but is considerably less hard than dentin. It has not been found to be softened on periodontally involved teeth.

Gingival Sulcus

A clinically normal marginal gingiva is held in close apposition to enamel by its turgor, by the native firmness of its lamina propria, by circumdental bands of connective tissue, and by adhesion of junctional epithelium through hemidesmosomes and by a basal lamina. This adhesion is quite tenuous. The marginal gingiva can be detached from the enamel by careful insertion of thin strips of metal or plastic. However, adhesive contact reestablishes promptly after removal of the separating element. Frequently, junctional epithelial cells do not directly contact enamel or cementum. Instead, they abut the *secondary dental cuticle,* an acellular coat 2 to 10 μm thick that is composed of acidophilic protein, carbohydrate, and some protein-bound lipid. Its origin remains uncertain. The functional epithelium seems to adhere to this cuticle on the tooth surface by means of extracellular protein–polysaccharide complexes. The junctional epithelium is constantly in an active state of renewal and possesses great powers of repair and adaptation. In fact, junctional epithelium renews itself in approximately 3 to 6 days, compared with 8 to 12 days for oral epithelium.

Sulcular exudate can be collected readily on strips of filter paper or in micropipettes inserted in the sulcus. With clinically normal gingiva the flow is negligible. However, it increases in chronic gingivitis, approximately in proportion to the severity of inflammation. This gingival exudate contains globulins, albumin, fibrinogen, and other plasma proteins. The potassium–sodium ratio of this fluid is three to seven times that of plasma. Its composition indicates that gingival fluid is not a simple filtration product but, in part, an inflammatory exudate.

The gingival sulcus seems to be the principal source of oral leukocytes. In stained sections of gingiva, neutrophilic granulocytes abound interstitially in junctional epithelium. They constitute 20% to 80% of the tissue cells in scrapings from the gingival sulcus, compared to 1.6% obtained from six other areas of the oral mucosa. Leukocytes constitute 79% (range, 67% to 95%) of the cells in sulcular exudate from clinically normal gingiva, compared to 92% (range, 81% to 99%) in those with chronic gingivitis. In edentulous mouths without gingival sulci, the salivary leukocyte count is very low. With the aid of a special technique to protect leukocytes from the lytic effect of saliva, it has been found that at least 100,000 leukocytes enter the oral cavity every second. This steady supply of phagocytic cells and the resulting increase in lysozyme in gingival fluid, plus antibodies in the exudate, contribute to the oral defenses against bacteria.

Classification of Inflammatory Periodontal Disease

No universally recognized classification of inflammatory periodontal diseases currently exists. Prior to the systematic study of the microbiology and host response associated with periodontal diseases, the range of gingivitis through severe periodontitis was thought to be a continuum of the same disease process. Recent evidence suggests that these may be separate disease entities characterized by differing clinical, microbiological, and host response parameters. The following classification is arbitrary but serves as a guide for later discussions of the bacteriology and immunological considerations of each disease.

Gingivitis

Chronic gingivitis, which ranges in degree from mild to severe, is characterized by inflammation confined to the gingival tissue that does not involve the alveolar bone or periodontal ligament. Clinically, the gingiva may appear erythematous and swollen, with a tendency to bleed on mild provocation. Plaque is always present and calculus may sometimes be observed. Gingivitis occurs in all age groups. Acute necrotizing ulcerative gingivitis (ANUG) (Vincent's infec-

tion) is distinguished by necrosis and ulceration of the interdental gingiva, with marked soreness and bleeding tendency. A gray pseudomembranous slough forms superficially and oral fetor is pronounced. If neglected, the infection may spread to the fauces (Vincent's angina). Prodromal episodes of debilitating disease, physical and emotional stress, dietary irregularity, excessive smoking of tobacco, and gross neglect of oral hygiene have been related to the onset of ANUG. This infection is not communicable. Epidemic outbreaks in populations living under uniform conditions should be attributed to a common traumatic experience.

Periodontitis

Chronic adult periodontitis is characterized by gingival inflammation, loss of connective tissue attachment to cementum of the tooth, alveolar bone loss, and apical migration of the junctional epithelium leading to pocket formation. Plaque is always present, and both supragingival and subgingival calculus are usually abundant. Suppuration exuding from the periodontal pocket may be seen. The tissue-destructive processes usually proceed slowly, beginning in early adulthood and culminating in complete loss of tooth support in 20 or more years. Recent evidence suggests that periodontal tissue destruction proceeds as short periods of acute exacerbation followed by periods of quiescence, rather than as a continuum.

Rapidly progressive or aggressive adult periodontitis differs from chronic adult periodontitis primarily in rate of progression. Severe bone loss affecting many teeth in an individual usually between 20 and 35 years of age is characteristic of this disease process. Suppuration is usually present, though supragingival plaque may be minimal. Abundant calculus is rarely found.

Localized juvenile periodontitis (periodontosis) is seen in adolescents and is characterized by rapid vertical bone loss affecting the first molar and incisor teeth. Plaque is usually minimal and calculus is absent. When other teeth are affected besides the first molars and incisors, the term *generalized juvenile periodontitis* is more descriptive. Individuals affected by these diseases are usually in good systemic health.

Progression of Periodontal Disease

Current concepts of the pathogenesis of inflammatory gingival and periodontal diseases are based in large extent on histopathological and ultrastructural analysis of the lesion. Recently, understanding of progression of the periodontal lesion from health through periodontal breakdown has been facilitated by subdivision of the lesion into four histopathological classifications: the initial, early, established, and advanced stages.

Initial Lesion. In experimental situations with teeth maintained plaque free by mechanical or antimicrobial means, absolute gingival health can be established. On histological examination, small numbers of neutrophils are seen migrating toward the gingival sulcus and within the junctional epithelium (Fig. 52.5, A). Few lymphocytes and plasma cells are observed within the connective tissue, and no pathological tissue alterations are seen. If plaque is then allowed to accumulate, the initial lesion develops within 2 to 4 days.

The initial lesion remains localized to the junctional epithelium and the most coronal aspect of the connective tissue. The vessels of the gingival plexus become engorged and dilated, and large numbers of emigrating neutrophils can be observed. Perivascular collagen disappears and serum proteins, especially fibrin, are seen extravascularly, in addition to an exudation of fluid from the gingival sulcus. The initial lesion is characteristic of an acute exudative inflammatory response.

Early Lesion. After 4 to 7 days of plaque accumulation, the early lesion develops. It is characterized by the formation of a dense lymphoid cell infiltration. Immunoblasts are frequently seen. Within the infiltrated tissue more than 60% of the collagen is lost and the remaining fibroblasts show significant alterations (Fig. 52.5, B). The exudative response expands and increased migration of leukocytes and gingival fluid flow is evident. The lesion appears characteristic of cellular hypersensitivity reactions.

Established Lesion. This lesion develops within 2 to 3 weeks of plaque accumulation and is consistent with the clinical features of chronic gingivitis. The distinguishing characteristic of the established lesion is the predominance of plasma cells within the connective tissue prior to significant bone loss (Fig. 52.5, C). Most of the plasma cells produce IgG, a lesser number produce IgA, and a few produce IgM. Immunoglobulins are present extravascularly in the connective tissue and junctional epithelium, and there is evidence of deposition of antigen–antibody complexes and complement around blood vessels. Loss of connective tissue substance continues and the junctional epithelium proliferates laterally and apically. It is not presently known under what circumstances the established lesion progresses to the advanced lesion.

Advanced Lesion. The advanced lesion represents overt periodontitis. There is loss of alveolar bone, fibrosis and scarring of the gingiva, and widespread manifestation of inflammatory and immunopathological tissue damage. The inflammatory infiltrate of plasma cells, lymphocytes, and macrophages extends into the alveolar bone and the periodontal ligament (Fig. 52.5, D). Periods of acute exacerbation, with pus and abscess formation, occur but can be followed by periods of quiescence.

Currently it is impossible to distinguish between established lesions that remain stable and those that become aggressive. Whether a progressively destructive lesion results from activation of additional destructive host mechanisms or from a change to a more pathological bacterial flora is unclear. Studies of the natural history of periodontitis in human populations demonstrate that in those who receive regular dental care and maintain fairly good plaque control, the average rate of attachment loss is less than 0.1 mm per year. However, in populations with limited access to dental care and poor plaque control, the rate of attachment loss occurs at least three times more rapidly. From these results it is clear that, in the presence of plaque, chronic destructive periodontitis will occur in a population. However, on an individual basis, it is unclear which mechanisms are responsible for the conversion of the stable established lesion into the advanced destructive lesion.

Microbiology of Inflammatory Periodontal Disease

Nonspecific Plaque Hypothesis of Periodontal Disease

During this century, continuing evidence has established the bacterial etiology of inflammatory periodontal disease. A direct relationship between the accumulation of oral debris and periodontal destruction has been recognized for some time. In the late 1950s, careful epidemiological studies found a strong association between the effectiveness of oral cleaning methods and the amount of alveolar bone loss. During the early 1960s, elegant experiments clearly demonstrated that the accumulation of dental plaque at the gingival margin caused gingival inflammation. When this plaque was removed on a daily basis, the gingival tissues quickly returned to a state of health. Further evidence to establish the microbial etiology of inflammatory periodontal disease was provided by observing the effect of antimicrobial agents. Both oral antiseptics and antibiotics prevented the establishment of gingivitis in animal models that received no mechanical cleansing. Germ-free rodents exhibited little periodontal breakdown but showed rapid periodontal bone loss when monoinfected with certain oral microorganisms. Based on the above evidence, bacterial

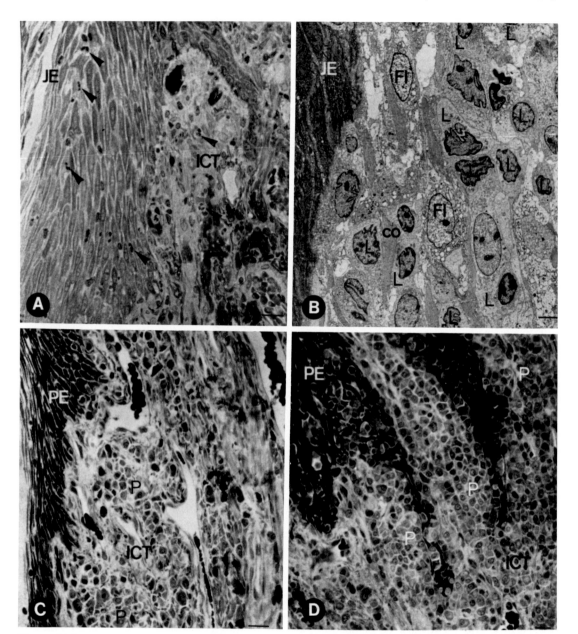

Figure 52.5: Electron micrographs of the progressive stages of periodontal disease. (**A**). The initial lesion seen in a beagle dog with experimentally induced gingivitis. Note the presence of neutrophils (*arrows*) in the infiltrated connective tissue (*ICT*) and junctional epithelium (*JE*). (**B**) The early lesion in a human biopsy. Pathologically altered fibroblasts (*FI*), numerous lymphocytes (*L*) and remnants of collagen (*CO*) can be seen. (**C**) The established lesion in a human biopsy. Note pocket epithelium (*PE*) and numerous plasma cells (*P*). (**D**) The advanced lesion in a human biopsy. The infiltrated connective tissue (*ICT*) adjacent to the pocket epithelium (*PE*) consists primarily of plasma cells (*P*). The *bar* represents 10 μm in **A, C,** and **D,** and 1 μm in **B.** (Reproduced with permission from R. C. Page and H. E. Schroeder: Pathogenesis of Inflammatory Periodontal Disease. A Summary of Current Work. *Lab Invest,* **33,** 235, 1976. © 1976, U.S.-Canadian Division, International Academy of Pathology.)

plaque appears to be the only factor that can initiate inflammatory periodontal disease.

Until the 1970s it was generally accepted that dental plaque had a relatively complex but constant composition of microorganisms and their products. Although microscopic studies in the 1940s and 1950s showed an increased percentage of gram-negative organisms and spirochetes in inflamed sites when compared to healthy sites, the differences were unimpressive. When plaque from either healthy or diseased sites was injected subcutaneously into guinea pigs, similar inflammatory reactions developed, suggesting equal pathogenic potentials. The first comprehensive cultural studies of bacterial plaque, conducted in the early 1960s, tended to confirm the notion that dental plaque had a consistent composition. When pooled supra- and subgingival plaque samples from healthy and periodontally diseased sites were compared, marked differences in composition were not found. Other studies have shown that the accumulation of plaque at a previously healthy site always caused gingivitis, and that the bacterial composition of the plaque shifted to one with more gram-negative and motile organisms with time. However, this change in bacterial composition could not be related to the onset of inflammation (Fig. 52.6).

From this information it was assumed that a quantitative increase in plaque rather than a qualitative change in microorganisms was the major cause of periodontal disease. However, this *nonspecific plaque hypothesis* failed to explain the fact that individuals with large plaque accumulations often have little destruction, while some individuals with little plaque have severe periodontitis. This hypothesis also could not account for the localized nature of periodontal destruction. Frequently individuals with an equal distribution of plaque throughout the mouth have destruction localized to only a few teeth.

In the 1970s, improvements in technique led to new findings. Difficulties that had plagued previous studies, such as inadequate sampling methods, poor dispersion of plaque, inadequate techniques to prevent loss of oxygen-sensitive organisms, and incomplete media for growth of fastidious organisms, have been substantially overcome. Today, considerable evidence supports the conclusion that certain microbial species are associated with different types and severities of periodontal disease.

Specific Plaque Hypothesis

Following various improvements in technique, a clearer understanding of the composition of dental plaque is now available. Although technical difficulties remain and present knowledge is incomplete, some conclusions about the nature of the bacteria associated with periodontal disease can be made. However, it has not been proved that any specific organism causes periodontal disease, only that its presence is associated with a given type or severity of disease. To date, the specific organism or group of organisms that actually initiates periodontal tissue destruction remains conjectural.

Microbial Flora Constituents

Periodontal Health. Electron microscope studies of in situ plaque at healthy gingival sites reveal a thin layer of gram-positive coccal bacteria adherent to the tooth surface. In culture streptococci, mainly *Streptococcus sanguis* and species of *Actinomyces,* predominate. Motile forms and spirochetes are uncommon, and few differences between subgingival and supragingival plaque are evident.

Gingivitis. Sites of gingivitis contain 10 to 20 times more organisms than healthy sites. All of the species present in healthy sites seem to be present in gingivitis. *Actinomyces* and streptococci each constitute one fourth of the flora. Gram-negative anaerobic rods make up another 25% of the flora. The majority of these species include *Bacteroides intermedius, Fusobacterium nucleatum,* and other *Bacteroides* species. *Veillonella* species are present in low numbers, and spirochetes can be found.

Chronic Adult Periodontitis. Gram-negative anaerobic rods (mostly asaccharolytic) constitute about 75% of the subgingival flora in adult periodontitis. The most common isolate is *Bacteroides gingivalis* (formerly called *Bacteroides asaccharolyticus* and *B. melaninogenicus* subspecies *asaccharolyticus*). *F. nucleatum, Selenomonas sputigena, Eikenella corrodens,* and *Capnocytophaga* species are usually seen. *Actinomyces* accounts for the majority of the gram-positive isolates.

Adult Aggressive Periodontitis. Although few patients with rapidly progressive adult periodontitis have been studied, *B. gingivalis, Actinobacillus actinomycetemcomitans,* and *Eubacterium* species are often recovered in large numbers. However, more saccharolytic gram-negative anaerobic rods are found than in chronic adult periodontitis.

Juvenile Periodontitis (Periodontosis). Little plaque is seen attached to the tooth in juvenile periodontitis. Many unclassified saccharolytic organisms have been recovered. The most common identifiable species are *Capnocytophaga* and *A. actinomycetemcomitans. B. gingivalis* is rarely found.

The above discussion of organisms associated with periodontal disease does not do justice to the complexities of the subgingival microflora. As techniques improve, new species of bacteria are being isolated and classified. The information available is based on a

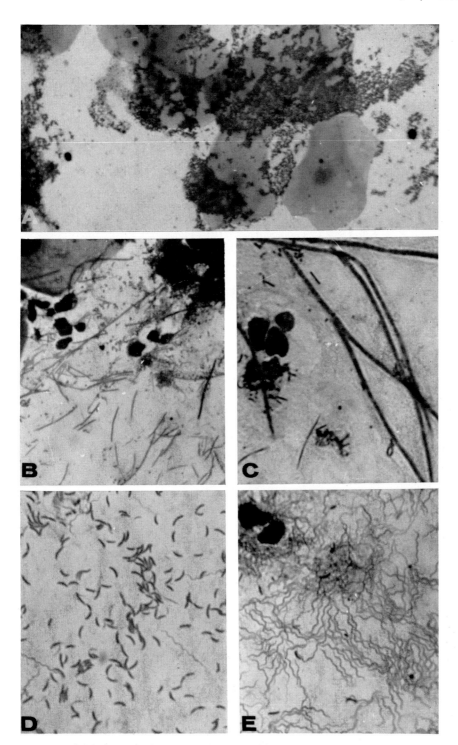

Figure 52.6: The changing microbiota at the gingival margin during a period of no oral hygiene. Impression preparations, crystal violet stain. (**A**) Predominantly coccoid bacteria and desquamated epithelial cells in early phase (×460). (**B**) Filamentous organisms and leukocyte accumulations after 7 days of no oral hygiene (×730). (**C**) Higher magnification of filaments and fusobacteria from preparation shown in **B** (×1,150). (**D**) Concentration of vibrios in same preparation as **E. (E)** Spirochetes and vibrios predominate after 2 weeks of no oral hygiene and 3 days before gingivitis could be diagnosed clinically (×1,150). (Reproduced with permission from H. Löe, E. Theilade, and S. B. Jensen: Experimental Gingivitis in Man. *J Periodontol,* **36,** 177, 1965.)

Table 52.1: Prominent Cultivable Microorganisms Associated with Various Periodontal Conditions*

Periodontal Condition	No. of Samples	% Gram-Negative Anaerobic Rods	% Gram-Negative Facultatively Anaerobic Rods	% Gram-Negative Anaerobic Cocci	% Gram-Negative Facultatively Anaerobic Cocci	% Gram-Positive Anaerobic Rods	% Gram-Positive Facultatively Anaerobic Rods	% Gram-Positive Anaerobic Cocci	% Gram-Positive Facultatively Anaerobic Cocci
Healthy periodontium	7	12.7	Not detected	2.0	0.3	9.5	35.1	0.8	39.6
Gingivitis	9	25.0	14.8	4.3	Not detected	9.2	16.9	3.0	26.8
Advanced periodontitis	8	74.3	Not detected	0.6	Not detected	15.1	3.9	Not detected	6.2
Juvenile periodontitis:									
Deep pockets	8	59.3	4.5	1.8	Not detected	15.3	3.1	6.1	10.2
Normal pockets	8	27.4	8.4	2.9	0.7	7.3	11.8	4.3	37.2

*Reproduced with permission from J. Slots: Subgingival Microflora and Periodontal Disease. *J Clin Periodontol,* **6**, 351, 1979. © 1979 Munksgaard, Copenhagen.

Table 52.2: Change in Cultivable Subgingival Flora during Ligature-Induced Periodontitis in Monkeys*†

	Stage I (Time = 0)	Stage II (1–3 weeks)	Stage III (4–7 weeks)
N‡	7	4	7
Total count (× 10⁶)§	7.78	11.05	5.48
	(2.6 − 73.6)	(0.5 − 27.6)	(0.8 − 11.4)
Gram-positive cocci‖	25.9 ± 7.7	14.9 ± 11.8	7.1 ± 7.1
Anaerobic	12.3 ± 12.7	6.9 ± 7.4	3.0 ± 5.1
Facultative	13.6 ± 10.9	8.0 ± 7.1	4.1 ± 3.2
Gram-positive rods	17.8 ± 12.7	18.9 ± 5.8	5.3 ± 6.3
Anaerobic	4.3 ± 10.5	7.2 ± 12.5	3.9 ± 6.4
Facultative	13.5 ± 10.1	11.7 ± 11.4	1.4 ± 3.4
Gram-negative cocci	2.2 ± 3.8	3.2 ± 3.6	4.1 ± 10.0
Gram-negative rods	49.0 ± 14.6	56.8 ± 30.7	77.1 ± 14.2
Anaerobic	31.4 ± 7.5	28.8 ± 9.1	61.9 ± 15.3
B. melaninogenicus ss. intermedius	17.2 ± 9.5	6.8 ± 10.1	0.9 ± 1.3
B. asaccharolyticus (B. gingivalis)	1.3 ± 3.5	5.3 ± 9.2	34.2 ± 15.7
Fusobacterium species	8.2 ± 6.4	8.3 ± 3.5	14.8 ± 5.0
Facultative	17.6 ± 8.2	28.1 ± 5.2	15.2 ± 14.6
Motile and surface translocating gram-negative rods	6.6 ± 2.9	20.0 ± 3.5	14.3 ± 20.9

*Reproduced with permission from K. S. Kornman, S. C. Holt, and P. B. Robertson: The Microbiology of Ligature-Induced Periodontitis in the Cynomolgus Monkey. *J Periodont Res*, **16**, 363, 1981.

†Stage I represents spontaneously occurring gingivitis prior to ligature placement, while Stage III represents periodontitis and Stage II represents a transitional phase. G = gram stain reaction. Values within box are significantly different ($p < 0.01$, Student *t*-test) from Stage I values in row.

‡Number of sample sites.

§Mean total colony-forming units with range of counts in parentheses.

‖Mean percentage of total cultivable flora ± standard deviation.

small number of patients who have been completely studied. However, the evidence suggests several conclusions. As periodontal disease increases in severity, a shift from gram-positive aerobic bacteria to gram-negative anaerobic bacteria occurs (Table 52.1). The microflora of adult periodontitis differs enough from that observed in gingivitis and juvenile periodontitis to suggest that these are separate disease entities. *B. gingivalis* is associated with destructive disease in adults while *A. actinomycetemcomitans* is linked with destructive disease in juveniles. However, no cause-and-effect relationship has yet been conclusively established for any specific microbial species. Nevertheless, with the available circumstantial evidence, many periodontal biologists of the 1980s suggested that periodontal disease should be treated as a specific infection by specific microorganisms such that the end point of therapy would be the elimination of those microorganisms. New techniques such as DNA hybridization and monoclonal antibodies now allow rapid detection of specific microorganisms in plaque samples without the difficult and laborious need to culture these organisms on artificial media. In the future, it may be possible to monitor changes in the microbial flora in the dental office and base therapy on the result of such assessments.

Pathogenic Potential of Specific Periodontal Pathogens

Bacteroides gingivalis. Sufficient microbiological evidence exists to state that *B. gingivalis* is associated with destructive periodontitis in humans. In monkeys, when a silk ligature is placed subgingivally, *B. gingivalis* increases from a few percent to nearly one third of the flora (Table 52.2). This increase in *B. gingivalis* parallels the loss of periodontal attachment and pocket formation. Further, implantation of *B. gingivalis* into a gingival site in monkeys is followed by bone loss at that site. These longitudinal studies in monkeys support the role of *B. gingivalis* as an important pathogen in periodontitis.

Other findings substantiate the pathogenicity of *B. gingivalis*. This organism is required in the transmission of mixed anaerobic infections and will cause significant bone loss when inoculated into germ-free animals. Some strains of *B. gingivalis* are encapsulated and resist phagocytosis and killing by neutrophils. *B. gingivalis* also elaborates various cytotoxic and proteolytic substances, including a potent collagenase. Endotoxin from this species will stimulate bone resorption in vitro. This organism can affect the phagocytic function of neutrophils in mixed infections. In addition, *B. gingivalis* stimulates a potent immune response in the host. Both high antibody titers and significant numbers of sensitized T-cells reactive with antigens of this organism are found in patients with severe periodontitis.

Actinobacillus actinomycetemcomitans. *A. actinomycetemcomitans* is found in high numbers in patients with juvenile and aggressive adult periodontitis. This species causes severe bone loss when inoculated into gnotobiotic rats. Both whole organisms and some extracts of this organism are directly toxic to neutrophils (PMNs). This toxin, termed a leukotoxin, is not lethal to most other cell types. This effect on local PMNs at the site of the lesion coupled with a systemic PMN defect in juvenile periodontitis may cause loss of protective neutrophil function at the disease site. Antibodies that neutralize the leukotoxin have been found in the serum of localized juvenile periodontitis patients but not in those with generalized juvenile periodontitis. It has been hypothesized that the disease does not go beyond involvement of the first molars and incisors in individuals who can respond with significant antibodies. In those who do not make antibodies, however, localized disease may become generalized.

Direct Effects of Bacterial Products on Host Tissues

Bacteria damage tissue directly by exotoxins, endotoxins, and histolytic enzymes. They also harm the tissue indirectly by triggering excessive inflammatory reaction of the tissue itself in response to toxins, to products of tissue breakdown, or as a result of specific hypersensitivity to bacterial antigens. Several reports show that gingival plaque accumulations contain filterable, relatively heat-stable factors toxic to human and animal cells. Cytotoxicity of plaque is indicated by the degenerative changes induced in cultured mammalian cells by debris, or bacteria-free filtrates of debris, from either normal sulci or periodontal pockets. No oral microorganisms have been shown to produce significant exotoxins, but a number of them contain endotoxins, liberate histolytic enzymes, and initiate the inflammatory process.

Endotoxins

Glycolipid endotoxins have been isolated by a conventional two-phase extraction procedure from representative strains of the principal bacteria that have been implicated in periodontitis, namely *F. nucleatum*, *Bacteroides* species, *Treponema vincentii,*

Treponema buccale, small oral treponema (*Treponema microdentium*), *Selenomonas sputigena,* *Veillonella* species, and *Leptotrichia buccalis,* but not from an oral viridans streptococcus. They have also been obtained in solution by autolysis or tryptic digestion of fusobacteria and veillonellae but not of oral diphtheroids or anaerobic streptococci. Toxicity was demonstrated by production of intracutaneous inflammatory necrotic lesions, preparation of cutaneous and oral mucosal sites for the local Shwartzman phenomenon, enhancement of cutaneous reactivity to epinephrine, pyrogenicity in rabbits, and lethality for mice. When applied to superficially denuded human skin beneath coverslips, single doses induce an acute inflammatory response persisting for as long as 16 hours with increased migration of neutrophils into the area. A similar result can be induced by repeated application of 0.2-µg doses every second hour. Presumably under the influence of the endotoxin, the mobilized neutrophils exhibit increased phagocytic activity. Additionally, endotoxin activates the alternate pathway of complement, which generates inflammatory mediators.

Histolytic Enzymes

Among the many enzymes produced by oral bacteria, hyaluronidase, chondrosulfatase (chondroitinase), neuraminidase, miscellaneous proteases, and collagenase attack substrates that form structural elements of the periodontium. Coagulase and streptokinase affect the fluid portion of blood; lysins attack the cellular components of blood; deoxyribonuclease and lecithinase disrupt component parts of cells.

Hyaluronidase is present in most human salivas, and its concentration is greater in subjects with gingivitis and poor oral hygiene. When injected into monkey interdental papillae, it produces histological changes resembling those seen in human gingivitis. The instillation of hyaluronidase into the gingival sulcus of humans causes a loss of intercellular substance from the junctional epithelium, with dilation of vessels, vacuolization, and disorganization of subjacent connective tissue. However, the hyaluronidase content per milligram of gingival accumulations has been found to be identical in normal subjects and those with periodontitis.

Hyaluronidase is produced by some pure cultures of viridans streptococci and diphtheroids isolated from dental plaque, but not by fusobacteria and spirochetes. The main source of oral bacterial hyaluronidase is the streptococci. Chondrosulfatase is present regularly in mixed cultures of sulcal contents. Neuraminidase, which hydrolyzes sialic acid polymers, is usually found in broth cultures inoculated with human subgingival plaque.

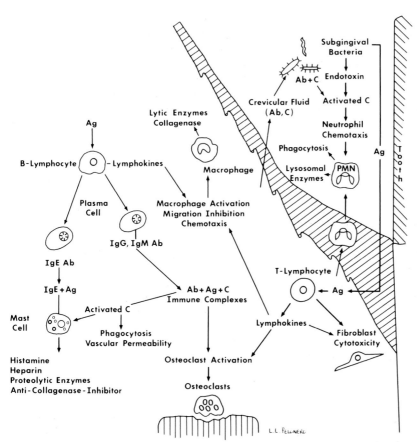

Figure 52.7: Schematic representation of host-mediated mechanisms that may be operative in periodontal disease. (Reproduced with permission from R. J. Nisengard: The Role of Immunology in Periodontal Disease. *J Periodontol,* **48,** 505, 1977.)

Gingival debris, salivary sediment, and pure cultures of various oral bacteria attack a variety of proteinaceous substrates, including collagen preparations. Ground substance of connective tissue is disaggregated by proteases, as well as by mucopolysaccharases. A majority of broth cultures inoculated with human gingival plaque digest reconstituted, presumably undenatured, collagen gel. *B. gingivalis* is known to produce collagenase. Because of the abundance of this organism in the gingival sulcus and its indispensability in certain experimental mixed anaerobic infections, its role may be particularly significant in the pathogenesis of periodontitis. In addition, *B. melaninogenicus* digests proteins other than collagen and, in exudates of experimental infections, produces ammonia to the extraordinarily high and possibly toxic concentration of 0.1M.

Cytotoxic Substances

Soluble materials can be extracted from dental plaque that are toxic to cells both in vivo and in vitro.

The specific bacteria that elaborate these substances are unknown, as is their role in periodontal tissue destruction.

Immune Mechanisms in Periodontal Disease

The components and products of the microbiota of dental plaque are major factors in the pathogenesis of periodontal disease. Some of these components contribute to the development of periodontal disease by direct action on appropriate substrates in periodontal tissues. On the other hand, as the plaque microbiota products often penetrate the epithelium of the gingival sulcus and even the deeper tissues of the periodontium, they stimulate the immune mechanism of the host and elicit immunological responses that are involved in the pathogenesis of periodontal disease (Fig. 52.7).

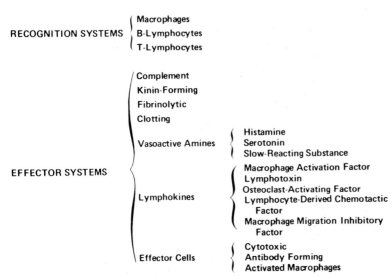

RECOGNITION SYSTEMS
- Macrophages
- B-Lymphocytes
- T-Lymphocytes

EFFECTOR SYSTEMS
- Complement
- Kinin-Forming
- Fibrinolytic
- Clotting
- Vasoactive Amines
  - Histamine
  - Serotonin
  - Slow-Reacting Substance
- Lymphokines
  - Macrophage Activation Factor
  - Lymphotoxin
  - Osteoclast-Activating Factor
  - Lymphocyte-Derived Chemotactic Factor
  - Macrophage Migration Inhibitory Factor
- Effector Cells
  - Cytotoxic
  - Antibody Forming
  - Activated Macrophages

Figure 52.8: Recognition and effector systems involved in the human immune mechanism. (Reproduced with permission from J. E. Horton, J. J. Oppenheim, and S. E. Mergenhagen: A Role of Cell-mediated Immunity in the Pathogenesis of Periodontal Disease. *J Periodontol,* **45,** 351, 1974.)

Human Immune Mechanism

The human immune mechanism consists of a recognition system and an effector system (Fig. 52.8). The recognition system involves macrophages and lymphocytes that interact with appropriate foreign antigens (Fig. 52.9). One lymphocyte that accepts such antigens is the immunocompetent, nonsensitized type that is thymus-derived and is termed thymus-dependent or the T-lymphocyte. The other lymphocytes are derived from bone marrow and are termed B-lymphocytes. Other lymphoid tissues, such as those associated with the intestinal tract, may also influence the differentiation of B-lymphocytes.

During differentiation, T- and B-lymphocytes become sensitive to antigens. When an antigen is initially introduced into the body it enters the lymphatics, passes to adjacent lymph nodes, and is then absorbed on the surface of cortical dendritic macrophages. The absorbed antigen is presented to resting T-lymphocytes via receptors on the lymphocytes specific for the antigen-DR histocompatibility complex on the surface of a macrophage (see Fig. 52.9). In response to antigenic stimuli and interleukin-1 (IL-1) released by the macrophage, the small lymphocytes undergo blastogenesis and become large lymphoblastic cells (activated T-cells). Following activation, the T-cells release a variety of lymphokines, including γ-interferon (γ-IFN), interleukin-2 (IL-2), interleukin-3 (IL-3), interleukin-4 (IL-4), B-cell differentiating factor (BCDF), and granulocyte–macrophage colony-stimulating factor (GM-CSF) and undergo numerous cell divisions. Under stimulation by antigen, IL-2, IL-4, γ-IFN, and

BCDF, B-cells differentiate into plasma cells that secrete specific antibody. Additionally, hemopoietic bone marrow stem cells are stimulated by IL-3 and GM-CSF released by activated T-cells.

The effector systems then amplify the host response by eliciting inflammatory and immune reactions. Components of the effector systems include complement, kinin formation, and the clotting system. Biologically active molecules are also involved, including vasoactive amines derived from basophils, mast cells, and platelets, and lymphokines derived from the sensitized T-lymphocytes. Also, several other effector cells are involved, including T-cells that are directly cytotoxic, antibody-killer cells that are T-lymphocyte dependent, B-lymphocytes, and plasma cells that produce antibodies. The differentiated small lymphocytes (sensitized T-cells) are essentially responsible for cell-mediated immunity (delayed hypersensitivity). Some of the plasma cells derived from the large lymphoblasts localize in the intestinal tract or lung and produce antibodies that are involved in immune reactions in tissues. Plasma cells that inhabit the lymph nodes produce most of the circulating antibodies involved in humoral immunity. Both types of immunity elicit the acute inflammatory response and maintain it, and both may operate in acute and chronic periodontal diseases.

Human Immunity in Periodontal Disease

There is considerable evidence that soluble substances applied to the gingiva can stimulate specific antibody production by the host. When cotton pellets

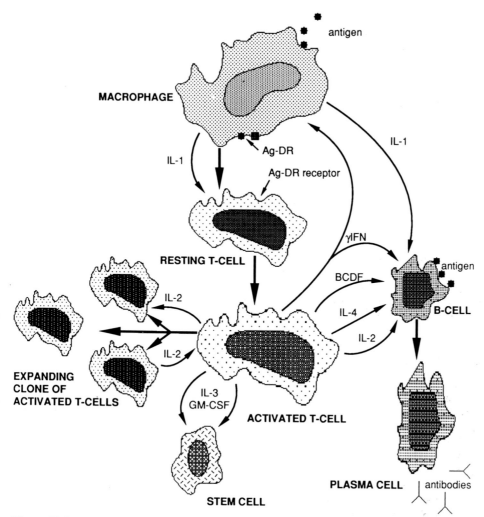

Figure 52.9: Schematic representation of the role of lymphokines (cytokines) during antigenic challenge. Processed antigen is presented to the resting T-cell under the influence of interleukin-1 (IL-1). The T-cell becomes activated and produces γ-interferon (γ-IFN), interleukins 2, 3, and 4, and B-cell differentiating factor (BCDF). T-cell proliferation leads to an expanded clone, while B-cells become antibody-secreting plasma cells following interaction with antigen, γ-IFN, IL-1, IL-2, IL-4, and BCDF. Hematopoiesis is stimulated by the T-cell products IL-3 and granulocyte–macrophage colony stimulating factor (GMCSF), which affect bone marrow stem cells.

containing the antigen egg albumin were inserted into the gingival sulcus of rabbits, antibody reactive with the antigen was evident 2 weeks after initial gingival immunization. On repeated challenge, gingival inflammation developed at the gingival challenge site, while little change occurred in rabbits similarly treated with saline. Similar results were seen in monkeys challenged with antigen-soaked threads placed in the gingival sulcus after systemic immunization with the same antigen. These and other similar studies clearly show that immunization can be attained through the gingiva and that inflammation develops on challenge with antigen when specific antibody titers exist.

Antibodies. Using several assays to measure specific antibodies such as immunofluorescence, hemagglutination, and precipitation in gel, antibodies to many periodontal microorganisms have been observed in humans. Antibodies in human serum have been detected to *L. buccalis, Fusobacterium, T. microdentium, Actinomyces, Veillonella,* and *B. melaninogenicus.* While some studies have found a relationship between antibody titer and disease, others have not. Use of a sensitive enzyme-linked immunosorbent assay (ELISA) demonstrated that subjects with chronic adult periodontitis were found to have significantly higher antibody titers reactive with *B. gingivalis* than subjects with gingivitis or juvenile

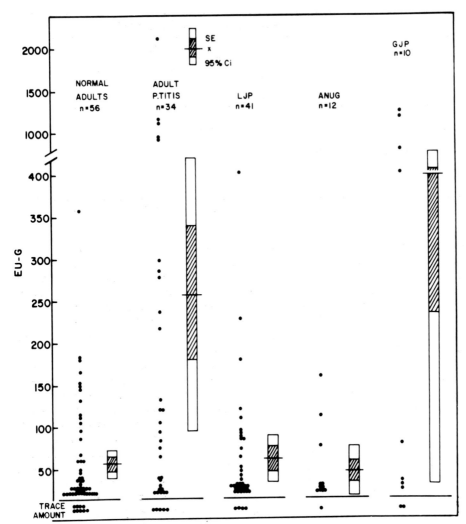

Figure 52.10: Levels of IgG specific for oral *Bacteroides asaccharolyticus* (*B. gingivalis*) in various periodontal conditions. Each point represents the antibody activity level of an individual serum sample. Shown for each group is the mean ± standard error (*SE:* □) and ± the 95% confidence interval (*CI:* □). *ANUG,* acute necrotizing ulcerative gingivitis; *P. TITIS,* periodontitis; *LJP,* localized juvenile periodontitis; *GJP,* generalized juvenile periodontitis. (Reproduced with permission from C. Mouton, et al.: Serum Antibodies in Oral *Bacteroides asaccharolyticus* (*Bacteroides gingivalis*): Relationship to Age and Periodontal Disease. *Infect Immun,* **31,** 182, 1981.)

periodontitis (Fig. 52.10). On the other hand, higher antibody titers to *A. actinomycetemcomitans* were seen in juvenile periodontitis patients than in subjects with chronic adult periodontitis. It is not surprising that these findings correlate with the microbiological findings in these disease states.

Evidence exists that microbial antigens enter the gingival tissue. Therefore, interaction of these foreign substances with specific antibody may occur in the gingiva. Immunofluorescent studies of inflamed gingiva have demonstrated the presence of antigen–antibody complexes and C3 deposition in the gingival tissue. These interactions could activate complement

as well as stimulate other tissue destructive mechanisms described in Table 52.3. On the other hand, antibodies may exert a protective effect by neutralizing bacterial toxins or enzymes as well as by enhancing the phagocytosis and killing of plaque microorganisms (see Table 52.3).

Complement and Periodontal Disease. Recent evidence suggests that complement (C′) activation may be an important mechanism in the local inflammatory process occurring in periodontal disease. Activation of the classical pathway by antigen–antibody complexes or of the alternate pathway by such substances as endotoxin leads to the generation

Table 52.3: Possible Role of Gingival Antibodies in Periodontal Disease*

Reaction or Process	Effects
1. Activation of C′ by Ag-Ab complexes	Protective early changes in inflammation
2. Phagocytosis of Ag-Ab complexes by PMNL with release of lysosomes	Destructive
3. Enhanced lymphocyte stimulation by Ag-Ab complexes	Release of lymphokines with protective and destructive effects
4. Blocking of lymphocytes by free antibody or by Ag-Ab complexes	Suppression of cell-mediated immune reactions
5. Neutralization of bacterial allergens, toxins, or histolytic enzymes	Protective
6. Enhanced opsonization or bacteriolysis of plaque bacteria	Protective

*Reproduced with permission from R. Genco, et al.: Antibody Mediated Effects on the Periodontium. *J Periodontol,* **45,** 330, 1974.

of complement fragments with potent biological activity. Activation of either pathway produces C3a and C5a, which have been shown to increase vascular permeability; in addition, C5a is chemotactic for neutrophils and monocytes. Other tissue destructive mechanisms in which complement components may play a significant role include the release of lytic enzymes from neutrophils, stimulation of lymphokine release by B-lymphocytes, and activation of prostaglandin-mediated bone resorption. The generation of these inflammatory mediators, as well as others listed in Table 52.4, may contribute significantly to the chronic inflammation and tissue destruction associated with periodontal disease.

The potential for complement activation to occur in the periodontal lesion by the classical pathway is associated with the presence of antigen and specific antibody of the IgG or IgM class. It is clear that foreign substances of potent antigenicity can enter the gingival tissue and sensitize the host to produce specific antibodies. Bacterial antigens have been shown to be present in inflamed periodontal tissues. There is also considerable evidence that humans have significant titers of antibody to many bacterial antigens derived from the periodontal microflora. Interaction between these specific antibodies and bacterial antigens, either within the gingival tissue or in the periodontal pocket, may cause activation of the classical complement pathway and the elaboration of inflammatory mediators.

Activation of the alternate pathway may also occur in periodontal disease. Gram-negative bacteria, which predominate in lesions of periodontitis, contain endotoxins in their outer membrane. Endotoxins have been shown to be potent activators of the alternate pathway. Products of certain gram-positive organisms, including actinomycetes and streptococci, can also activate complement in the absence of specific antibody. Activation by the alternative pathway will generate similar inflammatory mediators as those produced from classical pathway activation, including C3a and C5a.

Much of the direct evidence concerning the role of C′ in periodontal inflammation has been gathered in the study of the local exudate of the periodontal lesion, gingival fluid. Gingival fluid arises from the gingival capillaries as a transudate of serum and is modified by the inflammatory process as it exits into the oral cavity through the orifice of the gingival sulcus or pocket. Studies of the cellular, protein, carbohydrate, and enzymatic constituents of gingival fluid from inflamed periodontal lesions show it to be an altered inflammatory exudate. Although there is controversy as to whether gingival fluid flow occurs in periodontal health, it is known that the rate of fluid flow increases with inflammation. Analyses of the protein constituents of gingival fluid have shown that gingival fluid represents a 15% to 30% dilution of serum. However, native C3 has been shown to be reduced to 25% of the serum level, suggesting the possibility of

Table 52.4: Biological Effects of Components of the Complement System*

Activity	Complement Components
Cytolytic and cytotoxic damage to cells	C1–9
Chemotactic activity for leukocytes	C3a, C5a, C5, 6, 7
Histamine release from mast cells	C3a, C5a
Increased vascular permeability	C3a, C5a
Kinin activity	C2, C3a
Lysosomal enzyme release from leukocytes	C5a
Promotion of phagocytosis	C3, C5
Enhancement of blood clotting	C6
Promotion of clot lysis	C3, C4
Inactivation of bacterial lipopolysaccharides from endotoxin	C5, C6

*Reproduced with permission from R. J. Nisengard: The Role of Immunology in Peridontal Disease. *J Periodontol,* **48,** 505, 1977.

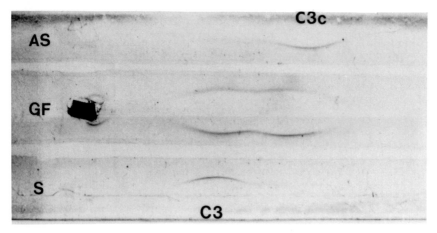

Figure 52.11: Immunoelectrophoretic pattern obtained when anti-human C3/C3c is reacted with zymosan-activated serum (*AS,* positive control with C3c, *top*), gingival fluid (*GF*) from a lesion of gingivitis (C3 + C3c, *middle*), and fresh serum (*S,* negative control, C3 only, *bottom*). The gingival fluid shows a pattern indicative of a complement activation. (Adapted with permission from M. R. Patters, H. A. Schenkein, and A. Weinstein: A Method for Detection of Complement Cleavage in Gingival Fluid. *J Dent Res,* **58,** 1620, 1979.)

its utilization by complement activation. Further studies confirmed that C3 is cleaved in gingival fluid derived from severe periodontal lesions, as the terminal cleavage products C3c and C3d are present (Fig. 52.11). Recent studies have found a strong correlation between the extent of complement cleavage in gingival fluid and the severity of periodontal inflammation and tissue destruction. Lastly, it has been shown that the extent of complement cleavage in gingival fluid is significantly reduced following periodontal therapy of patients with periodontitis.

To determine if components of the classical and/or alternate complement pathways were utilized in gingival fluid, both C4 (classical pathway component) and B (alternate pathway component) were assessed for cleavage. Cleavage of B to the active enzyme Bb was uniformly found in all fluids from lesions of both adult and juvenile periodontitis. However, cleavage of C4 occurred rarely in adult periodontitis, but was commonly observed in gingival fluid from juvenile periodontitis lesions.

These alterations in C′ components in gingival fluid might occur due to the action of nonspecific bacterial proteases rather than classical or alternate pathway activation. However, the available direct and indirect evidence suggests that activation of the complement system may play an important role in periodontal inflammation.

Immediate Hypersensitivity and Periodontal Disease

As described later, one of the immunological responses to the entrance of the bacterial antigens of dental plaque into the tissues of the periodontium is the development of cell-mediated immunity or delayed hypersensitivity, an important factor in the pathogenesis of periodontal disease. Depending on the nature of the bacterial antigen, however, the host may develop another immunological response that results in the formation of humoral antibodies and an immediate hypersensitivity, which is also called atopic allergy, anaphylactic reaction, or reagin-dependent allergy. Even a single pathogenic bacterial species, e.g., *Mycobacterium tuberculosis,* will induce both delayed and immediate types of hypersensitivity, with delayed hypersensitivity predominating over immediate hypersensitivity. All of the elements necessary for the formation of an immediate type of hypersensitivity are present in the tissues of the oral cavity of a human host. Though its exact role has not been entirely defined, this mechanism undoubtedly functions in the pathogenesis of periodontal disease.

The mediator of immediate type hypersensitivity is the reaginic or humoral antibody designated as IgE. The plasma cells that form IgE are found principally in respiratory and gastrointestinal mucosa and in regional lymph nodes. They are also present in the gingiva. IgE is formed in tissues and, even though it is present in low concentrations, its participation in the allergic reactions is critical. IgE does not ordinarily activate complement by the classical pathway. It does react with specific receptor sites in the membranes of tissue cells. Mast cells and basophilic leukocytes have specific receptor sites for IgE on their cell membranes, and IgE is homocytotropic for these cells. These cells are a source of the inflammatory agents histamine, serotonin, and heparin when properly stimulated by bacterial antigens.

Immediate hypersensitivity is mediated by the interaction of a specific antigen with IgE fixed to tissue cells. In this interaction, alterations occur in the Fc portion of the IgE antibodies. This reaction activates energy-dependent reactions that release histamine, bradykinin, and slow-reacting substance of anaphylaxis (SRS-A). While serotonin is involved in this type of hypersensitivity in animals, it has not been found to be released in human immediate hypersensitivity reactions. Histamine's pharmacological action increases capillary permeability, contracts smooth muscle, stimulates exocrine glands, causes dilation of blood vessels, and increases venule permeability. In the skin it causes a wheal and erythema response. SRS-A causes smooth muscle contraction and increases vascular permeability. Bradykinin is involved with smooth muscle contraction, vasodilation, capillary permeability, and migration of leukocytes; it also causes pain.

The mast cells seen in biopsies of inflamed gingiva have a similar ultrastructural appearance as mast cells in immediate hypersensitivity reactions. Following an immediate hypersensitivity reaction, or as seen in gingival inflammation, the granules of mast cells are enlarged and their perigranular membranes are ruptured; the contents of the ruptured granules tend to mix together in the cytoplasm.

Other changes in inflamed gingival tissue also indicate that immediate hypersensitivity may be involved in the pathogenesis of periodontal disease. The histamine levels are increased in inflamed gingival tissues in comparison to normal gingiva, as indicated by analysis of biopsied tissues. One of the clinical responses indicative of immediate hypersensitivity is the wheal-and-flare reaction when a susceptible individual is challenged with an antigen. A significant correlation exists between the incidence of immediate hypersensitivity to plaque bacterial antigens and the severity of periodontal disease.

Cell-Mediated Immunity and Periodontal Disease

Cell-mediated immunity seems to be an important factor in the pathogenesis of periodontal disease. In the early gingival lesions, the cellular response is characterized by a predominance of small or medium-sized lymphocytes, together with blastogenic lymphocytes. This cellular response is typical of delayed hypersensitivity. In chronic periodontal lesions, antibody-producing plasma cells predominate and T-lymphocytes are also present.

Cell-mediated immunity is initiated by T-lymphocytes. When immunocompetent lymphocytes are initially exposed to an appropriate antigen, it sensitizes them and they transform and replicate. The

---

Table 52.5: Some of the Biological Activities of Mediators of Cell-Mediated Immunity (Lymphokines)*

Inhibition of macrophage migration (MIF)
Chemotactic for macrophages
Activation of macrophages
Inhibition of leukocyte migration
Chemotactic for neutrophils, basophils, and eosinophils
Act as mitogens inducing blast formation of nonsensitized lymphocytes
Transfer cell-mediated immunity
Cytotoxic for fibroblasts
Osteoclast activating factor (OAF)

*Reproduced with permission from R. J. Nisengard: The Role of Immunology in Periodontal Disease. *J Periodontol,* **48,** 505, 1977.

---

transformed T-cells continuously recirculate in lymphatic and vascular channels to other tissues and organs. If transformed cells intercept their specific antigen, they produce substances called lymphokines that can directly destroy tissues. The lymphokines may also activate other monocyte-derived cells to destroy tissues (Table 52.5). Host cells that have antigens on their surface may be subject to direct cell-mediated cytotoxic reactions.

Cell-mediated immunity has been studied by culturing lymphocytes from peripheral blood, spleen, or lymph nodes. An appropriate antigen stimulates these cultured lymphocytes to transform and proliferate if such lymphocytes were sensitized before culturing. In periodontal disease, bacterial antigens which have entered through the gingiva interact with immunocompetent lymphocytes, and this clone of specifically sensitized cells expands by cell division and circulates throughout the body (Fig. 52.12). When these specifically sensitized lymphocytes are cultured in vitro with specific antigen, these cells synthesize and release lymphokines and then proliferate. In vitro assays to determine if an individual shows significant sensitization to a specific antigen generally measure either lymphokine release or subsequent cell division. Assessment of lymphokine release requires an assay to measure the biological activity of these substances, such as fibroblast killing by lymphotoxin or macrophage migration inhibition by migration inhibition factor. Measures of cell division are generally easier, as de novo synthesis of DNA can be assessed by incorporation of radiolabeled thymidine. Measurement of in vitro lymphocyte proliferation stimulated by specific antigen is termed "lymphocyte transformation" or "lymphocyte blastogenesis." These assays of cell-mediated immunity provide information similar to in vivo skin tests such as the tuberculin skin test for tuberculosis. If an individual has been significantly sensitized by previous exposure to a specific antigen,

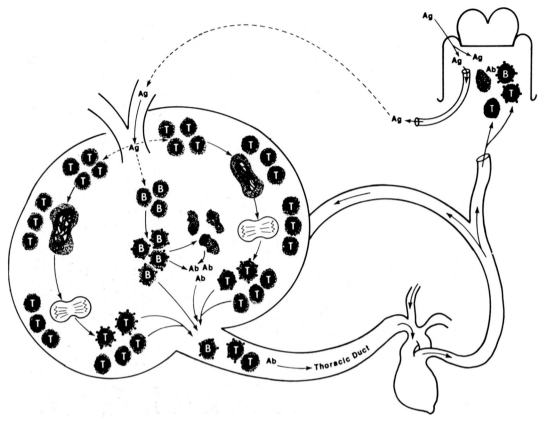

Figure 52.12: Lymphocyte recirculation from peripheral lymphoid tissues to organs and tissues via the vascular and blood channels. The initial exposure of immunocompetent lymphocytes to antigen (*Ag*) at the gingiva (or in other peripheral lymphoid tissue) results in sensitization of T-lymphocytes (*T*), which induces them to undergo transformation and replication. During this time the B-lymphocytes synthesize antibodies (*Ab*). (Reproduced with permission from J. E. Horton, J. J. Oppenheim, and S. E. Mergenhagen: A Role of Cell-mediated Immunity in Pathogenesis of Periodontal Disease. *J Periodontol,* **45,** 351, 1974.)

reexposure to this antigen, either in vivo by skin injection or in vitro by culturing lymphocytes with the specific antigen, will cause lymphokine release and proliferation. In vivo, these reactions cause a delayed (48 to 72 hours) skin reaction. In vitro, lymphocyte blastogenesis or lymphokine assays provide quantitative data as to the magnitude of sensitization of the individual to the antigen.

Studies of cell-mediated immunity by measurement of lymphokine release clearly show that lymphocytes from individuals with periodontal disease release lymphokines when cultured with plaque-related antigens. If this lymphokine release occurs in the gingival tissue when antigen and sensitized lymphocyte interact, the potential exists for cellular infiltration and tissue destruction. Lymphokines have many deleterious effects on tissue, including destruction of fibroblasts, dissolution of collagenous fibers, and stimulation of bone resorption. Lymphocytes produce a macrophage migration inhibitory factor that inhibits the migration of

macrophages. Lymphotoxin (LT) is produced by sensitized lymphocytes from persons with periodontal disease and is cytotoxic for cultured human gingival fibroblasts. LT is not produced by plaque-stimulated lymphocytes from persons without periodontal disease or from unstimulated lymphocytes from individuals with periodontal disease (Fig. 52.13).

Another lymphokine (cytokine), termed osteoclast activating factor (OAF), has been found in the culture fluid of leukocytes from persons with periodontal disease when such cultures were stimulated with human dental plaque extract. OAF induces osteoclastic activity in tissue cultures containing bone. OAF action is distinguishable from that of parathormone, an active metabolite of vitamin D, and from prostaglandins. Recent evidence suggests that OAF may be homologous to interleukin-1.

During the 1970s, considerable research into cell-mediated immunity provided a better but still incomplete understanding of its role in periodontal disease.

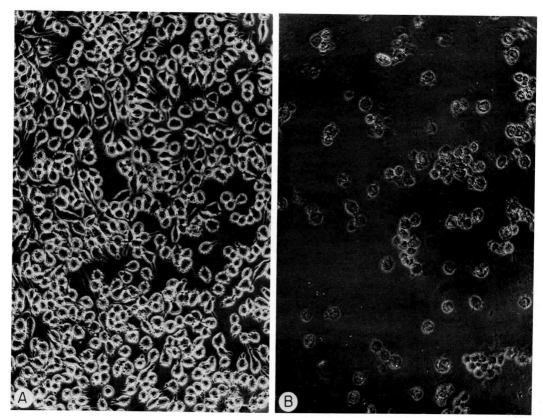

Figure 52.13: Effect of lymphotoxin on cultured human gingival fibroblasts. (**A**) Normal appearing fibroblasts exposed to cell-free supernatant from plaque-stimulated nonreactive leukocyte cultures from a clinically normal subject (× 160). (**B**) Damaged fibroblasts exposed to cell-free supernatant from plaque-stimulated reactive leukocyte cultures from a subject with periodontal disease (× 160). (Reproduced with permission from J. E. Horton, J. J. Oppenheim, and S. E. Mergenhagen: A Role of Cell-mediated Immunity in the Pathogenesis of Periodontal Disease. *J Periodontol,* **45,** 31, 1974.)

It is clear that the ability of dental plaque to stimulate lymphocyte transformation relates to a specific antigenic component rather than to a generalized reaction. At birth, lymphocytes obtained from cord blood are immunologically competent but do not respond to dental plaque antigens, indicating little or no previous exposure to them. Initial studies suggested that antigens from dental plaque stimulate lymphocytes to transform in proportion to the clinical severity of periodontal disease of the individual from which the cultured lymphocytes were derived. It was hypothesized that they became increasingly sensitized by exposure to the plaque antigens after birth, particularly if periodontal disease is present: the more severe the disease the more lymphocytes become sensitized. However, more recent studies have shown a specificity in the cell-mediated response that varies according to the specific organism from which these antigens are derived. As certain microorganisms are associated with different severities and types of periodontal disease, it would follow that individuals with

mild gingivitis might be sensitized to different bacterial antigens than individuals with severe periodontitis. Although only certain organisms have been tested for their ability to stimulate cell-mediated immunity reactions of individuals with varying severities of disease, certain patterns have emerged. Figure 52.14 shows the response of individuals with varying severities of periodontal disease (including edentulous subjects with a history of tooth loss due to periodontitis) to four different microorganisms. The first pattern is represented by the response to *Actinomyces*. This organism proved to be a potent stimulator of lymphocytes in most patients tested. Although this response pattern might appear to be similar to the response to a nonspecific mitogen, this preparation stimulates very few human fetal cord lymphocytes and therefore does not appear to be a nonspecific mitogen to human peripheral lymphocytes. This response pattern appears to reflect host sensitization caused by the ubiquitous presence of this organism in the oral cavities of humans.

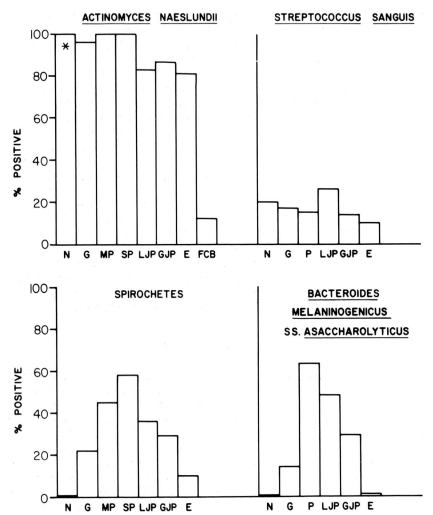

Figure 52.14: Percentage of subjects with positive lymphocyte blastogenic response to four oral organisms. *N*, normal; *G*, gingivitis; *MP*, moderate periodontitis; *SP*, severe periodontitis; *LJP*, localized juvenile periodontitis; *GJP*, generalized juvenile periodontitis; *P*, periodontitis; *E*, edentulous; *FCB*, fetal cord blood. (*) Although all normal patients were reactive to *Actinomyces naeslundii*, they responded at a significantly lower level than the other patient groups. *B. melaninogenicus* ss. *asaccharolyticus* is now called *B. gingivalis*.

Microbiological evidence suggests that actinomycetes are present in all dentulous subjects and that their numbers correlate with the presence of periodontal disease. This agrees with the lower blastogenic responses obtained from normal subjects who harbor fewer organisms than diseased subjects. The edentulous subjects who responded strongly may have been continually sensitized by the presence of actinomycetes on artificial dentures. Therefore, the measured response to actinomycetes appears to represent a naturally occurring cell-mediated immune response to a commensal organism which sensitizes the host primarily through the oral tissues.

In contrast to the *Actinomyces* response, all groups responded weakly to *Streptococcus sanguis*. Although a commensal organism, this species appears to be unable to stimulate a strong cellular immune response and has not been associated with periodontal disease in humans.

Finally, a different pattern of reactivity is shown by the blastogenic response to *Treponema denticola*, a spirochete, and *B. gingivalis*. Although these organisms appear to be capable of eliciting strong cellular immune responses, these responses seem to be limited to those individuals with destructive periodontitis. Recently, microbiological findings have related the presence of these organisms in subgingival plaque to destructive periodontitis in both humans and monkeys.

Although it is not clear that the magnitude of the

cellular immunity response to plaque microorganisms correlates with the severity of periodontal disease, the fact that individuals have sensitized lymphocytes to plaque microorganisms suggests a potential role for cell-mediated immunity in local tissue destruction. The understanding of this mechanism in the pathogenesis of periodontal disease might allow for the prevention of the development and continuation of the destructive phases of the inflammatory response.

Bone Destruction in Periodontal Disease

Destruction or resorption of alveolar bone is characteristic of the more advanced stages of periodontal disease. Whereas a definite relationship has been established between alveolar bone resorption and dental plaque, the manner in which the bone is resorbed has not been completely elucidated. Although plaque bacteria do not usually penetrate intact gingiva, their products do, and are involved in the pathogenesis of even the earlier stages of periodontal disease. In later stages, when there is pocket formation, plaque agents would more readily penetrate the tissues and cause bone resorption.

Several possible pathways have been described by which the products of the dental plaque could gain access to the alveolar bone and cause its resorption. Plaque products could stimulate progenitor cells in the periodontium to differentiate into osteoclasts. Complexing agents and hydrolytic enzymes from the plaque could act directly to decalcify bone and to hydrolyze its organic matrix. The products of plaque could stimulate gingival cells to produce mediators, which in turn would stimulate progenitor cells to form osteoclasts that destroy bone. Plaque products could stimulate gingival cells to produce substances that serve as cofactors to potentiate otherwise inactive bone resorptive agents, or gingival cell products could destroy bone by a direct action.

Using a model system of fetal bone in tissue culture, investigations of the various postulations for alveolar bone resorption have been made. Endotoxins from gram-negative bacteria, lipoteichoic acid (a glycolipid plus a glycerophosphate polymer) from gram-positive bacteria, such as lactobacilli, and a factor from *Actinomyces viscosus* stimulate osteoclastic destruction of bone. However, soluble products of plaque from adults with gingivitis and children without evidence of destructive periodontal disease also stimulate bone resorption by osteoclastic activity. Endotoxins, lipoteichoic acid, and extracts of dental plaque cause no release of calcium if the osteoclasts in the test bone have been heat-devitalized. This indicates

that these agents act by a direct action on osteoclasts rather than by a direct action on bone.

There is no question that gingival cells release or activate soluble mediators into periodontal tissues. Gingival mast cells release heparin and histamine. Heparin can act as a cofactor to potentiate bone resorption, but histamine has no demonstrable action on bone resorption. Although kinins are released into inflamed periodontal tissues, they have no action on bone resorption. Antigen–antibody complexes activate some component(s) of the complement system that stimulate prostaglandin-mediated bone resorption. Sensitized leukocytes release a factor (osteoclast-activating factor; Fig. 52.15) that stimulates bone resorption; prostaglandins also trigger bone resorption. Lysosomes, which contain many hydrolytic enzymes, have no known direct action on bone tissues. From such findings it is evident that alveolar bone resorption in periodontal disease is multifactorial, involving interactions between components of dental plaque and mediators in the periodontal tissues.

Role of Neutrophils

In response to chemotactic factors present in the gingival area, neutrophils constantly migrate from the gingival capillaries, through the connective tissue, epithelium, and gingival sulcus, and subsequently into the mouth. Several studies have revealed that the major source of oral leukocytes is the gingival sulcus, as few leukocytes can be recovered from the mouth when the orifices of the gingival sulcus are closed off with a plastic splint. Significantly more neutrophils are recovered from the mouth of individuals with inflamed gingiva than from a healthy mouth. In histological examinations of inflamed periodontal tissues, neutrophils are one of the major cell populations in the inflammatory infiltrate. Within the periodontal pocket, neutrophils appear to be associated with the tissue surface of the plaque mass and often contain phagocytized bacteria.

Numerous endogenous and exogenous chemical attractants (chemotactic factors) for neutrophils are present in the periodontal lesion. Many plaque microorganisms are known to produce low molecular weight substances that are strongly chemotactic for neutrophils. Additionally, activation of the alternate pathway of complement by bacterial endotoxin or other bacterial products generates chemotactic complement fragments such as C5a. Complement activation may also occur by the classical pathway following interaction of specific host antibodies with plaque bacterial antigens. Lymphocyte-derived chemotactic factors (lymphokines) may be elaborated by lymphocytes after interaction with specific bacterial antigens.

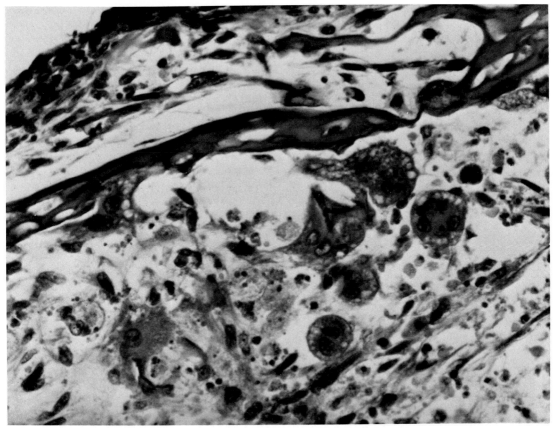

Figure 52.15: Histological appearance of a resorbing rat fetal bone shaft cultured for 96 hours with supernatant fluid from dental plaque-stimulated leukocyte cultures. Note the presence of numerous active osteoclasts as well as the loss of bone matrix (× 400). (Reproduced with permission from J. E. Horton, J. J. Oppenheim, and S. E. Mergenhagen: A Role of Cell-mediated Immunity in the Pathogenesis of Periodontal Disease. *J Periodontol,* **45,** 31, 1974.)

These and other chemotactic factors probably account for the presence of significant numbers of neutrophils in the periodontal tissues.

Neutrophils may also contribute to tissue damage. These cells contain lysosomal enzymes with which they digest phagocytized matter. Upon the ingestion of bacteria or other debris, these enzymes often leak into the surrounding tissue. Also, interaction of neutrophils with many bacterial products, including endotoxin and products of *Actinomyces,* can cause release of these tissue-destructive enzymes. Neutrophils contain collagenase, which will degrade collagen and thus lead to loss of integrity of the connective tissue. Also present in neutrophils are other histolytic and proteolytic enzymes that can digest host tissue substance. The tissue-destructive capacity of neutrophils has been demonstrated in leukopenic animals that failed to develop the usual abscesses seen in normal animals after injection of plaque into skin sites.

Although the tissue-destructive capacity of neutrophils has received considerable attention, recent research has focused on the host-protective aspects of neutrophil function. It has been known for many years that the neutrophil is the first line of defense against infection. It is therefore not surprising that the neutrophil might play an important role in protection from periodontal infection. In the last 50 years, numerous case reports have been published describing patients with systemic neutrophil disorders, including such conditions as agranulocytosis, cyclic neutropenia, "lazy leukocyte syndrome," Chediak-Higashi syndrome, etc. A consistent clinical finding in these cases has been exfoliation of permanent teeth, erythematous lesions of the gingiva, and spontaneous gingival bleeding. Careful clinical study of these patients revealed that many had extremely severe periodontitis at a very young age, often in childhood. Additional evidence that impaired systemic neutrophil function is associated with severe periodontitis is seen in the study of juvenile diabetes. Young diabetic patients often have unusually severe periodontitis. Often these patients have systemic neutrophil disorders as well.

Although the relationships between juvenile diabetes and periodontitis remains unclear, neutrophil disorders in some of these patients may be the link between these disorders.

The relationships between systemic neutrophil dysfunction and unusually severe periodontitis has led researchers to study neutrophil function in patients with an atypical severe periodontal disease, juvenile periodontitis (periodontosis). Juvenile periodontitis is characterized by rapidly progressive bone loss affecting the first molars and incisors in otherwise healthy, young individuals. Although inflammation is present, large quantities of bacterial plaque or calculus are not consistently seen. Recent evidence shows that the microflora associated with juvenile periodontitis lesions

differs markedly from chronic periodontitis. Nevertheless, there has been no clear understanding of this disease process.

The possibility that this severe form of periodontitis might be associated with a neutrophil disorder has been the object of intense investigation. It is clear that if a systemic neutrophil disorder exists, it would have to be mild, as these patients have no systemic disease. Using an in vitro assay of neutrophil chemotaxis, it has been demonstrated that peripheral blood neutrophils of subjects with juvenile periodontitis often have reduced neutrophil chemotaxis when compared to periodontally healthy subjects or subjects with chronic adult periodontitis. An example of such data is presented in Figure 52.16, where reduced chemotaxis

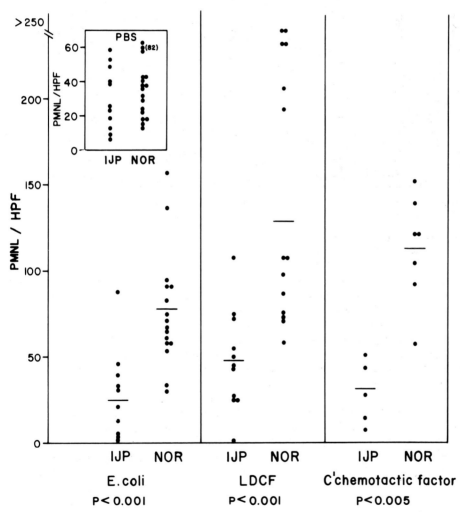

Figure 52.16: The chemotactic response of peripheral neutrophils (PMNL, polymorphonuclear leukocytes) from individuals with idiopathic juvenile periodontitis (*IJP*) and normal subjects (*NOR*) to filtrate of a culture of *Escherichia coli,* leukocyte-derived chemotactic factor (LDCF), and (*C'*) chemotactic factor and buffer control. *HPF,* high power field; *PBS,* phosphate-buffered saline. Reduced response is seen in the IJP population. (Reproduced with permission from L. J. Cianciola, et al.: Defective Polymorphonuclear Leukocyte Function in a Human Periodontal Disease. *Nature,* **265,** 445, 1977.)

Table 52.6: Number, Viability, and Phagocytic Capacity of Gingival Neutrophils Recovered from Lesions of Gingivitis, Chronic Adult Periodontitis, and Rapidly Progressive Periodontitis*

	Age Range	Cells/Site†	% Viable†	% PMN†	% Phagocytosis†
Gingivitis (N = 9)	21–30	$7.3 \pm 1.7 \times 10^3$‡	82 ± 2	90.0 ± 1.5	74.8 ± 2.6
Chronic periodontitis (N = 8)	49–62	$3.7 \pm 0.9 \times 10^4$	84 ± 2	86.0 ± 1.0	83.7 ± 4.8
Rapidly progressive periodontitis (N = 14)§	13–34	$3.1 \pm 0.2 \times 10^4$	79 ± 3.4	88.5 ± 1.5	12.9 ± 2.1‖

Note: PMN = polymorphonuclear leukocyte.

*Reproduced with permission from P. A. Murray and M. R. Patters: Gingival Crevice Neutrophil Function in Periodontal Lesions. *J Periodont Res,* **15,** 463, 1980.

†Mean ± standard error.

‡Significantly different from periodontitis groups ($p < 0.01$).

§A marked reduction in phagocytic capacity is seen in cells recovered from rapidly progressive lesions.

‖Significantly different from gingivitis and chronic periodontitis groups ($p < 0.001$).

was observed when neutrophils from juvenile periodontitis subjects migrated toward a bacterial factor derived from *Escherichia coli,* the chemotactic factor released by mitogen-stimulated lymphocytes (LDCF) and the chemotactic factors generated by activation of complement. Current evidence suggests that this defect is not associated with serum inhibitors of chemotaxis but appears to be a cell defect associated with a reduced number of membrane receptor sites for chemotactic molecules rather than a defect in locomotion. Also, evidence suggests that this systemic neutrophil dysfunction may be preexisting rather than induced by the disease process, and does not recover after the patients are successfully treated. A genetic cause of neutrophil dysfunction may explain the familial tendency of juvenile periodontitis.

Although the presence of a subtle systemic neutrophil defect in chemotaxis in patients with juvenile periodontitis is now well documented, no evidence exists to suggest that systemic cell defects occur in other forms of rapidly progressive periodontitis. However, information has been obtained to support the concept of locally induced neutrophil dysfunction within the periodontal lesion. When neutrophils recovered from the gingival sulcus of rapidly progressing lesions were compared with cells recovered from chronic long-standing lesions, impaired phagocytosis was seen in the former. No differences in number, viability, or percentage of neutrophils in the recovered cells were noted (Table 52.6). This reduction in phagocytosis was also evident when gingival neutrophils from progressive lesions were compared with noninvolved sites in the same mouth (Table 52.7), suggesting that this functional abnormality was the result of factors operating within the periodontal pocket. A hypothesis to explain these findings is that healthy neutrophils are exposed to products from specific microorganisms associated with progressive disease and are rendered dysfunctional by these substances. There is evidence that *Capnocytophaga* species and *A. actinomycetemcomitans* (organisms associated with juvenile periodontitis) and *B. gingivalis* (associated with adult periodontitis) produce substances that can seriously affect neutrophil function. The loss of function of these protective cells within the periodontal pocket may alter the environment of the pocket such that pathogenic bacteria may be able to become established, leading to rapidly progressive disease.

The current body of evidence suggests both a possible tissue-destructive as well as a protective role of

Table 52.7: Comparison of Gingival Polymorphonuclear Leukocytes from Periodontally Involved and Uninvolved Sites in Eight Patients with Localized Periodontitis*

Site	Cells/Site†	% Viable†	% Phagocytosis†
Diseased	$3.6 \pm 0.3 \times 10^4$‡	77.1 ± 2.8	10.9 ± 1.9‡
Nondiseased	$4.0 \pm 0.3 \times 10^3$	84.3 ± 2.0	72.2 ± 3.3

*Reproduced with permission from P. A. Murray and M. R. Patters: Gingival Crevice Neutrophil Function in Periodontal Lesions. *J Periodont Res,* **15,** 463, 1980.

†Mean ± standard error.

‡Significantly different ($p < 0.001$).

neutrophils. However, it appears that the protective aspects of neutrophil function have major consequences in the progression of periodontal disease.

Dental Calculus

Dental calculus is the concretion that accumulates on the teeth and on associated prostheses and restorations by calcification of dental plaque. It normally occurs infrequently or scantily in children under 10 years of age and is steadily more prevalent thereafter. The calculus index correlates closely with the periodontal disease index, but an etiological relationship is not clearly defined.

Calculus occurs in two main clinical types: supragingival, above the free margin, and subgingival, below the free margin of the gingiva, especially in the periodontal pocket. Though discrete foci of the two types are not uncommon, dental calculus seems to originate most often in plaque in cervical areas of the teeth and to form a continuum coronally and apically. Physical differences in color, texture, hardness, and adhesiveness have engendered the persistent but probably not very consequential designation of supragingival calculus as salivary in origin and subgingival calculus as serumal in origin. Supragingival calculus undoubtedly derives its inorganic and probably some of its organic matter constituents from saliva. The sulcular exudate almost certainly contributes similarly to subgingival calculus, which to some degree is kept from contact with saliva by its protected position in the gingival pocket. The final result, however, is essentially the same: an organic matrix consisting mostly of microorganisms with granular intermicrobial material, all mineralized predominantly with calcium and phosphate. Mineralization seems to be spotty, since the hardness index may vary threefold in different areas of a single specimen. The mean index is about twice that of cementum.

Mature calculus contains from 1.5% to 20% water and about 20% organic material. It contains, on average, about 30% calcium and 16% phosphorus, with ratios ranging from 1.66 to 2.31. Calculus also contains, on average, 1% magnesium, 2% sodium, and up to 5.3% carbonate. The inorganic part of calculus is a mixture of calcium phosphates (hydroxyapatite, $Ca_{10}(PO_4)_6 \cdot (OH)_2$; octacalcium phosphate, $Ca_8H_2(PO_4)_6 \cdot (5H_2O)$; whitlockite, $Ca_3(PO_4)_2$; and brushite, $CaHPO_4 \cdot (2H_2O)$. The organic matrix of calculus contains mucopolysaccharide and a variety of sugars and proteins in addition to the remains of bacterial cell walls.

Rates of calculus accumulation vary from person to person and in the same person in successive periods. In those who form calculus rapidly, plaque becomes as thick as 0.1 mm and begins to calcify within 3 days; mineralization is maximal (80% ash) in 2 weeks. Apatite crystals generally appear first between and on surfaces of the bacteria nearest the teeth. Later, the crystals appear inside them until the matrix is uniformly mineralized. Meanwhile, fresh bacterial growth accumulates on the surface. Mature calculus attaches to the tooth in four ways: to a cuticle layer on enamel or cementum, to minute irregularities in cementum, by penetration of plaque organisms into cementum, and by mechanical locking in undercut areas of cementum resorption. Plaque is considered to play an active role in calculus formation by providing nucleation sites where calcium, phosphate, and ancillary ions accumulate in the configuration of hydroxyapatite, thus initiating crystal growth. Such crystal nucleation by foreign substances is known as epitaxy.

Although bacteria are normally integral to dental calculus, they are not indispensable. The familiar calculi occurring in salivary glands and ducts are apparently bacteria free. Also, calculus forms on the teeth of germ-free animals. Generally, however, dental calculus forms more abundantly in conventional rats, particularly in those fed soft, sticky diets conducive to plaque accumulation. Even though bacteria are not essential to formation of dental calculus, they evidently enhance it under normal conditions.

Diet influences calculus formation in certain strains of experimental animals. Coarse, rough, abrasive diets are preventive, whereas fine, sticky, tenacious diets are conducive. The nutritional effects of varying the kinds and amounts of protein and carbohydrate in the diet are difficult to dissociate from their effects on dietary consistency. Certain altered calcium–phosphorous ratios and increased bicarbonate in the diet favor calculus formation in experimental animals. Variations in ordinary dietary factors have not convincingly shown an effect on calculus formation in man.

Calculus prevention has been attempted, without much success, by several mechanisms: 1) by preventing the attachment of plaque through repellent coatings on the teeth; 2) by altering the nature of plaque or reducing its accumulation through antibacterial agents, hydrolytic enzymes, or detergents; and 3) by dissolving the mineral salt of calculus with decalcifying or complexing agents. Regular, efficient toothbrushing and interdental hygiene to remove plaque before it mineralizes remain the only effective regimen.

The opinion has been accepted that subgingival calculus irritates the gingiva by its roughness. If it is sufficiently jagged, calculus can traumatize the tissue mechanically during mastication and toothbrushing. On the other hand, the junctional epithelium adapts readily and forms a normal contact with roughened enamel and various artifacts, *provided that bacteria are excluded.* The principal contribution of calculus to the progress of chronic periodontitis seems, therefore, to be due to its bacterial components, not as a mechanical irritant.

Predisposing Factors

A wide variety of factors are believed to predispose to or aggravate the degree to which periodontitis develops. Such factors are classified as local or systemic, but this distinction is not very meaningful. Predisposing factors may also be grouped according to their modes of action. Many simply worsen oral hygiene and augment bacterial plaque accumulations. A second group consists of some nutritional deficiencies, hormonal imbalances, and systemic disorders, which may either lower local tissue resistance or modify the oral microflora. A third group, including vitamin C deficiency and heavy metal or drug intoxications, induce distinct periodontal pathoses that might lower the resistance of the periodontium to infection. Owing to the preponderant effect of plaque, the significance of other predisposing factors unfortunately is not clear.

Oral Hygiene

It is difficult to distinguish effects mediated by worsened oral hygiene from effects seemingly due to other mechanisms. Even the age effect may be attributable in part to the concomitant rapid and progressive increase in the fraction of persons having extremely bad oral hygiene (see Fig. 52.3). The increased severity of periodontal disease associated with unfavorable socioeconomic conditions or psychosomatic disturbances is so closely correlated with poorer oral hygiene that concomitant lowering of local tissue resistance has not been ascertained.

Age

The reason why periodontitis becomes more prevalent and destructive with increasing age, even in a given oral hygiene group (see Fig. 52.2), remains unclear. It might be simply the consequence of prolonged exposure to plaque. Pocket formation, the first clinical evidence of destructive change, is normally rare before age 15 but becomes more frequent after age 30. Similarly, gingival and alveolar bone recession are only moderately prevalent before age 30 regardless of the degree of plaque control, even in a population practicing little oral hygiene. Recession remains moderate until age 40 in those with only slight plaque and calculus, but increases markedly thereafter in proportion to the amount of plaque. The accumulated evidence strongly indicates that bacterial plaque is responsible for the degeneration of the periodontium with age.

Since calculus is uncommon during childhood despite an abundance of plaque, some change of oral physiology may occur during puberty that favors calcification of plaque. Conceivably, oral physiology in the older persons also favors increased bacterial accumulations.

Whatever the factors adverse to the periodontium that develop with age may be, their consequences seem to be secondary to those of oral uncleanliness. Most persons can reasonably expect to keep a healthy functioning periodontium if they always maintain good oral hygiene.

Diet

Modern civilized diets have been implicated as predisposing to periodontal disease, partly because they lack detergency and partly because their consumption does not entail sufficient masticatory stimulation. Contemporary people subsisting on primitive diets comprised of raw, fibrous, coarse foods seem to have no better periodontal health. Some investigators concluded from a study of stain removal that vigorous mastication of coarse foods could *not* be expected to prevent accumulation of plaque in cervical areas of the teeth except in the maxillary palatal gingiva.

Persons with extreme deficiencies of vitamins and probably deficiencies in protein exhibit severe periodontal pathosis, part of which is independent of local infection. Available data are insufficient to determine if borderline dietary deficiencies prevailing in large areas of the world predispose to inflammatory periodontal disease.

Consequences of pronounced vitamin A deficiency include keratinizing metaplasia of epithelium, xerosis, disturbed osteogenesis, and lowered resistance to infection. A variety of periodontal abnormalities in epithelium, connective tissue, and bone have been discerned in vitamin A–deficient rats. Inflammation and pocket formation occur only in the presence of local irritation, such as that caused by bacteria and calculus. Associated deficiency of lysozyme may contribute to reduced resistance to infection.

Glossitis, glossodynia, cheilosis, gingivitis, and generalized stomatitis have been attributed to deficiency of the vitamin B complex (thiamine, riboflavin, niacin, pantothenic acid, pyridoxine, biotin, *p*-aminobenzoic acid, inositol, choline, folic acid, and cyanocobalamin). Individual deficiency of riboflavin or niacin produces such symptoms in humans. Severe gingivitis develops in animals deficient in folic acid.

Lack of vitamin C (ascorbic acid) impairs a variety

of biochemical functions, most notably synthesis of collagen and metabolism of mucopolysaccharides. Important consequences include loss of intercellular substance, edema, degeneration of collagen fibers, decreased osteoblastic function, increased osteoclastic function, and structural weakness and loss of contractility of peripheral blood vessels. Particularly in stressed areas, tissue integrity fails. The clinical result is known as scurvy, characterized by edema, marked tendency to perivenular hemorrhage, retarded wound healing, increased susceptibility to infection, and asthenia. The oral manifestations of edema, hemorrhage, "gangrene" of gingiva, and exfoliation of teeth, seem to be rare today. A local irritant such as bacterial accumulation seems to be necessary in addition to the ascorbate deficiency for the fully developed pathosis. The severe periodontal symptoms historically associated with scurvy nevertheless fostered widespread suspicion that chronic borderline ascorbate deficiency might be a frequent predisposing factor. The majority of modern clinical trials, however, have not found significant benefit from vitamin C therapy of periodontal patients.

Occlusal and Other Trauma

Adequate mechanical stimulation from mastication is thought to be necessary for structural maintenance of the periodontal ligament and alveolar bone. Clinical experience indicates that in individual cases or in particular sites, occlusal forces may exceed the adaptive capacity of the periodontium. The resulting "trauma from occlusion" may act synergistically with coexisting inflammation to increase destruction of the periodontium. Such trauma may result from innate malocclusion, disharmony from missing teeth, high restorations, bruxism, and clenching. On the other hand, it is clear that trauma from occlusion in the absence of bacterial plaque cannot initiate periodontitis.

Other sources of trauma implicated as secondary factors in periodontal disease include dental calculus (see above), a wide variety of dental procedures, mouth breathing, tongue thrusting, excessive smoking of tobacco, betel nut chewing in large regions of Asia, chemical irritation as from strong mouthwashes, too vigorous toothbrushing, and allergic reactions of the oral mucosa.

Hormones

An excess or deficiency of hormones has been considered responsible for an exaggerated reactivity of the periodontium to local irritation in a minor fraction of persons. Familiar examples are gingivitis associated with puberty, menstruation, or pregnancy. A chronic desquamative type of gingivitis occurs occasionally during and after menopause. For pregnancy only, the data are adequate to validate an exacerbation of gingivitis not attributable to increased plaque accumulation. Recent studies have found a qualitative change in plaque during pregnancy: a large increase in *Bacteroides intermedius*. This subsides postpartum, leaving no permanent alteration.

It is a prevalent clinical impression that diabetes predisposes to periodontal disease, but careful clinical investigations have not always established a correlation between these two disorders. In animal diabetes induced by alloxan, no distinctive periodontal changes have been reported. On the other hand, a hereditarily diabetic strain of Chinese hamster develops severe periodontal disease with pocket formation, inflammation, and alveolar bone resorption. Calculus is reported to be abnormally abundant in human diabetics. The extensive periodontal destruction seen in many diabetic children also indicates that uncontrolled diabetes does have some direct or indirect action on the periodontium, probably by affecting the protective function of neutrophils.

Large doses of corticosteroids depress resistance to infection. Smaller but significantly increased amounts of corticosteroids are secreted during emotional stress and may aggravate periodontal lesions. Stress results also in production of epinephrine from adrenals and norepinephrine from sympathetic nerve endings. Since both of these hormones produce severe necrotic hemorrhagic lesions when injected into tissues sensitized by minute amounts of endotoxins, they might exacerbate periodontal lesions in emotionally disturbed persons.

Concurrent Pathoses

Blood dyscrasias, such as leukemia, neutropenias, purpuras, and anemias, are frequently accompanied by characteristic and rather extensive changes in the periodontium, often alleviated by control of the dyscrasia. In most instances the periodontal changes are associated with a lowering of the resistance of the periodontal tissues to infection.

Intoxication by heavy metals and a variety of drugs seems to lower the resistance of mucous membranes to infection, leading to gingival disturbances in some cases. Arsenic, bismuth, and mercury may be derived from drugs containing them or, like lead and other heavy metals, may be acquired by occupational exposure. Bismuth, lead, and mercury are deposited particularly around the blood vessels beneath the epithelium and can be seen as darkly pigmented gingival areas. Mercury is also secreted in the saliva and may then act on the gingival mucosa. Dilantin sodium, used to control epilepsy, promotes gingival hyperplasia in a fraction of cases, sometimes complicated by secondary inflammatory changes.

Noma (cancrum oris) is essentially a gangrenous extension of Vincent's infection with destruction of facial soft tissues and bone, and usually a fatal outcome if untreated. Penicillin terminates this infection dramatically. Noma seems to be associated with severe general nutritional deficiency, particularly of protein. There is frequently a history of prodromal infection; measles, herpes simplex, smallpox, diphtheria, scarlet fever, typhoid fever, whooping cough, kala azar, and malaria have been cited.

Genetics

Epidemiological surveys have revealed no differences in periodontal experience attributable to racial characteristics. Inbred strains of mice, however, vary distinctively in the type and severity of the spontaneous periodontal pathosis they develop. In one study, gingivitis was slightly but significantly more frequent in inbred children in two Japanese cities, possibly due to greater susceptibility to infection. Acatalasemia, hypophosphatasia, and cyclic neutropenia, rare human syndromes attributable to respective single mutant genes, are regularly accompanied by severe periodontal disease in all environments. Down's syndrome individuals, whose condition results from an extra chromosome, experience an abnormally high incidence and severity of periodontitis.

The accumulated evidence suggests that some factors of genetic origin predispose to periodontal disease. Under present conditions their influence is very subordinate to that of poor oral hygiene and age.

Relationship of Periodontal Disease to Focal Infection

The concept of focal infection means simply that microorganisms or their toxic products disseminate from a primary localized infection and initiate secondary loci of infection or tissue damage in distant parts of the body. For many years, an astonishing variety of ailments, mostly inflammatory, were attributed to such oral foci as periapical abscesses, chronic pulpitis and periodontitis, and tonsillitis. Tonsillectomy and extraction of periapically involved or pulpless teeth enjoyed a great vogue, whether infection at these foci was proved or only suspected. These practices were considered justifiable because 1) typical oral bacteria could be isolated regularly from certain nonoral lesions, where they undoubtedly were etiological, 2) inoculation of animals with bacteria from oral foci was reported to produce the systemic conditions seen in

humans, 3) eradication of real or suspected oral foci was widely reported to alleviate presumably associated systemic ailments, and 4) it was reported that operative trauma at primary oral sites exacerbated secondary lesions. Microorganisms derived from the periodontium have been implicated etiologically in lung abscesses, subacute bacterial endocarditis, rheumatic fever, rheumatoid arthritis, neuritis, gastrointestinal disease, ocular diseases, skin diseases, prostatic diseases, and general malaise. Definitive evidence of a regular direct connection between oral infections and such systemic ailments is still lacking, and today clinical management of the oral phase is generally less drastic. This does not mean unconcern with oral infections; rather it accords with the realization that these infections do not often have the momentous systemic consequences once attributed to them.

ADDITIONAL READING

Attstrom, R. 1970. Presence of Leucocytes in Crevices of Healthy and Chronically Inflamed Gingiva in Humans. J Periodont Res, **5**, 42.

Attstrom, R., Laurell, A. B., Larsson, U., and Sjoholm, A. 1975. Complement Factors in Gingival Crevice Material from Healthy and Inflamed Gingiva in Humans. J Periodont Res, **10**, 19.

Baehni, P., Tsai, C. C., McArthur, W. P., Hammond, B. F., and Taichman, N. S. 1979. Interaction of Inflammatory Cells and Oral Microorganisms: VIII. Detection of Leukotoxic Activity of a Plaque-derived Gram-Negative Microorganism. Infect Immun, **24**, 233.

Cianciola, L. J., Genco, R. J., Patters, M. R., McKenna, J., and Van Oss, C. J. 1977. Defective Polymorphonuclear Leukocyte Function in Human Periodontal Disease. Nature, **265**, 445.

Clark, H., Page, R. C., and Wilde, G. 1977. Defective Neutrophil Chemotaxis in Juvenile Periodontitis. Infect Immun, **18**, 694.

Dinarello, C. A., and Mier, J. W. 1987. Current Concepts: Lymphokines. N Engl J Med, **317**, 940.

Ebersole, J. L., Frey, D. E., Taubman, M. A., and Smith, D. J. 1980. An ELISA for Measuring Serum Antibodies to *Actinobacillus actinomycetemcomitans*. J Periodont Res, **15**, 621.

Fearon, D. T., and Austen, K. F. 1980. Alternative Pathway of Complement: A System for Host Resistance to Microbial Infection. N Engl J Med, **303**, 259.

Forster, O. 1972. Nature and Origin of Proteases in the Immunologically Induced Inflammatory Reaction. J Dent Res, **51**, 257.

Genco, R. J., and Krygier, G. 1973. Localization of Immunoglobulins, Immune Cells and Complement in Human Gingiva. J Periodont Res Suppl, **10**, 30.

Gibbons, R. J., Socransky, S. S., DeAranjo, W. C., and Van Houte, J. 1964. Studies of the Cultivable Microbiota of Plaque. Arch Oral Biol, **9**, 365.

Gibbons, R. J., Socransky, S. S., Sawyer, S., Kapsimalis, B., and MacDonald, J. B. 1963. Microbiota of the Gingival Crevice Area of Man: II. The Predominant Cultivable Organisms. Arch Oral Biol, **8**, 281.

Hellden, L., Lindhe, J., Attstrom, R., and Sundin, Y. 1973.

Neutrophil Chemotactic Factors in Gingival Crevice Material. Helv Odontol Acta, **17**, 1.

Horton, J. E., Oppenheim, J. J., and Mergenhagen, S. E. 1973. Elaboration of Lymphotoxin by Cultured Human Peripheral Blood Leukocytes Stimulated with Dental Plaque Deposits. Clin Exp Immunol, **13**, 383.

Horton, J. E., Oppenheim, J. J., and Mergenhagen, S. E. 1974. A Role for Cell-mediated Immunity in the Pathogenesis of Periodontal Disease. J Periodontol, **45**, 351.

Horton, J. E., Raisz, L. G., Simmons, H. A., Oppenheim, J. J., and Mergenhagen, S. E. 1972. Bone Resorbing Activity in Supernatant Fluid from Cultured Human Peripheral Blood Leukocytes. Science, **177**, 793.

Ivanyi, L., and Lehner, T. 1970. Stimulation of Lymphocyte Transformation by Bacterial Antigens in Patients with Periodontal Disease. Arch Oral Biol, **15**, 1089.

Karring, T. 1973. Mitotic Activity in the Oral Epithelium. J Periodont Res, **8**, Suppl. 13.

Kelstrup, J., and Theilade, E. 1974. Microbes and Periodontal Disease. J Clin Periodontol, **1**, 15.

Kornman, K. S., Holt, S. C., and Robertson, P. B. 1981. The Microbiology of Ligature-induced Periodontitis in the Cynomolgus Monkey. J Periodontol Res, **16**, 363.

Lang, N. P., and Smith, F. N. 1977. Lymphocyte Blastogenesis to Plaque Antigens in Human Periodontal Disease: I. Populations of Varying Severity of Disease. J Periodontol Res, **12**, 298.

Lehner, T. 1982. Cellular Immunity in Periodontal Disease: An Overview. In *Host-Parasite Interaction in Periodontal Disease,* pp. 202–216, edited by R. J. Genco and S. E. Mergenhagen. American Society for Microbiology, Washington, D.C.

Lindhe, J., and Hellden, L. 1972. Neutrophil Chemotactic Activity Elaborated by Human Dental Plaque. J Periodontol Res, **7**, 297.

Listgarten, M. A. 1976. Structure of the Microbial Flora Associated with Periodontal Health and Disease in Man: A Light and Electron Microscopic Study. J Periodontol, **47**, 1.

Löe, H., and Silness, J. 1963. Periodontal Disease in Pregnancy: I. Prevalence and Severity. Acta Odontol Scand, **21**, 533.

Löe, H., Theilade, E., and Jensen, S. B. 1965. Experimental Gingivitis in Man. J Periodontol, **36**, 177.

Manson, J. D., and Lehner, T. 1974. Clinical Features of Juvenile Periodontitis (Periodontosis). J Periodontol, **45**, 636.

Mouton, C., Hammond, P. G., Slots, J., and Genco, R. J. 1981. Serum Antibodies to Oral *Bacteroides asaccharolyticus (Bacteroides gingivalis):* Relationship to Age and Periodontal Disease. Infect Immun, **31**, 182.

Murray, P. A., and Patters, M. R. 1980. Gingival Crevice Neutrophil Function in Periodontal Lesions. J Periodont Res, **15**, 463.

Newman, M. G., and Socransky, S. S. 1977. Predominant Cultivable Microbiota in Periodontosis. J Periodont Res, **12**, 120.

Niekrash, C. E., and Patters, M. R. 1985. Simultaneous Assessment of C3, C4 and B Cleavage in Human Gingival Fluid: II. Longitudinal Changes during Periodontal Therapy. J Periodont Res, **20**, 268.

Niekrash, C. E., and Patters, M. R. 1986. Assessment of Complement Cleavage in Gingival Fluid in Humans with and without Periodontal Disease. J Periodont Res, **21**, 233.

Nisengard, R. J. 1977. The Role of Immunology in Periodontal Disease. J Periodontol, **48**, 505.

Page, R. C., and Schroeder, H. E. 1976. Pathogenesis of Inflammatory Periodontal Disease: A Summary of Current Work. Lab Invest, **33**, 235.

Patters, M. R., Chen, P., McKenna, J., and Genco, R. J. 1980. Lymphoproliferative Responses to Oral Bacteria in Humans with Varying Severities of Periodontal Disease. Infect Immun, **28**, 777.

Patters, M. R., Schenkein, H. A., and Weinstein, A. 1979. A Method for Detection of Complement Cleavage in Gingival Fluid. J Dent Res, **58**, 1620.

Patters, M. R., Sedransk, R. N., and Genco, R. J. 1977. Lymphoproliferative Response during Resolution and Recurrence of Naturally Occurring Gingivitis. J Periodontol, **48**, 373.

Payne, W., Page, R. C., Ogilvie, A. L., and Hall, W. B. 1975. Histopathologic Features of the Initial and Early Stages of Experimental Gingivitis in Man. J Periodont Res, **10**, 51.

Polson, A. M., Meitner, S. W., and Zander, H. A. 1976. Trauma and Progression of Marginal Periodontitis in Squirrel Monkeys: IV. Reversibility of Bone Loss due to Trauma Alone and Trauma Superimposed upon Periodontitis. J Periodont Res, **11**, 290.

Raisz, L. G., Sandberg, A. L., Goodson, J. M., Simmons, H. A., and Mergenhagen, S. E. 1974. Complement-Dependent Stimulation of Prostaglandin Synthesis of Bone Resorption. Science, **185**, 789.

Ranney, R. R. 1978. Immunofluorescent Localization of Soluble Dental Plaque Components in Human Gingiva Affected by Periodontitis. J Periodont Res, **13**, 99.

Ranney, R. R., and Zander, H. A. 1970. Allergic Periodontal Disease in Sensitized Squirrel Monkeys. J Periodontol, **41**, 12.

Rizzo, A. A., and Mitchell, C. H. 1966. Chronic Allergic Inflammation Induced by Repeated Deposition of Antigen in Rabbit Gingival Pockets. Periodontics, **4**, 5.

Russell, A. L. 1956. System of Classification and Scoring for Prevalence Surveys of Periodontal Disease. J Dent Res, **35**, 350.

Schenkein, H. A., and Genco, R. J. 1977. Gingival Fluid in Serum in Periodontal Diseases: I. Quantitative Study of Immunoglobulins, Complement Components, and Other Plasma Proteins. J Periodontol, **48**, 772.

Schenkein, H. A., and Genco, R. J. 1977. Gingival Fluid in Serum in Periodontal Diseases: II. Evidence for Cleavage of Complement Components C3, C3 Proactivator (Factor B) and C4 in Gingival Fluid. J Periodontol, **48**, 778.

Schroeder, H. E. 1970. The Structure and Relationship of Plaque to the Hard and Soft Tissues: Electron Microscopic Interpretation. Int Dental J, **20**, 353.

Shurin, S. B., Socransky, S. S., Sweeney, E., and Stossel, T. P. 1979. A Neutrophil Disorder Induced by *Capnocytophaga,* a Dental Microorganism. N Engl J Med, **301**, 849.

Silness, J., and Löe, H. 1964. Periodontal Disease in Pregnancy: II. Correlation between Oral Hygiene and Periodontal Condition. Acta Odontol Scand, **22**, 121.

Slots, J. 1976. The Predominant Cultivable Organisms in Juvenile Periodontitis. Scand J Dent Res, **85**, 1.

Slots, J. 1977. Microflora in the Healthy Gingival Sulcus in Man. Scand J Dent Res, **85**, 247.

Slots, J. 1977. The Predominant Cultivable Microflora of Advanced Periodontitis. Scand J Dent Res, **85**, 114.

Slots, J. 1979. Subgingival Microflora and Periodontal Disease. J Clin Periodontol, **6**, 351.

Slots, J., and Hausmann, E. 1979. Longitudinal Study of Experimentally Induced Periodontal Disease in *Macaca arctoides:* Relationship between Microflora and Alveolar Bone Loss. Infect Immun, **23**, 260.

Slots, J., Moenbo, D., Langebaek, J., and Erandsen, A. 1978. Microbiota of Gingivitis in Man. Scand J Dent Res, **86**, 174.

Socransky, S. S. 1977. Microbiology of Periodontal Disease: Present Status and Future Considerations. J Periodontol, **48**, 497.

Socransky, S. S., Gibbons, R. J., Dale, A. C., Bortnick, L., Rosenthal, E., and MacDonald, J. H. B. 1963. The Microbiota of the Gingival Crevice Area of Man: I. Total Microscopic and Viable Counts and Counts of Specific Organisms. Arch Oral Biol, **8,** 275.

Socransky, S. S., Tanner, A. C. R., Haffajee, A. D., Hillman, J. D., and Goodson, M. J. 1982. Present Status of Studies on the Microbial Etiology of Periodontal Disease. In *Host-Parasite Interaction in Periodontal Disease,* pp. 1–12, edited by R. J. Genco, and S. E. Mergenhagen. American Society for Microbiology, Washington, D.C.

Suomi, J. D., and Doyle, J. 1972. Oral Hygiene and Periodontal Disease in an Adult Population in the United States. J Periodontol, **43,** 677.

Taichman, N. 1970. Mediation of Inflammation by the Polymorphonuclear Leukocytes as a Sequela of Immune Reactions. J Periodontol, **41,** 228.

Tanner, A. C. R., Hoffer, C., Bratthal, G. T., Visconti, R. A., and Socransky, S. S. 1979. A Study of the Bacteria Associated with Advancing Periodontitis in Man. J Clin Periodontol, **6,** 278.

Theilade, E., Wright, W. H., Jensen, S. B., and Löe, H. 1966. Experimental Gingivitis in Man: II. A Longitudinal Clinical and Bacteriological Investigation. J Periodont Res, **1,** 1.

Van Dyke, T. E., Horoszewicz, H. U., Cianciola, L. J., and Genco, R. J. 1980. Neutrophil Chemotaxis Dysfunction in Human Periodontitis. Infect Immun, **27,** 124.

Van Dyke, T. E., Levine, M. J., and Genco, R. J. 1980. Periodontal Disease and Neutrophil Abnormalities. In *Host-Parasite Interaction in Periodontal Disease,* pp. 235–245, edited by R. J. Genco, and S. E. Mergenhagen. American Society for Microbiology, Washington, D.C.

53

Endodontic Disease

Eugene A. Pantera, Jr.

Introduction

Within the confines of the tooth and about its periapical regions are tissues and structures that are subject to infection. These tissues and their morphology are unique, as is the response of the region to infection. Localized infection is common and can constitute a site from which infection spreads to other parts of the body. For a complete understanding of the course of infection of these structures, a knowledge of their gross and microscopic anatomy is essential. For this the reader should review the various texts on anatomy and histology of the teeth and supporting structures.

To appreciate the interaction between the pulp, bacteria, and inflammation, it is necessary to examine the microbiology of endodontic disease in relation to pulpal histopathology.

Pulpal Pathophysiology

Dental pulp is a unique formative organ with limited capacity to heal following repetitive bacterial, mechanical, and chemical insults. Although the pulp has mechanisms for regeneration and repair, it is essentially a reactive tissue with elevated periods of activity proportional to the degree of external stimuli. Lesions of endodontic origin develop from the progressive coronal–apical necrosis of pulpal tissue, eventually infecting periapical structures. As the result of bacteremia, direct invasion through tissues, and microthrombi, periapical infections can lead to such grave complications as cavernous sinus thrombosis and Ludwig's angina. These infections can also exacerbate existing conditions in patients with impaired immunity, organ transplants, implanted circulatory devices, and congenital or acquired heart defects.

As fluid leaves the microvasculature during inflammation, there is a rise in interstitial pressure within the pulp. The unyielding wall of dentin prevents this pressure from dissipating (as in soft tissue edema) and the ensuing pressure increase may cause a local collapse of the microvasculature. This collapse can result in additional necrosis with release of tissue breakdown products, elevating the pulpal interstitial concentration of osmotically active protein molecules. This osmotic attraction draws more fluid from the circulation with an expectant rise in pulpal interstitial pressure. Vascular permeability increases with fluid outflow and increase in pressure. Reversing this process becomes futile with the formation of inflammatory exudate. From a single point source of inflammation or infection, a circumferential spread of necrosis occurs in proportion to the degree and repetition of the insult; furthermore, necrotic spread can start at any point in this "pressure cycle."

Bacteria are deterrents to pulpal repair, as almost any microorganism in the oral cavity, nasopharynx, or gastrointestinal tract can infect the pulp. Yet pulpal breakdown and necrosis may still occur without viable bacteria where toxins may be the source of repetitive irritation or where trauma severs vascular bundles to the pulp. Constant toxin irritation leaves little opportunity for pulp tissue to "catch up" with repair. The degree to which bacterial infection contributes to pulpal degeneration and periapical destruction is not fully understood, though various disease-inducing microbiological factors and mech-

anisms of host resistance to these factors do contribute to the process. With pulpal degeneration, antigens collect within the root canal system. They can be viable or nonviable bacteria, bacterial toxins, necrosing pulp tissue, medicaments, and pulp tissue altered by medicaments.

Immunocompetent cells are present in normal human pulp and, as caries approaches the pulp, there is a progressive increase in inflammatory cells, exudate, and immunoglobulin-containing cells. Bacteria and bacterial antigens have been identified in association with antibodies and frequently in association with complement in tissue sections of pulp from teeth with advanced caries. Immunoglobulins and complement have been detected in odontoblast cytoplasm as well. Once a severe inflammatory state has been established, pulpal healing cannot take place, since the protective effects of the host pulpal immune response cannot prevent spread to the radicular tissues. Thus the host immune response itself contributes to the pathogenesis of periapical lesions.

As antigens move from the root canal into periapical tissues, granulation tissue proliferates, ultimately

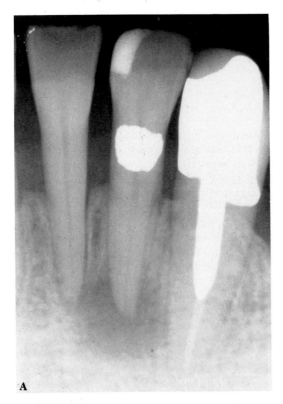 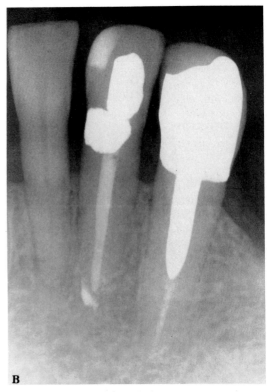

Figure 53.1: (**A**) Patient presented with a pulpal diagnosis of necrosis and a periapical diagnosis of chronic apical periodontitis associated with the lateral incisor. A periapical radiolucency can be seen extending mesially to include the central incisor. (**B**) At the 18-month recall visit, complete healing of the apical lesion is seen after thorough cleaning, shaping, and canal obturation of the lateral incisor.

replacing normal tissue. Pathological changes associated with periapical tissue result from activation of nonspecific inflammatory reactions as well as specific immunological responses. Nonspecific inflammatory mediators identified with pathogenesis of these lesions include complement components, vasoactive amines, kinins, and arachidonic acid metabolites. The presence of IgG, IgA, IgM, IgE, and immunologically competent cells suggests participation by specific immunological responses in initiation and perpetuation of the pathological process. The immunologic response in periapical tissue, then, is a combination of protective and allergic reactions.

Endodontic Success

The dental pulp and periapex form a connective tissue continuum. This continuum differs from other connective tissue by the interposition of an unyielding wall of dentin, which has an effect on the pulpal inflammatory response to physical and bacterial injury. Endodontic treatment is successful because of the chemomechanical elimination of microorganisms from the canal system, a reduction in microbial numbers so that growth is no longer possible, and the creation of a hermetic seal in the canal system that prevents exit of any remaining organic substrate into the periapical tissues (Fig. 53.1). Extraction of a tooth is proof of the potential success of endodontic treatment. That is, when a tooth is removed, there is complete elimination of the root canal system that contains the toxins that precipitate pulpal and periapical disease. With elimination of the root canal system, disease of endodontic origin heals. The goal in endodontic treatment, then, is elimination of the contents of canal systems without extracting the tooth.

Endodontic Failure

Endodontic failure results from the persistence of the disease process attributable to incomplete removal or suppression of the microbial etiology within a canal system. Although recent studies suggest that bacterial plaque formation on cemental surfaces of root apices may contribute to some failures, most failures occur from the lack of a hermetic seal and the presence of canal organisms or canal antigens (Fig. 53.2).

Bacteria as a Pulpal Irritant

In 1965, the results of a pulpal histological study were reported by Kakehashi, Stanley, and Fitzgerald. Their experiment compared the degree of pulpal injury in normal and gnotobiotic rat populations following me-

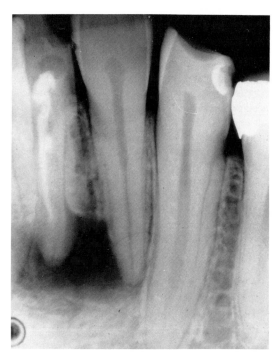

Figure 53.2: Patient presented with symptoms of chronic apical periodontitis. The periapical radiolucency was being sustained through failed endodontic treatment of the central incisor that neither eliminated the canal antigens nor provided a hermetic seal. The lateral incisor, a normal vital tooth, was being displaced by the expanding lesion.

chanical pulpal exposures that were left open to the oral fluids. In timed observations these investigators saw that pulpal necrosis and periapical disease only appeared in normal animals; the gnotobiotic animals exhibited minimal inflammation. Additionally, in the gnotobiotic population, repair occurred in the form of secondary dentin formation. Later experiments supported these findings and showed further that the degree of pulpal inflammation is directly proportional to the degree of bacterial infection and that pulpal repair (bridging) is indirectly proportional to the degree of bacterial infection. These observations established that microbes have a pathological effect on pulpal health.

Early studies reported the prevalence of α-hemolytic streptococci associated with endodontic disease. These studies were restrictive since only aerobic microbiological techniques were used. Studies completed since the early 1970s have demonstrated that, with appropriate techniques, anaerobes are the predominant bacteria associated with pulpal and endodontic periapical disease. Anaerobic bacteria recovered from endodontic lesions exhibit the same characteristics associated with other human anaerobic infections: inhibition of neutrophil chemotaxis and phagocytosis and interference with antibiotic sensitivity; production of endotoxins and enzymes that affect inflammatory responses; and the association of specific anaerobic bacteria with persistent painful periapical lesions. Pulpal infections are associated with a compromised blood supply with antecedent aerobic infections (caries), both of which result in a lowered oxidation–reduction potential (E_h). Anaerobic pathogenicity is dependent on the level of oxidation within the pulp. When the E_h falls, the saprophytic anaerobes can invade the pulp and multiply. Maintenance of E_h is thought to be the body's main defense against pathogenetic proliferation of endogenous anaerobes. Anaerobes therefore are hypothesized to be secondary invaders and not primary pulpal pathogens.

Bacterial Pathways to the Pulp

Caries

The most obvious and typical source of endodontic pathogens is the carious lesion. Bacteria (size ≈ 0.3 μm) can be found in dentinal tubules (size ≈ 1 to 3 μm) and advance by reproduction rather than motility (Fig. 53.3). They progress toward the pulp while their toxic byproducts are transported to the pulpal intersti-

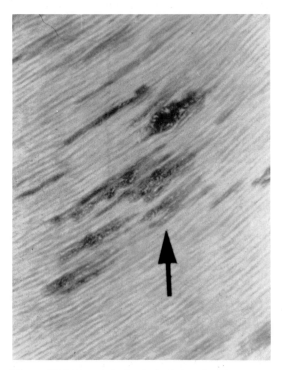

Figure 53.3: Bacteria in dentinal tubules advancing toward the pulp by replication. (Courtesy of Dr. Ralph V. McKinney, Jr., Medical College of Georgia, Augusta.)

tial fluid by the dentinal fluid transport system. These toxins affect the pulp in advance of the physical presence of bacteria. The degree of pulpal response, then, depends on the remaining dental thickness and the function of the meshed microanatomy of the dentinal tubule system. The progress of incipient caries creates the aciduric environment favorable for a lowered E_h, while enzymes such as catalase destroy the intracellularly produced peroxides. This environment is now ideal for anaerobic organisms to supplant whatever aerobic progenitor organisms were present.

The bacteria penetrating the dentin before carious pulpal exposure are undoubtedly some of those involved in the carious process. Streptococci, staphylococci, lactobacilli, and filamentous microorganisms have been isolated from deep carious dentin. Of this group, streptococci are found most consistently as the causative agents of pulpitis arising from deep dentin caries not exposing the pulp. In such circumstances, staphylococci and filamentous microorganisms are also occasional causes of pulpitis.

Periodontal Disease

There is no question that endodontic disease can induce or aggravate periodontal disease. However, since there is seldom loss of epithelial attachment from endodontic disease, this pattern of periodontal disease is reversible following removal of the endodontic irritant. (This is not true if there is a communication between a true endodontic lesion and a true periodontal lesion.)

There has been some debate as to whether or not periopathogens precipitate endodontic disease. This question must be interpreted in light of the anatomical relationship between the pulp and the periodontium, the level of epithelial attachment, and the course of periodontal treatment. A study by Czarnecki and Schilder examined serial histological sections of human teeth with varying degrees of periodontal disease. These teeth did not have any previous periodontal or endodontic treatment. It was found that pulps remained within normal limits regardless of the severity of the periodontal disease. Additionally, they found that very deep caries or extensive coronal restorations initiated pulpal changes independent of the degree of periodontal involvement. Others have reported that there is no apparent relationship between the number of immunocompetent cells in pulp tissue and the periodontal status of teeth. Therefore, endodontic disease occurs independent of periodontal disease but may occur 1) secondary to periodontal treatment that cuts vascular bundles traversing accessory canals or 2) secondary to the egress of bacteria through denuded dentin tubules following periodontal scaling.

Anachoresis

Another means of bacterial colonization within the pulp chamber is through anachoresis. Anachoresis is the localization of blood-borne microbes or their products to an inflamed area. Animal studies show that blood-borne bacteria can be recovered from root canal fluids. A study by Sundqvist examined teeth with a history of trauma and were clinically diagnosed as nonvital but intact. That is, these teeth were free of fractures, caries, restorations, and periodontal disease. When the canal contents were examined bacteriologically using anaerobic techniques, a preponderance of anaerobic bacteria was found. When the earlier studies of Kakehashi regarding pulpal necrosis are compared with the findings of Sundqvist, anachoresis (in the presence of pulpal inflammation) becomes a reasonable explanation for initiation of the endodontic disease process that leads to pulpal necrosis.

Fractures and Cracks

Crown fractures that expose dentin to the oral environment cause only insignificant pulpal inflammation. If unprotected, however, toxins and pathogens can penetrate the exposed dentin tubules and precipitate inflammation in the underlying pulp. Deep dentinal exposures that remain unprotected for long periods of time will result in pulp necrosis.

As a result of a crack, the pulp tissue and the periodontal attachment apparatus become inflamed from the trauma and mechanical movement of the segments. Breakdown progresses rapidly when a communication develops between the coronal extent of the crack and the periodontal sulcus. With this development, there is an accelerated ingress of oral flora and bone loss. The condition worsens with pulpal and apical extension of the crack. If not already damaged from the initial trauma, the pulp can secondarily become infected and necrose as the crack progresses toward the chamber or canals. Characterizing these lesions are a vertical loss of bone and sometimes sinus tracts that result from the action of the host bacteria.

Trauma

Traumatic displacement of a tooth is another obvious route for microbial ingress to the pulp through a damaged periodontal ligament or frank exfoliation. Violent disruption of pulpal blood supply results in ischemia with breakdown of the pulpal capillary structure, hemorrhage into the interstitial tissue, and necrosis of the pulpal cellular elements. The breakdown products of these necrotic tissues can diffuse through the apex and induce periapical disease.

Compound Etiology

Any combination of events, if severe enough, can lead to pulpal disease and necrosis. Although treatment in many circumstances is the same—root canal therapy or extraction—understanding the etiology is more than of academic interest in the presence of multiple lesions. These lesions may exist as a result of failed endodontic treatment, severe infection, metastatic tumors, or an irreparable split tooth.

Bacterial Pathways from the Pulp

Bacteremia

Bacteremia may or may not occur as a result of endodontic treatment. Whether bacteremia occurs depends on the presence of bacteria in the pulp canal system, or bacteria that are introduced to the canal system during treatment. During a pulpotomy or treatment of a vital pulp, the potential for bacteremia is low. If there is necrosis with bacteria present, or if the canal system becomes contaminated during endodontic treatment, then the chance of bacteremia developing increases. Overinstrumentation or violation of the apical constriction during cleaning, shaping, and obturation procedures will initiate bacteremia. Control of endodontic instrumentation procedures in order to keep within the anatomical apex becomes important to decrease the incidence or degree of bacteremia (Fig. 53.4). In healthy patients, bacteria are cleared within 10 minutes by various systemic mechanisms. In medically compromised patients this clearance may take longer or may not occur at all. Although any number of precautions can be taken

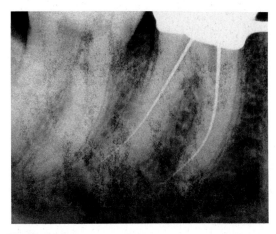

Figure 53.4: During endodontic treatment, care should be taken to confine instruments within the canal. In this length determination radiograph, the file in the distal canal is within acceptable limits. The file in the mesial buccal canal is long and should be adjusted.

during endodontic procedures, it should be assumed that bacteremia will occur and appropriate precautions should be taken in susceptible patients.

Septicemia

Septicemia is invasion of the bloodstream by microbes, their toxins, or both. Septicemia is a grave condition that can occur in compromised patients or secondary to an overwhelming infection such as the inability of an acute periapical abscess to drain. Septicemic meningitis is documented as having occurred during endodontic treatment.

Infective Endocarditis

Infective endocarditis can occur secondary to endodontic treatment. However, the number of reported cases of infective endocarditis following endodontic treatment is minimal when compared with exodontia and operative procedures. Nonetheless, the risk cannot be ignored. Regardless of the condition of the pulp or periapex or the method of treatment, all patients at risk should be given prophylactic antibiotics as recommended by the American Heart Association and the American Dental Association.

Focal Infection

A relationship between teeth and the theory of focal infection was propagated from 1910 to the 1940s. Focal infection is defined as sepsis arising from a focus of infection, such as abscessed teeth, that initiates a secondary infection in a nearby or a distant tissue or organ. In other words, an anachoretic effect is created with a diseased tooth as the nidus. It was believed that many systemic diseases resulted from odontogenic infections, which resulted in the unnecessary removal of countless teeth with little or no scientific or medical evidence to support or refute various claims. Secondary infection *can* arise following pulpal disease. Documented reports include cavernous sinus thrombosis, cerebral abscesses, endophthalmitis, osteomyelitis of the tibia, and bacterial myocarditis, which have led to death or serious impairment. These incidents, however, were secondary to longstanding, untreated, and acute abscesses of endodontic origin that had progressed far beyond the usual course for these lesions. Ludwig's angina, a grave complication of endodontic lesions, arises from the direct extension of a periapical abscess across fascial planes rather than as a secondary site of infection.

Hollow Tube Theory

At one time it was thought that periapical fluids collected in unfilled canals, the cellular constituents

lysed, and these toxins maintained or exacerbated the inflammatory response. Animal studies show that this does not occur.

Diagnosis of Endodontic Disease

To date there has been no direct correlation between the clinical diagnosis of endodontic pulpal and periapical disease and the histological makeup of pulpal and periapical lesions. Clinical symptoms of teeth presenting with pulpitis often have no association when compared to histological serial sections of these same teeth. Tables 53.1 and 53.2 review the terminology and descriptions characterizing clinical and histological endodontic disease.

Lesions of Endodontic Origin

Lesions of endodontic origin refer to periapical and soft tissue lesions that result solely from the sequelae of pulp necrosis. Though lesions of endodontic origin are odontogenic infections, "lesions of endodontic origin" more precisely states the etiology. The term also implies a particular course of treatment, that is, elimination of the noxious pulpal irritant either through extraction or endodontic therapy. Lesions of endodontic origin can be definitively diagnosed only through histological examination. Nonetheless, certain patterns of clinical signs, symptoms, and pulpal responses to thermal and mechanical stimuli can suggest whether a lesion is or is not of endodontic origin. This becomes significant in differentiating lesions of endodontic origin from such pathology as metastatic carcinoma, periapical cemental dysplasia, or developmental cysts, all of which can appear radiographically similar (Figs. 53.5 and 53.6).

Granulomas and Cysts

Granulomas and cysts constitute most periapical lesions of endodontic origin, in about equal numbers. Differentiating these lesions can only be done through histological examination since there are no radiographic differences or distinguishing clinical signs and symptoms. When of endodontic origin, these lesions resolve following extraction or competent nonsurgical endodontic treatment.

Abscesses

Abscesses that occur in the oral tissues most often are in, or originate in, periapical regions (Fig. 53.7). The abscess contains a central area of microorganisms and disintegrating polymorphonuclear leukocytes,

Table 53.1: Endodontic Diagnosis: Pulpal Disease

Diagnosis	Clinical Signs and Symptoms	Histologic Description
Normal	Asymptomatic Moderate response to stimuli (thermal and/or electric); response subsides when stimulus is removed No radiographic signs of pulpal calcification, internal resorption, or periapical changes	Specialized connective tissue, with a dense intercellular ground substance supporting mineralizing cells, the odontoblasts, arranged as a pseudomembrane at the pulp dentin interface, and encased by noncompliant hard tissue, dentin
Reversible pulpitis	Asymptomatic unless provoked by stimuli Moderate to sharp response to thermal, sweet, or sour stimuli; response subsides when stimulus is removed Pain is *not* spontaneous Etiology is usually caries, defective restoration, restorative procedures, toothbrush abrasion, tooth fracture, or recent prophylaxis No radiographic evidence of pulp calcifications, internal resorption, or periapical changes	Dilation of blood vessels Minimal disruption of odontoblastic layer of cells Possible extravasation of red blood cells and/or diapedesis of white blood cells Changes are localized in pulp at the base of involved dentin tubules and are generally considered reversible
Irreversible pulpitis	May have acute or chronic symptoms Sharp, painful response to thermal stimulus; pain lingers after stimulus is removed Pain may be spontaneous; may be past repeated episodes of pain Electric pulp testing may give conflicting results Radiography may reveal normal pulp, calcifications, narrow pulp chamber, "calcified" canals, deep caries and/or restorations, evidence of previous pulp cap, or condensing osteitis; an enlarged PDL may also be present The disease process is initiated when a vital pulp is exposed by caries; also present with hyperplastic pulpitis or internal resorption May or may not be sensitive to percussion	Severe tissue damage and inflammation Carious exposure and egress of bacteria into pulp cavity common Advanced vascular dilation and pooling of edema fluid surrounding the blood vessels Pavementing of PMNs which migrate into the interstitial tissues Heavy leukocyte infiltration, particularly proximal to the site of exposure Formation of microabscesses and subsequent liquefaction necrosis
Necrosis	Usually asymptomatic; pain emanates from periapical tissues Crown may be discolored No response usually to electric pulp tester; usually no response to cold test. May have exaggerated response to heat May or may not have evidence of periapical disease Multirooted teeth *may* have necrosis in one canal and vital tissue in the other canal(s), presenting confusing pulp testing results; occurs infrequently	A circumferential progression of the above events resulting in massive liquefaction necrosis Zones of chronic inflammation may be found adjacent to areas of liquefaction necrosis Intact and altered neural tissues may still be present in degenerating and any remaining healthy tissue Occasional appearance of dry necrosis or "sicca" described as a pulp space containing particulates of debris or no pulpal material at all

Table 53.2: Endodontic Diagnosis: Periapical Disease

Diagnosis	Clinical Symptoms	Histologic Description
Normal	Asymptomatic Not sensitive to percussion No radiographic change in the periapical tissues No draining sinus tract present	A rich combination of cellular and extracellular components containing blood and lymphatics, motor and sensory fibers to the pulp and periodontium Structural elements include ground substance, fibroblasts, cementoblasts, osteoblasts, clastic cells, histiocytes, undifferentiated mesenchymal cells, and the epithelial cells organized as the Rests of Malassez
Acute apical periodontitis	Tooth is sensitive to percussion or palpation Tooth may be vital or nonvital Radiographs may appear normal or show a thickening of the periodontal ligament *space*	Localized inflammation of the periodontal ligament at the apical region Infiltration and localization of PMNs and macrophages in apical area Liquefaction necrosis may be present Bone resorption may be present
Chronic apical periodontitis	Etiology may be an extension of pulp disease into periapical tissue, endodontic procedures, or occlusal trauma	*Periapical granuloma:* Replacement of alveolar bone and periodontal ligament with granulation tissue; chronic infiltration of plasma cells, lymphocytes, and phagocytes, with occasional multinucleated foreign body giant cells and foam cells Varying amounts of islands of epithelial proliferation *Periapical cyst:* A central cavity of stratified squamous epithelium surrounded by varying amounts of connective tissue
Acute periapical abscess	No response to pulp vitality check Often asymptomatic May be slightly tender to percussion Sequela of pulp disease or endodontic therapy Radiographic evidence of periapical radiolucency (lesions do not become radiographically visible until there is resorption of cortical bone) There is *no* radiographic distinction between a granuloma or a cyst May be tender to palpation with resorption of cortical plate May have draining sinus tract	Cavity contains necrotic debris and an infiltrate containing macrophages, lymphocytes, plasma cells, and occasional PMNs A central area of liquefaction necrosis; within are disintegrating neutrophils and other cellular debris surrounded by macrophages; may be some lymphocytes and plasma cells present as well Viable and nonviable bacteria may be present

surrounded by viable leukocytes and some lymphocytes. Clinical features include pain, swelling, fever, and sometimes regional lymphadenitis, which is usually confined to the immediate region of the source of infection. However, microbial byproducts and tissue breakdown products may produce systemic illness. A periapical abscess may remain limited to the osseous structures or, through bone resorption, may follow the path of least resistance, breaking through the periosteum and invading the soft tissues. During abscess formation there may be regional cellulitis. The infection then becomes well circumscribed, producing a localized collection of suppuration in a cavity, which is the true abscess.

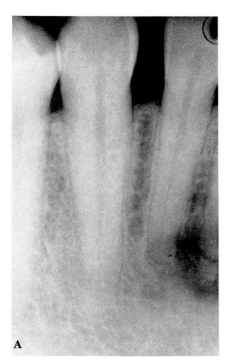
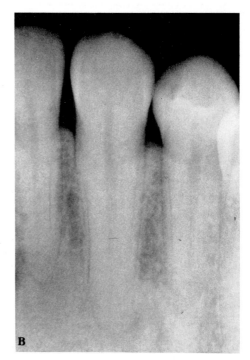

Figure 53.5: In the absence of pulpal disease or obvious bacterial etiology, careful diagnosis is necessary before one assumes radiopaque or radiolucent periapical lesions are endodontic in origin. These radiographs, from the same patient, indicate the benign presence of periapical osseous dysplasia.

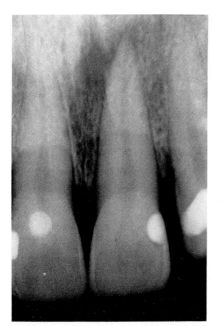
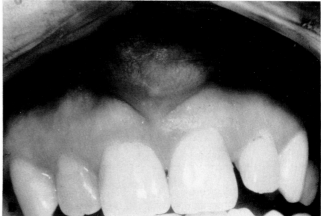

Figure 53.6: Patient presented with fluctuant midline swelling and a periapical radiolucency associated with the left central incisor. Pulpal diagnostic tests indicated that the pulp was vital and could not have contributed to such a periapical response. Surgical biopsy showed that the bony radiolucency was secondary to pressure of the soft tissue lesion, which was completely in soft tissues and not of endodontic origin.

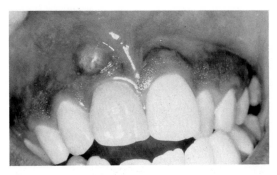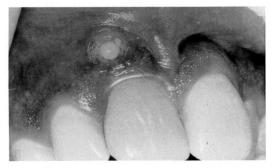

Figure 53.7: Endodontic abscesses can present in different patterns. This patient had a suppurative lesion secondary to failed endodontic treatment of the right central incisor. Simple drainage and antibiotic treatment were used as immediate care until nonsurgical endodontic retreatment could be initiated.

Abscesses of the head and neck are caused by aerobic and anaerobic microorganisms. Studies disagree on which organisms are most associated with such infections. In some studies, when only one type of organism was recovered, α-hemolytic streptococci were more common, with the remaining infections attributable to *Staphylococcus aureus* or *Staphylococcus epidermidis* in about equal proportions. Other studies reported that staphylococcal infections were more common. Single organism infections have also been attributed to *Actinomyces* species; enterococci, *Proteus* species; *Branhamella catarrhalis;* and pleomorphic gram-positive, irregularly arranged organisms classified as *Corynebacterium* species.

Gram-positive and gram-negative anaerobes have been isolated from head and neck abscesses. The gram-positive anaerobes most frequently isolated include *Peptostreptococcus* species, *Peptococcus* species, and *Eubacterium* species. The gram-negative anaerobes were black-pigmented *Bacteroides* species, some *Fusobacterium* species, and *Veillonella* species. Several studies indicate that anaerobic infections tend to be a mixture of organisms. Indeed, some investigations suggest that many of the species isolated, such as the *Bacteroides* species, are incapable of producing abscesses by themselves.

There is disagreement about the role of various bacteria in abscesses of the head and neck region. Some of the differences may be due to sampling procedures, such as how soon after the infection began, how far it had progressed, and what other factors were superimposed (e.g., therapeutic attempts) at the time of sampling. Also there may be a shift in the type of microorganisms isolated due to the increased technical ability to recognize and cultivate others.

Actinomycosis

Actinomycosis is a fastidious, noncontagious, slowly growing, chronic suppurative infection. The uncontrolled actinomycotic infection is characterized by peripheral spread to contiguous tissue without the limitation normally imposed by anatomical barriers. There is usually formation of sinus tracts with purulent drainage. Actinomycosis occurs in cervicofacial, abdominal, and pulmonary forms, the cervicofacial being the most common. Periapical actinomycosis, once considered rare, is usually diagnosed only when persistent periapical lesions are biopsied since these organisms are generally not reported in routine culture surveys. Periapical actinomycotic lesions often present as failed nonsurgical endodontic treatment having multiple sinus tracts. *Actinomyces israelii* is the principal species implicated in these lesions. There is some feeling that periapical actinomycosis may be a distinct form of actinomycosis since clinical signs may differ from typical actinomycotic symptoms. There appears to be a correlation between endodontic treatment and periapical actinomycosis. It may be possible that endodontic procedures introduce the *Actinomyces* organisms into the periapical tissues, or that secondarily the organism enters through a root canal left open to oral fluids, or as a direct extension of the carious process. Alternatively, this may only be an observational anomaly since biopsies of periapical lesions are not routinely done unless there is nonresolution of the lesion. Treatment for periapical actinomycosis usually involves surgical excision of the suspected lesion and a 4- to 6-week regimen of antibiotic therapy.

Cellulitis

Cellulitis is a diffuse inflammatory reaction in which the host defenses are unable to contain the infection to one area. Instead, it progresses through the surrounding tissues and along fascial planes to areas away from the original site of infection (Fig. 53.8). Cellulitis of the face and neck can result from periapical infection, can be secondary to endodontic treatment, or can follow periodontal infection. The tissues involved show separation of muscle or connective tissue. There is a nonspecific inflammation with exudation of polymorphonuclear leukocytes, lymphocytes, serous fluid, and fibrin. Clinically there is firm, painful swelling of the involved tissues and usually regional lymphadenitis. If the superficial tissues are involved, the overlying skin appears inflamed or even purple in color. The diffuse spread of infection may involve considerable areas of the face and neck. Aerobic organisms, principally α-hemolytic streptococci, are commonly associated with endodontic cellulitis in the orofacial region.

Cellulitis readily resolves with treatment. It can become localized, forming an abscess that may break through skin or mucous membrane and drain spontaneously. Suppurative drainage will take the path of least resistance and may occur into the oral vestibule, floor of the mouth, nose, maxillary sinus, face, or the infratemporal fossa. Extension can also occur into the cranial vault by bony resorption or to the base of the skull through foramina.

Ludwig's Angina

A particularly severe form of cellulitis is Ludwig's angina, which often begins in the submandibular space, then invades other tissue spaces bilaterally. The source of infection is often a mandibular tooth, but it may result from a fracture or penetrating injury. The clinical features of Ludwig's angina include rapid development of a boardlike swelling in the floor of the mouth, which becomes elevated. The tongue protrudes, and swallowing and respiration are difficult. The swelling does not localize. It spreads to involve the neck, the peripharyngeal spaces, and other regions (Fig. 53.9). If the larynx becomes edematous,

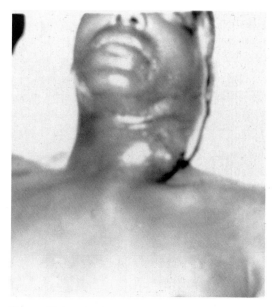

Figure 53.9: Ludwig's angina can become life-threatening. This patient required hospitalization to control the odontogenic infection.

the patient may suffocate. Streptococci are commonly involved in Ludwig's angina, but usually it is a mixed infection. A variety of gram-positive and gram-negative aerobic and anaerobic bacteria have been implicated, including fusiforms, spirochetes, diphtheroids, staphylococci, *Bacteroides, Klebsiella, Escherichia coli, Pseudomonas aeruginosa, Haemophilus influenzae,* and *Branhamella catarrhalis.*

Osteomyelitis

Osteomyelitis is an acute, subacute, or chronic inflammation of bone and bone marrow that may develop as a result of odontogenic or other infections. Acute osteomyelitis often results in a diffuse spread of infection throughout the medullary spaces, with necrosis of bone. A variety of bacteria are associated with osteomyelitis. Staphylococci and a few strains of *Streptococcus* are the most common, although actinomycetes and anaerobic bacteria are not uncommon. Other infections, such as tuberculosis or syphilis, also may produce osteomyelitis.

Condensing Osteitis

Unlike most lesions of endodontic origin, which appear as radiolucent areas, condensing osteitis is radiopaque on radiographs. It is thought to be a low-grade, subclinical response to chronic pulpal inflammation. Little is known about this lesion but it is generally felt that endodontic treatment is indicated if signs and symptoms of endodontic disease are present.

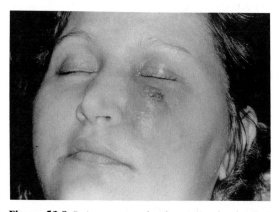

Figure 53.8: Patient presented with an acute alveolar abscess that developed into a cellulitis that expanded into the canine space. The lesion eventually drained suborbitally. Elimination of the bacterial etiology resolved the problem through antibiotic coverage and the removal of the maxillary second premolar. (Courtesy of Dr. Kenneth T. King, Charleston, South Carolina.)

Foreign Body Reaction

Any number of substances can cause foreign body reactions. Multinucleated giant cells surrounding a foreign material characterize these lesions histologically. Clinically, a foreign body reaction can occur during or subsequent to endodontic treatment if materials such as paper points or cotton pellets are forced through the apex and remain in the periapical tissues. Fibers from cotton sponges used to wipe endodontic instruments or powder from rubber gloves may also be carried into the apical tissues. Such a foreign body reaction can appear clinically as an abscess with draining sinus tracts that resist nonsurgical endodontic treatment and antibiotic therapy. The problem will resolve only when the foreign body has been removed.

Endotoxin and Endodontic Disease

Gram-negative anaerobic bacteria are most often associated with severe periapical lesions of pulpal origin. The gram-negative lipopolysaccharide cell walls are nonspecific antigens that are poorly neutralized by antibodies. These antigens can activate the complement cascade without antibody through the classical pathway (C1) or the alternate pathway (C3). These cell wall endotoxins can result in mast cell degranulation and the release of collagenase from macrophages, and can enhance neutrophil-mediated injury through the release of oxygen radicals and proteases, leading to tissue injury. They are nonspecific B-lymphocyte stimulators and resist phagocytosis through inclusion in the capsule. Endotoxins have been identified in necrotic pulp tissue and have been proportionately correlated with the quantity of anaerobic organisms recovered from these same canals. Additionally, cell wall material from anaerobic bacteria recovered from root canals has generated acute pulpitis and produced periapical lesions in primate animal models. However, endotoxin in and of itself may not be the significant factor in pulpal disease. It is the repetitive assault on a damaged pulp's ability to heal and withstand a chronic onslaught of antigens that induces the inflammatory reactions that lead to necrosis. Table 53.3 lists pathological mechanisms identified with *Bacteroides* species, which are common endodontic pathogens.

Host Defense

Specific and nonspecific host factors affect the capacity of bacteria to initiate endodontic disease.

Specific host factors involve antibody production

Table 53.3: Potential Pathogenic Mechanisms of Black-Pigmented *Bacteroides* Species*

Bacterial Products or Action	Effect
Abscess formation	Destruction of tissue
Capsule	Inhibition of phagocytosis
Lipopolysaccharide	Bone resorption
Enzymes	
Collagenase	
Trypsin	
Fibrinolysin	
Hyaluronidase	
Heparinase	
Ribonuclease	
Deoxyribonuclease	
Cytotoxic substances	Destruction of tissue
Indole	
Ammonia	
Hydrogen sulfide	
Methylmercaptan	
Fatty acids	
Immunopathology	Destruction of tissue
Humoral	
Cellular	

*Adapted with permission from Slots, J.: Importance of black-pigmented *Bacteroides* in human periodontal disease. In *Host-Parasite Interactions in Periodontal Diseases*, edited by R. J. Genco and S. E. Mergenhagen. American Society for Microbiology, Washington, D.C., 1979.

and the elements of cellular immunity. All cells normally and usually associated with inflammation and immunity are found within the pulp during inflammation. There is no reason not to expect the immune process to function as it does in other connective tissue.

Nonspecific host factors include the production of reparative dentin and macrophage phagocytosis of bacteria. The degree to which reparative dentine can act as a buffer to the ingress of bacteria and their byproducts is dependent on the rate of mineralization, the remaining dentin thickness, and the pace of decay. With compromised circulatory structures, as is seen in the capillary beds during pulpal inflammation, there is a reduced ability to transport away contents of necrosed macrophages, the products of which continue to contribute to the pulpal inflammatory response. In response to injury, granulation tissue proliferates periapically and replaces normal tissue. Compared with pulpal tissue, periapical tissues are highly vascularized. Pathological changes occur from activation of both the nonspecific and specific immune responses to the point where the periapical immunological response to pulpal disease is a combination of protective and allergic reactions.

Immunology and Lesions of Endodontic Origin

Inflammation is a complex vascular, lymphatic, and local tissue reaction of higher organisms to injury, to irritants, or both. Progression of inflammation is dependent on the presence or absence of vascular leakage. Simon outlined four sources of vascular leakage:

1. Application of heat, chemicals, bacteria or their toxins. This can result in delayed capillary leakage that lasts for several hours, the so-called "delayed–prolonged response."
2. Direct vascular injury, which occurs from all vessels—arterioles, capillaries, and venules.
3. Histamine-type leakage, which occurs mainly from the venule. Bradykinin and serotonin (from platelets) can also produce vascular leakage.
4. Leakage from a regenerating capillary. (This is a characteristic of granulation tissue.)

Nonspecific Inflammatory Reactions in Development of Periapical Lesions

Nonspecific inflammatory reactions may contribute to enigmatic pathways which lead to formation of initiators, mediators, or augmenters of endodontic periapical diseases. Biochemical systems of nonspecific periapical inflammation include the vasoactive amines, the kinin system, the complement system, and the arachidonic acid metabolites.

Vasoactive Amines. Mast cells have been identified in human endodontic periapical lesions. These cells release histamine following mechanical or chemical injury to the periapical tissues. Mast cell degranulation can occur following the physical damage from cleaning, shaping, or obturation of the root canal system if instruments or materials are extended beyond the root apex.

Kinin System. The kinin or kallikrein system is activated by the Hageman factor through its release from physical damage done to vascular basement membranes of periapical tissues. Bacterial endotoxins seeping from a diseased canal system also activate the Hageman factor. Kinin activities such as chemotaxis, smooth muscle contraction, arteriole dilation, and increased capillary permeability contribute to periapical inflammation and its consequences, which are pain and edema.

Complement System. Complement C3 components have been found in periapical endodontic lesions. Activation of the complement system, through classical or alternate pathways, can occur from a wide number of stimuli, including IgM, IgG, bacteria, bacterial metabolites and endotoxins, lysosomal enzymes, and clotting factors. These activators are all found in pathological periapical tissue. Periapical bone resorption occurs either through inhibition of new bone formation or destruction of bone present. This occurs through activation of the complement system in periapical tissues. The activated complement system also stimulates phospholipid metabolism and the release of lipids from cell membranes providing a source for arachidonic acid, the prostaglandin precursor.

Arachidonic Acid Metabolites. Complement activation stimulates cyclooxygenase metabolism of arachidonic acid, thereby generating PGE_2 from neutrophils and macrophages. Studies have confirmed that significant amounts of PGE_2 are present in periapical endodontic lesions. Torabinejad suggests that the presence of complement components and a high concentration of PGE_2 activate the complement system and stimulate bone resorption by increasing PGE_2 formation as well as inhibiting collagen formation via a PGE_2-independent mechanism.

Acquired Immunity in Development of Periapical Lesions

Immediate Hypersensitivity Reactions (Type I). Type I reactions are characterized by basophil and mast cell degranulation following IgE attachment with later release of chemical mediators such as histamine, leukotrienes, prostaglandins, eosinophil chemotactic factor, platelet-activating factor, and heparin. There is also activation of the Hageman factor following endothelial damage. All the components for type I reactions, namely IgE-containing plasma cells, mast cells, basophils, and allergens, can be found *within* periapical lesions of endodontic origin. Bacteria, endotoxins, and medicament-altered host pulp tissue can serve as antigen sources that cause host sensitization. Patients presenting with acute apical abscesses have demonstrated elevated levels of serum IgE, which suggests that some endodontic flareups may be mediated by IgE and as a result are refractory to antibiotics. Atopic and nonatopic patients often have different clinical reactions to endodontic problems. Elevated IgE levels characterize atopic individuals, suggesting an increased ability to produce IgE in response to canal antigens. These patients are more likely to experience a type I reaction after endodontic procedures.

Cytotoxic Reaction (Type II). It is theorized that periapical lesions of endodontic origin can be maintained through type II reactions in which cell lysis is IgG or complement dependent.

Antibody-dependent, Cell-mediated Cytotoxicity. These reactions are characterized by the binding of bacterial cells from diseased canal systems to IgG, which in turn is bound by the Fc region to Fc receptors on effector cells, the macrophages, and PMN leukocyte membranes. Furthermore, there is additional attraction of PMNs and macrophages to formed complexes and a subsequent increase in phagocytosis, release of lysosomal enzymes, and an increase in vascular leakage, all contributing to abscess formation. The presence of IgG molecules, killer cells such as PMN leukocytes and macrophages, and complement fragments in human periapical lesions indicates that type II reactions occur in this region.

Complement-dependent Antibody Lysis. Diseased root canal antigens such as bacteria, bacterial endotoxins, or bacterial metabolic products may interact with tissue components or cell membranes and either IgG or IgM to form immune complexes. These complexes bind to the platelets, resulting in the release of vasoactive amines, increased vascular permeability, and chemotaxis of PMN leukocytes. The binding of immune complexes to PMN leukocytes can lead to the release of lysosomal enzymes and pathological sequelae of immune complex deposition in periapical tissues. Immunoglobulin G, immune complexes, and C3 complement component have been identified in lesions of endodontic origin and detected in elevated systemic levels in patients with acute periapical lesions as compared with patients with chronic lesions. These findings suggest that, although immune complex formation is a protective mechanism for neutralization and elimination of antigen, this phenomenon can also initiate or perpetuate the development of human periapical lesions.

Antigen–Antibody Complex Reaction (Type III). Intense inflammation and pain can result from activation of the complement system through the formation and binding of soluble antigen–antibody complexes to granulocytes, macrophages, platelets, and endothelial cells. Components associated with these reactions are present in periapical tissue biopsied from some endodontic lesions.

Cell-mediated Immune Reaction (Type IV). Delayed-type hypersensitivity results from antigen-induced activation of cytotoxic T-cells, the release of lymphokines, or both. Pan-B-lymphocytes, pan-T-lymphocytes (T11), helper (T4), and suppressor (T8) T-lymphocytes have been identified in pulp tissue. In normal pulp tissue, there are scattered T8-lymphocytes with a few B-lymphocytes. As the pulp regresses from normal to irreversible pulpitis (clinical classification), greater numbers of both T- and B-lymphocytes are seen, T-cells make up 90% of the cells present, T4 begins to outnumber T8-cells, and B-cells begin to outnumber T1-cells.

Studies of chronic periapical lesions of endodontic origin demonstrate the presence of T-lymphocytes, including T-suppressor cells, T-helper cells, and T-natural killer cells; B-cells; and macrophages. Macrophages and lymphocytes make up most of the cells in these lesions, with T-cells significantly outnumbering B-cells. There is a high T4/T8 ratio. As would be expected, in AIDS and ARC patients, the T4/T8 ratio is reduced so that most of the cells present are T8. Osteoclast-activating factor (OAF), a lymphokine, has been identified in periapical lesions, lymphocytes containing OAF were identified, and PGE_2 in significant quantity as well. The presence of these components suggests that cell-mediated immunological reactions play a significant role in periapical pathology. It has been proposed that prostaglandin production is necessary for the development of bony endodontic lesions in periapical tissues since, in addition to the above findings, the use of a prostaglandin inhibitor in animal models blocks formation of these lesions.

Microbiology of Endodontic Disease

Bacteria from diseased teeth were observed soon after development of the microscope. There are many reports from many investigators describing flora identified in necrotic pulp systems and endodontic lesions (Table 53.4). To date there is no clear consensus on any one causative species, the most numerous species, or the most pathological species. One can only speculate on which organisms are the principal members of microbial climax communities in infected pulp tissue.

The microorganisms found in soft tissue infection of endodontic origin may be the same as those precipitating pulpal infection or might be secondarily opportunistic during the necrotic process. If a multiple bacterial flora were originally present, the pulp could favor one species while the soft tissues could favor another or a co-infector. Differences in isolates may result from fluctuations in the proportion of organisms over a given time period or through the course of the disease and treatment attempts.

The following discussion will consider some of the problems in the study of endodontic microbiology and some of the major bacterial species associated with endodontic disease. Hopefully, it will be impressed upon the reader the importance of recognizing when the bacteriology of endodontic disease transcends academic interest and becomes of clinical importance.

Interpretation of Clinical Studies

Periodontal research suggests that distinct forms of periodontal disease exist, each having unique etiological pathogens. Popular concepts of endodontic

Table 53.4: Bacteria Reported from Endodontic Abscesses and Perimandibular Space Infections

Spirochetes

Treponema
  T. macrodentium, T. microdentium
  T. vincentii

Spiral and Curved Bacteria

Campylobacter
  C. sputorum

Gram-Negative Facultatively Anaerobic Rods

Actinobacillus
  A. actinomycetemcomitans
Klebsiella
  K. pneumoniae
Enterobacter
  E. cloacae

Gram-Negative Anaerobic Bacteria

Bacteroides
  B. asaccharolyticus, B. bivius, B. capillosus, B. clostridiformis, B. corrodens, B. coagulans, B. distasonis, B. endodontalis, B. fragilis, B. fragilis ss. diastasonis, B. furcosus, B. gingivalis, B. intermedius, B. melaninogenicus, B. nodosus, B. ochraceus, B. oralis, B. pneumosintes, B. ruminicola, B. ruminicola ss. brevis, B. thetaiotaomicron, B. ureolyticus, B. uniformis, B. vulgarus
Capnocytophaga
  species reported
Fusobacterium
  F. fusiforme, F. necrophorum, F. nucleatum, F. russi, F. varium
Leptotrichia
  L. buccalis
Eikenella
  E. corrodens
Wolinella
  W. recta, W. succinogenes

Genera of Uncertain Affiliation

Selenomonas
  S. sputigena
Mycobacterium
  M. leprae, M. tuberculosis

Gram-Negative Cocci and Coccobacilli

Neisseria
  N. flava, N. sicca
Branhamella
  B. catarrhalis

Gram-Negative Anaerobic Cocci

Veillonella
  V. alcalescens, V. parvula

Gram-Positive Cocci

Micrococcus
  species reported
Streptococcus
  S. constellatus, S. epidermidis, S. faecalis, S. faecium, S. hemolyticus, S. intermedius, S. liquefaciens, S. milleri, S. mitis, S. mitior, S. morbillorum, S. mutans, S. pneumoniae, S. pyogenes, S. salivarius, S. sanguis, S. zymogenes
Staphylococcus
  S. aureus, S. citreus, S. epidermidis

Peptococcus
  P. asaccharolyticus, P. constellatus, P. intermedius, P. magnus, P. morbillorum, P. micros, P. prevotii, P. saccharolyticus, P. variabilis
Peptostreptococcus
  P. anaerobius, P. intermedius, P. micros, P. minus, P. parvula, P. productus

Endospore-Forming Rods

Bacillus
  B. subtilis, B. cereus

Gram-Positive, Asporogenous Rod-shaped Bacteria

Lactobacillus
  L. acidophilus, L. caseii var rhamnosus, L. catenaforme, L. cellobiosus, L. crispatus, L. fermentum, L. lactis, L. plantarium
Sporulating organisms
  species reported

Actinomycetes and Related Organisms

Corynebacterium
  C. pseudodiphtheriticum, C. xerose
Actinomyces
  A. bovis, A. israelii, A. naeslundii, A. odontolyticus, A. viscosus, Streptobacillus monoiliformus, Bacterionema matruchotii
Norcardia
  N. asteroides
Arachnia
  A. propionica
Eubacterium
  E. alactolyticum, E. lentum, E. limosum, E. ventriosum
Propionibacterium
  P. acnes, P. avidum
Bifidobacterium
  B. adolescentis, B. bifidum, B. dentum, B. ruminicola ss. ruminicola
Mycoplasmas
  Mycoplasma
    M. salivarium

Gram-Negative, Nonsporulating, Facultative Anaerobic Rods (the Enterobacteriaceae)

Aerobacter aerogenes
Escherichia coli
Klebsiella pneumoniae
Proteus vulgaris
Salmonella typhi
Alcaligenes faecalis
Pseudomonas aeruginosa
Haemophilus influenzae
Mima polymorpha
Campylobacter sputorum
Enterobacter agglomerans

Yeasts

Saccharomyces sp.
Cryptococcus sp.
Candida
  C. albicans, C. guilliermondi, C. krusei, "C. mortifera"

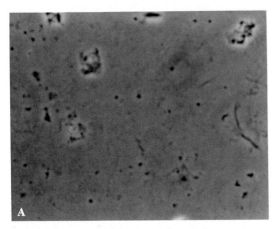

Figure 53.10: Immunofluorescence microscopy is more sensitive than culture technique for identification of microorganisms from clinical samples. A polyclonal antibody specific for *Bacteroides gingivalis* is used to identify the organism in a smear of mixed organisms. (**A**) View with phase-contrast microscopy. (**B**) Same field under ultraviolet illumination.

disease embrace one pathological process, pulpal necrosis, that manifests in diverse patterns of periapical destruction.

Although it is recognized that bacterial microorganisms are central to the pulpal pathologic process, few advances have been made in the application of current techniques for the identification of etiological endodontic pathogens. Similarly, when various identification methods are evaluated, the sensitivity of the identification technique is a critical factor in recognizing the presence of these organisms. Recovery of these bacteria from endodontically diseased teeth is difficult. This is especially true for fastidious anaerobes. Several variables can affect any microbial survey: differences in culture technique, prior treatment, time of sampling, provision of antibiotic therapy, quantity of viable organisms, thoroughness of sampling technique, and appropriate media. These factors, together with the skill of the investigator, can influence the incidence and proportion of organisms recovered by culture and consequently can influence the perceived relationships of any pathogens that may be present. Variations in bacterial survival in vivo imply differences in the ability of bacterial species to evade host defense mechanisms. Several techniques are available for the identification of specific bacteria from clinical specimens, including culture, microscopy, DNA probes, and immunofluorescence assays. These methods may be applied to specimens from endodontic disease as well, expediting identification of organisms and their origins.

An example of an alternative technique is indirect immunofluorescence microscopy. When used as specific staining reagents for antigens in tissues or cells, antibodies are not visible unless combined with a dye or isotope used as an indicator. The principles behind indirect immunofluorescence involve two antigen–antibody reactions. Specific bacterial antigens react with antibodies directed to these antigens. A second antibody, conjugated with fluorescein isothiocyanate, is directed against the first antigen–antibody complex and observed using a fluorescence microscope (Fig. 53.10).

There are significant clinical advantages to this technique: labeled bacterial cells can be rapidly detected, usually within 2 to 3 hours from time of initial sampling; the morphology of positive cells can be distinguished, avoiding false positive reactions; and the fluorescing cells can be quantified as a proportion of the total cell count. With indirect immunofluorescence, low bacterial cell counts can be quantified, with no need for cell viability. Additionally, obtaining bacterial samples through the root canal is consistent with nonsurgical endodontic treatment as well as classic endodontic culture technique (Table 53.5).

Frequently, pure cultures are reported from clinical endodontic samples, that is, only one organism is cultured from a particular lesion or diseased tooth. It is debatable if sampling, culturing, and speciation techniques are adequate to ensure recovery and identification of all bacteria that are actually present, and that the single species isolated is the only species involved in the infection.

In 1983 Williams et al. examined the aspirants of 10 abscesses of endodontic origin that had produced fluctuant soft tissue swelling. In order to select representative colony types of all bacterial growth from these samples, the investigators randomly selected 100 colonies from each of the 10 samples, for a total of 1,000 isolates. For identification and speciation, each bacterial isolate required over 40 tests, representing over 40,000 diagnostic tests and observations for this one study. Yet even with this enormous undertaking, some of the recovered samples were not completely identified. Findings from this study are listed in Table 53.6.

A different study by Oguntebi et al., reported in 1982, was similar in that these investigators examined aspirants of 10 abscesses of endodontic origin also manifesting with fluctuant soft tissue swelling. However, different transport and growth media and different selection criteria were used. Complete identification of all recovered bacteria was reported. The results are shown in Table 53.6.

Fusobacterium nucleatum was the most frequent organism reported in the Williams study, while *F. nucleatum* and *Streptococcus mitis* were the most numerous organisms in the Oguntebi study. However, *S. mitis* was not reported as being present in the Williams study at all. Findings for the *Bacteroides* species are interesting also. Williams et al. reported six strains of *Bacteroides* species and four *Bacteroides* isolates they could not identify beyond genus. Oguntebi et al. only reported two bacterial strains identified as *B. intermedius,* while asaccharolytic *Bacteroides* strains were not reported at all. Such differences are not uncommon. These well done studies illustrate the difficulty in correlating endodontic research investigating etiological flora with the endodontic disease process.

Table 53.5: Detection of *Bacteroides* Species in Root Canals by Bacterial Culture and Immunofluorescence Microscopy*†

Organism	Culture Positive‡ No. (%)	Immunofluorescence Positive§ No. (%)
B. endodontalis	1 (1)	13 (16)
B. gingivalis	3 (4)	12 (15)
B. intermedius	9 (11)	35 (43)
Total Bacteroides‖	13 (20)	40 (49)

*Adapted with permission from E. A. Pantera, Jr., J. J. Zambon, M. Shih-Levine: Indirect Immunofluorescence for the Detection of *Bacteroides* Species in Human Dental Pulp. *J Endodont,* **14**, 218–223, 1988. © by *Journal of Endodontics.*

†Bacteria were recovered from 82 patient samples.

‡Number (%) of samples exhibiting the target organism in culture.

§Number (%) of samples exhibiting the target organism on indirect immunofluorescence.

‖Total number (%) of samples with target *Bacteroides* species.

Clinical Culture

The routine sampling of root canals during endodontic treatment is not recommended. Historically, microbiological culture was used as an end point indicator for endodontic treatment and as a method for evaluating cleaning and shaping techniques. Findings from routine cultures indicated when *not* to obturate, but reports suggested that negative culture was more likely dependent on methods and materials rather than on the presence or absence of organisms. Beginning in the 1970s the efficacy of culturing in endodontics was challenged, owing to the difficulties in culturing technique and lack of ready access to a microbiology laboratory service.

Should bacteriological sampling be indicated, it should be performed by personnel with appropriate background in clinical anaerobic recovery techniques. A suggested procedure is given in Table 53.7.

Endodontic Pathogens

Several bacterial species are discussed in the context of endodontic disease more often than others. Following is a brief summary of some of these organisms.

***Bacteroides* Species.** *Bacteroides* has routinely been associated with pulpal and periapical disease. The black-pigmented *Bacteroides* organisms are nonmotile, non-spore-forming, obligate anaerobes that produce black pigment and are found as a normal component of the oropharyngeal and urogenital flora. These gram-negative organisms are thought to play an important role in the etiology of specific human infections. The *Bacteroides* species can cause septicemia and severe infections in various parts of the body, including the liver, appendix, and brain. They are the predominant organisms found in aspiration pneumonia, chronic destructive pneumonia, primary lung abscess, bites, perimandibular space infections, and adult periodontitis. Studies also correlate the presence of *Bacteroides* species in human dental pulp with the severity of endodontic lesions and patient pain. Many studies have described the anaerobic black-pigmented *Bacteroides* species *B. melaninogenicus.* Over 30 reference strains from eight distinct species and a proposed ninth species have been classified from the single previous taxonomic group, *B. melaninogenicus.* Figure 53.11 shows the evolution of current taxonomy used for some of the *Bacteroides* species that were previously reported only as *B. melaninogenicus.* Characteristics of *B. gingivalis, B. intermedius,* and *B. endodontalis* include the production of a black hematin pigment when cells are grown on a blood-supplemented medium, the ability of colonies to fluoresce under long-wave ultraviolet light,

Table 53.6: Bacteriology of Individual Endodontic Abscess Specimens*

Sample No.†	Williams et al.	Oguntebi et al.
1	*Streptococcus milleri*	*Streptococcus mitis* *Peptostreptococcus anaerobius*
2	Anaerobic gram-positive cocci *Bacteroides* species *Fusobacterium nucleatum* *Bacteroides oralis* *Bacteroides melaninogenicus*	*Streptococcus mitis* *Fusobacterium nucleatum* *Bacteroides melaninogenicus* subsp. *intermedius* *Peptostreptococcus anaerobius*
3	*Fusobacterium nucleatum* *Fusobacterium* species *Streptococcus sanguis* *Staphylococcus epidermidis*	*Streptococcus mitis* *Actinomyces viscosus* *Fusobacterium nucleatum*
4	Anaerobic diphtheroids *Bacteroides* species *Fusobacterium nucleatum*	*Fusobacterium nucleatum* *Peptostreptococcus micros*
5	*Streptococcus intermedius* *Bacteroides melaninogenicus* *Bacteroides distasonis* *Bacteroides oralis* *Bacteroides corrodens* *Fusobacterium nucleatum*	*Streptococcus mitis* *Fusobacterium nucleatum* *Bacteroides melaninogenicus* subsp. *intermedius*
6	*Staphylococcus epidermidis* *Peptostreptococcus micros* *Fusobacterium nucleatum* *Bacteroides* species (2)	*Streptococcus faecalis* *Actinomyces viscosus*
7	*Peptostreptococcus micros* *Eubacterium lentum* *Bacteroides ruminicola* subsp. *brevis* *Bacteroides corrodens*	*Streptococcus faecalis* *Fusobacterium nucleatum*
8	*Peptostreptococcus micros* *Bacteroides* species (3) *Bacteroides melaninogenicus* *Bacteroides asaccharolyticus* *Fusobacterium nucleatum* *Lactobacillus* species	*Streptococcus faecalis* *Actinomyces viscosus*
9	*Peptostreptococcus micros* *Lactobacillus fermentum* *Bacteroides oralis* *Bacteroides ruminicola* subsp. *brevis*	*Streptococcus mitis* *Staphylococcus mitis* *Fusobacterium nucleatum*
10	*Peptostreptococcus micros* *Peptostreptococcus anaerobius* *Bacteroides corrodens* *Capnocytophaga ochracea*	*Streptococcus mitis* *Fusobacterium nucleatum*

*Adapted with permission from B. L. Williams, G. F. McCann, F. D. Schoenknecht: Bacteriology of Dental Abscesses of Endodontic Origin. *J Clin Microbiol,* **18,** 770, 1983; and B. Oguntebi, A. M. Slee, J. M. Tanzer, K. Langeland: Predominant Microflora Associated with Human Dental Periapical Abscesses. *J Clin Microbiol,* **15,** 964, 1982.

†Sample numbers are for comparative purposes only and do not reflect analysis done on the same bacteriological sample.

Table 53.7: Anaerobic Culturing for Endodontic Infections*

Equipment

1. Disposable aspirating syringe.
2. One and one-half inch 15- or 18-gauge sterile disposable beveled needle.
3. Sterile rubber stopper.
4. Anaerobic transport device.

Technique

1. Obtain anesthesia: a division block is preferred.
2. Delineate the area of fluctuance by palpating the swelling.
3. Disinfect the mucosa at the site of swelling by swabbing the area with an antiseptic solution such as povidone iodine. The antiseptic should be left in contact with the tissue for at least 1 minute.
4. Aspirate fluid sample from the swelling. Ideally, obtain 1 to 2 mL of aspirant.
5. Transport the specimen to the laboratory in the syringe if it can be delivered within 30 minutes. Expel all air from the syringe and cap the needle with a sterile rubber stopper.
6. Inject the specimen into an anaerobic transport device if transport time is more than 30 minutes.
7. Request the laboratory to determine microbial susceptibility and identify the anaerobic and aerobic microorganisms.

*Table provided courtesy of M. C. Eldridge and J. LaCombe, Naval Dental School, Bethesda, Maryland.

and the production of a strongly disagreeable odor, often associated with necrotic pulpal contents.

Intricate ecologies of bacteria may exist, contributing to pulpal necrosis and endodontic abscess. *B. melaninogenicus* was reported in appreciable numbers whenever infections due to mixed anaerobic bacteria were observed in both humans and other warm-blooded animals. It was previously believed that *Bacteroides* species were not pathogenic because of their inability to produce infection when injected subdermally. If other bacteria are present in an infection, required metabolites may be produced and a symbiotic relationship might develop. An early study demonstrated synergism in mixed bacterial infection by the production of necrotizing lesions of the abdominal wall of mice using *Bacteroides* species and other bacteria. This view is somewhat modified in that some strains of *B. gingivalis* have varying degrees of

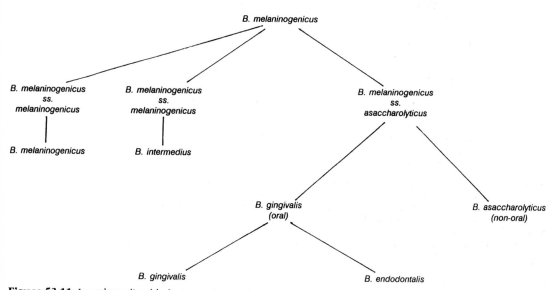

Figure 53.11: In early studies, black-pigmenting species were reported only as *B. melaninogenicus*. With revision of identification techniques, there is continued refinement of taxonomy.

pathogenicity and can seemingly produce abscesses without supporting organisms.

Spirochetes. Spirochetes is a term generally used when referring to members of the order Spirochaetales. Members of this order have been identified as causative organisms in such human disorders as syphilis and yaws, and their invasive nature is clearly seen in necrotizing ulcerative gingivitis. Culture and taxonomic identification of spirochetes is difficult. While complex media are used for successful recovery and identification of treponemes from periodontal disease, culture and specific identification have not been reported from endodontic specimens. Treponemes can be identified in endodontic samples with the use of dark-field microscopy. These organisms are generally considered nonpathogenic; however, the treponemes *T. denticola* and *T. socranskii* are now implicated as etiological pathogens in human adult periodontal disease.

The relationship between the spirochetes and endodontic disease has yet to be established. It is suggested that since treponemes are infrequently identified in teeth with endodontic disease, these organisms may serve as adjucators in distinguishing true endodontic lesions from true periodontal lesions. However, specific growth factors such as long or short chain fatty acids from animal sera or α-globulin are required for growth in culture and are seldom if ever included in media used for endodontic culture studies. The absence of these supplements may have hindered recovery of spirochetes from endodontic samples. Additionally, unlike samples of periodontal fluids, smears of endodontic canal contents often contain considerable debris that may muddle observations. An absolute determination as to the place spirochetes have in endodontic disease is yet to be done.

Streptococci (α-Hemolytic). Before anaerobic recovery techniques became available, α-hemolytic streptococci such as *S. mitis* and *S. salivarius* were considered the most numerous and the most prevalent bacteria identified in endodontic disease. Currently these organisms are thought to be either the initiators of an environment that enhances growth for the more anaerobic/pathogenic bacteria or else just contaminants of the sampling procedure.

Staphylococcus. *Staphylococcus epidermidis* is occasionally reported as the principal organism in endodontic cultures as well as being present in trace numbers. However, *Staphylococcus aureus,* the principal pathogen in the genus, often is not isolated. This suggests that staphylococci, while common in normal oral flora, are not that important in endodontic disease. Staphylococci have been recovered from normal flora as well as from abscess contents. Penicillin would not be as effective in the vast majority of oral infections if staphylococci were a critical pathogen.

Actinomyces Species. *Actinomyces* organisms are thought to be of low virulence but nonetheless are common saprophytes of the oral cavity in plaque and calculus. *Actinomyces* species are known to be inhabitants of deep carious lesions but were infrequently reported in association with diseased pulp tissue. In selected studies that used anaerobic methods of recovery and identification, these organisms have been reported in 10% or more of infected pulp tissue. As with deep carious lesions, there is no unanimity on which of the *Actinomyces* species is most prevalent. The role any *Actinomyces* species may have in the pulpal disease process is only speculative.

Peptococcus. *Peptococcus* species, anaerobic gram-positive cocci, have been reported in mixed periapical infections with *Bacteroides* species. The combination of these organisms may exacerbate chronic periapical lesions.

Peptostreptococcus. *Peptostreptococcus* organisms, which are anaerobic, have been reported. Their pathogenicity develops from being highly proteolytic and possessing an ability to proliferate in low E_h, which is typical of pulpal necrosis or a closed root canal. When subcutaneous pathogenicity was assessed in mice, *Peptostreptococcus* species were one of two organisms (*Fusobacterium nucleatum* was the other) that consistently created abscesses.

Actinobacillus actinomycetemcomitans. *A. actinomycetemcomitans* has been associated with juvenile periodontitis and has been identified within the gingival tissues. To date little correlation has been shown between this periodontal pathogen and endodontic disease, which accentuates the autonomous etiologies of the endodontic and periodontal disease process. It would probably be more promising to pursue this organism as an adjudicator in differentiating endodontic and periodontal diseases.

ADDITIONAL READING

Czarnecki, R. T., Schilder, H. 1979. A Histological Evaluation of the Human Pulp in Teeth with Varying Degrees of Periodontal Disease. J Endodont, **5,** 242.

Kakehashi, S., Stanley, H. R., Fitzgerald, R. J. 1965. The Effects of Surgical Exposure of Dental Pulps in Germ-Free and Conventional Laboratory Rats. Oral Surg, **20,** 340.

Oguntebi, B., Slee, A. M., Tanzer, J. M., Langeland, K. 1982. Predominant Microflora Associated with Human Dental Periapical Abscesses. J Clin Microbiol, **15,** 964.

Pantera, E. A., Jr., Zambon, J. J., Shih-Levine, M. 1988. Indirect Immunofluorescence for the Detection of *Bacteroides* Species in Human Dental Pulp. J Endodont, **14,** 218.

Simon, J. H. 1984. Periodontal-endodontic treatment. In *Pathways of the Pulp,* Ed. 3, edited by S. Cohen and R. C. Burns. C. V. Mosby, St. Louis.

Slots, J. 1979. Importance of Black-Pigmented *Bacteroides* in Human Periodontal Disease. In *Host-Parasite Interactions in Periodontal Diseases,* edited by R. J. Genco and S. E. Mergenhagen. American Society for Microbiology, Washington, D.C.

Sundqvist, G. 1976. *Bacteriological Studies of Necrotic Dental Pulps,* Dissertation 7. Umea, Sweden, University of Umea.

Torabinejad, M., Eby, W. C., Naidorf, I. J. 1985. Inflammatory and Immunological Aspects of the Pathogenesis of Human Periapical Lesions. J Endodont, **11,** 479.

Williams, B. L., McCann, G. F., Schoenknecht, F. D. 1983. Bacteriology of Dental Abscesses of Endodontic Origin. J. Clin Microbiol, **18,** 770.

Index